D1715905

BIOPHYSICAL PROPERTIES OF THE SKIN

A TREATISE OF SKIN

Harry R. Elden, *Series Editor*

Volume 1   Biophysical Properties of the Skin

Biophysical Properties of the Skin

Edited by

HARRY R. ELDEN

Barry College
Miami Shores, Florida

WILEY-INTERSCIENCE, a Division of John Wiley & Sons, Inc.

New York · London · Sydney · Toronto

Preface

This volume of A Treatise of Skin begins a new review series on the physics, chemistry, and biology of skin. The plan is to examine topics that are not usually covered in the literature on dermatology, surgery, or leather but nevertheless relate to skin and its components. For example, a professor of analytical mechanics could be expected to discuss the physics of nonlinear deformation of a heterogeneous model of hair; a mathematical physicist could discuss mechanisms of diffusion in a fluid-filled heterogenous fiber matrix (dermis); and radiation of energy or electrical conduction of skin could be discussed by a biophysicist. Physics and chemistry of keratin are other topics that are treated in depth, because a vast literature on wool exists in the textile field. This literature usually is not read by biological scientists, although it contains some of the most advanced work done on the structure and properties of a biological tissue (hair).

A very important goal is to show that chronological age is a significant factor in the design of experiments. The contributors are alerted to the importance of this aspect before writing begins, thus ensuring that the topic receives the necessary emphasis.

Duplication is minimized so that reviews supplement one another, but simultaneous appearance of more than one review on the same topic permits full expression of ideas by various experts. This plan also gives the reader a greater opportunity to appraise critically the research done by different experts when their findings converge to the same conclusion as well as when they diverge in conflict.

This volume on the physical properties of skin focuses attention on connective tissue components, hydration, and aqueous solutions. It is clear from the content of these chapters that extensive theoretical work has been done on components of skin, particularly the thermodynamics of melting, deformation, hydration, and properties of solutions. Such progress will aid the interpretation of experimental data, because the theoretician often has had to introduce models or mechanisms of action as a base for the theoretical analysis. It is hoped that theory and laboratory experimentation now will grow together. If this happens, we can anticipate rapid advances in the pursuit of mechanisms of aging in skin. I believe that this achievement will lead to solutions of other problems, that we now have little guidance for attacking—either deliberately or by secondary innovation.

An appraisal of success in achieving these goals cannot honestly be made by testing the contents of just one volume. The positive, critical, and interested reader, however, can help to ensure success for all by suggesting appropriate new subject matter for review, rather than by overly emphasizing an opinion on deficiencies in subject matter selected by others. You are cordially invited, therefore, to share in planning this continuous treatise on the basic properties of skin and its components.

HARRY R. ELDEN

Barry College
Miami Shores, Fla. 33161
January 1971.

Contents

BIOPHYSICAL PROPERTIES OF THE SKIN

1

Biophysical Analysis of Aging Skin

HARRY R. ELDEN, Ph.D.

Orentreich Foundation for the Advancement of Science, New York

Skin is composed of fibrous and amorphous components which impart unique physical properties to this tissue; namely, ease of deformation

1

varies with direction of elongation. Skin is taut on the body of young subjects, it hangs more loosely from old subjects, with folds and wrinkles accentuating the appearance of the aged skin [1, 2]. Very little is known about the molecular basis for these macroscopic properties of aging skin.

Chemical composition and physical properties of skin vary greatly with respect to anatomical location. It is difficult to find a series of reports in the literature on aging skin that uses the same organism and tissue site. This lack of uniformity in experimental design complicates a topic in physiology (aging) that already is exceedingly complex in itself. A uniform tissue site, or one whose variation can be measured, is needed to minimize the lack of uniformity that now exists in skin from various parts of the body.

It is proposed here that the rat tail is a structure in which tissue properties graduate according to linear position. Topology can be precisely expressed as fractional distance from a reference point such as tail tip or back of the animal.

The effect of age on physical properties of skin from the tail tip is presented in this chapter, and rings of tissue were used as described by Harkness and Harkness [3] and Fry et al. [4]. Data show that aging from 1 to 24 months changes the physical properties of nonmelted and melted skin. The primary site for these changes is judged to be the collagenous structures in the dermis.

Rheology of human skin is reviewed and evaluated with regard to composition, hydration, and models of mechanical deformation. An effort is made to correlate findings and concepts of what happens to skin during growth, maturation, and senescence. Findings show that the influence of age on skin can be determined by measuring certain physical properties; however, it is not comparatively easy to interpret these measurements in terms of biochemical or molecular processes.

1.1 METHODS

1.1.1 Animal Selection and Preparation of Tissues

Female (Wistar-derived) rats were obtained from the animal colony at the Gerontology Research Center, City Hospitals, Baltimore, Maryland, at ages of 1, 2, 4, 6, 12, 18, and 24 months (3 of each age) for precision collection of data in run 2. An earlier study used male and female rats (3 animals each) at ages of 1, 3, 6, 12, 18, and 24 months for run 1. Animals were dispatched with excess ether, they were weighed, and tails were amputated at the back with a pair of bone cutters. The

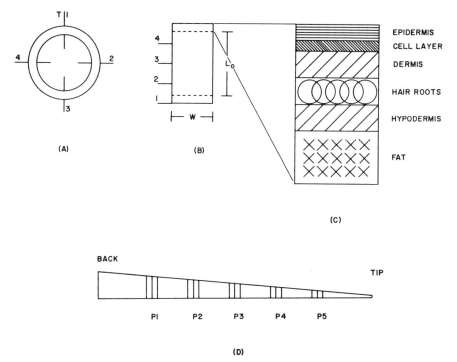

Figure 1.1 (a).   Mean thickness T determined from readings at four places.
Figure 1.1 (b).   Typical side view of a ring of skin. Mean width W determined from readings at four places. Sample length L_0 was determined during a stress-strain tensile test.
Figure 1.1 (c).   Idealized description of strata as seen in microscopic cross-section of skin.
Figure 1.1 (d).   Location of five positions (P1 to P5) where rings were isolated along a rat tail. Rings excised at P3 were used for tensile tests in Run 1, whereas rings obtained at P1 to P4 were used in Run 2.

tail length was measured and delineated into five equal segments (see Fig. 1.1). Rings were cut in duplicate at five sites numbered from the body to the tip as positions P1 to P5. Rings at position P3 only were used for run 1, but rings from sites P1 to P4 were used in run 2.

1.1.2 Histology and Microscopic Measurement of Rings

Rings of tissue from run 2 were placed immediately in formalin solution. After fixation overnight in formalin, samples were dehydrated serially with alcohol/water solutions. Paraffin-embedded samples were sectioned on a microtome, then transferred to glass slides. Stained sections then were examined with a Leitz polarizing microscope. A Filar-eyepiece micrometer was used to measure broadly demarcated regions called epidermis, cell layer, and dermis. This delineation oversimplified the microscopic histology of the tissue, but the approximation adequately reveals age effects. Thickness of skin also was measured on a gross scale. Rings of tissue from P3 in run 1, and for all tissues in run 2, were placed on the stage of a profile projector (Nikkon Optical Company). Thickness readings were taken at four quadrants around the circumference using a movable X-Y stage equipped with precision-graduated micrometers. The sample then was placed on its side, and width was read at four positions. Length readings were obtained during elongation of the sample. Figure 1.1 identifies where these measurements were made for rings of tail skin, and it also shows how cross-sectional area was calculated.

1.1.3 Dehydration of Strips of Skin

Strips of skin were isolated along the dorsal midline of the sacral region of rats in run 1. Pieces were cut in a rectangle (1 $\times$ 2 cm), scraped free of subcutaneous fat, then attached to a length of nichrome wire. Wire and sample were suspended from the lever arm of a Statham strain gauge in a zero-humidity atmosphere of flowing air. The apparatus shown in Fig. 1.2 illustrates the technique used to measure rate of desorption of water. Dehydration was continued until samples reached constant weight; 48 hours was sufficiently close to equilibration that it was routinely used as an endpoint. Sample weight readings from four strain gauges were automatically detected and serially monitored by the motor-driven switching mechanism. Output of the gauges was plotted by the recorder, while room air was dehydrated by pumping through concentrated sulfuric acid and then passed into the column of Drierite to indicate that water had been adequately removed. One switch of the timing mechanism was set so that it turned off the air pump during the weight reading cycle. This eliminated fluctuations in the sample weight induced by flowing air.

1.1.4 Physical Properties of Rings

The tensile properties of rings were measured on the Instron tensile testing apparatus with a special cell assembly shown in Fig. 1.3. Rings of tissue were weighed on a torsion micro balance to 0.0X mg after equilibration in 20°C phosphate buffer (pH 7.4), then placed on the

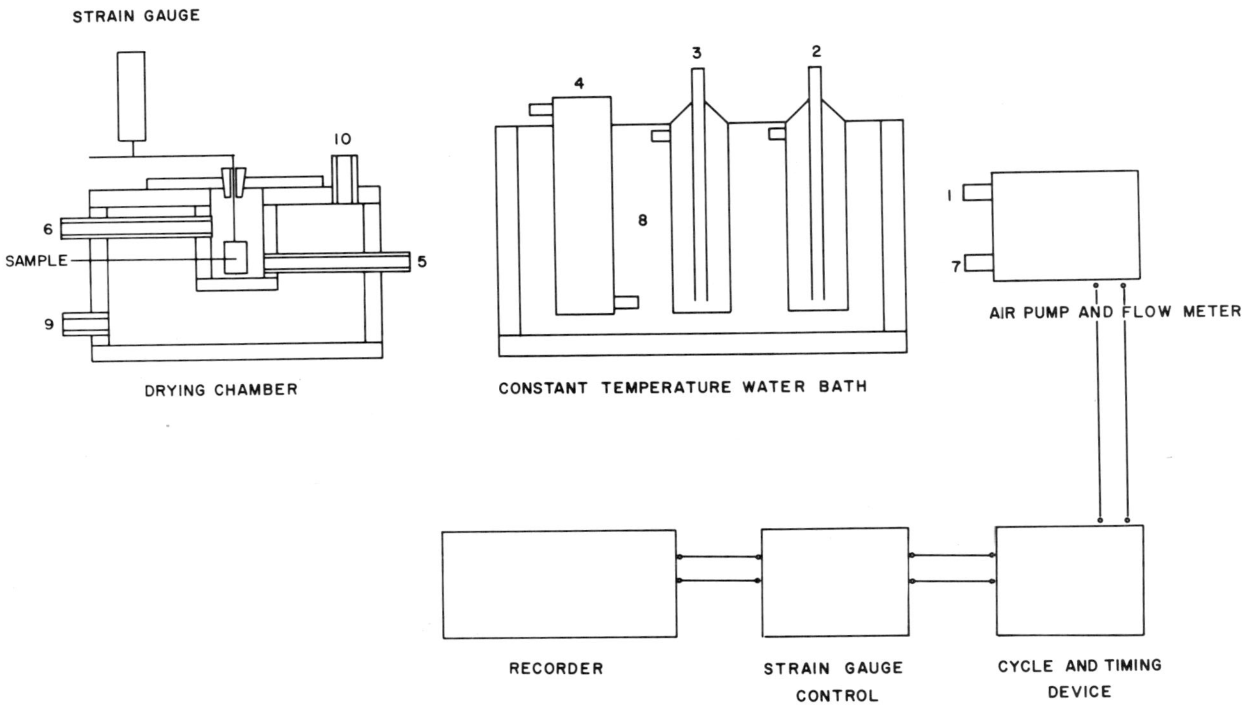

AIR PUMP AND FLOW METER

CONSTANT TEMPERATURE WATER BATH

STRAIN GAUGE

DRYING CHAMBER

RECORDER

STRAIN GAUGE CONTROL

CYCLE AND TIMING DEVICE

SAMPLE

Figure 1.2. Apparatus used to measure dehydration of skin. Air is pumped (1) through a sulfuric acid drying tube (2), a splash trap (3), and indicating column (4) before it enters (5) the drying chamber. Wet air exits from the drying chamber (6) and returns (7) to be pumped around the circuit again. Water circulates through the thermostated bath (8) and drying chamber (9 and 10). Sample weight is determined from outputs of strain gauges, while strain gauge controls are used to calibrate the recorder. Cyclical operation of all components is coordinated by motor-driven cams and microswitches of the cycle and timing device.

5

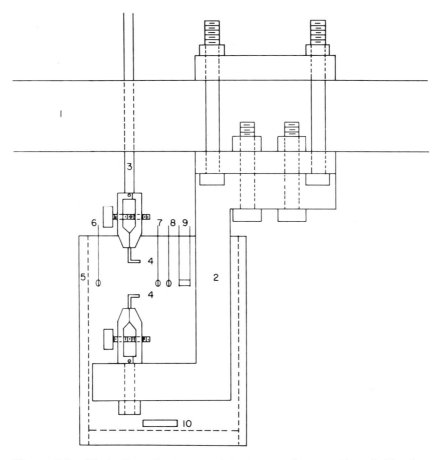

Figure 1.3. Illustration of set-up used to test tensile properties of skin rings. Lever arm (1) of tensile-testing apparatus moves the extension arm (2) in a vertical direction. Rings of tissue slip over hooks (4) and transmit force to strain gauge (3). All components are surrounded by plastic cylinder (5) containing phosphate buffer. Thermistor (6), thermoregulator (7), heater (8), cooling coil (9), and stirring bar (10) are used to read and regulate temperature.

hooks. Each sample was stretched five times for work conditioning, after which three succeeding cycles were analytically recorded. Maximum load was limited to 100 g. Temperature was raised to 30, 40, and 50°C, and stress/strain data were obtained at each step. After the 50° cycle, sample length was adjusted to that length which sustains a 10-g load. Temperature was then elevated to 60°C (linearly with respect to time), and every one degree was denoted manually on the recording of force versus time at constant sample length. Sample length then was shortened at 60°C until the force was reduced to zero; the sample then was stretched to rupture by one continuous process.

The wet weight of skin ruptured at 60°C was quickly determined after lightly blotting off the excess of phosphate buffer. Repeated acetone

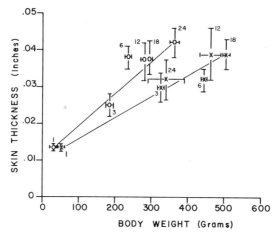

Figure 1.4. Macroscopic thickness of rings plotted against body weight (Run 1). Bar width expresses one standard deviation of mean (in this and subsequent graphs) at ages indicated in months for male (x) and female (o) rats.

extraction dried the sample and prepared it for chemical analysis. Collagen content was determined by the method of Neuman and Logan [5] and was expressed as mg 100 mg^{-1} of dried skin.

1.2   RESULTS

1.2.1   Morphology

Gross macroscopic thickness of skin at P3 (run 1) increased linearly with respect to body weight (Fig. 1.4) for 1- to 24-month-old rats. The rate of increase was greater in females than males, even though females did not attain the same (heavier) weight as did males. Skin thickness was the same for both sexes when compared at the same age.

Microscopic dimensions of strata in rings depend on position along the tail. The uppermost stratum, identified grossly as epidermis in Fig. 1.1, showed the least variation with respect to age and position (Fig. 1.5). Thickness of the midstratum, that which contained the hair roots and cells, decreased as the tip of the tail was approached. Figure 1.6 shows also that aging from 1 to 18 months increased the thickness of this stratum. Thickness of the balance of skin also depended on position and age, and Fig. 1.7 shows that enlargement occurred with aging primarily at P1.

These measurements are now reviewed with age as the independent variable. Gross epidermal thickness at P1 and P5 remained essentially constant between 1 and 24 months of age (Fig. 1.8), while cell layer

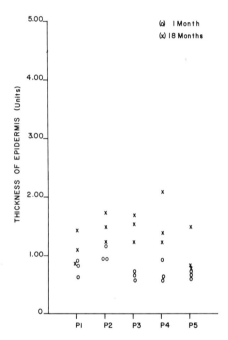

Figure 1.5. Mean thickness of epidermal layer plotted against position number along the tail for 1-month-(o) and 18-month-old-(x) rats (Run 2).

thickness increased continuously (Fig. 1.9) to reach a peak at 18 months at positions P1 and P5. Dermis showed a similar pattern of continuous enlargement with age at P1 and P5, but this stratum began to involute at 12 months in P5 and at 18 months in P1 (Fig. 1.10). Distal portions of the rat's tail, therefore, showed aging effects before those parts that were closer to the animal's body.

The collagen content of samples, irrespective of position, is shown in Fig. 1.11 as a function of age. It is essentially constant between 2 to 24 months of age at about 30 mg %. Insight into the compaction (density) of skin is obtained by comparing cross-sectional mass with geometrical cross-sectional area. Figure 1.12 shows that W_0, the mass/length ratio, increased linearly with respect to cross-sectional area. Wet weight of rings is plotted in Fig. 1.13 as a function of dry weight for 1- and 18-month-old rats. Ratio of wet weight/dry weight is independent of age (Fig. 1.14) for samples measured below and above the melting temperature of dermal collagen. The ratio tends to be higher for 1-month-old rats compared with other ages, and suggests that 1-month-old rats might have special water-binding properties.

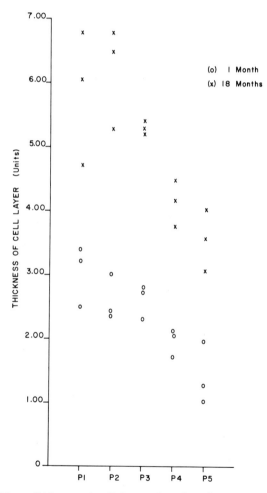

Figure 1.6. Mean thickness of cell layer plotted against position number along tail for 1-month-(o) and 18-month-old-(x) rats (Run 2).

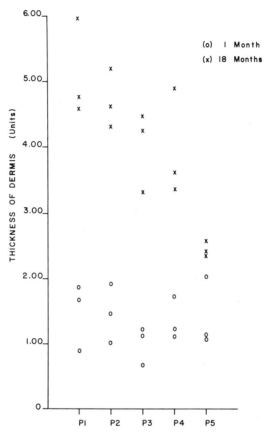

Figure 1.7.   Mean thickness of dermal layer plotted against position number along tail for 1-month-(o) and 18-month-old-(x) rats.

1.2.2   Dehydration

   Strips of skin taken from the back of the rat lost weight in the dessication chamber according to the curve illustrated in Fig. 1.15. An initially rapid rate of dehydration progressively slowed down, and samples reached a steady value at 48 hours. Initial wet weight (W_0), transient weight (W_t), equilibrium weight (W_{48}), and half-life were used to describe the process of dehydration. Fractional water content is plotted in Fig. 1.16 against time and shows that tissue from 1-month-old rats loses water at a slower rate than that from the 18-month-old rats. This is an unexpected finding since water content of isolated tissue is higher in the younger than in the older rat. Figure 1.17 shows that water content of isolated tissue decreased continuously with respect to increasing body

weight for rats between the ages of 1 and 24 months. Half-life of dehydration also decreased with increasing body weight (Fig. 1.18) indicating that water volatility decreases with increasing age.

It was not possible to show a simple mathematical formulation between experimental variables. However, velocity of dehydration was
plotted against the water content for all samples that were 3 months
of age and older. Figure 1.19 illustrates that velocity of dehydration
decreased in proportion as water content decreased (for 3- to 24-month-
old rats). One-month-old rats lost water at a uniquely slower rate than
the 3- to 24-month-old group. It is evident that water in 1-month-old
rats (male and female) is in a different state, that is, less volatile even
though more abundant, than it is in tissues of rats 3 to 24 months
of age.

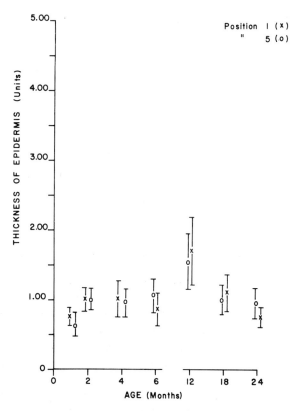

Figure 1.8.   Thickness of epidermal layer for P1 (x) and P5 (o) plotted against
age (Run 2).

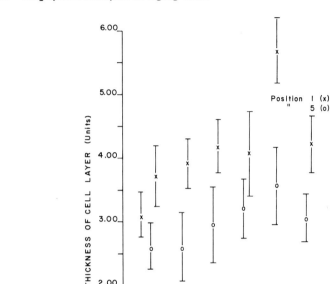

Figure 1.9.   Thickness of cell layer for P1 (x) and P5 (o) plotted against age.

1.2.3   Mechanical Properties of Rings of Tail Skin

A typical plot of force versus extension is shown in Fig. 1.20. Length
(L) and force (F) coordinates were obtained at initial (0), yield (Y),
and break (B). Coordinates for cyclical stress/strain data were identified
further as extension (E) and retraction (R). Cycle number N is not
a factor in this report, since findings are based only on the sixth ($N = 6$)
cycle. The immediately preceding five cycles were used to work-condition
the sample.

The ratio $L(O, R, N = 6)/L(O, E, N = 6)$ plotted against body
weight in Fig. 1.21 shows that extension of rings does not eliminate
plastic flow. A constant value of about 1.20 indicates that sample length

stretched about 20% during the sixth cycle of loading to 100 g. Except for an individual variation of length ratio, such as occurred in 4-month-old female rats at the y-axis = 1.35, there is no correlation with age or body weight.

A previous study by Elden [6] reported that work-conditioned skin deformed according to Equation 1.

$$\text{Stress} = \frac{K_c'}{2} \times \left[\left(\frac{L}{L_0} \right) - 1 \right]^2 \tag{1}$$

This equation was used to compute an index of elastic stiffness ($K_c'/2$) for the sixth cycle of stress/strain. Figure 1.22 shows that K_c ($= K_c'/2$) increased rapidly during growth, except for the unexplained spurious excursion of 3-month-old rats. When the abscissa for 24-month-old male rats

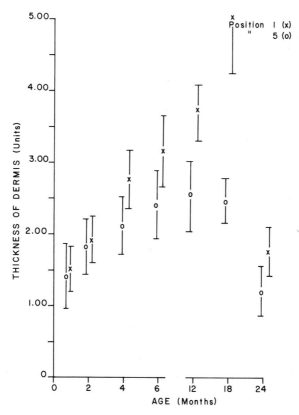

Figure 1.10. Thickness of dermis layer for P1 (x) and P5 (o) plotted against age.

is shifted to the value estimated for a rat of that age, the ordinate comes nearly in line with the anticipated value of K_C. However, the y-value shown could be high at the stated x-value, because physiological stress accompanying weight loss increases cohesion of collagen fibers. Yield stress (Fig. 1.23) and break stress (Fig. 1.24) also increased continuously with respect to body weight for run 1. A relationship existed between yield and break stress (Fig. 1.25) such that one increased linearly with respect to the other.

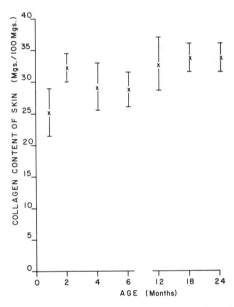

Figure 1.11.   Collagen content of P1 to P4 rings plotted against age (Run 2).

Melting temperature was estimated by replotting force-time data recorded during the rise of temperature from 50 to 60°C (Fig. 1.26). Straight lines were drawn through data obtained between 50–55 and 60–65°. The point of intersection between extrapolations of these lines determined T_s, the melting temperature, even though data curved in this vicinity. Figure 1.27 shows that melting temperature of collagen, that is, the shrinkage temperature of skin (T_s), varied between 56.5 and 55.5°C through ages of 1 to 24 months. Shrinkage temperature, therefore, did not change significantly with respect to body weight or age. The isometric force produced at 60°C by the melted sample restrained to constant length was calculated relative to that produced at 52°C of the nonmelted sample. This ratio increased exponentially with respect to body weight (and age) as shown in Fig. 1.28. Isotonic contraction of melted skin, defined as $L_{0,60°}/L_{0,50}$, decreased exponentially with respect to increasing body weight and age (Fig. 1.29). Stress required to break melted collagen, however, increased continuously and

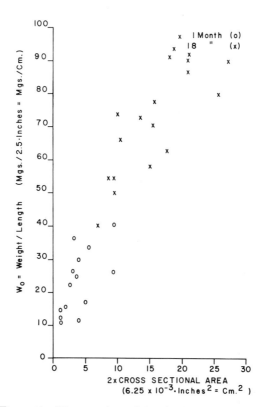

Figure 1.12. The ratio W_o, sample weight (mg) length cm^{-1}, plotted against $2 \times$ cross-sectional area of sample. Multiplicative constants (2.5 × in. and 6.25 × 10^{-3} × in.^{2}) convert original data to metric units. Slope is ratio of cross-sectional mass/cross-sectional area and equals density of the sample. Same slope for data selected at 1 (o) and 18 (x) months shows that tissue density is independent of age (Run 2).

nonlinearly with respect to body weight as shown in Fig. 1.30. Notice also that the strain required to break melted skin (Fig. 1.31) increased with respect to body weight and age. These tests thus show a variegated response of dermal connective tissue to aging.

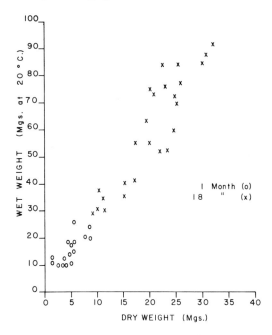

Figure 1.13. Wet weight of skin (equilibrated at 20°C) plotted against dry weight for typical samples at 1 (o) and 18 (x) months of age (Run 2).

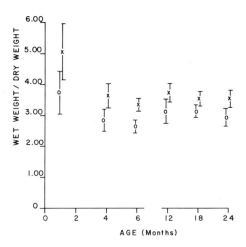

Figure 1.14. Ratio of wet weight/dry weight plotted against age (Run 2) for samples equilibrated before tensile test at 20°C (o) and after tensile test at 60°C (x).

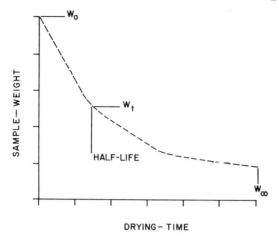

Figure 1.15. Typical plot of sample weight versus time for strips of skin suspended in the drying chamber.

1.3   DISCUSSION

1.3.1   Biological Structure of Rat Tails

Topology of skin on the main part of the body is highly diverse. This limits the extent of serial replicate sampling that can be done in a single animal or at a specific site. Tail skin is relatively uniform, on the other hand, and it has two additional features as a result of

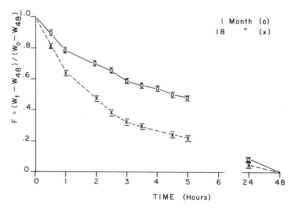

Figure 1.16. Ratio of transient water content/total water content plotted against drying time for 1-(o) and 18-(x) month-old rats (Run 1). Equilibrium dessication occurs in approximately 48 hr.

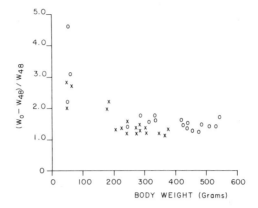

Figure 1.17.   Total water content per unit dry weight of samples plotted against body weight for male (x) and female (o) rats (Run 1).

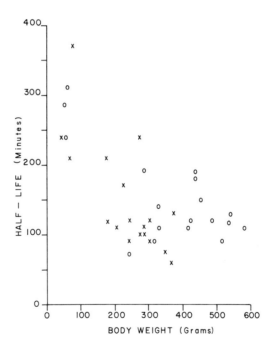

Figure 1.18.   First half-life of dessication rate plotted against body weight of male (x) and female (o) rats (Run 1).

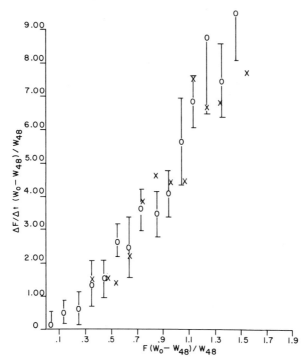

Figure 1.19. Velocity of dehydration, calculated as rate of change in fraction (f) $\times$ total water content per unit dry weight, plotted against water content (Run 1). Data for 1-month-old rats fall below the trend shown here for 3- to 24-month-old rats.

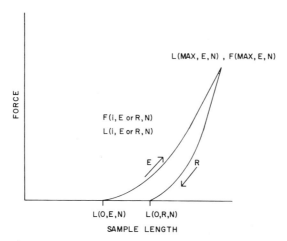

Figure 1.20. Illustration of typical relationship between force and length of nonmelted skin. Coordinates F and L are identified further according to extension E or retraction R of which i number of coordinate values may be transcribed from instrumental graphs of F versus L. N is the number of repetitive cycles for stretching nonmelted tissue.

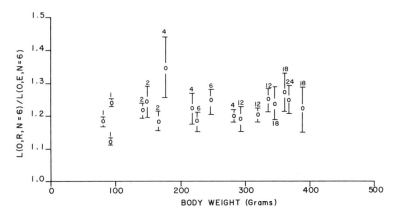

Figure 1.21. Drift in zero-length of test sample, computed as ratio of initial sample lengths for R and E at $N = 6$, plotted against body weight (Run 2). Mean value of four rings are shown for each animal as a function of body weight while age is listed next to data points. Notice that hysteresis is independent of age when tissues are stretched at 40°C.

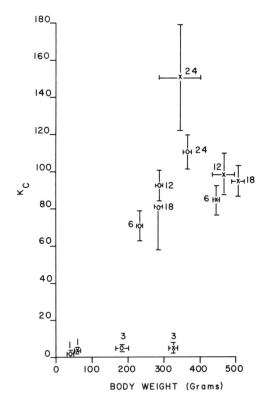

Figure 1.22. Elastic stiffness of skin (K_c) in units of 10^3 g in.$^{-2}$ plotted against body weight of male (x) and female (o) rats (Run 1). See text for comments on reliability of 3- and 24-month (x) data.

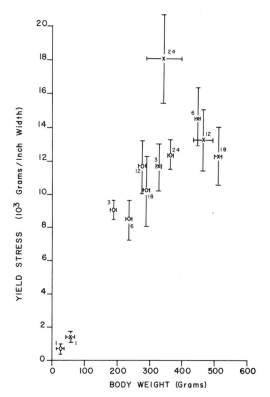

Figure 1.23. Yield stress of nonmelted skin plotted against body weight for aging rats (Run 1).

its anatomical location. That variation which is present can be mapped out topologically along a linear projection (the distance along the tail). This feature greatly simplifies serial testing of skin in the same animal. The second feature is that the tail is an appendage, or extension, of the body which can be isolated regionally. This permits the investigator to limit certain physiological factors that influence skin.

Development of techniques for regulating the *in vivo* melieu of tail skin will help to decipher biological mechanism of aging therein. Current research on connective tissue reflects an increasing regard for biochemical and physiological factors. It is appropriate to emphasize a few details that could generate new ideas on how physical properties of aging skin are regulated by endogenous processes.

The tail consists of a vertebral column, tendons, arterial-venous blood systems, and skin. Muscle bundles are attached to the body skeleton

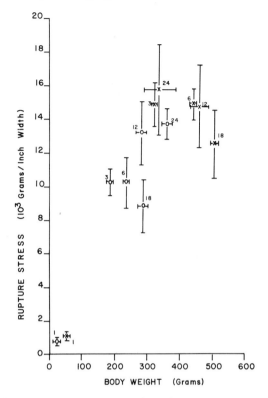

Figure 1.24. Rupture strength of nonmelted skin plotted against body weight for aging rats (Run 1).

(outside the tail), and they move the tail by pulling tendons that interdigitate with vertebrae. The tip is a growing bud with high cell density and vascularity. Since there is a change in thickness of skin layers along the tail, the translation toward the body could reiterate the chronological sequence of postnatal growth and development.

It has been suggested that physiological and biochemical reactions of inaccessible organs influence skin. Conversely, the analysis of skin could reveal some aspects of these internal reactions. The rat tail may be an excellent structure for testing this hypothesis, because many physiological systems are contiguous therein and with inaccessible organs.

Collagen fibers are deposited in tendons when there is active mechanical tension between muscles and skeleton to which the tendons are attached [7]. This resembles fibroblastic proliferation and deposition of collagen that is stimulated by physical stress in the rat uterus [8].

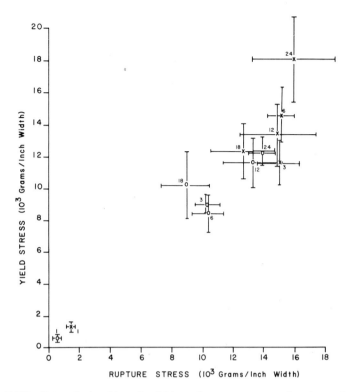

Figure 1.25. Interrelationship of yield and rupture strengths for aging rats (Run 1).

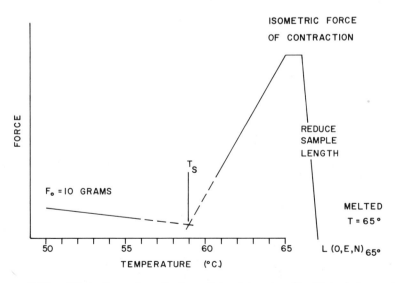

Figure 1.26. Illustration of method used to determine T_S. Data between 50–55°C and between 60–65°C were used to establish two linear functions which intersect at T_S by linear extrapolation.

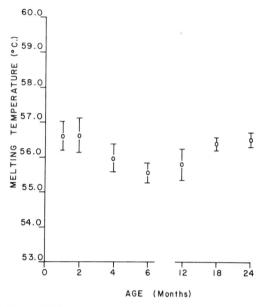

Figure 1.27.   Melting temperature T_s plotted against age (Run 2).

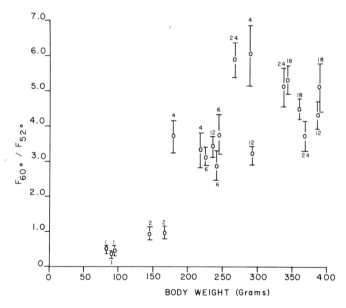

Figure 1.28.   Isometric elevation of force at 60°C relative to that at 52°C for melted-skin collagen plotted against body weight. Mean values for four rings are shown for each animal and age is listed next to data points (Run 2).

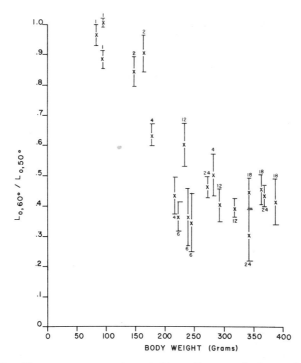

Figure 1.29. Percentage contraction of skin collagen melted at 60°C relative to that at 50°C plotted against body weight (Run 2).

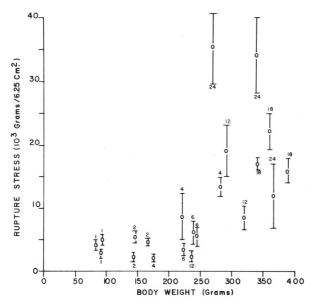

Figure 1.30. Rupture stress of skin collagen melted at 60°C plotted against body weight (Run 2).

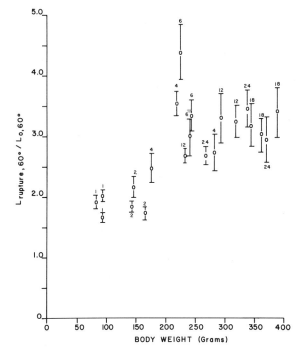

Figure 1.31. Rupture strain of skin collagen melted at 60°C plotted against body weight (Run 2).

Tail skin could proliferate in a similar fashion by responding to the physical stress of a longitudinally expanding vertebral column. Supporting evidence for this is the fact that destruction of epiphyseal cartilage cells terminates growth of the tail [9].

Thermal regulation of the body is mediated partly by conductive dissipation of heat through the skin. This is particularly important for the rat. Whole-body calorimetry and volumetric collection of heat flowing from an encapsulated limb have been used [10] to measure heat exchange between a physiological system and the environment. Heat loss from the tail also can be thermally isolated from the rest of the body by inserting the tail into an insulated and thermoregulated chamber. Mechanisms of peripheral heat regulation, therefore, can be delineated experimentally from the "core" of the body.

This technique was used by Proskauer et al. [11] to show that cutaneous temperature strongly regulated blood pressure in the tail. Blood pressure varied with respect to core (rectal) temperature, while the cardiac rat rose and fell with changes in tail blood pressure. Other reports show that the tail can be used to follow changes in the peripheral vascular system. Wu and Visscher [12] constructed a plethysmograph to measure pulsatile volume dilatations in the tail, and blood flow was stopped by raising pressure to the systolic level in an occlusive cuff. Shuler et al. [13] used an optical monometer and this plethysmographic method to compare direct and indirect blood-pressure readings in the tail. Friedman et al. [14] perfused the vascular bed in the intact rat tail with media of different ionic composition, while sodium and potassium electrodes were used to monitor cation concentrations of solutions flowing in a closed system that forced ionic fluxes within perivascular tissue. A ligature at the base of the tail prevented flow of ionic solutions through the skin from the tail to the body. Volume distensibility of the rat-tail artery already had been measured by Hinke and Wilson [15].

Physical resemblance of the rat tail to the anatomy of the human finger may be sufficient to consider it an experimental model of finger joints. Flexibility of the tail could be studied with devices that were constructed [16] to test flexibility of human-finger joints. Along the same line, Peacock [17] suggested that deposition of new collagen in constrained joints accounted for their increased stiffness during immobilization. These studies on joint stiffness pose questions which cannot be investigated easily with human-finger joints, but they might be studied in the rat tail as an experimental model. One such point is whether or not collagen fibers in skin and tendon of the same gross structure change similarly with respect to age.

The rat tail, therefore, is an anatomical structure in which the relationship between skin, arterial-venous blood supply, skeleton, and tendon can be studied comparatively. Blood flow to the tail can be controlled easily, while the external temperature is maintained at set values with little technical difficulty. These and other manipulations are possible because the tail extends from the animal body like a digital appendage. This unique geometry is particularly valuable in studying the biophysical properties of skin, because one can precisely demarcate the anatomical site (position along the tail) where test samples are obtained.

1.3.2 Morphology of Tail Skin

Thickness of rat-tail skin can be expressed in two ways: namely as a geometrical dimension or as the collagen content/surface area. Tail skin is 0.50 to 1.50 mm thick, according to data shown in Fig. 1.4, while the collagen content of rat tail skin per surface area increases with respect to body weight [4]. A plot of log collagen content (mg cm^{-2})

versus log body weight (g) increased linearly from about 0.50 mg cm^{-2} at 25 g (21 days old) to 5.0 mg cm^{-2} at 500 g (60 days old). Geometrical thickness of skin also increased with respect to body weight (Fig. 1.4), but calculations by Fry et al. [4], using a fixed density of 1.05 for wet whole skin, yielded constant values of thickness (about 0.20 mm).

The plot shown in Fig. 1.12 deals with the compaction (density) of rat tail skin. A slope of about 0.28 equals density as defined by Equation 2.

$$W_0 = \text{weight/length} = \frac{\text{cross-sectional area} \times 2L_0 \times \text{density}}{L_0} \quad (2)$$

$$= \text{cross-sectional area} \times 2 \times \text{density}$$

Corrections were made to express density as weight/cm of circumference/unit cross-sectional area. The much lower value of density, compared with that of Fry et al. [4], indicates that dehydrated whole skin contains voids or low density components that are not obvious. Constant level of slope as shown in Fig. 1.12 for 1- and 18-month-old rate indicates that compaction, or voids, at least is not greatly influenced by age. This supports the assumption made by Fry et al. [4], even though our values for density are not the same. In addition to having an interest in density of skin, these calculations were made originally to correlate mass/circumference and geometrical cross-sectional area. If density had not been constant, tensile properties of tissue would need to be expressed both as load/quantity of tissue and load/geometrical area. Fry et al. [4] did this with their data in their definition of surface mechanical resistance.

The ratio of wet/dry weights for rat-tail skin (Fig. 1.14) is about 3.0 at 20°C. Since L_0 did not change greatly with changing temperature (20–50°C), a correction can be made to $d = 0.28$ for water content of samples. Accepting that $\frac{2}{3}$ of the cross-sectional area is filled by water, whose removal does not disturb the geometry, a new density (d_2) of $0.28 \times \frac{3}{2} = 0.42$ is obtained for dry skin.

This value of density represents weights and volumes of collagenous (C) and noncollagenous (NC) components according to Equation 3.

$$d_2 = \frac{W_C + W_{NC}}{V_C + V_{NC}} = 0.42 \quad (3)$$

If d of collagen is 1.33, then $V_C = W_C/1.33$. Inspection of Fig. 1.11 shows that the concentration of collagen in rat-tail skin (about 30 mg %) yields a ratio of W_C/W_{NC} of $\frac{3}{7}$, or $W_{NC} = \frac{7}{3} W_C$.

Inserting real numbers for appropriate values in Equation 3, therefore, yields a ratio of 4 for V_{NC}/V_C. The very low value for density, therefore, is due to the high effective volume of NC components in rat-tail skin relative to that of collagen (C). These are visualized as thick epidermal layer, thick subdermal layer plus fat deposits, blood vessels, cells, and hair roots. Data showing thickness of dermal stratum in skin corroborate the level of collagen found by chemical analysis, if it is assumed that collagen is not present elsewhere in the cross-section. At age 12 months, for example, the three strata add up to 7.25 units, namely, 1.50 for epidermis $+3.20$ for cell layer $+2.50$ for dermis at P5. The dermal layer, therefore, is $2.50/7.25 = 34.5\%$ of the sample strata. This is not a bad comparison with the 30% value based on chemical determination.

Decline in thickness of skin layers commencing between 12 and 18 months in the rat tail is an important finding. This shows that the tail continuously adjusts to chronological events in the physiology and biochemistry of aging. Early onset in thinning of P5 at 12 months, followed by involution in P1 at 18 months, demonstrates a gradient in refractivity along the tail. The distal portion (P5) responds faster than the proximal position (P1) for at least two possible reasons. The distal portion (P5) is the growing bud, and it may be physiologically younger than proximal P1. The response to a "signal to involute" could be faster in the young growing tissue than in the chronologically older tissue. On the other hand, the distance between P5 and central organs, that is, brain, heart, liver, and so on, might predispose it to an enhanced rate loss of function compared with proximal P1. More detailed explanations are not warranted. However, if this feature of tail skin is reproducible and consistent, it could be used to study an important problem in human gerontology—thinning of skin with aging in certain areas of the body [18].

1.3.3   Dehydration

Kinetic mechanisms for dehydrating skin involve (1) changing surface area of aqueous phase exposed to the flowing air stream; (2) vapor pressure of water (hence temperature); (3) energy flux for heat of vaporization; and (4) concentration gradient of water molecules across the vapor/liquid interface. The setup used here attempted to reduce experimental influences on 2, 3, and 4. Temperature of flowing air was fixed at 40°C which should volatilize liquid water bound to tissue. Constant temperature also forced the vapor pressure of tissue water to depend only on chemical potential of water molecules in the liquid state. Concentration gradient across the vapor/liquid interface was regulated in part by recirculating air through the drying tube. This produced a flowing air stream of constant relative humidity (approximately zero). Even though surface area and vapor pressure of water were independent of experimental factors, they were not constant during the course of dehydration.

Vapor pressure and surface area of water at the tissue/air interface depend on the net flux of molecules at the surface. If diffusion to the interface from within fibrous tissue balances efflux into the air stream, the surface area should remain constant. However, this need not be expected to hold throughout complete dehydration, because the structure of fibrous connective tissue changes with loss of plasticizing water [19]. A time will be reached when evaporation is limited by diffusion of water up to the surface. The curve of weight versus time abruptly changes slope at this point as dehydration shifts to a new mechanism of evaporation.

Dehydration of skin may be compared to dehydration of hydrophilic fabrics. Rate of evaporation of hydrated fabrics [20] is linear so long as "free" water exists in interfibrous spaces. Evaporation rate abruptly slows down, however, when free water is depleted leaving bound water exposed at the surface. Plots of water content versus drying time thereby begin and remain linear throughout the region of free water, but they become nonlinear abruptly when free water is completely volatilized.

Experimental data shown here do not reveal a discrete compartment of free water in skin. If there is free water in skin, it quickly evaporates and reverts to nonlinear decline such as shown in Fig. 1.16 for plots of F versus time. The initial linear rate of dehydration, which appears to be constant for a short period, increased during growth (1 to 3 months), but aging beyond 3 months to 24 months did not unequivocally change the initial linear rate. However, first half-life of dehydration declined with increasing body weight (and age) continuously throughout 1 to 24 months age span. Young (1-month-old) skin, therefore, has a lower rate of dehydration than older (3 to 24 month) skin, but its water content is greater relative to that of older skin as shown in Fig. 1.17. The increased linear rate of dehydration might represent an increase in surface area of free water. However, these data cannot be interpreted only in terms of changing surface area.

A number of computations were made to facilitate interpretation. Ultimately, F data were expressed as velocity of dehydration (y-axis) versus water content (x-axis) as shown in Fig. 1.19. Dehydration thus commences at positive x-y-values and proceeds to zero at the origin. Evaporation rate is related to volatility, or vapor pressure, of water in the drying tissue.

Data shown in Fig. 1.19, therefore, pertain to a very complex system where high velocity of evaporation occurs with high water content. The plot of velocity versus water content indicates that evaporation rate decreases as loosely held water is successively depleted, leaving water molecules that are bound with increasing affinity. The abrupt change in slope of data beyond 1 month indicates that something happens to water binding with completion of early growth. Surface area or volatility of water could be reduced by metabolic processes associated with onset of maturation of connective tissue per se. It also is possible that total body water is depressed thermodynamically by changes in endocrine control of fluid-electrolyte balance. Another possibility is that collagen and polysaccharide biopolymers begin to interact with water to form structured macromolecules which entrap the aqueous phase.

Numerous reports show that water does exist in discrete compartments of tissue [21, 22]. Widdowson and Dickerson [23] showed that water segregates into cellular and extracellular spaces of human skin. Flemister [24] introduced the idea that only a part of total water is mobilizable. Nonmobile water is not static, although it exchanges more slowly than mobile water. Static water, however, may be an essential component of macromolecular and tissue structures. This topic is reviewed by Millero and by Joseph in Chapters 9 and 16.

Structure or composition of connective tissue may determine the absorption, liberation, and fixation of water [25]. If hyaluronic acid is principally responsible for tissue water level [26], water content then should change in linear proportion to concentration, or molecular weight, of tissue hyaluronic acid. Hvidberg [27] showed that the water content of rats decreased from 6 to 2.5 g per 1 g of fat-free dry tissue between birth and 2 months of age; hexosamine content decreased nearly in linear proportion to this water reduction. Boas and Foley [28] also showed a concurrent reduction in hexosamine and water during growth of rat skin.

Water is bound so tightly by skin that it resists very high hydrostatic pressure [29]; only 60% of water in skin can be removed by compression under 3 kg cm^{-2} pressure. The remaining 40% can not be displaced even at 211 kg cm^{-2} pressure. About one third of the total water content, relative to fat-free and dry solids, is retained by strong molecular forces. Mobility of loose water under low pressure is comparable to that of water in the bulk liquid state. Tregear and Dirnhuber [30] showed, however, that rate of compression of skin under constant hydrostatic pressure was limited by radial flow of water toward the periphery through the subcutaneous tissue. Plots of sample thickness under a constant load versus time agreed with a mathematical relationship derived for this system. Even though tissue water is assumed to be fluid in this theoretical mechanism, the high coefficient of viscosity of water calculated from data and the model shows that mobility is greatly impeded.

Water can be injected into skin to form a bullae, but this is different from water that is incorporated into skin *in vivo*. Hall [31] showed that plots of log $a/(a-x)$ versus time were linear, where a is the maximum percentage (x) of injected saline lost in time t. Slope (K) of this plot was negative and related linearly to body weight of aging animals. Slope (K) declined with increasing body weight [32], thereby indicating that evaporation of injected water slowed down with aging. This is opposite to the influence of age on rate of evaporation shown here in Fig. 1.1.

Collagen fibers in skin are associated molecularly with polysaccharides, and glycoproteins [33], albumin [34], and other noncollagenous proteins [35] also are present and probably contribute to cohesion of collagen fibers as well as binding of water. There is little consistent agreement on the hexosamine content of aging dermis, mainly because methods vary. Sobel et al. [36] showed a decrease in concentration of hexosamine in gluteal dermis that was accompanied by an increase in collagen content. Collagen and hexosamine of rat skin were reported to increase during growth [37], but Houck and Jacob [38] showed that hexosamine content of fresh whole skin changed very little during growth from 0 to 450 g body weight of rats. Nitrogen and hydroxyproline increased, thus reducing the ratio of hexosamine/hydroxyproline. Recalculating their data on the basis of nitrogen, these authors showed that hexosamine decreased but so did collagen after it attained a peak value at about 200 g body weight of the growing rat. These computations supposedly obviated the need to extract fat and dehydrate samples prior to chemical analysis. However, when nitrogen and hexosamine were analytically determined on fat-free dry rat dermis [39], nitrogen content declined continuously with increasing age from 1 to 5 days and 30 to 36 months while total hexosamine fluctuated with a tendency to decline.

Analysis of ventral thoracic skin in rats [40] also showed relatively little tendency for hexosamine to change in fat-free dry tissue, while collagen abruptly increased after 100 days of age. Smith [41] showed that the hexosamine/collagen ratio is low in old compared with young animals, because collagen increased faster than hexosamine. Clausen [42] showed that hexosamine decreased with age in human-abdominal skin, while collagen increased. Even though a variety of tissues have been examined, there is little agreement on the way findings are reported. The hexosamine/collagen ratio does tend to decline during growth, and this could shift the hydration in favor of binding water to collagenous fibers. A shift toward domination of tissue water by collagen, even if it might be slight, could greatly reduce mobility of water due to special properties of hydrated collagen. However, an excess of hyaluronic acid also could immobilize water in the presence of considerable amount of collagen. Albumin is another factor that needs to be considered as it is present in interfibrous space of connective tissue.

1.3.4 Hydration of Collagen

Collagen fibers actively interact with water at low and high vapor pressure. Plots of water adsorbed versus equilibrium relative humidity [43] can be used to compute free energy, enthalpy, and entropy of adsorption [44]. Integral negative enthalpy of adsorption increased and entropy decreased rapidly when water formed a unimolecular layer on collagen fibers. Subsequent adsorption of water continued to release heat and lower entropy, but the rate of change was less. Negative entropy indicates that adsorbed water is constrained, while the magnitude of enthalpy change compares with that expected for van der Waals type of adsorption.

Bull's data [43] also obeyed the Brunauer, Emmet, and Teller [45] multilayer adsorption theory. The surface area of collagen covered by one molecular layer of water was estimated to be about 300 meters^2 g^{-1} of protein according to the BET theory. The quantity of water (x) adsorbed by collagen at equilibrium partial pressure is related to other parameters by the BET equation.

$$x = \frac{V_M CA}{1 - A} \times \frac{1 - (n + 1)A^n + nA^{n+1}}{1 + (C - 1)A - CA^{n+1}} \qquad (4)$$

The V_M is the volume of gas required to fill the first monolayer $(n = 1)$; A is the relative pressure (p/p_0) of water in the gas phase; n is the maximum number of layers that can be built up; and C is an energy term (exp (E/RT)), where E is the heat of adsorption of the first layer in excess of the latent heat of condensation). When there is no restriction on the number of monolayers, that is, when $n =$ infinity, Equation 4 becomes Equation 5 by simplification.

$$\frac{A}{x(1 - A)} = \frac{1}{V_M C} + \frac{(C - 1)(A)}{V_M C} \qquad (5)$$

Green [46] showed that the BET equation with $n = 5$ closely agreed with the experimental data obtained at relative humidity less than 0.40. The agreement between data and BET theory might be pushed to 0.75 relative humidity by increasing n to 6; however, the uptake of water above this partial pressure rapidly exceeds that predicted by the theory even with $n = $ infinity [47].

This departure can be viewed as representing a different type of interaction of collagen with water for which a new model was proposed by Kanagy [47]. If the ends of collagen fibers are assumed not to react with water, the measured surface area may be equivalent to that of a continuous fiber. The hypothetical area S is $2\pi rL$ and its volume V is $\pi r^2 L$. The ratio of $S/V = 4/2r$ from which the diameter $(2r)$ of the hypothetical fiber can be calculated. Using 0.70 as the volume/gram (V) and 290×10^4 cm^2 g^{-1} as the surface area (S), a radius of 94 Å is obtained. This contains about 100 tropocollagen particles assuming a 10 Å diameter for each tropocollagen particle. Since the surface area used herein represents the binding of water to the first monolayer, the interior of the Kanagy model is not permeated by water according to the model. This is reasonable because surface area was estimated by extrapolating data over regions obtained at low water content. Higher vapor pressure and water content, however, either force water molecules to penetrate the Kanagy fibers or lead to a long-range interaction that influences the interfibrillar spacings on the order of 10 Å.

Even though data on adsorption of water agree with the BET theory in the range of low adsorption, data obtained from the region of high adsorption agree better with condensation in capillary channels. Using the Kelvin equation, namely, $\ln p/p_0 = -2\ yV/rRt$, Kanagy [47] calculated the channel radius r as a function of water adsorbed at various p/p_0. It turns out that one third of water in equilibrium at 0.90 p/p_0 could fit in 20 Å radius capillary channels; two thirds of the water adsorbed at 0.90 p/p_0 could fit into 100 Å capillaries. Capillary channels could be made of voids by longitudinal dislocation of Kanagy (94 Å diameter) fibers whose existence is postulated by data obtained in the region of low water content.

It is appropriate to consider other facets of the interaction of collagen and water based on precise relationships between fiber structure, water content, and x-ray scattering data. Dry fibers scatter x-rays incoherently when they are finely segregated and contracted; wet fibers, on the other hand, scatter coherently because they are extended and uniformly compounded into about 1000 Å diameter bundles [48, 49]. Changes in organization proceed in steps as one adds water to dry fibers. The first monolayer of water slightly increases the lateral dimension at constant longitudinal molecular dimension. Further addition of water vapor near saturation increases both longitudinal and lateral dimensions. Lateral order develops strongly when the limit of agreement between BET theory and data is reached. This also is the same region where capillary condensation becomes plausible. The increase in equatorial spacing of fibers from 10.6 to 14.5 Å may be due to specific penetration of water which also increases the meridional spacing from 600 to 800 Å. Adsorption of water begins as a multilayer buildup possibly on Kanagy-type fibers, but water adsorbed at high content takes place by condensation in capillary spaces. The Kanagy-type fiber (100 Å diameter) is part of the hydrated fiber of 1000 Å diameter. Water molecules, therefore, actively bind tropocollagen particles or plasticize fibers so that they flow together into coherently aligned cylinders.

A number of other studies show that water interacts with fibrous collagen in a specific manner. The dynamic electrical capacitance of hydrated skin was measured by Compton [50], Weir [51], Witnauer [52], and Milch et al. [53]. Selected conditions of frequency, temperature, and water content revealed that water molecules were bound to collagen although they could rotate. A highly specific interaction was discovered by Berendsen [54] using NMR spectroscopy. Interpretation of data led to the proposal that a chain of water molecules spirals around and is attached to the collagen fiber. Later Berendsen and Migchelsen [55] showed that the chain breaks up at elevated temperature. Chapman and McLauchlan [56] confirmed the ordering of water near collagen fibers; however, it is not certain whether these waters are bound regularly to collagen. They propose that collagen induced water to orient into chains without specific attachment. A recent report by Ramachandran and Chandrasekharan [57] mentions specific chemical sites within a tropocollagen particle where water molecules form hydrogen bonds and stabilize the structure.

It is abundantly clear, therefore, that water is bound to collagen at levels of structure ranging from molecular to macroscopic. Rate of dehydration of macroscopic skin would be expected to disturb structures at these various levels in addition to changing hyaluronic acid and numerous other components. Interpreting the data on the influence of aging on rate of dehydration, shown in Figs. 1.16 to 1.19 and by reference to the literature, obviously is a complicated matter. If the correspondence between hyaluronic acid and water content holds even approximately, it would be the simplest basis for interpreting data on hydration of aging skin. More than likely this is not the only molecular basis for regulating water content of dermal connective tissue.

1.3.5 Mechanisms of Deformation

The mechanisms of elastic, viscous, and plastic deformation of skin can be analyzed two ways: one can compare stress/strain data with equations derived for theoretical models of homogeneous and continuous structures or one can relate stress/strain data of real tissue to histological features which give rise to heterogeneous and discrete physical properties. Both approaches are required to interpret the numerous mechanical properties of skin.

The one-dimensional (large) deformation of soft tissue was analyzed by Fung [58] in terms of nonlinear equations. Analysis was restricted to elastic deformation assumed to be independent of time. This is justifiable since 80 to 90% of the total stress response is independent of time. Fung [58] showed that the slope (dP/dL) of a plot of force (P) versus length (L) increased linearly with respect to force for rabbit mesentery. This empirical relationship was then used to develop a stress/strain equation based on analytical mechanics of elasticity. Fung's analysis for elasticity of skin concurred with data obtained by Ridge and Wright [59], even though the latter found it necessary to separate their data into two groups.

Ridge and Wright [59] described the stiffness of skin by plotting extension (E) versus load (L) for a uniaxial elongation. Initial zero length of the sample progressively increased with repetitive stretching, but the curves approached the linear relationship of data obtained in the first cycle. Extension and load below 100 g were related according to the following equations:

$$E = x + y \log L \qquad (6)$$

where x and y are constants; extension versus load above 200 g obeyed,

$$E = c + KL^b \qquad (7)$$

where c, K, and b are new constants. Inspection of graphs, however, shows that data are not discontinuous in the region of 100 to 200 g, nor is there an abrupt change in slope. The slope of force versus length increases rapidly and continuously throughout the 0 to 1000 g range, but there is no obvious reason for segregating data into the two groups defined by the equation.

Biaxial deformation more closely approximates the real function of skin as it is seen *in vivo*. Hildebrandt et al. [60] devised an experimental technique to compare data with theory for two-dimensional stretching of sheets of soft tissue. These authors showed that soft tissues deform analogously with rubbery material; however, a multiplicative factor converts specific deviations of tissue from the idealized behavior of the model rubber. Uniaxial and biaxial linear deformation of rubbers obeys the following equations:

$$s = G\left(L^2 - \frac{1}{L}\right) \qquad \text{uniaxial} \qquad (8)$$

$$s = G\left(L^2 - \frac{1}{L^4}\right) \qquad \text{biaxial} \qquad (9)$$

where s is stress, G is the elastic modulus, and L is length. Multiplicative functions of length $F(L)$ and $G(L)$, respectively, adapt the uniaxial and biaxial equations to the data for specific tissue.

Biaxial stress in skin also can be measured by deforming strips in two orthogonal directions. Ridge and Wright [61, 62] showed that biaxial deformation of isolated strips was asymmetric. Deformation in parallel with Langer's lines required greater force than that at right angles. Since collagen fibers are oriented parallel to Langer's lines in dermis, this mapping of asymmetric deformation follows the pattern of collagen deposition. Gibson et al. [63] also showed that biaxial deformation could be measured *in vivo* on human subjects. They constructed a simple device which rests and records the force required to stretch a rectangular segment of skin. A topological map of biaxial deformation is obtained by measuring two uniaxial deformations in orthogonal directions. The distribution of biaxial elastic stiffness over the skin determines the area of an open wound just after incision. Asymmetric stress patterns deform wounds, or they can be used to enforce wound closure by making an incision with proper regard for the influence of Langer's lines. Relative orientation of a skin sample with respect to body axis must be known in tensile deformation tests. One cannot compare data obtained from samples excised without regard for their orientation. Fortunately, this source of error can be minimized by using rings of skin excised from the rat tail. If the ring is cut at right angles to the longitudinal axis of the tail, the topological location is completely defined if its position along the tail is known. Subsequent variation in physical properties of this prescribed sample then indicates an intrinsic modification of collagen fibers.

The biaxial rheology of human skin can be measured *in vivo* by deforming a circular plate of tissue. Grahame and Holt [64] used reduced atmospheric pressure to deform a circular plate of skin into a spherical surface. Volume of the spherical surface was measured as a function of pressure in order to compute a stress/strain function. Geometrical analysis of this mechanical situation leads to a working equation of elastic stiffness [65]. Tension/strain diagrams of rubbery material were used to show agreement between data and a linear elastic model of deformation implied in this simplified treatment of the problem. The ratio of tension/strain was used to compute Young's modulus of elastic stiffness.

Biaxial deformation of skin also was studied in compression [30]. This system represents viscous and plastic deformation, where the rate at which a circular plate of skin reduces its thickness under a steady load was measured as a function of time. Mathematical analysis of this model yielded an equation for thickness versus time which agreed well with data. The model supposed that water rapidly exuded out of the compressed layers by a diffusion-limited process. The rate of compression, therefore, was set by the viscosity of water held in the fibrous connective tissue.

A number of biomechanical tests of skin deformation rely on compression [66–69]. The pinch test of Hollingsworth et al. [69] falls into this category, while it also depends on elastic deformation of skin. Thus the early invention of the penetrometer by Schade [70] has been followed and modified by current investigators until the technique of compression has almost become a universal test of skin rheology.

Further insight into the biological mechanisms of stiffness must be accompanied by detailed measurement and analysis of uni-, bi-, and triaxial deformation. The anisotropic uniaxial deformation of skin was measured and theoretically analyzed by Veronda and Westman [71] who also assumed a model that was independent of time. Uniaxial force versus elongation data were converted to stress and strain based on initial cross-sectional area. When L_1 is defined as the relative length in the direction of loading, L_2 is the relative width, and L_3 is relative thickness, it was found that L_2 decreased from 1.0 to 0.3 as L_1 was increased from 1.0 to 2.1 during elongation. However, L_3 increased from 1.0 to a maximum of 1.20 when L_1 was increased from 1.0 to 1.9; L_3 then declined to 1.15 as L_1 approached 2.1. Normalized volume of test samples increased from 1.0 to 1.30 as L_1 increased from 1.0 to 1.55, but volume then declined to 0.81 at $L_1 = 2.1$. Gibson et al. [72] also showed that skin expands volumetrically when stretched. Uniaxial extension of skin thus generates considerable force in the remaining two orthogonal directions. Volume expansion during L_1 elongation is due to changes in fiber architecture along the L_1 axis, because L_2 and L_3 decreased during elongation. The three orthogonal dimensions, therefore, should be measured during a tensile test of skin. Because this was not done, valuable information is missing from most studies reported in the literature.

Mechanical properties of skin also depend on rate of loading, or rate of elongation, and this limits the use of models based entirely on time-independent elasticity. Witnauer and Palm [73] measured the vibration of strips of animal hide at various frequencies and showed that low-frequency oscillation of strips of animal hide exhibited a maximum amplitude at about 17 Hz. Real and imaginary parts of the dynamic modulus also were calculated from vibration data. Analysis showed that the dynamic elastic modulus is nonlinear, but it decreased when the driving frequency was increased (this increased the amplitude of vibration). Tests also showed that the resonance curve is reproducible, even when the sample is manipulated extensively. Nonlinearity of the dynamic modulus was not due to nonlinearity of ordinary stress/strain characteristics of hide. The authors proposed instead that changes in the number of fiber/fiber contacts during elongation caused dynamic nonlinearity. At sufficiently low frequency of vibration, there should be no change in number of fiber/fiber contacts, and linear dynamic elasticity should appear. This prediction was verified for amplitude of vibration below 0.1% strain. The dynamic modulus at low strain (low amplitude) agreed with the static modulus of elasticity determined by a torsion test [74].

Higher frequencies of deformation can be obtained by driving the sample with a sonic pulse. Kanagy and Robinson [75] showed that the sonic modulus of elasticity of hide is higher than that obtained by static tests, but it agreed favorably with that measured on isolated fibers.

Sonic propagation in hide appears to occur by fiber/fiber contact. This supports the interpretation of nonlinear dynamic elasticity presented by Witnauer and Palm [73]. If fiber/fiber contact are required for transmission of sonic pulses, then the velocity of propagation should depend on fiber orientation in samples. Elongation of hide markedly increased the velocity of sonic propagation; however, the increase in transmission velocity exceeded that expected for the proportional elongation of the sample. Transmission velocity increased rapidly at low stress, but the rate of increase slowed down with further elongation. Transmission velocity should vary with respect to location of samples. The direction of transmission also should influence the velocity of propagation over the same general area. Sonic propagation, therefore, could be used to map out Langer's lines of fiber orientation.

The study of deformation of skin must be pursued further in terms of analytical mechanics. There are many bioengineering aspects of skin [71, 72] which involve the rheology of connective tissue. However, the hope for controlling aging skin ultimately rests with regulating physiological aspects of collagen deposition, orientation, and cross-linking. Thus we need to relate the macroscopic deformation of skin to properties of dermal connective tissue, particularly collagen, elastin, and water. Since collagen fibers of tendon have been used traditionally as models of connective tissue, the rheology of tendon collagenous fibers will now be discussed as a basis for considering the physiology and biochemistry of aging skin.

Deformation of collagen fibers was measured as a function of temperature and evaluated in terms of thermodynamics by Hall [76]. Force F on a sample of length L at temperature T is determined by energy E and entropy S changes during deformation according to a fundamental equation.

$$F = -T\left(\frac{dS}{dL}\right)_T + \left(\frac{dE}{dL}\right)_T \qquad (10)$$

Both thermodynamic terms can be measured in terms of F, L, and T:

$$-\frac{dS}{dL} = \frac{dF}{dT} \quad \text{and} \quad \frac{dE}{dL} = F - T\frac{dF}{dT} \qquad (11)$$

The energy term can be corrected for volume changes during elongation;

$$\frac{dE}{dL} = F - T\frac{dF}{dT} - MBTA \qquad (12)$$

where V = volume of test sample, P = hydrostatic pressure, B = thermal coefficient of linear expansion at constant deformation and zero pressure, and A is an anisotropy factor $(3V/L)(dL/dV)$. However, the correction due to $-MBTA$ amounts to 10^{-3} units which is too small to be significant.

Summation of differential E and S increments with respect to L quantitatively shows how entropy and energy contribute to elastic deformation. Findings indicate that elongation of nonmelted collagen fibers raises the energy content very rapidly. Its nonlinear rise with respect to elongation closely resembles the force elongation curve. Entrophy also increases with elongation, but the magnitude is about two-thirds that of the energy change.

An increase in energy suggests that deformation of crystalline collagen fibers distorts molecular structure. Entropy increase indicates that organization of structure has decreased. The rise in energy is expected, but it is surprising to find a considerably increased entropy with elongation. However, one must remember that polysaccharides, calcium phosphate, and water are present in collagenous fibers of tendon. Alteration in their structure or their interaction with collagen also contributes to E and S terms of the macroscopic sample. This shows that molecular structure of collagen must be related to macroscopic properties of fibers in gross tissue.

Macroscopic histology of connective tissue shows that orientation of collagen fibers does change when tissues are stretched. Viidik and Eckholm [77] used light and electron microscopy to observe the surface of collagen fibers in tendon that were stretched in a rigid frame. The corrugated surface of zero-load tendons smoothly disappeared with elongation, while it reappeared when deformation was eliminated. Corrugations exist in the zero-load state, because fibers tend to undulate in the longitudinal direction. Rigby et al. [78] also showed that waved fibers in rat tail tendon unfolded with elongation. Their presentation most vividly showed the wave pattern of fibers.

Mobility of collagen fibers is greater in skin than it is in tendon, because they are highly disoriented at zero-load. An imposed stress moves fibers in the direction of elongation. Various orientation of collagen fibers are clearly revealed by scanning electron micrographs [79]. Large bundles comprise many fibers which were better oriented among themselves than were the large bundles; however, distribution of bundles is not totally random. Restrictions on random orientation are not obvious at zero-load, but they appear when the sample is formed. Since undeformed skin *in situ* is under positive tension, the orientation of collagen fibers of an excised sample is not the same as when the sample is *in situ*. Thus the rheological properties of skin in the laboratory situation must be evaluated with due consideration for anatomical location and relationship with respect to Langer's lines in the body.

Molecular dimensions of collagen fibers also are altered by elongation of tissue. Schmitt et al. [80] showed by electron microscopy that the principal (640 Å) dimension is the mode of a statistical distribution ranging between 360 and 960 Å in a sample of freshly precipitated fibers. Some preparations showed spacings that reached 6000 Å. A force-elongation curve was computed from the electron micrographs by relating spacing and cross-sectional diameter (D). Cross-sectional area (D^2) was proposed to have decreased in linear proportion to rising force along a fibril which exhibited different spacings. A plot of $1/D^2$ versus spacing, therefore, is analogous to plotting force versus elongation. This plot indicated that elastic stiffness, defined as the slope of force versus length, increased continuously with respect to elongation. Maximum extendability of molecular fibers was above $5\times$ that for macroscopic fibers.

Any satisfactory theory of collagen structure must account for this fact. Most models of collagen structure, however, permit only a limited degree of extension without rupture. The counterpoint to this proposal is that the electron micrographic technique damaged the collagen fibers which presumably allowed their increased extensibility. Even if this were true, extensibility of macroscopically melted tendon is limited in comparison with that of molecular fibers. In lieu of a satisfactory explanation for the excessive extendability of Schmitt's fibers, perhaps it is best to withold further evaluation until new facts are obtained.

Deformation of structural units in tendon also has been determined by measuring the scattering of x-rays [81]. High-angle scattering increased linearly with respect to elongation, but the sample could be stretched only about 3% before meridian spacings changed. Low-angle meridian spacing increased linearly with respect to fiber length commencing at the origin. These measurements show that macroscopic sample elongation influences molecular dimensions of collagen fibers on the order of 10 and 600 Å. Schwartz et al. [82] found that elongation of collagen fibers, experimentally attached to mylar film, preferentially stretches in the polar regions. Micro densitometric tracings of electron micrographs of PTA-stained collagen showed that a_1a_2, b_1b_2, and c_1c_2 polar regions extended in proportion to overall stretching of fibers. They also noted that fibers "necked down" at the point of rupture. Polypeptide chains, therefore, appear to draw out with elongation to rupture, but this is confined to the terminus of the fiber. Structure of collagen fibers not deformed to the point of rupture is stabilized by water molecules. They increase crystallinity and extend the fiber by coalescing the randomly oriented polypeptide chains [83].

Analysis of the elastic properties of skin comes down to considering various ways of disturbing the orientation of collagen fibers. A basis for the elastic stiffness of skin is developed by analyzing the stress/strain data of rat tail tendon. Relatively few attempts have been made to mathematically analyze the stress/strain properties of tendons. Empirical descriptions have been reported in the literature, but few models have been worked up analytically. An early report by Hall [84] showed that load-elongation curves did not agree with most equations derived for synthetic amorphous polymers. A time-dependent model proposed by Viidik [85] suggests that collagen fibers have different lengths projected on the longitudinal axis of tendon. Fibers unfold independently as the sample is stretched to a critical length; the uncurled fibers resist further stretching due to their high modulus of linear elasticity. Nonlinear stress/strain properties of macroscopic tendons thus arise because low-modulus curled fibers are converted to high-modulus uncurled fibers. A distribution of waviness is thus redistributed among fibers of the tendon by elongation; stretched fibers are more uniformly dispersed than are nonstretched fibers in the same tendon.

This suggests that one ought to find a relationship between strain rate of loading, that is, dF/dL, and either force F or length L. Fung

[58] plotted dF/dL versus F and found that it was linear for mesentery tissue. Stromberg and Wiederhielm [86] showed that a linear plot also worked for tail tendons of mice. They verified the fact that collagen fibers are curled at zero-load, and become oriented in parallel with direction of elongation.

The relationship described by Fung was implicit in a model used to describe the influence of age on elasticity of rat-tail tendon [87]. It is possible that the latter is a special case in Fung's analysis [58].

The stress/strain relationship of rat-tail tendons was measured in an apparatus similar to that used here for rat-tail skin. Cross-sectional mass (W_0) was used to compute stress (F/W_0) instead of (geometrical) cross-sectional area. The weight/length ratio (W_0) in mg cm^{-1} equals cross-sectional area $\times$ density. Plots of F/W_0 versus strain ($L/L_0 - 1$) suggested a parabolic relationship which was verified by plotting F/W_0 versus $(L/L_0 - 1)^2$. The slope was called K_C and defined a specific index of elastic stiffness. Furthermore, a linear relationship with negative slope existed between $\log K_C$ and $\log W_0$. These measurements focus attention on two features of elastic stiffness of collagenous fibers in tendon, namely a parabolic dependence of stress on strain and further dependence of stiffness on size of fibers.

The second-degree equation (1) can be derived by assuming that discrete collagen fibers, or bundles of fibers, are curled to varying extent in a tendon. Some will be highly curled, a few will be nearly straight, while the remainder are distributed statistically between the two limits. Elongation of a gross sample straightens out the curled elements while it elongates the straight elements. It takes relatively little force to uncurl elements, but a large force is required to elongate straight elements which are assumed to be linearly elastic. Force rises during elongation by a function which uncurls the elements. This is assumed to be related linearly with strain as stated in Equation 13.

$$\frac{d(F/W_0)}{d(L/L_0)} = K_C \left(\frac{L}{L_0} - 1 \right) \tag{13}$$

Integration between appropriate boundaries, namely,

$$\frac{1}{W_0} \int_0^F dF = \frac{K_C}{L_0} \int_{L_0}^L \left(\frac{L}{L_0} - 1 \right) dL \tag{14}$$

yields Equation 15 that was discovered empirically (Equation 1).

$$\frac{F}{W_0} = \frac{K_C}{2} \left(\frac{L}{L_0} - 1 \right)^2 \tag{15}$$

Higher-order dependence of K_C on W_0 shows that large fiber bundles are intrinsically softer than small fiber bundles. Chemical composition or structural perfection changes with respect to increasing cross-sectional mass so that large bundles are less perfectly constructed. Stress/strain data for rings of rat-tail skin approach Equation 15 when they are stretched repetitively. Consequently, the stress/strain data of skin rings were reduced to K_c values for the study reported here.

Data reported for the elasticity of mouse tail tendon [86] show that $d(\text{stress})/d(\text{strain})$ increases linearly with respect to stress, but not strain as proposed in Equation 13. This derivitive cannot be related linearly to both stress and strain, although they did show a relationship between strain and log stress that refers back to the analysis of Fung [58].

Fung's theoretical analysis of elasticity is based on properties of soft connective tissue (rabbit mesentery) that stretched about 100% at practically zero force before high-modulus elasticity commenced. Dynamic stress/strain curve was converted to a static curve by multiplying force by the ratio (stress-relaxed force/peak force). Force data also were related to the transient cross-sectional area of the sample rather than the initial cross-sectional area at zero load. Findings of Stromberg and Wiederhielm [86] are based on instantaneous length change of mouse tendon when force was applied in discrete steps. They also found a linear relationship between stress and velocity of stress with respect to elongation. These legitimate and appropriate corrections nevertheless modify the data so that they are not comparable with those used to derive Equation 1. The rationale for the influence of force or length on velocity of stress with respect to length is not obvious. The model used here to derive Equation 13, however, is inherent in all discussions of deformation of connective tissue, and it was proposed also by Viidik [85].

Further work is needed to elucidate the theoretical mechanics of deformation of collagenous tissue, where discrete pattern and structure are included. The dynamic rheology of connective tissue is a fact of reality that also must be taken into consideration. Most reports show that fiber orientation contributes to rheology [63, 77, 78, 86–88], while techniques also have been described for measuring and evaluating dynamics of deformation [89–93]. Deformation of tissue now can be measured precisely, and theoretical evaluations should help to further delineate the influence of aging on physical properties of skin.

1.3.6 Aging and Physical Properties of Nonmelted Skin

Elasticity, plasticity, and viscosity are rheological parameters of crystalline collagen fibers that can describe the effect of age on skin. The "pinch" test of Hollingsworth, et al. [69], that is, the time required for an elevated fold of skin to recover its initial conformation when it is released, is an example of a useful rheological parameter. This test is easy to perform, can be instrumented to give precise data, and is strongly age dependent. Immediate indentation and rebound of a weighted fixture is a test of skin that decreased nonlinearly with respect to age [66]. The rate at which compressive thickness declined with time for a fold of skin maintained under constant force also changed with age in human subjects [67]. The slope of a semilogarithmic plot of thickness versus time also varied with site and sex. The rate of compression as defined by this slope was high in young subjects and low in older subjects. Skin compressibility in the scapular region declined most rapidly with age, while it was slowest in the neck region for men and women. These findings were generally confirmed by Brozek and Kinzey [68]. It is evident, therefore, that elastic, viscous, and plastic deformation (rheology) of skin depends sensitively on anatomical and physiological factors.

A recent study by Grahame and Holt [64] determined elastic deformation of aging skin (*in situ*) by using suction to stretch a circular sheet into a hemisphere. Stress/strain data obtained by this mode of deformation [65] yielded a modulus of elastic stiffness which increased linearly (about $3\times$) with respect to age (20 to 85 years). Elastic stiffness thus increased linearly with respect to age while viscoplastic deformability declined exponentially [66]. Separate values of elastic and viscoplastic rheology thus show a complicated nonlinear response to age when measured *in vivo*.

These findings on deformation of skin tested *in vivo* do not agree with data obtained on skin tested *in vitro*. In a study reported by Jansen and Rottier [95] on excised skin, no mention was made about the skin being tested wet or dry. Their apparatus did not provide for testing in water, so it is assumed that samples were tested in air. A Young's modulus calculated from low-stress region did not change continuously with respect to age as was observed by Grahame and Holt [64]. Instead, the elastic stiffness showed a tendency to increase transitionally between 40 and 60 years of age, while otherwise remaining on plateaus. Water and hexosamine contents also did not change. Elongation to rupture declined after 30 years, but rupture stress fluctuated about a fixed mean value. On the other hand, reports by Ridge and Wright [61, 62] showed that mechanical properties of excised human skin tested in water did change with age. They did not reduce their tensile data to a Young's modulus, but instead calculated constants of empirical equations used to fit curves to data. Their study shows that extensibility constant (b) increased between ages of 0 to 40 years, but it declined continuously thereafter with aging to 90 years. Another constant (k) which is related (inversely) to Young's modulus declined linearly with respect to age from 0 to 90 years. This indicates that Young's modulus increased with respect to age.

Results from these *in vitro* studies tend to agree with data obtained on skin tested *in vivo*. However, data of Jansen and Rottier [95] clearly do not agree. The constant level of collagen in human skin with respect to age [61, 62] emphasizes the fact that observed changes are independent of collagen content. It is possible that rheology of skin tested *in vivo* depends on water content and hydration of connective tissue, in addition to the chemical composition (collagen content) of fibrous and nonfibrous components.

Recall that tensile data reported here were obtained *in vitro* by immersing samples in buffer. Figure 1.21 shows that viscoplastic flow of initial sample length is about 20% of all ages for a fixed mode of deformation at 40°C, and Fig. 1.14 shows that maximum uptake of water is constant. However, the *in vivo* water content of dorsal rat skin decreased with age (Fig. 1.15). If the *in vivo* water content of rat tail skin also had declined with age, it is possible that rheology of tail skin, too, would have changed had it been measured *in vivo*. Constant values of test parameter as shown in Fig. 1.21, therefore, might be due to the artificial effect of a constant water level that is produced experimentally by immersing the sample to saturation in buffer.

The elastic stiffness of hydrated rat-tail skin, defined by empirically relating stress and strain with K_C, increased rapidly during the period of early growth (1 to 6 months), but it increased more slowly thereafter (6 to 24 months). If the elastic deformation and the viscoplastic deformation of hydrated rat skin are grouped together, we can detect changes in nonmelted skin most easily during the period of early growth. Expropriation to rats of findings on human skin, however justifiable, leads us to expect a continuous change in these parameters throughout life. Other test data such as yield and rupture stress and strain (Figs. 1.23 and 1.24) indicate that cohesion of fibrous components has increased, but age-dependent changes in compressibility of human skin tested *in vivo* do not reach these *in vitro* levels of rupture stress. Physiological data (64, 66–68), therefore, differ from tensile data of rat tail skin tested *in vitro*.

Fry et al. [4] present comprehensive *in vitro* data on skin taken from the rat leg which relate to the findings reported here. The fractional increase in circumference of tissue per unit time, defined as extensibility, decreased continuously with respect to age. The viscoplastic creep, shown in Fig. 1.21 for rat-tail rings, should also have changed with age. If rat-*leg* skin saturated with water has an age-dependent viscoplastic creep, then it might not be necessary to relate all rheological properties of rat-*tail* skin simply to *in vivo* water content of tissue. The semilogarithmic correlation of extensibility and tensile strength for hydrated leg skin of rats [4] suggests that hydration alone is not responsible for all changes seen in physical properties of rat-tail skin. A report by Hall [96], however, emphasizes that hydration of skin *in vivo* is strongly dependent on age.

This report shows that the water content of human plasma decreased to a minimum at 45 years of age after which it increased to values at 80 years that greatly exceeded the initial level. Absolute minimal water concentration at 45 years corresponds to the age at which Ridge and Wright [61, 62] showed a change in the direction of their b-term of elastic deformation in human excised skin. Hall [96] attributes special significance to this age, the hypoentropic point, as the time when rate of cross-link formation (decreasing entropy) equals rate of degradation of collagen (increasing entropy). Age at which water content of plasma is minimal might have fortuitously coincided with the abrupt change in rheology of skin; or there might be a direct dependence of physical properties of dermal connective tissue on water content of plasma. This point needs to be explored further.

Tensile strength of rat tail skin increased with age and body weight, Fig. 1.24, just as it did for leg skin [4]. Fluctuations in data of both studies are comparable. The collagen content of leg skin increased from 3.7 to 19.7 per 100 g of skin between 21 and 272 days. However, the content at 101 days was 15.1, while at 601 days it was 13.7. The low rate of change in leg skin compares favorably with that measured in tail skin. The difference in collagen contents of tail and leg skin is not unexpected, since the chemical composition of skin varies greatly with topology. Fry et al. [4] also showed that collagen/area of skin and body weight were correlated logarithmically, while circumference and body weight varied semilogarithmically. Empirical relationships of test parameters with respect to body weight also were recognized and emphasized in the data presented here on rat tail skin.

1.3.7   Aging and Physical Properties of Melted Skin

Fibrous collagen is composed of molecular particles (tropocollagen) whose high geometrical asymmetry forces them into parallel alignment. The three polypeptide chains of each tropocollagen coil in a specific pattern that produces intramolecular regions of crystallization. Nonpolar residues, such as glycine, proline, and hydroxyproline, form a linear sequence of crystallites among the three chains [97]. These in turn produce a linear-cylindrical core that is ordered and rigid. Polar residues with reactive chemical groups extend laterally as appendages from the cylindrical core. They are not ordered in a crystalline lattice, but they do form intra- and intermolecular chemical linkages. Regions near crosslinkages may be ordered by these chemical reactions, which could further influence the mutual alignment of tropocollagen particles. Thus crystallization and ordering of asymmetric macromolecules is a very complex matter as pointed out by Cassel, Ciferri, and Cooper (Chapters 2, 3, and 17).

It has been shown theoretically [98] that asymmetry alone will force rodlike molecules to become oriented in parallel when their concentration is raised sufficiently. Electrostatic interactions increase the likelihood of perfecting the molecular alignment. Volume/mass of crystalline macromolecules decreases in proportion to the degree of ordering. Thus density can be used to measure extent of ordering and the transition of structure between crystalline, glass, and amorphous states.

A first-order phase transition is depicted by an abrupt decrease in density; a second-order phase transition changes the slope of density with respect to temperature. Melting of crystalline collagen [99, 100] is accompanied by an abrupt decrease in density, whereas the glass transition [99] changes the derivative of density with respect to temperature. Fibrous collagen, therefore, contains both crystalline and glass regions of rigid structure in addition to amorphous regions of flexible structure.

Stability of fibers can be analyzed in terms of equilibrium thermodynamics [76, 98]; however, the influence of age on thermostability usually has been based on data obtained under transient conditions where force, volume, and temperature change with respect to time. Melting of fibrous collagen, like that of any polymer, can be studied many ways. The x-ray diffraction study of Wright and Wiederhorn [101] shows most clearly what happens to the ordered structure. Diffraction patterns of tendon collagen were measured as a function of sample length and temperature. Relative degree of crystallinity was defined as the summed intensity of scattering for all peaks relative to the summed intensity of background scattering. Relative crystallinity of the low-angle scattering decreased at constant length when temperature was raised and also at constant temperature when sample length was reduced. The fundamental spacing was calculated to be about 660 Å. The high-angle pattern of melted samples did not change significantly from that of the non-melted material. Complete disorientation of collagen was shown to exist when the melted fibers had contracted to about 25% of the initial length.

Length and temperature data also were shown to be compatible with a model consisting of crystalline segments in a linearly contiguous array. Widerhorn and Reardon [102] then showed that stress/strain data for melted collagen were consistent with that expected for a cross-linked rubber (amorphous polymer) according to Equation 16.

$$f = \frac{RT}{M_C} \times dv_2^{1/3}(a - a^{-2}) \tag{16}$$

M_C is the molecular weight per cross-link, R is the gas constant, T is the absolute temperature, d is the density of the dry sample, v is the volume fraction of melted polymer, and a is the extension ratio. This equation represents purely entropic contributions to elastic deformation, since energy terms decrease rapidly with loss of crystalline structure.

Thermal shrinkage of hide was shown to depend on a first-order phase transition of collagen fibers [103]. The temperature at which shrinkage commenced abruptly was measured as a function of solvent composition that acted as inert diluent. Data obeyed the equation derived by Flory [104] to account for depression of melting points of crystalline polymers where amorphous phase alone reacted with solvent.

$$\frac{1}{T_m} - \frac{1}{T_m^0} = \frac{R}{\Delta H_u} \frac{V_u}{V_1} v_1 - X_1 v_1^2 \tag{17}$$

T_m is the actual melting temperature; T_m^0 is the melting temperature of pure sample; V_u and V_1 are molar volumes of polymer and diluent, respectively; X_1 is the interaction parameter of solvent with polymer; R is the gas constant; and ΔH_u is the heat of fusion of crystallites.

These studies show that collagen fibers are interdigitated lengthwise, and that the molecular structure of native material is partly crystalline. Contiguity still exists in melted collagen, which implies the presence of interchain attachments outside the crystalline region.

The thermodynamics of phase change and elasticity of fibrous macromolecular structure were discussed by Ciferri and Smith [105] and Smith et al. [106]; the helix/coil transformation of tropocollagen solutions [107] and fibers [108–110] also were considered in detail (see a discussion of these topics by Ciferri in Chapter 3). These authors proposed that collagen molecules exist in fibers as an aggregate (C) of crystalline tropocollagen particles, and in solution as tropocollagen helices (H) and (melted) random coils (RC). The three states can be interconverted:

(I) $\qquad\qquad\qquad\qquad C \rightarrow RC$

(II) $\qquad\qquad\qquad\qquad H \rightarrow RC$

(III) $\qquad\qquad\qquad\qquad H \rightarrow C$

Processes I and II occur by raising the temperature and result in loss of crystalline structure. Process III takes place by lowering the temperature and represents disaggregation of intermolecular fibrous structures without melting of intramolecular crystallites. Reactions that lead to fibrous aggregates (C) of crystalline tropocollagen (H) could be responsible for the changes observed in connective tissue with respect to aging. Intermolecular crosslinkages via reaction of functional groups in side chains of collagen would increase the contiguity of tropocollagen particles and also increase ordering of the fibrous state. Special experimental techniques are needed to prove this point, especially if the findings are to relate molecular reactions of collagen with physiological aspects of aging in complex tissues such as tendon and skin.

Melting of crystalline collagen fibers also can be analyzed as a rate process. Disruption of crystallites within tropocollagen particles involves separating three polypeptide chains at a point. This is subjectively akin to formation of a vapor bubble in a superheated liquid; for example, it is a phase transformation that requires concurrent events of atoms that make up the crystallite. The entire molecule undergoes a phase transition by propagation of the isolated reaction. One can follow the overall rate of transformation by measuring the end-to-end length of the macromolecule as a function of time. Steven and Tristram [111] showed that calf skin collagen in dilute acetic acid undergoes a phase transition when urea is added. Viscosity decreases immediately upon adding urea and reaches a minimum at 4.75 M concentration; optical rotation remains constant until 3 M is exceeded, then it declines rapidly until 4.75 M is attained. These reactions indicate that the extent of melting, namely, the degree of end-to-end length reduction measured by viscosity, strongly depends on the urea concentration at 18°C and pH 3.5 when 24 hours are allowed for equilibration at serial steps of urea addition. A report by Engel [112] delineates the breakdown of crystalline collagen into at least two steps. Light scattering data shows that the end-to-end length of crystalline collagen molecules rapidly declines at the melting temperature, while the molecular weight remains constant (first step). Molecular weight then declines (second step) at a rate which is very strongly dependent on temperature. The weight-average molecular weight of products decreases according to a first-order rate law that has an activation energy of 108 kcal mole^{-1}. Disintegration of crystallites per se is rapid, whereas separation of polymeric chains is relatively slow. Changes in macroscopic sample dimension, that is, thermal shrinkage, reflect the reduction in molecular dimension of melted collagen provided there is sufficient interchain attachment to maintain a contiguous system. It is apparent intuitively that transient isometric force, or isontonic length accompanying melting, will depend on relative rates of chain contraction and separation. Interchain attachments help to transmit stress as well as reduce the rate of interchain slippage. Macroscopic dimension of melting collagenous tissue, therefore, can be used to measure the overall rate of chain configuration that changes during melting.

It has been reported by several authors that rates of macroscopic parameters of melting collagenous tissue change greatly with respect to age. The first report dealing with kinetics of thermal shrinkage was issued by Weir [113]. He showed that contraction of melted tendon obeyed Equation 18.

$$\log (l - l_\infty) = \log (l_0 - l_\infty) - Kt \qquad (18)$$

Here l is the sample length at time t; l_∞ is the length of the fully contracted sample; l_0 is the initial sample length; and K is a specific rate constant. The enthalpy of activation was of the order of 10^2 kcal mole^{-1} for thermal contraction of kangaroo tail tendon.

Macroscopic collagenous tissue not only contracts when it melts, but also reextends after attaining a maximum in isotonic (or isometric) contraction. The overall two-step process of macroscopic melting was studied by Elden and Cassac [114] and Elden [115]. Equation 19 describes the net velocity of isotonic (or isometric) contraction.

$$\log \left[\frac{dL}{dt} - \left(\frac{dL}{dt} \right)_\infty \right] = \log \left[\left(\frac{dL}{dt} \right)_0 - \left(\frac{dL}{dt} \right)_\infty \right] - K_{cr}t \qquad (19)$$

The dL/dt is the transient velocity at time t; dL/dt_0 is the initial and dL/dt_∞ is the terminal velocity, and K_{cr} is a specific rate constant. This velocity equation shows that two rate steps are involved in melting of macroscopic collagenous tissue. This is a limiting case for samples that are loaded to a sufficiently high stress. A more complex process develops when the stress is reduced. Chvapil and Zahradnik [116] proposed that a three-step serial process is required to account for length-time data obtained with tendons loaded to a low stress. They simplified the mathematics of this serial reaction by considering the last step as rate limiting. Unreported studies by Elden and Gregory (1966) showed that progressively reducing stress prolonged successive stages of melting in the Chvapil-Zahradnik mechanism. The time required for a tendon to reach a particular stage in the contraction-relaxation process can be used as a test parameter of that particular preparation.

An unequivocal test parameter based on the concept discussed is the time required for a tendon to contract, relax, and degrade until it no longer remains contiguous under the stress—it breaks. The time-to-break of tendons melting in 5 M urea was originally devised by Elden and Boucek [117] as an efficient method for detecting changes in cohesion of collagenous fibers. A study by Boros-Farkas and Everitt [118] compared time-to-break with several other test parameters of cohesion in aging connective tissue. The ratio of time-to-break at 40 months relative to that at 1 month was 100, whereas the ratio of maximal tension at 40 months of isometric thermal contraction relative to that at 1 month was only 16. Time-to-break rises with respect to age by a rate that changes with stress. Low stress gives a high time-to-break that increases nonlinearly with aging; high stress speeds up the reaction as indicated previously resulting in lower time-to-break but this rises linearly with aging. The test parameter, therefore, is not only efficient, but has a sensitivity that accelerates with increasing age.

This digression into theoretical aspects of melting relates to the studies reported here on melting of collagen in skin of aging rats. Data were obtained on melted skin in order to delineate the influence of cross-link formation on rheology of nonmelted skin. Much of what has been said about physical properties of connective tissue in aging skin pertains either to hydration, tensile properties, or cross-link formation of collagenous fibers. Measurements have been made on both nonmelted and melted samples. Quite frequently investigators relate changes observed in tensile properties of nonmelted skin with aging to cross-link formation. However, few investigators show a correlation of data obtained on the same animal tissue for both phases of collagen.

The melting point of collagen, that is, the first-order phase transition temperature, is defined as the temperature at which crystalline and amorphous phases coexist. The melting temperature of rat tail skin was determined here as the temperature at which shrinkage abruptly commenced (Fig. 1.26). Figure 1.27 shows that melting temperature of fully hydrated skin did not change appreciably with respect to age (1 to 24 months). Notice that the enthalpy of fusion (ΔH_u) in Equation 17 is determined by the slope of plots of $1/T_m$ versus a function of diluent volume fraction ($v_1 - X_1 v_1^2$). Experimental determination of melting temperature, even when the tissue is saturated with diluent, does not a priori express the stability of crystallites; the change in $1/T_m$ with respect to diluent fraction ($v_1 - X_1 v_1^2$) also must be known. A precise statement of crystalline stability can be made only by the enthalpy of fusion (ΔH_u). An appropriate determination of changes in stability can be made by measuring $1/T_m$ only if the diluent fraction of melted collagen remains constant with respect to age. Figure 1.14 shows that the water content of nonmelted and melted skin is constant; consequently, the heat of fusion probably is constant.

This implies that the structure of crystallites does not change during growth, development, and aging from 1 to 24 months. Changes observed in tensile properties of skin collagen with aging, therefore, probably occur at sites other than the primary crystalline region of tropocollagen particles.

Qualitative interpretation of Fig. 1.28 to 1.31 suggests that polypeptide chains are interconnected more tightly in aged skin than in young skin, even though thermal stability of primary crystallites has not changed. The process of melting removes contributions of crystallites to tensile properties while revealing the interchain connections of amorphous collagen. Notice that rupture stress (Fig. 1.30) of melted collagen is considerably lower than it is for crystalline fibers. Also notice that isometric contraction force and isotonic contraction (fractional length) change markedly with respect to age.

Is it possible that the number of cross-linkages/mass of collagen fibers increases with age, or is there a shift in the orientation of cross-linkages while not necessarily changing the total number? The former would raise the melting temperature at constant ΔH_μ (heat of fusion) by reducing the diluent volume fraction. The latter also could take place at constant melting temperature if intramolecular cross-linkages of young collagen became oriented intermolecularly. The effect would be to further interdigitate tropocollagen particles that initially were independent units.

Evidence in favor of the latter point is based on data of Heikkinen et al. [119] who showed that the stress/strain curve of melted skin did not change greatly with age, while it did obey the theoretical stress/strain equation for amorphous polymers (Equation 16). Veis and Anesey [120] suggested that intramolecular cross-linkages of young collagen shift their orientation to form inter molecular cross-linkages with aging. Data presented by Rasmussen et al. [121] showed that melting temperature of human skin did not change greatly with ages between 20 to 90 years, but the isometric force of contraction steadily increased over this age span. Thus it is tentatively concluded that intramolecular cross-linkages shift their orientation to intermolecular, while the total number remain constant.

There are exceptions to the statement that thermal stability of collagen fibers is independent of age, but they are legitimately rationalized. Nordschow [122] reports that the shrinkage temperature of aging Achilles tendon varies with pH. It has a strong dependence for young (7-year-old) tissue, while it is practically independent of pH in old (80-year-old) tissue. The isoelectric melting temperature [123] was 58°C from 0 to 10 years of age; it increased to 63°C between 20 and 40 years of age; but it did not change thereafter to 95 years of age. Since the melting temperature greatly depends on interaction of collagen with diluents, it is possible that chemical components of Achilles tendon specifically influence the test. This is not a great problem in rat-tail tendon, however, because very little noncollagenous components are present. Melting temperature of human skin [121] was 60°C at 10 years of age and increased to 62°C at 30 years of age where it remained until at least 90 years of age. Spread of the data allows for about a 1°C rise in melting temperature during growth, but this also could be due to changes in chemical composition. A review of melting temperatures of rat-tail tendon [124] shows that growth of rats is primarily responsible for a slight (about 0.5°C) elevation.

A final point must be made regarding age changes in tensile properties of crystalline and amorphous collagen in skin. Notice that the age at which tensile properties changed with the greatest rate depends on the test parameter. Elastic stiffness of nonmelted collagen increased rapidly during early growth while isotonic contraction decreased. Tensile strength of nonmelted collagen increased rapidly during growth, while isometric force, isotonic contraction, and strain to rupture of melted skin also changed. The tensile strength of melted skin, however, increased slowly during growth and then rapidly when growth was completed. The time course of tests is not the same for each. This suggests that reactions which influence tensile properties (cross-link formation) probably occur at different levels of structure. Also, they begin at different ages and proceed with independent velocity. These test parameters, therefore, may provide a differential analysis of an age-dependent cohesion of fibers in dermal connective tissue.

1.3.8 Physiological Regulation of Aging Connective Tissue

Some information has been acquired on physiological processes that either lead to or result from changes observed in physical properties of aging connective tissue. Rheology of nonmelted skin probably is determined by plasticizers such as water and polysaccharides that soften the high elastic stiffness of crystalline collagen fibers. However, there are other components such as serum albumin whose function has yet to be delineated. Albumin present in interfibrous space of connective tissue could influence the flexibility of collagen-polysaccharide aggregates. Since albumin of interfibrous space is in equilibrium with vascular serum, this macromolecule could bridge some processes that otherwise seem to be independent of connective tissue. As an example, consider the fact that concentration of serum albumin is a negative feedback signal for proliferation of liver cells [135]. Since serum albumin is present extensively in connective tissue [34], binding of serum albumin by polysaccharides or collagen could influence the feedback mechanism for proliferating liver cells.

Even though albumin is excluded from the domain of hyaluronic acid in model *in vitro* systems [126], evidence supports the view that plasma proteins are present in interfibrous space of connective tissue [127]. *In vivo* hyaluronic acid, however, could be different from the model experimental system. Sobel et al. [128, 129] found that both tissue albumin and hyaluronic acid increased in skin following estrogen treatment. Estradiol increased the molecular weight of polysaccharides of rat skin [130], while aging, severe dehydration, and cortisone decreased polymerization. Interaction of hyaluronic acid with collagen [131], or the specific interaction of hormones and other systemic agents, could modify the exclusion of albumin by this polysaccharide. The number of possible regulating routes for connective tissue increases rapidly when other known control systems are called to mind; for example, fluid and electrolyte balance and pituitary-adrenal-thyroid endocrine systems.

Dependence of connective tissue on fluid-electrolyte control would provide a regulatory system for moderating the rheology of nonmelted skin. Changes observed in flexibility of skin [59, 61, 62, 64, 66, 68, 69] then would be a consequence of changes originating in distant parts of an overall control grid for connective tissue.

Pituitary, thyroid, and adrenals are specific hormonal systems which regulate cohesion of connective tissue]132]. Direct administration of growth hormone to middle-age rats does not prolong life or even alter the expected course of their aging [133], but this need not imply that loss of pituitary function is not a factor in degradation of connective tissue in the aged rat. A recent study by Pecile et al. [134] showed that transplants to young hypophysectomized rats of pituitary tissue from rats of 1, 3, and 24 months showed progressively reduced levels of growth-promoting ability. There is no evidence of decreased growth hormone levels in aging animals to explain this finding as a decreased function of pituitary gland with respect to age. However, secretion, utilization, and target-organ response to pituitary hormones are highly unique reactions. These specificities may have prevented Everitt [133] from detecting a response to exogenous growth hormone. Pituitary tissue of aging rats might also contain an antigrowth hormone that suppresses growth of young rats. An endogenous antigrowth hormone could have impeded the response of old rats to administration of exogenous hormone in the Everitt [133] experiment.

A very early report by Wolfe et al. [135] showed by histological means that collagen fibers infiltrate the uterus, cervix, and vagina of virgin female rats between ages of 5 to 832 days. Changes were observed primarily in mucosa, but muscle also was infiltrated by fibrous tissue. Schaub [136] measured the collagen content of rat uterus and showed that aging steadily increased the amount of fibrous tissue. The percentage of collagen which could be extracted declined continuously with aging, thereby showing a conversion of soluble to insoluble collagen. The pregnant uterus acquires additional collagen that is more soluble than that present before conception. This fraction is rapidly depleted during involution, but insoluble collagen of the previously nonpregnant uterus is not removed. The collagen content of rat ovaries and testes also increase with conversion of soluble to insoluble fibers [137]. No information is available about the influence of collagen accumulation on the endocrine function of ovaries and testes. However, some information exists on the influence of endocrine systems on cohesion of collagen fibers in rat-tail tendon.

The rate of loss of water injected into skin to form a bullae was used by Hall [138] to show that hypophysectomy retarded the influence of aging. Olsen and Everitt [139] found that hypophysectomy of young rats retarded the elevation of time-to-break of rat-tail tendon analyzed at a much later age. Steinetz et al. [140] showed that hypophysectomy of young rats raised the time-to-break compared to controls when analyzed shortly after the endocrine disturbance was imposed. Everitt et al. [141] compared the response of hypophysectomy in young rats by measuring time-to-break shortly and a long while following the endocrine disturbance. They confirmed the finding of Steinetz et al. [140] and their work [139], while they described a different time course in response of control and hypophysectomized rats (at 45 days of age) under 6 months of age (70, 135, and 240 days of age).

Whether or not hypophysectomy retards aging of connective tissue depends on how the data are interpreted. Loss of pituitary function does reduce the cohesion of collagen fibers as judged by time-to-break tests. Reduction in cohesion of aging animals to that of animals chronologically younger need not imply retardation of aging processes. A special study designed to evaluate the influence of hypophysectomy on time-to-break [132] showed that many factors contribute to cohesion of collagen fibers. Some are age-dependent while others are linked to stress, hormones, and endocrine systems other than the pituitary. Recent reports by Giles and Everitt [142, 143] show that thyroid gland influences cohesion of collagen fibers.

It is clear, therefore, that endocrine systems are linked to cohesion of collagen fibers in aging rats. Using rat tail tendon and time-to-break as a test model, progress has been made in determining the influence of age on the endocrine control of cohesion in collagen fibers. Physical properties of skin in aging rats now need to be investigated with respect to endocrine control. Theory, techniques, and data presented here and elsewhere in this volume should help to plan specific experiments along this line.

ACKNOWLEDGMENTS

The experimental part of this report was conducted between 1964 and 1968 when the author was at the University of Miami School of Medicine (Miami, Florida), and the NIH Gerontology Research Center (Baltimore, Maryland). Partial financial support was provided by the Florida Heart Association, the Maryland Heart Association, and the Warner-Lambert Research Institute (Morris Plains, New Jersey). Initial experimental work also was supported by a U.S. Public Health Service Grant HD-01066-01 while the final part was supported by intramural programs of the NICHHD through the Gerontology Research Center.

REFERENCES

1. M. M. C. Lee, *Anat. Record*, **129**, 473 (1957).
2. R. Evans, E. V. Cowdry, and P. E. Nielson, *Anat. Record*, **86**, 545 (1943).
3. R. D. Harkness and M. L. R. Harkness, *Proceedings of the Fourth International Congress on Rheology*, A. L. Copley, Ed., Interscience Publishers, John Wiley and Sons, New York, 1965, p. 477.
4. P. Fry, M. L. R. Harkness, and R. D. Harkness, *Amer. J. Physiol.*, **206**, 1425 (1964).
5. R. E. Neuman and M. A. Logan, *J. Biol. Chem.*, **184**, 299 (1950).
6. H. R. Elden, *Advan. Biol. Skin*, **10**, 231 (1970).
7. D. H. Elliot, *Biol. Rev.*, **40**, 392 (1965).
8. B. M. Cullen and R. D. Harkness, *Quart. J. Exptl. Physiol.*, **53**, 33 (1968).
9. B. Dixon, *Intern. J. Radiation Biol.*, **15**, 215 (1969).
10. R. A. Little and H. B. Stoner, *Quart. J. Exptl. Physiol.*, **53**, 76 (1968).
11. G. G. Proskauer, C. Neumann, and I. Graef, *Amer. J. Physiol.*, **143**, 290 (1945).
12. H. C. Wu and M. B. Visscher, *Amer. J. Physiol.*, **153**, 330 (1948).
13. R. H. Shuler, H. S. Kupperman, and W. F. Hamilton, *Amer. J. Physiol.*, **141**, 625 (1944).
14. S. M. Friedman, M. Nakashima, and C. L. Friedman, *Circulation Res.*, **13**, 223 (1963).
15. J. A. M. Hinkle and M. L. Wilson, *Amer. J. Physiol.* **203**: 1153 (1962).
16. V. Wright and R. J. Johns, *Arthritis Rheumat.*, **3**, 328 (1960).

17. E. E. Peacock, *Ann. Surg.*, **164**, 1 (1966).

18. B. McConkey, K. W. Walton, S. A. Carney, J. C. Lawrence, and C. R. Ricketts, *Ann. Rheumat. Diseases*, **26**, 219 (1967).

19. M. A. Rougvie and R. S. Bear, *J. Amer. Leather Chemists' Assoc.*, **48**, 735 (1953).

20. L. Fourt, A. M. Sookne, I. Frishman, and M. Harris, *Textile Res. J.*, **21**, 26 (1951).

21. W. Bondareff, *Gerontologia*, **1**, 222 (1957).

22. I. Gersh and H. R. Catchpole, *Perspectives Biol. Med.*, **3**, 282 (1960).

23. E. M. Widdowson and J. W. T. Dickerson, *Biochem. J.*, **77**, 30 (1960).

24. L. J. Flemister, *Amer. J. Physiol.*, **135**, 430 (1941).

25. E. Hvidberg, *Acta Pharmacol. Toxicol.*, **16**, 55 (1959).

26. A. G. Ogston, *Federation Proc.*, **25**, 986 (1966).

27. E. Hvidberg, *Acta Pharmacol. Toxicol.*, **16**, 55 (1959).

28. N. F. Boas, and J. B. Foley, *Proc. Soc. Exptl. Biol. Med.*, **86**, 690 (1954).

29. E. Hvidberg, *Acta Pharmacol. Toxicol.*, **16**, 245 (1960).

30. R. T. Tregear and P. Dirnhuber, *J. Invest. Dermatol.*, **45**, 119 (1965).

31. M. C. Hall, *Can. J. Biochem. Physiol.*, **39**, 915 (1961).

32. M. C. Hall and E. J. Macfarlane, *Gerontologia*, **7**, 181 (1963).

33. B. P. Toole and D. A. Lowther, *Biochim. Biophys. Acta*, **121**, 315 (1966).

34. A. Neuberger, *Connective Tissue*, R. E. Tunbridge, Ed., Blackwell Scientific Publications, Oxford 1957, p. 35.

35. K. Y. T. Kao and T. H. McGavack, *Proc. Soc. Exptl. Biol. Med.*, **101**, 153 (1959).

36. H. Sobel, S. Gabay, E. T. Wright, I. Lichtenstein, and N. H. Nelson, *J. Gerontol.*, **13**, 128 (1958).

37. H. Sobel and J. Marmorston, *J. Gerontol.*, **11**, 2 (1956).

38. J. C. Houck and R. A. Jacob, *Proc. Soc. Exptl. Biol. Med.*, **97**, 604 (1958).

39. G. Prodi, *J. Gerontol.*, **19**, 128 (1964).

40. D. H. Murray, W. R. Watts, and J. R. Ring, *J. Gerontol.*, **16**, 17 (1961).

41. Q. T. Smith, *J. Invest. Dermatol.*, **42**, 353 (1964).

42. B. Clausen, *Lab. Invest.*, **12**, 538 (1963).

43. H. Bull, *J. Amer. Chem. Soc.*, **66**, 1499 (1944).

44. S. Davis and A. D. McLaren, *J. Polymer Sci.*, **3**, 16 (1948).

45. S. Brunauer, P. H. Emmett, and E. Teller, *J. Amer. Chem. Soc.*, **60**, 309 (1938).

46. R. W. Green, *Trans. Roy. Soc. New Zealand*, **77**, 24 (1948).

47. J. R. Kanagy, *J. Res. Nat. Bur. Stand.*, **38**, 119 (1947).

48. O. E. A. Bolduan and R. S. Bear, *J. Polymer Sci.*, **6**, 271 (1951).

49. O. E. A. Bolduan and R. S. Bear, *J. Appl. Phys.*, **20**, 4267 (1956).

50. E. D. Compton, *J. Amer. Leather Chemists' Assoc.*, **39**, 74 (1944).

51. C. E. Weir, *J. Res. Nat. Bur. Stand.*, **48**, 349 (1952).

52. L. P. Witnauer, *J. Amer. Leather Chemists' Assoc.*, **56**, 343 (1961).

53. R. A. Milch, L. J. Frisco, and E. A. Szymkowiak, *Biorheology*, **3**, 9 (1965).
54. H. J. C. Berendsen, *J. Chem. Phys.*, **36**, 3297 (1962).
55. H. J. C. Berendsen and C. Migchelsen, *Federation Proc.*, **25**, 998 (1966).
56. G. E. Chapman and K. A. McLauchlan, *Proc. Roy. Soc.*, **B173**, 223 (1969).
57. G. N. Ramachandran and R. Chandrasekharan, *Biopolymers*, **6**, 1649 (1968).
58. Y. C. B. Fung, *Amer. J. Physiol.*, **213**, 1532 (1967).
59. M. D. Ridge and V. Wright, *Biorheology*, **2**, 67 (1964).
60. J. Hildebrandt, H. Fukaya, and C. J. Martin, *J. Appl. Physiol.*, **27**, 758 (1969).
61. M. D. Ridge and V. Wright, *Gerontologia*, **12**, 174 (1966).
62. M. D. Ridge and V. Wright, *J. Invest. Dermatol.*, **46**, 341 (1966).
63. T. Gibson, H. Stark, and J. H. Evans, *J. Biomechanics*, **2**, 201 (1969).
64. R. Grahame and P. J. L. Holt, *Gerontologia*, **15**, 121 (1969).
65. R. T. Tregear, *The Physical Functions of The Skin*. Academic Press, New York, 1966.
66. J. E. Kirk and M. J. Chieffi, *Gerontologia*, **17**, 373 (1962).
67. S. Parot and F. Bourliere, *Gerontologia*, **13**, 95 (1967).
68. J. Brozek and W. Kinzey, *J. Gerontol.*, **15**, 45 (1960).
69. J. W. Hollingsworth, A. Hashizume, and S. Jablon, *Yale J. Biol. Med.*, **38**, 11 (1965).
70. H. Schade, *Die physikalische Chemie in der inneren Medizin*, T. Steinkopf, Dresden and Leipzig, 1921.
71. D. R. Veronda and R. A. Westmann, *J. Biomechanics*, **3**, 111 (1970).
72. T. Gibson, R. M. Kenedi, and E. J. Craik, *Brit. J. Surg.*, **52**, 764 (1965).
73. L. P. Witnauer and W. E. Palm, *J. Amer. Leather Chemists' Assoc.*, **56**, 58 (1961).
74. L. P. Witnauer and W. E. Palm, *J. Amer. Leather Chemists' Assoc.* **59**, 246 (1964).
75. J. R. Kanagy and M. Robinson, *J. Amer. Leather Chemists' Assoc.* **51**, 174 (1956).
76. R. H. Hall, *J. Soc. Leather Trades' Chemists*, **36**, 137 (1952).
77. A. Viidik and R. Eckholm, *Z. Anat. Entwicklungsgeschichte*, **127**, 154 (1968).
78. B. J. Rigby, N. Hirai, J. D. Spikes, and H. Eyring, *J. Gen. Physiol.*, **43**, 265 (1959).
79. B. Finlay, *Bio-Med. Eng.*, July, 322 (1969).
80. F. O. Schmitt, C. E. Hall, and M. E. Jakus, *J. Cellular Comp. Physiol.*, **20**, 11 (1942).
81. P. M. Cowan, A. C. T. North, and J. T. Randall, *Symp. Exptl. Biol.*, **9**, 115 (1955).
82. Z. Schwartz, P. H. Geil, and A. G. Walton, *Biochim. Biophys. Acta*, **194**, 130 (1969).
83. M. A. Rougvie and R. S. Bear, *J. Amer. Leather Chemists' Assoc.* **48**, 735 (1953).
84. R. H. Hall, *J. Soc. Leather Trades' Chemists*, **35**, 195 (1951).
85. A. Viidik, *J. Biomechanics*, **1**, 3 (1968).

86. D. D. Stromberg and C. A. Wiederhielm, *J. Appl. Physiol.*, **26**, 857 (1969).

87. H. Elden, *Intern. Rev. Conn. Tissue Res.*, **4**, 283 (1968).

88. S. Glagov and H. Wolinsky, *Circulation Res.*, **14**, 400 (1964).

89. R. W. Lawton, *Circulation Res.*, **3**, 403 (1955).

90. D. H. Bergel, *J. Physiol.*, **156**, 458 (1961).

91. F. W. Cope, *J. Appl. Physiol.*, **14**, 55 (1959).

92. J. Apter and E. Marquez, *Biorheology.*, **5**, 285 (1968).

93. P. Mason, *Kollcid-Z. Polymer.*, **202**, 139 (1965).

94. J. C. Dick, *J. Physiol.*, **112**, 102 (1951).

95. L. H. Jansen and P. B. Rottier, *Dermatologica*, **117**, 65 (1958).

96. D. A. Hall, *Gerontol. Clin.*, **10**, 193 (1968).

97. J. Josse and W. F. Harrington, *J. Mol. Biol.*, **9**, 269 (1964).

98. P. J. Flory, *Proc. Roy. Soc. London*, **A234**, 73 (1956).

99. P. Mason and B. J. Rigby, *Biochim. Biophys. Acta*, **66**, 448 (1963).

100. P. J. Flory and R. R. Garrett, *J. Amer. Chem. Soc.*, **80**, 4836 (1958).

101. B. A. Wright and N. W. Wiederhorn, *J. Polymer Sci.*, **7**, 105 (1951).

102. N. W. Wiederhorn and G. V. Reardon, *J. Polymer Sci.*, **9**, 315 (1952).

103. L. P. Witnauer and J. G. Fee, *J. Polymer Sci.*, **26**, 141 (1957).

104. P. J. Flory, *Principles of Polymer Chemistry,* Cornell University Press, Ithaca, New York, 1953, p. 458.

105. A. Ciferri and K. J. Smith, Jr., *J. Polymer. Sci.*, **2** Part A, 731 (1964).

106. K. J. Smith, A. Ciferri, and J. J. Hermans, *J. Polymer Sci.*, **2** Part A, 1025 (1964).

107. E. Bianchi, G. Conia, and A. Ciferri, *Biopolymers*, **4**, 957 (1966).

108. L. V. Rajagh, D. Puett, and A. Ciferri, *Biopolymers*, **3**, 421 (1965).

109. D. Puett, A. Ciferri, and L. V. Rajagh, *Biopolymers*, **3**, 439 (1965).

110. A. Ciferri, L. V. Rajagh, and D. Puett, *Biopolymers*, **3**, 461 (1965).

111. F. S. Steven and G. R. Tristram, *Biochem. J.*, **85**, 207 (1962).

112. J. Engel, *Arch. Biochem. Biophys.* **97**, 150 (1962).

113. C. E. Weir, *J. Res. Nat. Bur. Stand.*, **42**, 17 (1949).

114. H. R. Elden and B. Cassac, *J. Polymer Sci.*, **59**, 283 (1962).

115. H. R. Elden, *Biochim. Biophys. Acta*, **75**, 48 (1963).

116. M. Chvapil and R. Zahradnik, *Biochim. Biophys. Acta*, **40**, 329 (1960).

117. H. R. Elden and R. J. Boucek, *Biological Aspects of Aging*, N. W. Shock, Ed., Columbia University Press, New York, 1962, p. 34.

118. M. Boros-Farkas and A. V. Everitt, *Gerontologia*, **13**, 37 (1967).

119. E. Heikkinen, L. Mikkonen, and E. Kulonen, *Exptl. Gerontol.*, **1**, 31 (1965).

120. A. Veis and J. Anesen, *J. Biol. Chem.*, **240**, 3899 (1965).

121. D. M. Rasmussen, K. G. Wakin, and R. K. Winkelmann, *J. Invest. Dermatol.*, **43**, 341 (1964).

122. C. D. Nordschow, *Exp. Mol. Pathol.*, **5**, 350 (1966).

123. C. D. Nordschow and E. B. Marsolais, *Arch. Pathol.*, **88**, 65 (1969).

124. H. R. Elden, *Perspectives in Experimental Gerontology,* N. W. Shock, Ed., Charles C Thomas Publishers, Springfield, Illinois, 1966, p. 83.

125. A. D. Glinos, *Ann. N. Y. Acad. Sci.,* **90,** 592 (1960).

126. A. G. Ogston and B. N. Preston, *J. Biol. Chem.,* **241,** 17 (1966).

127. R. H. Pearce and B. J. Grimmer, *Advan. Biol. Skin,* **10,** 89 (1970).

128. H. Sobel, A. M. Kovacevic, and G. Ramelli, *Proc. Soc. Exptl. Biol. Med.,* **119,** 358 (1965).

129. H. Sobel, K. D. Lee, and M. J. Hewlett, *Biochim. Biophys. Acta,* **101,** 225 (1965).

130. E. Hvidberg and C. E. Jensen, *Acta Chem. Scand.,* **13,** 2047 (1959).

131. J. H. Fessler, *Biochem. J.,* **76,** 124 (1960).

132. H. R. Elden, *Trans. N. Y. Acad. Sci.,* **31,** 855 (1969).

133. A. V. Everitt. *J. Gerontol.,* **14,** 415 (1959).

134. A. Pecile, E. Muller, and G. Falconi, *Arch. Intern. Pharm.,* **159,** 434 (1966).

135. J. M. Wolfe, E. Burack, W. Lansing, and A. W. Wright, *Amer. J. Anat.,* **70,** 135 (1942).

136. M. C. Schaub, *Gerontologia,* **10,** 137 (1964).

137. I. Takacs, *Gerontologia,* **14,** 174 (1968).

138. M. C. Hall, *Can. J. Biochem.,* **39,** 1525 (1961).

139. G. G. Olsen and A. V. Everitt, *Nature,* **206,** 307 (1965)

140. B. G. Steinetz, V. L. Beach, and H. R. Elden, *Endocrinology,* **79,** 1047 (1966).

141. A. V. Everitt, G. G. Olsen, and G. R. Burrows, *J. Gerontol.,* **23,** 333 (1968).

142. J. S. Giles and A. V. Everitt, *Gerontologia,* **13,** 65 (1967).

143. A. V. Everitt, J. S. Giles, and A. Gal, *Gerontologia,* **15,** 366 (1969).

2

Aggregation Phenomena of Collagen

J. M. CASSEL

National Bureau of Standards, Washington, D.C.

Collagen, in the form of insoluble fibers or fibrous aggregates, represents the major proteinaceous constituent of most vertebrates and many invertebrates. The properties of collagen fiber are closely related to the nature and mode of attachment of its constituting subunits. That the collagen fiber represents an end product in a series of interrelated steps is obvious. That this process begins extracellularly with a macromolecular unit of well-characterized dimensions have been recognized only since the early 1950s.

An early indication that insoluble collagenous tissue was indeed derived from a more soluble precursor came from the observation by Zachariades [1] that tendon of rat tail, suspended in very dilute formic or acetic acid, swelled markedly and then began to dissolve. This dissolution of collagenous tissue, particularly the tail tendon of rat, was studied in great detail by other French workers, Nageotte [2–10], Leplat [11, 12], and Faure-Fremiet [13, 14].

On dialyzing the collagen solution against distilled water, a gel was formed if the pH was above 5.0 [5, 15]. Addition of sodium chloride in high concentration produced a massive precipitation, but at low ionic strengths the precipitation was in the form of fibrils, the size and shape of which appeared to vary with salt concentration and probably with pH [2–5]. Some of the fibrils had a crystalline appearance and were birefringent [2, 3, 13, 14]. The reconstituted fibrils closely resembled the native collagen fibers observed in sections of connective tissue, and their staining characteristics were those of collagenous tissue—indeed similar to those of native, intact, mammalian collagenous tissue [16]. A further development came when electron microscopy revealed the same ordered morphology, namely, the repeated axial period of about 640 Å and detailed fine structure, in both the reconstituted fibrils and the native fibrils [17, 18].

Early in the study of the structure of the collagen fibril, the term "protofibril" was coined [19] to connote the smallest columnar array capable of carrying the characteristics of collagen, the lateral aggregates of which were postulated to produce the collagen fibril visible in the electron microscope. Orekhovitch [20] applied the term "procollagen" to the solubilized collagen product obtained by citrate-buffer treatment of rat skin in the belief that it was a precursor of fibrous collagen. It has since become apparent that such a definition must be restricted to certain preparations of soluble collagen. The term "tropocollagen" was applied by Gross et al. [21] to define a unit particle capable of being converted into collagen. Concurrent research [22, 23] identified the tropocollagen unit to be the molecular unit of the collagen structure and not an aggregate of units which participates (in observed reactions) as a kinetic unit.

Piez [24] has observed that application of the term "tropocollagen" to soluble collagen preparations regardless of their source and nature is not completely satisfactory, since the intent of the original designation was to distinguish the monomer from the fibrous form. Because "collagen" is now a better defined term meaning the protein and not the

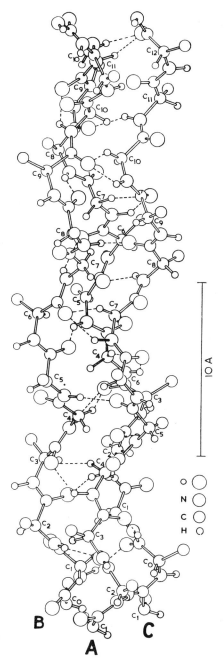

Figure 2.1. Perspective view of the collagen structure for a height of about 30 Å. The α-carbon atoms along each of the three chains (A, B, C) of the triple helix are numbered (from Ref. [28] with permission).

fiber, it appears preferable to use the terms "soluble collagen" or "fibrous collagen" to indicate the physical state of the collagen molecule.

The size and shape of the collagen molecule in solution has been determined by various means. Reviews of that work have been provided by Harrington and von Hipple [25] and by Veis [26]. Some representative recent measurements on native vertebrate and invertebrate collagens appear in the review of von Hipple [27].

The common structural unit of collagen consists of three polypeptide chains (α chains) of approximately one thousand amino acid residues each. The individual chains are in the form of left-handed helices with a pitch of about 9 Å. The triad of these is further twisted around a common axis to form a superhelix with a pitch of about 100 Å (Fig. 2.1) [28]. The basic, rather steep, threefold, left-handed helix characteristic of these individual chains also occurs in the water-soluble form

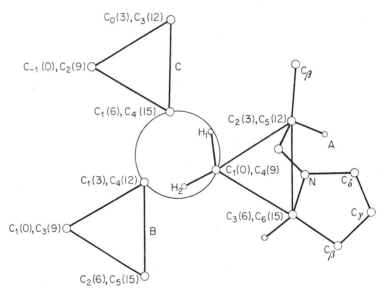

Figure 2.2. The projection of the prototype triple helical structure on a plane perpendicular to the fiber axis. The peptide units out of which the chains are built are shown as rods joining the α-carbon atoms. The numbers indicate the heights of the α-carbon atoms in Angstroms in the three chains A, B, and C. Only hydrogens (marked H_1, H_2) can occur attached to the α-carbon atoms C_1, while β-carbon atoms in the L-configuration (marked C_β, C_β) can readily be attached to the α-carbon atoms C_2 and C_3. The five-membered ring of a proline residue is also shown attached to the atom C_3 in one of the chains (marked C_β, C_α, C_δ, N). The carbon atoms are indicated by big circles and the hydrogens by small circles (from Ref. [28] with permission).

of poly-L-proline (the poly-L-proline II structure) and in polyglycine cast from an aqueous solution (polyglycine II) [29, 30].

The supercoiling requires that every third residue in each chain be glycine and that the glycine residues on adjacent chains be out of phase with each other, since these positions fall along the axis of the molecule where there is no room for a side chain (Fig. 2.2) [28]. The main stabilization interaction in the superhelix or tertiary structure is derived from the cooperative system of lateral hydrogen bonds between the component polypeptide helices, whereas the secondary structure of the individual chains is maintained by the rigidity conferred by the rotational restrictions which exist at the α carbon to carbonyl-carbon bonds of pyrrolidine residues and the partial double-bond character of all the peptide bonds. The decreases in the denaturation temperature of acid-soluble collagen caused by addition of alcohols has been interpreted by Schnell [31] as being evidence that hydrophobic interactions also contribute to collagen intramolecular stabilization. Stabilization by means of intramolecular hydrophobic interaction does not appear likely, however, in view of the fact that projection of the amino acid side chains outward from the central axis of the extended, rigid, triple-chain conformation makes it difficult to achieve close proximity of apolar residues on any adjacent pair of component α chains.

In almost all collagens analyzed [24] two of the chains appear to have essentially identical amino acid contents, a result which has led to the shorthand notation $(\alpha 1)_2 \alpha 2$. The designations used to specify chains involved in intramolecular covalent cross-linking, that is, between chains of a collagen molecule, are β_{11} and β_{12} for the dimeric forms and γ_{112} for the trimetric form. These dimers and trimers are chromatographically separable following denaturation and dissociation of the native helical structure.

The sequence of the amino acid residues along the rodlike unit is such that regions containing polar and apolar side chains are distributed nonuniformly giving an asymmetric or polarized structure. This distribution is assumed to play a dominant role in the modes of aggregation evidenced by the rodlike collagen units.

2.1   THE COLLAGEN SOLUTION

The mode of preparation and the standards of purification of such solutions have varied with the goal of the investigation. Investigation of the amino acid composition and sequence requires removal of all detectable noncollagenous impurities. Customarily, treatment of the soluble collagen extract with relatively mild reagents is pursued until the composition of the product is altered little by additional procedure or until it approaches a predetermined standard. Final estimates of purity have been based on the extent to which known contaminants (such as hexosamine-containing polysaccharides) are minimized and on analytical values for hydroxyproline, glycine, and tyrosine in particular. Studies *in vitro* formation of collagen aggregates as model systems to reveal information on *in vivo* synthesis require stable solutions of native collagen monomers. Comparative studies of aggregation phenomena may (but not always) require less emphasis on complete removal of impurities, but do demand a greater concern for minimizing subtle partial denaturation and for the state of dispersity in the initial system.

2.1.1   Aspects of Solubilization Procedures

The two main procedures applied to extract undenatured collagen from tissues employ dilute organic (usually citric or acetic) acids, free or in buffer form, and neutral salt solutions; the extractions are performed in the cold. These preparations are referred to as acid-soluble and neutral salt-soluble collagen, respectively. The efficacy of the extraction procedures can be judged in several ways: (1) the similarity in amino acid composition of the soluble portion to that of the parent materials (except for relatively minor differences in tyrosine content, where differences that do exist in amino acid composition between insoluble and soluble collagens may be a question of purification); (2) the viscosity and optical rotation of the soluble collagen solution ($[\eta] \cong 12 - 16$ dlg^{-1}; $[\alpha]_D = -330$ to $-370°$); (3) the resistance of the extracted material to attack by proteolytic enzymes under conditions which in themselves do not induce loss of helical structure; and (4) the capability of the solubilized material to be reconstituted to an aggregated form which displays organization under the electron microscope very similar to that of the original parent substance.

There is considerable evidence that the ease of extraction of soluble collagen using neutral salt or weak acid solutions is determined primarily by the state of the collagen in the tissue rather than by inherent differences in the protein extracted. Gross et al. [32] proposed that the collagen extractable from connective tissue by neutral or slightly alkaline solutions of phosphates and other salts is present as a component of the ground substance, an omnipresent viscous gel of the extracellular phase of tissue. Gross [33] subsequently suggested loose, less mature fibrillar aggregates of the tissue as the source of neutral salt-extractable collagen. Such structures were presumed "young" in the sense that they had not had time to establish a more stable, sterically organized aggregate characterized by an increased number of secondary cross-links. Cold, neutral-salt solutions, being weaker dispersing agents than acidic media, are presumed to extract collagen from the more recently formed and poorly integrated fibrils, whereas acid solutions solubilize collagen from older fibrils as well. By chromatographically determining the distribution of α, β, and γ components in the collagen preparations from pig, rat, and human skin, Piez and co-workers [34–36] have shown that the degree of intramolecular cross-linking of acid-extracted material is significantly greater than that which has been extracted with neutral salt. Similar results with calfskin were reported by Engel and Beier [37].

A property of soluble collagen preparations that may be expected to be of particular importance in studies of the kinetics of fibril formation is the degree of monodispersity. That collagen solutions are difficult to prepare in monodisperse form was shown by Boedtker and Doty [22] who found it necessary to apply prolonged and repeated ultracentrifugation with sufficiently dilute solutions. Solutions not treated in this way contained small amounts of aggregated material which, they concluded, could consist of clusters of collagen molecules or end-to-end non-linear aggregates of collagen molecules. Additional evidence for the presence of aggregated forms in collagen preparations was provided by Hodge and Schmitt [38] who noted that ultracentrifugation significantly narrowed the distribution of the length of the collagen molecule as assessed by electron microscope observations of the segment-long-spacing (SLS) forms that are precipitated on addition of adenosinetriphosphate to acidified solutions of collagen.

Despite the conclusion of Engel and Beier [37], based on sedimentation, viscosity, and light scattering measurements, that there was no difference in the size and shape parameters of neutral salt-and-acid-extracted collagens, the degree of dispersity of a collagen solution appears dependent on the mode of extraction [24, 39]. The intrinsic viscosity of acid-soluble collagen is normally 10–15% greater than that of neutral salt-soluble material. Proteolytic enzyme attack, under nondenaturing conditions, reduces the intrinsic viscosity of the two types of preparations to essentially the same value [25]. These treatments are assumed to cleave a portion of the collagen molecule at the N-terminal region which is in a nonhelical configuration (approximately fifteen amino acids in each of the α chains) as well as cross-links between adjacent collagen molecules. From their sedimentation and viscosity data Veis and Drake [40] concluded that the solutions prepared by weak acid extraction of fish swim bladder tunics, that is, ichthyocol collagen preparations, contained an average of approximately 20% of the dimer.

Even within the collagen extracted by neutral-salt solutions Fessler [41, 42] observed a heterogeneity not explicable on the basis of the physical methods he employed to characterize his fractions. He distinguished three fractions: A, which formed fibers at 37°C that completely dissolved on cooling; B, which did not precipitate at 37°C; and C, which irreversibly formed fibers at 37°C. Since B could be precipitated by going to higher ionic strengths, Fessler pointed out that this might indicate the presence of an impurity whose capacity for interfering in the precipitation was reduced by the high ionic strength. Piez [24] has suggested as alternative explanations, heterogeneity in cross-linking and in the amount of lysine-derived aldehyde component, as well as the possibility of a partially denatured species, perhaps involving subtle alterations.

Candlish [43], in chromatographic experiments in which he eluted acid-soluble calfskin collagen from Sephadex columns in the presence of 3 M KI (a concentration sufficient to promote complete breakdown of the triple helix), found that approximately two tenths of the nitrogen applied to the column was not recovered. He assumed that the Sephadex gel permitted elution of α, β, and γ components only (the elution pattern suggested the presence of three components) and attributed the nonelution of a sizable proportion to be a consequence of a spectrum of hydrogen-bonded aggregates in the native soluble collagen preparation. Jackson and Bentley [44] had earlier expressed similar support for the concept that soluble collagen systems contain "a continuous spectrum of aggregates with various degrees of molecular cohesion (or crosslinking), the degree of which depends upon the biological age of the constituted molecules." A greater degree of aggregate formation would then be expected in the extraction of the more mature collagen molecules with dilute organic acids than in the neutral-salt extraction of biologically younger material.

2.1.2   NonCollagenlike Components

The presence of noncollagenlike peptides has attracted considerable interest in recent years. These are peptides that have smaller than characteristic proportions of proline and glycine and little or no hydroxyproline, but are rich in tyrosine and are acidic in nature. Such peptides were revealed by proteolytic enzyme treatment of collagen preparations under conditions deemed normally not to cause loss of helical structure. Schmitt and co-workers [45–49] suggested that these peptides, termed "telopeptides," are derived from appendages that play a particular role in a number of processes including fibril formation, immunological reactions of collagen, and covalent cross-linking. The original concept [50] of native fibril formation involving the interacting, taillike properties accounted for the formation of a columnar array of collagen units, called protofibrils, as precursors to a lateral aggregation process in which neighboring protofibrils were displaced relative to one another by one fourth of the macromolecular length (the quarter-stagger hypothesis). This concept required modification in light of electron microscope evidence that the ends of collagen molecules in the native fibril are generally separated longitudinally by several hundred angstroms [51, 52].

A number of researchers [53–56] have held the view that these non-collagenlike peptides were in the category of impurities. The fibril-forming abilities of collagen preparations subjected to extensive precipitation and resolution purification procedures were shown to be like those of preparations subjected to enzyme treatment such as trypsin, pepsin, or ficin, because, provided that all traces of residual enzyme were removed, the kinetics of fibril formation and the morphology of the precipitated forms obtained by the two types of preparation were comparable.

On the basis of extensive sequence studies [24] Piez has suggested that instead of multiple peptides which branch away from the helical body of the molecules there exists a nonhelical region involving 10 to 15 amino acid residues per α chain at the N-terminal end continuous with the helical portion. It is in this N-terminal region that intramolecular cross-linking has been shown to occur [24, 57].

2.2   FIBRILLAR FORMS DERIVABLE FROM DILUTE COLLAGEN SOLUTIONS

Various types of aggregates or fibrillar forms can be derived from dilute collagen solution. Their detailed structural differences observed with the electron microscope depend on the conditions by which they are precipitated. By appropriate manipulation of pH, ionic strength, and temperature or by adding certain nonspecific agents, such as ATP (adenosine triphosphate) or chondroitin sulfate, collagen may be precipitated in a number of different fibrous modifications [58]. They have substantially aided in the interpretation of fibrous-collagen structure at the molecular level.

An early concept of the interconvertibility of the various precipitated forms is illustrated in Fig. 2.3. The fact that all the different ordered forms of precipitated collagen observed by electron-microscopy staining techniques are associated with the apposition of polar regions of different molecules and that the mode of precipitation depends strongly on ionic strength, pH, and the presence of highly charged polyanions such as

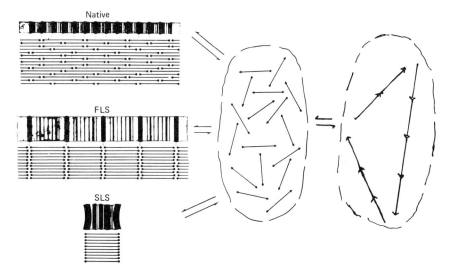

Figure 2.3. Schematic representation of four of the modes of aggregation of monomeric collagen units. Native-type fibrils are formed by dialysis of an acid solution of collagen versus 1% NaCl. The SLS-type precipitate is produced by addition of ATP to an acidified collagen solution. Addition of substances such as α-1 acid glycoprotein, chondroitin sulfate, hyaluronic acid, or heparin to an acid solution of collagen followed by dialysis yields the FLS form. Dialysis of a dilute solution of collagen from a dilute acetic acid medium to distilled water generates the protofibrillar type aggregate shown in the right-hand area of the figure (from Ref. [59] with permission).

ATP, suggested that the mode of precipitation is determined predominantly by electrostatic forces [59]. The nature of the polar groups of the collagen that play the dominant role has been intensively studied. Martin et al. [60] implicated the imidazole groups, a conclusion subsequently questioned by Bensusan et al. [61] who, in turn, postulated an important role for the arginyl residues. Earlier work of Bensusan and Scanu [62] indicated that ionization of the tyrosyl residues was an important step in native-fibril formation. Kahn et al. [63] have suggested a specific role for the inorganic ions in the aggregation media through ion binding with its consequent alteration of surface-charge pattern.

It has been clear since the work of Gross, Highberger, and Schmitt [21, 58] that the electron-microscopically observed, polarized-band pattern of the SLS precipitated-form of soluble collagen represents a molecular map or "fingerprint" of the distribution of both polar and nonpolar side chains along the length of the rodlike collagen molecule. Hodge

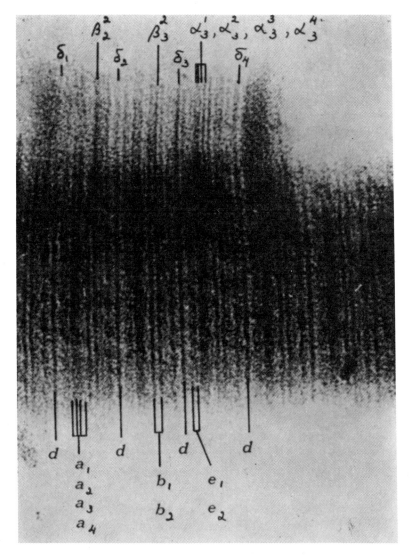

Figure 2.4. Dimorphic-ordered aggregates of collagen produced by exposing native-type fibrils to a solution of collagen molecules and ATP at a pH favoring the formation of SLS. The Greek and English letters designate characteristic bands of the SLS and native-fibril forms respectively (from Ref. [64] with permission).

and Schmitt [64] reasoned that in principle the band patterns of other aggregation states should be obtainable by multiple photographic exposure of the SLS pattern with appropriate longitudinal displacements and with due regard for centrosymmetry or the lack of it. In the case of the native-type fibril, an optical synthesis resulted in a band pattern in qualitative agreement with the observed native-type pattern when the successive displacement approximated one fourth of the length of the collagen molecule as depicted by the SLS precipitated form. Additional evidence in support of the quarter-stagger array in native fibrils was provided by experiments in which SLS crystallites were grown under appropriate conditions on native-type collagen fibrils (Fig. 2.4). The "obviousness" of the continuity of bands in these "dimorphic" aggregates claimed by Hodge and Schmitt [64] has more recently been questioned [65].

The original quarter-stagger concept of the native collagen fibril which was based on positive-staining techniques required modification with the introduction of evidence derived with negative-staining methods. Negative-staining techniques showed that the length of the SLS unit as determined by positive staining was in fact underestimated by 10%. Olsen [66, 67] after analysis of electron micrographs from negatively stained preparations postulated that the mechanism of linear polymerization of the collagen molecules to form protofibrils was by an overlapping of the terminal 10% of the molecule. Hodge and Petruska [52] came to a similar conclusion, and in 1965 Hodge, Petruska, and Bailey [68] altered the original concept of quarter-stagger packing by postulating that the "protofibril has an intrinsic periodicity of 4 D, where D refers to the repeat period within which is observed a major light- and a major dark-band on electron-microscope examination of negatively stained collagen. Petruska and Hodge [69] had determined the length of the collagen molecule by a negative contrast technique to be 4.4 D. On close examination of the band pattern of the fibrous form of SLS (F-SLS) generated by dialysing an acid solution of collagen against water prior to the addition of ATP, it was observed that all the D distances, including that across the junction between longitudinally adjacent molecules of the protofibril, were equal to 1.0 D [52]. From this result and the value of 4.4 D for single SLS segments, they postulated the formation of protofibrils must involve a specific end-to-end overlap of 0.4 D, that is, about 10% of the molecular length. The same degree of overlap was presumed to be present in native-type fibrils. It was further postulated [68] that in the hydrated structure of native-type fibrils, there must be holes or pores about 0.6 D (400 Å) in length with an effective cross-sectional diameter about that of the collagen

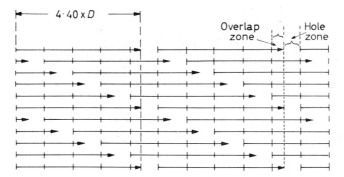

Figure 2.5. A two-dimensional representation of the packing arrangement of collagen molecules in native-type fibrils. Longitudinal displacement of nearest neighbors by a distance D results in formation of a fibril of period D, with each period comprising an overlap zone of $0.4D$ and a hole zone of $0.6D$ (from Hodge et al. [68] with permission).

molecule. A two-dimensional representation of the packing arrangement of collagen molecules envisioned in the native-type fibril is shown in Fig. 2.5. Similar adjustments in the mode of packing of FLS structures from that shown in Fig. 2.3 have been postulated by the same authors [68].

While the proposed overlap explanation by Hodge and Petruska of the packing of collagen molecules in a native fibril very plausibly explains the cross-striation pattern seen in a two-dimensional pattern, the transition to a three-dimensional arrangement which maintains a quarter-stagger relationship between all nearest neighbor monomer units has been difficult to perceive. Smith [70] deduced that only two thirds of monomer contacts in the native structure could be in quarter-stagger agreement.

Cox, Grant, and Horne [65] have been critical of the central role assigned in the modified quarter-stagger theory to the formation of a long linear protofibril, and they have questioned whether such protofibrils as depicted in the overlap hypothesis could be packed by a process of quarter-stagger to form native-collagen fibers. They have proposed a mechanism of aggregation in which the formation of long linear protofibrils becomes unimportant. They postulate a collagen molecule that can be divided longitudinally into five main bonding zones (0.4 D each) separated by four nonbonding zones (0.6 D each) (Fig. 2.6). The bonding zones are thought to contain amino acids arranged in a mutually specific manner so that when two such bonding zones approach each other closely

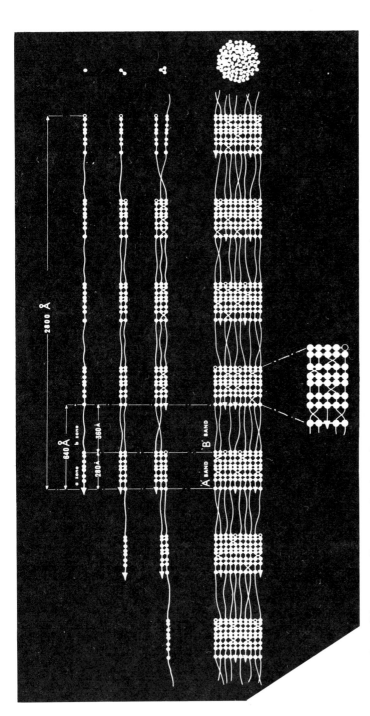

Figure 2.6. Diagram to illustrate the formation of a native-collagen fibril with 640 Å periodicity from collagen molecules of length 2800 Å. The collagen molecule is divided into five main bonding or a zones (approximately 280 Å) separated by 4 main nonbonding or b zones (approximately 360 Å). Some of the bonding sites within the main bonding zones are represented by asymmetrically arranged white dots. By virtue of this asymmetry the collagen molecules are polarized. The white arrow heads and black dots at the ends of the molecules are inserted merely to emphasize this polarity. For the sake of clarity, minor bonding sites within the four main nonbonding zones are omitted.

When such collagen molecules are assembled so that a main bonding zone on one molecule is given an initial random choice in laterally cross-linking, in a structurally complementary manner, with a main bonding zone on another molecule the various stages depicted in the formation of the native fibril occur.

The morphological flexibility of the collagen molecules is emphasized and their ability to cross one another in both the A and B bands is illustrated. The ratio of the number of collagen molecules in the B band to the number in the adjacent A band approaches 4:5 (from Ref. [65] with permission).

in proper alignment, a strong lateral attraction results from the formation of many intermolecular electrostatic and hydrogen bonds. The structurally complementary bonding groups are distributed around the molecule in bonding zones giving the three-dimensional result. The absence of a detectable ordered-electron microscopic pattern in early stages of native fibril formation suggested to these authors that the process was fundamentally random. It was postulated that native-collagen fibrils with 640 Å periodicity (D) were formed by allowing a main bonding zone on one collagen molecule an equal probability of initially cross-bonding in a structurally complementary manner with any of the five main bonding zones on a different macromolecule. The combining molecules are oriented in the same direction. This method of aggregation enables a fibril to be formed by repetition of a single process and permits individual collagen molecules or aggregates of such molecules to be added to a growing fibril.

Doubt has been expressed that a theory of essentially random accretion can in fact account for the formation of the native fibril *in vivo* [71, 72]. Bard and Chapman [71] prefer a mechanism involving very specific interactions precisely located on the collagen molecule. Alterations in the environment lead to a loosening of this specificity with the subsequent formation of structures which show abnormal properties of growth and aggregation.

Veis et al. [72] have objected to representations which treat the collagen monomer as a rigid rod with radial symmetry of its properties at any particular point along the rod. They point to the fact that while two of the component polypeptide chains of the collagen molecule (α1) are essentially identical, the third peptide strand (α2) has a different composition. To achieve fibril stability through a packing arrangement which maximizes electrostatic interactions between rods, Veis et al. [72] propose that a rotational phasing perpendicular to the collagen molecular long-axis must exist in addition to the axial quarter-stagger. Evidence to support this hypothesis is drawn from earlier work which showed (1) that no molecular weights intermediate between the γ components (3×10^5) and the δ components (1.2×10^6) could be detected among the intermolecular polymers derivable from denatured collagen [73] and (2) that addition of salt-free ATP to γ_{111} solutions, renatured by cooling to 4°C, produced copious amounts of monomeric SLS whereas the same procedure when applied to γ_{222} produced fibrous precipitates with native-type periodicity. They concluded that while α1 chains can be aligned and intermolecularly cross-linked *in vivo* with their lengths in register, α2 chains are aligned and intermolecularly cross-linked in the quarter-stagger array. The aggregated structure proposed by Veis et al. [72]

for the native fibril then is a right-handed helical arrangement of four collagen molecules displaced successively from the origin by 0, 1, 2, and 3 fundamental repeat distances, D, along the axis and 90° about the axis. A second tetramer of the rodlike molecules fits directly into the first tetramer, leaving a 0.6 D unit hole and a 0.4 D overlap, and the process may continue to make microfibrils of indefinite length in which each monomer is in quarter-stagger with respect to its neighbors. The model in the view of those proposing it is in accord with observed physicochemical behavior of native collagen fibers.

2.3   KINETICS OF COLLAGEN PRECIPITATION

In preceding sections collagen molecules were described as existing at low temperatures in dilute solutions as highly asymmetric, internally ordered structures. Dilute solutions of such molecules are known to be stable. However, because of the space-filling problem that is encountered with highly asymmetric macromolecules of any type, isotropic solutions can only exist at extremely high dilution [74–76]. As the solute concentration is increased, phase separation must occur as a consequence of the asymmetry of the large collagen molecules. In the absence of any intermolecular interactions, both phases that result are predicted to be dilute with one being isotropic and the other anisotropic. However, supplementation of the consequence of high asymmetry with a comparatively low-interaction energy is predicted to cause the formation of a concentrated phase with the near depletion of solute from the dilute phase. The change from a dilute isotropic solution to a dense ordered phase should occur reasonably abruptly and possess the general characteristics associated with a phase transition. It was therefore logical to see if experimental observations of the precipitation of native-type collagen fibrils were indeed consistent with the general theory just outlined.

2.3.1   Fibril Formation as a Nucleation and Growth Process

Precipitation of native-type collagen fibrils can be studied isothermally [77–84] or by raising the temperature at some selected rate [85, 86]. Early isothermal studies [78–80] revealed that the rate of fibril formation (determined by measuring the turbidity of collagen solutions) was dependent on pH, ionic strength, and temperature and could be sensitive to the presence of specific ions in the aggregating media. Wood and

Keech [83] in an electron microscope study examined the distributions in fibril diameter produced in native-type fibrils which were precipitated isothermally. These fibrils were formed in pH 6–8 buffer solutions of collagen at selected temperatures in the range 21–37°C. Large fibrils and a greater range in diameter were favored by precipitation at low temperature and pH, but high ionic strength at neutral pH also promoted formation of large fibrils.

Isothermal studies demonstrated that native-type collagen fibril formation took place in two steps; a lag or induction period, followed by a period of rapidly increased precipitation. Such kinetics indicated that nucleation and growth processes were involved. Nucleation processes possess certain unique features which distinguish them from the usual chemical and physical processes. Cassel et al. [84] reasoned that verification of a nucleation act in the isothermal precipitation of native fibrils would indeed permit the conclusion that a phase change was involved and would allow the formal physical chemical classification of the phenomenon along the lines previously discussed.

Mathematical analyses of the rate of fibril formation were given by Wood [80] and by Cassel et al. [84]. Wood, assuming that reaction of the soluble collagen particles with the surface of growing fibrils controlled the rate of growth and employing the nucleation-growth concept, as applied by Waugh [87] to the precipitation of insulin fibers, derived equations which qualitatively accounted for (1) the occurrence of a lag period in precipitation during which nucleation predominates over growth, (2) the time course of precipitation after the lag period, and (3) the observation that the final distribution of fibril width is determined during the lag period.

Cassel et al. [84] observed the kinetics of native-type fibril formation over a wide range of collagen concentrations (0.001–0.40%) at temperatures of 16–40°C. The magnitude of the very strong, positive temperature coefficient of the precipitation was noted as not being reconcilable with that associated with normal chemical reactions. A dependence of the rate of precipitation on concentration, while not nearly as dramatic as that of temperature, was demonstrated, the more concentrated systems precipitating at a more rapid rate. Defining the relative extent of the precipitation X as

$$X = \frac{C_0 - C}{C_0 - C_s}$$

where C_0 is the initial collagen concentration, C the concentration of collagen in the supernatant at the time t, and C_s the corresponding quantity at the termination of the process, it had been shown earlier

[77] that

$$X = \frac{E}{E_\infty}$$

where E is the extinction at time t and E_∞ the corresponding quantity upon completion of the precipitation. Defining a "half-time" for the process, $t_{1/2}$, as the time required for half the maximum value of the extinction coefficient to be achieved, the rates of precipitation were quantitatively

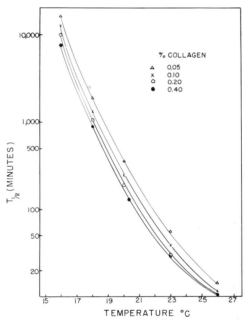

Figure 2.7. Semilog plots of precipitation half-times ($t_{\frac{1}{2}}$) versus temperature for aggregating solutions of varying collagen concentration at constant ionic strength 0.5 and pH 7.5 [84].

compared in plots such as that shown in Fig. 2.7. The logarithmic plot is necessitated by the broad time scale encompassed by the measurements. The shapes of these time-temperature curves are quite similar for each concentration and if rescaled, utilizing a fictitious temperature for each concentration, will result in a single curve.

Plots of the extent of precipitation, X, as a function of time, t, were made, a typical one being that of Fig. 2.8. As illustrated in the right-hand

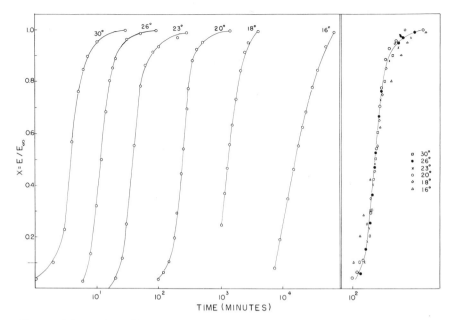

Figure 2.8. *Left:* Effect of temperature on extent of precipitation X at time t for 0.1% collagen solutions at constant ionic strength 0.5 and pH 7.5. *Right:* Superposition of isotherms to the isotherm at 20°C [84].

box of the figure, at temperatures above 16°C the curves are superposable to $X = 1$ merely by shifting each an appropriate distance along the horizontal axis. This superposability permitted the conclusion that the kinetics of the process were indeed explicable by a reduced variable involving time and temperature.

According to nucleation theory for precipitation [88–90], the rate of nucleation can be expressed by

$$N = N_0 \exp\left[\frac{-b\sigma^3}{RT(\Delta F_A)^2}\right]$$

where N_0 is a term dependent on the concentration of solute molecules and the activation energy for the growth of a nucleus, b is a geometrical factor describing the shape of the nucleus, σ is the interfacial energy per unit area between a nucleus and the mother liquor, and ΔF_A is the free energy involved in the transfer of a participating molecule between two macroscopic phases. At constant temperature, ΔF_A will be proportional to the logarithm of the supersaturation ratio, and at constant composition there will be proportionality with the difference in the temperature from that at equilibrium. In effect, the term $\sigma^3/(\Delta F_A)^2$ is related to the size or the number of molecules required to form a nucleus of minimum-sized stability. This quantity is very sensitive to temperature and supersaturation ratio, and consequently the rate of nucleation is affected.

For a dilute system of nucleating particles, growth will be governed by processes occurring either at the particle-solution interface or in the diffusion of the solute component to the interface. Cassel et al. [84] treated these processes independently in the analysis of their data. The functional dependence of the extent of collagen fibril precipitation on a reduced time variable, κ, as deduced from equations derived from diffusion- and interface-controlled reactions is shown in Fig. 2.9. For the range 18–30°C, good agreement with interface control (assuming a fixed number of particles) is obtained for $X \geq 0.2$ in accord with

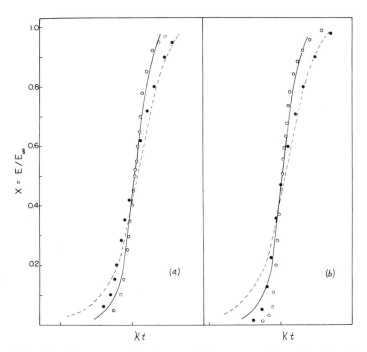

Figure 2.9. Fit of superposed isotherms of the extent of precipitation X against log time with calculated curves based on interface (continuous line in figure) or diffusion (dashed line in figure) controlled processes. Solid circles are experimental data obtained at 16°C. Open circles represent superposed isotherms (18°–30°C) of the type shown in Fig. 2.8. Graphs (a) and (b) are for 0.1% and 0.3% collagen solutions respectively [84].

the conclusion of Wood [80]. The data at 16°C however, are more adequately described by the equation for diffusion-controlled growth. Both Wood [80] and Cassel et al. [84] were in agreement that nuclei are not constant in number during the lag period but increase with time. The results of Wood [80] and of Cassel et al. [84] also clearly substantiated the concept that a phase transition is involved during the isothermal precipitation of native-type collagen fibrils, commonly referred to as "heat precipitation."

2.3.2   Role of Polyanions in Collagen Precipitation

It has been indicated that, since soluble collagen can be reconstituted to native-type fibrils in the absence of added polyanions, mucopolysaccharides are unlikely to play any direct role in the *in vivo* fibril forming process [79, 91, 92]. Lowther [93] suggested an indirect role through the formation of an extracellular viscous gel which may play the role of confining collagen molecules near a cell surface and thus by a concentration effect assist in their aggregation to fibrils.

It has been known for some time [94, 95] that mucopolysaccharides cause precipitation of collagen from tissue extracts over a pH range 3–4. The probability that these precipitations were a demonstration of the nonspecific coprecipitation of oppositely charged colloids was pointed out by Jackson and Bentley [96]. In many cases the fibrils precipitated under these circumstances were either devoid of structure or showed spacings other than the 640 Å spacing associated with native fibers [94].

The first observations of the effect of polyanions such as chondroition sulfate, hyaluronic acid, keratin sulfate, and heparin sulfate in a neutral pH range indicated little or no effect on the rate of native-type collagen fibril formation. Wood [81], however, using the more discriminatory temperature of 25°C in a careful study of the effect of such polyanions, showed that very low concentrations of chondroitin sulfates A and C and keratosulfate accelerated the nucleation phase and rate of fibril development, whereas heparin, deoxyribonucleic acid, and a series of dextran sulfates of different molecular weights and degrees of sulfation had an opposing effect. Such effects were eliminated by prior dialysis of the collagen solution against phosphate buffer. On the other hand, chondroitin sulfate B and hyaluronic acid were without effect on the fibril formation. The electron microscope observations of Keech [97] indicated that precipitation-accelerators produced thinner fibrils, whereas the presence of inhibitors provided thicker fibrils.

For compounds to have an accelerating effect on fibril formation, the structural requirements are apparently severe, since compounds as closely related as chondroitin sulfates A and B have different effects. Evidence of similar sensitivity is provided by the results of Caygill [98] who observed that while ascorbic acid delays or, depending on concentration, prevents native-type fibril formation under conditions similar to those expected *in vivo*, dehydroascorbic acid is without effect. Trnavska et al. [99], examining the effect of certain intermediary metabolites of the aldehyde and benzoquinone type on the kinetics of fibril formation at 30°C in neutralized, acid-soluble collagen preparations of rat skin, found homogentistic acid to be much more potent than gentistic acid in its ability to decrease the lag phase, that is, in enhancing the nucleation process.

From measurements of the rate of turbidity developed at 25°C in neutralized, acid-soluble collagen extracts of skin, Németh-Csóska and Kaiser [100] concluded that the effect of chondroitin sulfate A on fibril formation was dependent on the age of the rat used as the source of the collagen. Addition of the chondroitin sulfate A was found to reverse the order as regards the relative rate of fibril formation observed in neutralized, acid-soluble skin collagens derived from young, middle-aged (the most rapidly precipitating form in the control experiment), and old rats (the most rapidly precipitating form in the presence of chondroitin sulfate A). While chondroitin sulfate A significantly accelerated fibril formation in the "young" and "old" collagen, it had a negligible effect—in fact, a slight inhibitory one on the "middle-aged" collagen. However, a factor of undetermined importance in these experiments is the presence of 20–30% of noncollagenous protein in these acid-soluble collagen preparations.

Toole and Lowther [101] have recently described precipitation of acid-soluble collagen by chondroitin sulfate protein. At 40°C, instantaneous precipitation occurred at physiological pH and ionic strength involving approximately two thirds of the total collagen, and electron microscope examination indicated that native-type fibrils were precipitated. Further addition of chondroitin sulfate protein did not give added precipitate. Heating the supernatant at 37°C caused precipitation after a lag period dependent on the concentration of the components. The lag period observed in the fibril formation of the supernatant was four to five times that observed on a portion of the untreated solution (not containing chondroitin sulfate protein) diluted to comparable concentration. These authors suggested that the original collagen solution contained two fractions differing both in ability to react with chondroitin sulfate protein and to form fibrils at 37°C. Toole and Lowther's [101] schematic representation of the interactions between components of a collagen solution and chondroitin sulfate protein are shown in Fig. 2.10.

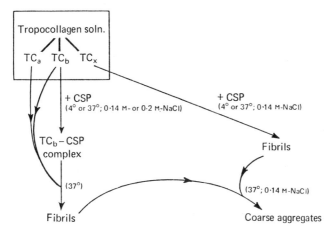

Figure 2.10. Schematic representation of the interactions between components of a collagen solution and chondroitin sulfate-protein. Abbreviations TC_a and TC_b refer to "growth" and "nucleus-forming" collagen monomers respectively; TC_x refers to an aggregate of collagen; CSP is chondroitin sulfate protein (from Ref. [101] with permission).

2.4   SOME THERMODYNAMIC ASPECTS OF COLLAGEN AGGREGATION

2.4.1   Phase Diagram Determinations

In collagen precipitation the free energy of forming a critical-size nucleus will be dependent on the undercooling and supersaturation, and the steady-state rate of nucleation will be similarly affected [84]. It is important, therefore, that the equilibrium phase line, or solubility curve, be established, because it is from this curve that nucleation rates must be reckoned. A schematic representation of the transitions and phase equilibria involving collagen molecules is given in Fig. 2.11. The aggregation process, which is the subject of this review, involves transition from phase II to phase III. In Fig. 2.11 the boundary between these phases is shown by a solid line. In agreement with the positive temperature coefficient of the aggregation process (Fig. 2.7), this line has a negative slope rather than the positive slope of the dashed line. (Transitions to phase I represent denaturation processes and are not of concern in the present review. It is to be noted that an isotropic solution of rodlike collagen molecules can be converted directly by appropriate temperature increase into either an ordered anisotopic phase or a disordered phase containing denatured molecules. Conversion into the

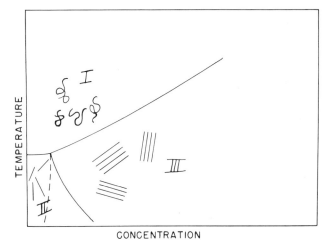

CONCENTRATION

Figure 2.11. Schematic representation of the transitions and phase equilibria involving collagen molecules. Temperature and collagen concentration are the variables plotted.

latter phase may also occur via the anisotropic phase with sufficient increase in temperature. A specific phase diagram would depend on the conditions of pH, ionic strength, and salt types present.

Pseudophase diagrams with temperature and salt concentration as variables have been determined by Bianchi et al. [85, 86]. From their work, a systematic overview of the effects of salt concentration, salt type, and pH on transformation temperatures can be obtained. Freshly prepared rat-tail-tendon-collagen solutions of a given pH and salt concentration were equilibrated in the cold for at least 12 hours after which the temperature was gradually increased. From visual observation and viscosity measurements, the nature of the physical state of the collagen molecules under a specific set of conditions was determined; these data, plotted as pseudophase diagrams, are given in Fig. 2.12. The authors concluded that the variety of effects investigated could be most usefully rationalized by the assumption of one primary mechanism of interaction between salts and protein, namely a binding of the ions with the collagen substrate. The adsorption of cations was envisaged as increasing the stability of the helical form in isotropic solution relative to that in the ordered native-fibril form. Adsorption of anions produces the reverse stability relationship.

2.4.2 Hydrophobic Bonding Aspects

Hydrophobic bonding is the term used to describe the tendency of nonpolar groups to adhere to one another in an aqueous environment.

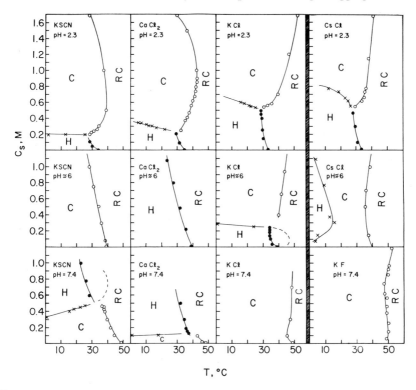

Figure 2.12. Pseudo-phase diagrams for ternary water–collagen–salt solutions. The temperature of the transformations of the helical monomers H, aggregates C, helical monomers H, randomly coiled forms RC and aggregate C to randomly coiled forms RC are plotted as a function of salt concentration C_s. Collagen concentration is near 0.05% (from Ref. [86] with permission).

The aversion of the apolar side chains of globular proteins for water results in the tendency for these residues to be in the interior of these rather compact spherelike conformations, an arrangement responsible for the hydrophobic bond stabilization of these structures [102].

Evidence of a role for hydrophobic bonding in native-type collagen fibril formation has been presented by Cassel [103] who determined the temperature coefficients of the proportions of collagen aggregated in the three processes: native-type fibril formation as induced in the heat precipitation process, ATP-induced lateral aggregation giving the SLS form, and the end-to-end aggregation that occurs on dialysis of weakly acidified, dilute collagen solutions against distilled water [64]. The endothermicity of the native-type fibril formation was in strong contrast to the exothermic character of each of the other aggregation processes.

The opposing effects of temperature along with the contrasting effect of ionic strength on the aggregations were interpreted by Cassel [103] as evidence against any interpretation that the forces governing the native-type fibril formation are a simple composite of those directing the other two aggregations. Despite the role of electrostatic forces in the highly specific alignment of collagen units in the native aggregate, it was concluded that the greatest stabilizing contribution was that achieved through entropy-driven hydrophobic bonding. The thermodynamics of this type of bond have been discussed by Kauzmann [102] in some detail. Cassel [103] and Bianchi et al. [85] independently postulated that the required entropy gain in transferring collagen molecules from the isotropic phase to the ordered anisotropic phase of native-type fibrils was provided by a disruption of water structure around the individual rodlike collagen molecules. The nonhelical end regions of the collagen molecules were not considered to play a dominant role in this aggregation although intermolecular cross-links involving these regions could presumably be responsible for diminished reversibility of the aggregation noted with time.

Supporting the interpretation that disruption of water structure plays an important role in native-type fibril precipitation is the fact that the energy of activation for this process decreases with increased addition of various alcohols known to act as breakers of water structure [104]. Cassel and Christensen [105] reasoned that an aggregation process placing apolar side-chain groups in contact would diminish the organized water structure around such surfaces and should, in accordance with measurements made on hydrocarbon-water systems [102], be accompanied by a net increase in volume. By precise dilatometric measurement, they observed a volume increase of 0.8×10^{-3} ml g^{-1}, of collagen in a system aggregating at neutral pH in phosphate buffer.

Fessler [106] concluded from apparent density measurements that nearly one fourth of the water "shell" is lost on formation of native-type fibril, for example, the water decreases from 19.0 to 14.5 mM g^{-1} collagen. Cassel and Christensen [105] estimated that agreement between this calculated "water loss" and their dilatometrically measured volume increase required a density 1% greater than normal in the water involved in the quasi-crystalline water sheath, hence concluded that the apparent density increase observed by Fessler was compatible with their finding of a volume increase.

It should be noted that other polymeric substances, for example, polyproline [107–110] and tobacco mosaic virus protein [111], exhibit aggregation phenomena very closely related to those of collagen in that they occur without change of polymer conformation and are favored by in-

creasing temperatures. The active role of solvent water has been implicated in these phenomena as well.

2.4.3   Time-Dependent Changes in the Reversibility of Native-Type Fibril Formation

Judging from x-ray diffraction and electron microscope evidence, the
native-type fibrils precipitated *in vitro* from collagen solutions are very
similar to the collagenous material observed in various tissues. However,
with the exception of rat-tail tendon, most collagenous tissue of mature
animals yields little, extractable, undenatured collagen without the aid
of enzymatic treatment.

The extent to which *in vitro*, heat-precipitated, collagen can be resolubilized by decreasing the temperature has been shown to depend on
(1) the mode of collagen preparation, that is, the resolubilization of
acid-soluble collagen preparations after heat precipitation is apparently
much less readily achieved than with neutral-salt soluble collagen precipitated in a similar manner [82]; (2) the ionic strength employed
during the heat precipitation [33]; (3) the relative extent to which a
particular heat precipitation has been allowed to proceed [33]; and
(4) the time lapse between complete precipitation and attempts at
resolubilization [33, 41, 112].

Fessler [41] observed that while one fraction of neutral-salt-soluble
rabbit-skin collagen was capable of repeated heat precipitation and resolution by cooling, a second fraction was relatively insoluble when subjected to similar temperature manipulation. Since the reversibly precipitated fibrils remained so after removal of the insoluble material from
the system, Fessler concluded the heterogeneity was a property of the
native, neutral, collagen solution and was not caused by the heat-precipi-
tation step. Of the two fractions, the one showing irreversible fiber formation was found by ultracentrifugation to have a significantly greater
portion of β component, the formation of which involves cross-linking
of any two of the α chains [82].

Gross [33] had suggested that the decrease in solubility of heat-precipitated collagen with time was due to a gradual attainment of a more
ordered arrangement and closer packing of the collagen molecules in
the precipitated fibrils under the influence of thermal motion. This re-
ordering, together with elimination of water molecules, was presumed
to produce stronger intermolecular attractions. Gross subsequently [113]
specified that among these stronger intermolecular attractions were those
which resulted in covalent cross-link formation. Supporting evidence for
the occurrence of intermolecular cross-linking between collagen molecules

resulting from the close proximity achieved in the heat precipitation step was provided by Bannister [114]. Salt-soluble, rat-skin collagen, precipitated from solution at neutral pH and 37°C, partly resolubilized in 24 hours at 4°C. After denaturing the collagen components of the dissolved and nondissolved phases, analysis of the aggregated forms was performed by starch-gel electrophoresis. Compared with the parent salt-soluble collagen, the material remaining insoluble after heat precipitation and subsequent cooling had significantly more of a component of low mobility, shown previously [115] to be an aggregate of collagen molecules.

Studies with *in vivo* altered collagens have provided an insight into the mechanism by which insolubility of collagen fibrils is developed both *in vivo* and *in vitro*. Animals in which lathyrism has been produced have been of particular value. Lathyrism, commonly induced experimentally by feeding the reagent β-aminopropionitrile, is characterized by mesenchymal deformities, loss of tensile strength in collagenous tissue, and dramatic increase in extractability of collagen from such tissues [116]. The molecular dimensions, conformation, and rate of fibril-forming ability of lathyritic collagen do not seem to be grossly altered [117] although there is evidence for reduced intramolecular cross-linking characteristics of the *in vivo* maturation process [35, 118, 119].

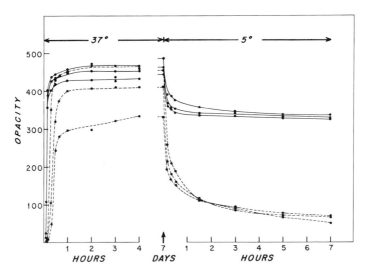

Figure 2.13. Opacity changes observed on heating and then cooling neutral solutions of collagen extracted from the skin of normal (———) and lathyritic (----) guinea pigs. Curves to the left represent aggregation, those to the right dissolution (from Ref. [117] with permission).

The fibrils precipitated at 37°C from neutral solutions of collagen derived from lathyritic animals do not develop the insolubility with time that is characteristic of collagen from normal animals (Fig. 2.13) [117]. The inability to develop insolubility in fibrils aged at 37°C was termed by Gross an "intermolecular defect." Subsequent investigators have correlated this defect with an aldehyde component of the collagen structure. The collagen of animals fed the lathyrogen β-aminopropionitrile apparently becomes extractable as a result of an inhibition of cross-linking that involves aldehydic forms derived *in vivo* from both lysine [120, 121] and hydroxylysine [122–124]. Blockage of cross-linking by lathyrogens is presumed to involve inhibition of the enzymatic oxidative deamination step in the conversion of lysyl residues to allysyl (α-amino-adipic-δ-semialdehyde). Penicillamine feeding, on the other hand, prevents utilization of these allysine residues in a subsequent step of the cross-linking procedure [125, 126]. When cross-linking of two α chains occurs within the collagen molecule—intramolecular cross-linking, that is—the β components that are formed can be readily characterized, since they are soluble following denaturation of the collagen and are separable from α chains on the basis of size and charge. However, when cross-links are formed intermolecularly, little of the collagen dissolves even under denaturing conditions and the products formed by such cross-linking are not readily characterized, hence the specific cross-linking mechanism is difficult to determine. It is generally assumed, however, that reactions similar to those involved in the intramolecular cross-linking occur. While there is strong evidence that intramolecular cross-linking occurs in the nonhelical N-terminal regions of the collagen molecule, intermolecular cross-linking is presumably not so restricted.

Tanzer et al. [127] in a study of the role of aldehydes in cross-linking, investigated the characteristics of a product produced by reaction of thiosemicarbazide (TSC) with embryonic calfskin collagen. Two moles of TSC were found to react per mole of collagen. The reaction was without effect on the intramolecular cross-linking structure as judged by carboxymethylcellulose chromatography and acrylamide gel electrophoresis of the thermally denatured TSC-collagen. While the rate of aggregation to fibrils at neutral pH and 37°C was unchanged from that of the control by the TSC treatment, the stability of the precipitated fibrils to a temperature of 5°C was markedly diminished. Electron microscopic examination of the TSC-collagen fibrils revealed the normal native-type pattern. The exact nature of the bond between TSC and collagen could not be determined, but on the basis of absorption spectra, it was suggested that thiosemicarbazones were formed by reaction with aldehydic carbonyl groups in collagen. The two moles of "aldehyde" per collagen molecule would provide one more than the minimum number required to form a continuous, covalently linked polymeric network between adjacent collagen molecules. The mechanism for intermolecular cross-linking was envisaged as a condensation of aldehyde and ε-amino group of either lysine or hydroxylysine residues to give a Schiff base. Support for this mechanism was provided in a subsequent paper by Tanzer [128] who found that treatment of precipitated collagen fibrils with sodium borohydride, a procedure designed to reduce Schiff bases, produced a firmly cross-linked species as determined by solubility, thermal shrinkage, and dissolution as well as by examination of the denatured protein by ultracentrifugation, gel filtration, polyacrylamide electrophoresis, and carboxymethyl cellulose chromatography.

Deshmukh and Nimui [112] demonstrated a correlation between thermally fractionated, neutral-salt-soluble collagen and the corresponding aldehyde content. The concentration of aldehyde present in the neutral-salt-soluble collagen before precipitation, as well as that found in the different fractions isolated by repeated thermal precipitation and cold dissolution, is shown in Table 2.1. The aldehyde concentration of the collagen remaining in the supernatant decreased after every precipitation. After the fourth precipitation, the aldehyde content of the collagen is approaching that observed in collagens extracted from the tissue of animals fed lathyrogens such as β-aminopropionitrile. Table 2.1 also demonstrates that the portion of collagen returning to solution after the gel-forming incubation period is enriched in β components. The change in α/β subunit ratio from approximately 4 to 1.8 is considerably greater than the approximately 5 to 4 ratio as detected after a similar incubation period by Wood [82] who employed ultracentrifugation as the analytical tool.

2.5   COLLAGEN AGGREGATION *IN VIVO*

A number of *in vivo* studies of fine structure have indicated that collagen precursors are secreted by the fibroblast [129]. Histological and electron-microscopic examinations of tissue sections have shown that although the fibers lie close to the cell surface, they are entirely outside the cell [130]. The extracellular aggregation hypothesis is strongly supported by the experiments of Fitton Jackson and Smith [131] and Kuwabara [132] who found in tissue cultures that during a period of active growth a soluble collagen was formed and secreted into the medium without the concurrent formation of collagen fibers. In older cultures, on the other hand, collagen fibers appeared without any further increase in the total collagen content.

Table 2.1 Aldehyde Content and Subunit Composition of Neutral-Salt-Soluble Collagen and Its Various Fractions Separated During the Process of Repeated Thermal Precipitation and Redissolution at 4°C [112][a]

Number of Thermal Precipitations	Total Collagen, mg		Acetaldehyde Content, μM/100 mg of collagen		Super-natant Collagen, α-Subunit/ β-Subunit Ratio
	Super-natant	Precip-itate	Super-natant	Precip-itate	
Original neutral-salt-soluble collagen	12.2	—	0.84	—	4.0
First precipitation	9.61	2.55	0.75	0.96	1.77
Second precipitation	8.53	1.14	0.71	0.77	1.81
Third precipitation	6.34	2.17	0.60	0.68	1.80
Fourth precipitation	4.58	1.66	0.53	0.59	1.82

[a] Neutral-salt-soluble collagen was incubated at 37° overnight, cooled at 4°, and centrifuged. The procedure was repeated four times. All precipitates and supernatants at every step were analyzed for their aldehyde content and subunit composition (α-subunit/β-subunit ratio).

That the collagen molecule as defined in Section 2.1.2 is the *in vivo* precursor of collagen fibers is largely deduced from turnover studies using isotopically labeled amino acids. Jackson and Bentley [44] injected C^{14}-glycine into guinea pigs and at various time intervals determined the specific activity of collagen extracted by successive increments in ionic strength at neutral pH. The most highly labeled fraction was initially extracted by 0.14 M NaCl, but within twenty-four hours the peak of the activity was obtained from fractions which could only be extracted with 0.45 M NaCl and 1.0 M NaCl. From these observations, these authors proposed the following hypothesis for collagen-fiber formation. Collagen fibrils are formed at the surface of the fibroblast. Further increase in size occurs by accretion from extracellular soluble collagen rather than by aggregation of fibrils. They propose two controlling processes: (1) the formation of new fibrils and production of soluble collagen in the cell to be added to the fibrils and (2) the increase of cross-linking activity with time. In this view, the deeper the collagen molecule in the fiber, the more firmly it will be cross-linked; conversely, the outer, loosely aggregated collagen will be more easily extractable.

The hypothesis of Jackson and Bentley [44] that growth of fibrils occurs by accretion to fibrils rather than by an aggregation of fibrils is in line with the view that fibrogenesis is a nucleation and growth process [80]. The size of fibrils formed *in vivo* in a particular tissue is considered a function of the amount of collagen synthesized with equal importance given the number of fibrils formed. Fitton Jackson [133] found in an electron microscopic study of fibrogenesis in embryonic avian tendon that the diameter of fibrils in any one bundle of fibrils had a rather narrow distribution and concluded that they were formed almost simultaneously at a very early stage. Analysis of the development of the avian tendon showed that the diameter of the collagen fibrils increased steadily with age and further that the enlargement was linearly correlated with a reduction in the relative amount of interfibrillar material (a material distinct from the more ubiquitous ground substance) detected with each fibril. Extrapolation indicated an initial fiber diameter between 20 and 30 Å, a result interpreted as indicative of the presence of a "central core" presumed to act as a nucleus and deposited by one process with subsequent addition of other collagen molecules occurring by a different method. Veis et al. [72] have proposed a similar central core. Their limiting microfibril model for the three-dimensional arrangement within collagen fibers consists of a helical arrangement of four collagen molecules displaced successively by a fundamental repeat distance D, defined electron-microscopically.

The *in vitro* studies of Wood [81] on fiber formation in the presence of chondroitin sulfate A suggest that a high proportion of this substance will increase the rate of formation of nuclei and retard the subsequent rate of fiber growth. Therefore, secretion by the cell of a limited amount of chondroitin sulfate A could produce thin uniform fibrils. It may be significant that cartillage with its high chondroitin sulfate A content has thin fibrils, whereas skin with a high proportion of chondroitin sulfate B, shown by Wood not to affect the nucleation step, has a much larger average fibril diameter.

In many studies [134–139] small extracellular fibrils have been observed in the early stages of *in vivo* collagen formation. There is little difficulty in detecting periodic banding in extracellular collagen fibrils greater than 100 Å in diameter. However, nonbanded fibrils approximately 100 Å in diameter or less are often also detected. Ross and Benditt [135] proposed that extracellular collagen fibrils 100 Å or less in diameter would not display the characteristic 650–700 Å periodicity associated with native collagen fibers. This suggestion was made on the basis of the dimensions of the collagen molecule and the possible ways in which these molecules could be packed together to form fibrils, assuming the quarter-stagger, side-to-side arrangement of molecules in a linear array as proposed by Hodge and Schmitt [64].

The question of whether the collagen fiber generating system *in vivo* is in fact a self-limiting system has been the subject of debate [140]. Chapman [141] has observed that if the structure achieved by a packing of rodlike units in staggered array is to be intrinsically self-limiting in diameter, so that a fibril is formed, the rodlike units can only be quasi-equivalently related and some measure of strain energy must be stored in a unit or assembly. He proposed a design for self-limitation in which bond sites are arranged so that the rods twist slightly together; this requires both radial and axial shifts of the sites from the positions they would occupy in a straight-rod structure. The minimum-energy conformation of a larger assembly of rods will then be a cylindrohelical structure with rod tilt increasing with radius. As more rods are added the tilt of the innermost rods decreases; the average strain energy per rod, hence the energy barrier opposing the incorporation of new rods, increases toward an assymptotic limit with the presumption that radial growth ceases when the energy barrier reaches a critical level. Chapman believes this model of the collagen-fiber forming system more readily explains the observed mechanical and thermal behavior of collagenous tissue.

The extrinsic factors which affect the precipitation of collagen fibrils from solution *in vitro* include pH, ionic strength, temperature, concentration of collagen, and the presence of various extraneous substances. Spontaneity of fibril formation has been demonstrated *in vitro*, but the molecular units used in these experiments of necessity have to be extracted from tissue. Indeed, whether these molecular units are in exactly the same state of molecular order as the cell's newly synthesized monomers destined to form fibrils *in vivo* has not been ascertained. Also unknown is whether, at the appropriate time in the sequence of events *in vivo*, the microenvironment of each fibril is altered to conditions similar to those which obtain when typical fibrils are formed *in vitro*.

REFERENCES

1. P. A. Zachariades, *Compt. Rend. Soc. Biol.*, **52**, 182 (1900).
2. J. Nageotte, *Compt. Rend. Soc. Biol.*, **96**, 172, (1927).
3. J. Nageotte, *Compt. Rend. Soc. Biol.*, **96**, 464 (1927).
4. J. Nageotte, *Compt. Rend. Soc. Biol.*, **96**, 828 (1927).
5. J. Nageotte, *Compt. Rend. Soc. Biol.*, **97**, 559 (1927).
6. J. Nageotte, *Compt. Rend. Soc. Biol.*, **98**, 15 (1928).
7. J. Nageotte, *Compt. Rend. Soc. Biol.*, **104**, 156 (1930).
8. J. Nageotte, *Compt. Rend. Soc. Biol.*, **113**, 841 (1933).

9. J. Nageotte and L. Guyon, *Compt. Rend. Soc. Biol.*, **113**, 1398 (1933).

10. J. Nageotte and L. Guyon, *Compt. Rend. Assoc. Anat.*, **29**, 408 (1934).

11. G. Leplat, *Compt. Rend. Soc. Biol.*, **112**, 1256 (1933).

12. G. Leplat, *Compt. Rend. Assoc. Anat.*, **28**, 404 (1933).

13. E. Fauré-Fremiet, *Compt. Rend. Soc. Biol.*, **113**, 715 (1933).

14. E. Fauré-Fremiet, *Compt. Rend. Assoc. Anat.*, **28**, 277 (1933).

15. L. Guyon, *Compt. Rend. Acad. Sci.*, **198**, 975 (1934).

16. R. W. G. Wycoff and R. B. Corey, *Proc. Soc. Exptl. Biol. Med.*, **34**, 285 (1936).

17. C. E. Hall, M. A. Jakus, and F. O. Schmitt, *J. Amer. Chem. Soc.*, **64**, 1234 (1942).

18. F. O. Schmitt, C. E. Hall, and M. A. Jakus, *J. Cellular Comp. Physiol.*, **20**, 11 (1942).

19. R. S. Bear, *Advan. Protein Chem.*, **7**, 69 (1952).

20. V. N. Orekhovich, *Second Intern. Cong. Biochem. Commun.*, 106 (1952).

21. J. Gross, J. H. Highberger, and F. O. Schmitt, *Proc. Nat. Acad. Sci.*, **40**, 679 (1954).

22. H. Boedtker and P. Doty, *J. Amer. Chem. Soc.*, **77**, 248 (1955).

23. C. E. Hall, *Proc. Nat. Acad. Sci.*, **42**, 801 (1956).

24. K. A. Piez *Treatise on Collagen I Chemistry of Collagen*, G. N. Ramachandran, Ed., Academic Press, New York, 1967, p. 207.

25. W. F. Harrington and P. H. von Hipple, *Advan. Protein Chem.*, **16**, 1 (1961).

26. Veis, A., *The Macromolecular Chemistry of Gelatin*, Academic Press, New York, 1964.

27. P. H. von Hipple, *Treatise on Collagen I Chemistry of Collagen*, G. N. Ramachandran, Ed., Academic Press, New York, 1967, p. 253.

28. G. N. Ramachandran, *Treatise on Collagen I Chemistry of Collagen*, G. N. Ramachandran, Ed., Academic Press, New York, 1967, p. 103.

29. P. M. Cowan and S. McGavin, *Nature*, **176**, 501 (1955).

30. F. H. C. Crick and A. Rich, *Nature*, **176**, 780 (1955).

31. J. Schnell, *Arch. Biochem. Biophys.*, **127**, 496 (1968).

32. J. Gross, J. H. Highberger, and F. O. Schmitt, *Proc. Nat. Acad. Sci.*, **41**, 1 (1955).

33. J. Gross, *J. Exptl. Med.*, **108**, 215 (1958).

34. K. A. Piez, P. Bornstein, M. S. Lewis, and G. R. Martin, *Structure and Function of Connective and Skeletal Tissue*, S. Fitton Jackson, R. D. Harkness, S. M. Partridge, and G. R. Tristram, Eds., Butterworths, London, 1965, p. 16.

35. K. A. Piez, M. S. Lewis, G. R. Martin, and J. Gross, *Biochim. Biophys. Acta*, **53**, 596 (1961).

36. K. A. Piez, E. A. Eigner, and M. S. Lewis, *Biochemistry*, **2**, 58 (1963).

37. J. Engel and G. Beier, *Z. Physiol. Chem.*, **334**, 201 (1963).

38. A. J. Hodge, J. H. Highberger, G. G. J. Deffner, and F. O. Schmitt, *Proc. Nat. Acad. Sci.*, **46**, 197 (1960).

39. Y. Nagai, J. Gross, and K. A. Piez, *Ann. N.Y. Acad. Sci.*, **121**, 494 (1964).
40. A. Veis and M. P. Drake, *J. Biol. Chem.*, **238**, 2003 (1963).
41. J. H. Fessler, *Biochem. J.*, **76**, 452 (1960).
42. J. H. Fessler, *Biochem. J.*, **76**, 463 (1960).
43. J. K. Candlish, *Biochim. Biophys. Acta*, **74**, 275 (1963).
44. D. S. Jackson and J. P. Bentley, *J. Biophys. Biochem. Cytol.*, **7**, 37 (1960).
45. F. O. Schmitt, *Connective Tissue, Thrombosis and Atherosclerosis*, I. H. Page, Ed., Academic Press, New York, 1959, p. 43.
46. A. J. Hodge and F. O. Schmitt, *Proc. Nat. Acad. Sci.*, **44**, 411 (1958).
47. F. O. Schmitt, *Federation Proc.* **23**, 618 (1964).
48. A. L. Rubin, D. Pfahl, P. T. Speakman, P. F. Davison, and F. O. Schmitt, *Science*, **139**, 37 (1963).
49. M. P. Drake, P. F. Davison, S. Bump, and F. O. Schmitt, *Biochemistry*, **5**, 301 (1966).
50. F. O. Schmitt, J. Gross, and J. H. Highberger, *Exptl. Cell Res. Suppl.*, **3**, 329 (1955).
51. A. J. Hodge and J. A. Petruska, *International Conference on Electron Microscopy, 5th*, S. S. Breese, Jr., Ed., **1**, Paper QQ-1 Academic Press, New York, 1962.
52. A. J. Hodge and J. A. Petruska, *Aspects of Protein Structure*, G. N. Ramachandran, Ed., Academic Press, New York, 1963, p. 289.
53. K. Kühn, K. Hannig, and H. Hörmann, *Leder,* **12,** 237 (1961).
54. K. Kühn, J. Kühn, and K. Hannig, *Z. Physiol. Chem.*, **326**, 50 (1961).
55. R. Hafter and H. Hörman, *Z. Physiol. Chem.*, **330**, 169 (1963).
56. R. Hafter, *Leder,* **15,** 237 (1964).
57. K. A. Piez, *Ann. Rev. Biochem.*, **37**, 547 (1968).
58. J. Highberger, *Chemistry and Technology of Leather*, F. O'Flaherty, W. Roddy, and R. Lollar, Eds., Rheinhold, New York, 1956, p. 65.
59. J. H. Highberger, *J. Amer. Leather Chemists' Assoc.*, **56**, 422 (1961).
60. G. R. Martin, S. E. Mergenhagen, and D. B. Scott, *Biochim. Biophys. Acta*, **49**, 245 (1961).
61. H. B. Bensusan, V. R. Mumaw, and A. W. Scanu, *Biochemistry*, **1**, 215 (1962).
62. H. B. Bensusan and A. W. Scanu, *J. Amer. Chem. Soc.*, **82**, 4990 (1960).
63. L. D. Kahn, R. J. Carroll, and L. P. Witnauer, *Biochim. Biophys. Acta*, **63**, 243 (1962).
64. A. J. Hodge and F. O. Schmitt, *Proc. Nat. Acad. Sci.*, **46**, 186 (1960).
65. W. Cox, R. A. Grant, and R. W. Horne, *J. Roy. Microscop. Soc.*, **87**, 123 (1967).
66. B. R. Olsen, *Z. Zellforsch.*, **59**, 184 (1963).
67. B. R. Olsen, *Z. Zellforsch.*, **59**, 199 (1963).
68. A. J. Hodge, J. A. Petruska, and A. J. Bailey, *Structure and Function of Connective Skeletal Tissue,* S. Fitton Jackson, R. D. Harkness, S. M. Partridge, and G. R. Tristram, Eds., Butterworths, London, 1965, p. 31.
69. J. A. Petruska and A. J. Hodge, *Proc. Nat. Acad. Sci.*, **51**, 871 (1964).

70. J. W. Smith, *Nature,* **205,** 356 (1965).

71. J. B. L. Bard and J. A. Chapman, *Nature,* **219,** 1279 (1968).

72. A. Veis, J. Anesey, and S. Mussell, *Nature,* **215,** 931 (1967).

73. A. Veis, and J. Anesey, *J. Biol. Chem.,* **240,** 3899 (1965).

74. L. Onsager, *Ann. N.Y. Acad. Sci.,* **51,** 627 (1949).

75. A. Isihara, *J. Chem. Phys.,* **18,** 446 (1950).

76. P. J. Flory, *Proc. Roy. Soc. London,* Ser. A, **234,** 73 (1956).

77. J. Gross, *Nature,* **181,** 556 (1958).

78. J. Gross and D. Kirk, *J. Biol. Chem.,* **233,** 355 (1958).

79. H. B. Bensusan and B. L. Hoyt, *J. Amer. Chem. Soc.,* **80,** 719 (1958).

80. G. C. Wood, *Biochem. J.,* **75,** 598 (1960).

81. G. C. Wood, *Biochem. J.,* **75,** 605 (1960).

82. G. C. Wood, *Biochem. J.,* **84,** 429 (1962).

83. G. C. Wood and M. K. Keech, *Biochem. J.,* **75,** 588 (1960).

84. J. M. Cassel, L. Mandelkern, and D. E. Roberts, *J. Amer. Leather Chemists' Assoc.,* **57,** 556 (1962).

85. E. C. Bianchi, Giuseppina, and A. Ciferri, *Biopolymers,* **4,** 957 (1966).

86. E. Bianchi, G. Conio, A. Ciferri, D. Puett, and L. Rajagh, *J. Biol. Chem.,* **242,** 1361 (1967).

87. D. Waugh, *J. Cellular Comp., Physiol.,* **49,** Suppl. 1, 145 (1957).

88. R. Becker, *Ann. Physik,* **32,** 128 (1938).

89. D. Turnbull and J. C. Fisher, *J. Chem. Phys.,* **17,** 71 (1949).

90. L. Mandelkern, Crystallization of Polymers, McGraw-Hill, New York, 1964, p. 215.

91. D. S. Jackson, *New Eng. J. Med.,* **259,** 814 (1958).

92. J. Gross, *Connective Tissue, Thrombosis and Atherosclerosis,* I. H. Page, Ed., Academic Press, New York, 1959, p. 77.

93. D. A. Lowther, *International Review of Connective Tissue Research,* D. A. Hall, Ed., Academic Press, New York, 1963, p. 63.

94. J. H. Highberger, J. Gross, and F. O. Schmitt, *Proc. Nat. Acad. Sci.,* **37,** 286 (1951).

95. J. T. Randall, R. D. B. Fraser, S. F. Jackson, A. V. W. Martin, and A. C. T. North, *Nature* **169,** 1029 (1952).

96. D. S. Jackson and J. P. Bentley, *Treatise on Collagen,* B. S. Gould, Ed., **2,** Academic Press, New York, 1968, p. 189.

97. M. K. Keech, *J. Biophys. Biochem. Cytol.,* **9,** 193 (1961).

98. J. Caygill, *Biochim. Biophys. Acta.,* **181,** 334 (1969).

99. Z. Trnavská, S. Sit'aj, M. Grmela, and J. Malinsky, *Biochim. Biophys. Acta,* **126,** 373 (1966).

100. M. Németh-Csoka and M. Kaiser, *Acta Morphol. tomus,* **13,** 119 (1965).

101. B. P. Toole and D. A. Lowther, *Biochem. J.,* **109,** 857 (1968).

102. W. Kauzmann, *Advan. Protein Chem.,* **14,** 1 (1959).

103. J. M. Cassel, *Biopolymers,* **4,** 989 (1966).

104. H. B. Bensusan, *J. Amer. Chem. Soc.,* **82,** 4995 (1960).

105. J. M. Cassel and R. G. Christensen, *Biopolymers,* **5,** 431 (1967).

106. J. H. Fessler, *Structure and Function of Connective and Skeletal Tissue,* G. R. Tristram, Ed., Butterworths, London, 1966, p. 80.

107. L. Mandelkern, *J. Polymer Sci.,* **49,** 125 (1961).

108. L. Mandelkern, *Crystallization of Polymers,* McGraw-Hill, New York, 1964, p. 66.

109. E. R. Blout and G. D. Fasman, *Recent Advances in Gelatin and Glue Research,* G. Stainsby, Ed., Pergamon Press, London, 1958, p. 122.

110. J. Kurtz, A. Berger, and E. Katchalsky, *Recent Advances in Gelatin and Glue Research,* G. Stainsby, Ed., Pergamon Press, London, 1958, p. 131.

111. A. T. Ansewin, C. L. Stevens, and M. A. Lauffer, *Biochemistry,* **3,** 1512 (1964).

112. K. Deshmukh and M. E. Nimni, *Biochem. J.,* **112,** 397 (1969).

113. J. Gross, *Science,* **143,** 960 (1964).

114. D. W. Bannister, *Biochem. J.,* **113,** 419 (1969).

115. T. Hollmen and E. Kulonen, *Biochim. Biophys. Acta,* **93,** 655 (1964).

116. C. I. Levine and J. Gross, *J. Exptl. Med.,* **110,** 771 (1959).

117. J. Gross, *Biochim. Biophys. Acta,* **71,** 250 (1963).

118. G. R. Martin, J. Gross, K. A. Piez, and M. S. Lewis, *Biochim. Biophys, Acta,* **53,** 599 (1961).

119. E. Schiffmann and G. R. Martin, *Arch. Biochem. Biophys.,* **138,** 226 (1970).

120. P. Bornstein, A. H. Kang, and K. A. Piez, *Proc. Nat. Acad. Sci.,* **55,** 417 (1966).

121. P. Bornstein and K. A. Piez, *Biochemistry,* **5,** 3803 (1966).

122. A. J. Bailey, L. J. Fowler, and C. M. Peach, *Biochem. Biophys. Res. Commun.,* **35,** 663 (1969).

123. A. J. Bailey and C. M. Peach, *Biochem. Biophys. Res. Commun.,* **33,** 812 (1968).

124. A. J. Bailey and L. J. Fowler, *Biochem. Biophys. Res. Commun.,* **35,** 672 (1969).

125. M. E. Nimni, *J. Biol. Chem.,* **243,** 1457 (1968).

126. K. Deshmukh and M. E. Nimni, *J. Biol. Chem.,* **244,** 1787 (1969).

127. M. L. Tanzer, D. Monroe, and J. Gross, *Biochemistry,* **5,** 1919 (1966).

128. M. L. Tanzer, *J. Biol. Chem.,* **243,** 4045 (1968).

129. R. Ross, *Treatise on Collagen,* B. S. Gould, Ed., Academic Press, New York, 1968, p. 2.

130. K. A. Porter and G. D. Pappas, *J. Biophys. Biochem. Cytol.,* **5,** 153 (1959).

131. S. Fitton Jackson and R. H. Smith, *J. Biophys. Biochem. Cytol.,* **3,** 897 (1957).

132. H. Kuwarbara, *Japan J. Exptl. Med.,* **29,** 627 (1959).

133. S. Fitton Jackson, *Proc. Roy. Soc.,* **B 144,** 556 (1956).

134. M. H. Ross, *Proceedings of Fifth International Congress for Electron Microscopy,* S. S. Breese, Jr., Ed., Academic Press, New York, 1962, p. T-13.

135. R. Ross and E. P. Benditt, *J. Biophys. Biochem. Cytol.,* **11,** 677 (1961).

136. R. Ross and E. P. Benditt, *J. Cellular Biol.,* **22,** 365 (1964).

137. J. A. Chapman, *J. Biophys. Biochem. Cytol.,* **9,** 639 (1961).
138. H. E. Karrer, *J. Ultrastruct. Res.,* **4,** 420 (1960).
139. R. Peach, G. Williams, and J. A. Chapman, *Amer. J. Pathol.,* **38,** 495 (1961).
140. C. Cohen, *Principles of Biomolecular Organization,* G. E. W. Wolstenholme and M. O'Connor, Eds., J. A. Churchill Ltd., London, 1966, p. 130.
141. J. Chapman, *Principles of Biomolecular Organization,* G. E. W. Wolstenholme and M. O'Connor, Eds., J. A. Churchill Ltd., London, 1966, p. 129.

3

Swelling and Phase Transition of Insoluble Collagen

A. CIFERRI

Research Laboratory for Polymer Technology and Rheology of the National Research Council, Naples, Italy

The swelling and shrinkage of collagen have been the subject of numerous investigations over the past decades. A review of the early literature can be found in Gustavson's book [1]. Veis has more recently reviewed the subject in connection with the physical properties of both gelatin [2] and intact collagen [3]. In this chapter emphasis is given to developments which have occurred over the last ten years with special regard to results of investigations carried out by the author and his co-workers using cross-linked rat tail tendons.

The body of data on swelling, melting, and ion binding of dermal collagen in whole-skin tissue is, of course, extensive. However, data derived from experiments with cross-linked tendons have an important advantage which may ultimately be useful in the study of dermal collagen. Due to the presence of the chemical cross-linkages, the product resulting from shrinkage (or melting) is an insoluble amorphous gel, allowing one to measure and to differentiate clearly between the swelling of the fibrous, native state and the swelling of the amorphous, denatured state. While not identical in all respects to dermal collagen *in situ,* data on cross-linked rat tail tendons may afford a reasonable model for both the highly organized (fibrouslike) and the highly disorganized (gelatinlike) macroscopic states of collagen, thus serving to provide better understanding of the more complex structure occurring in skin tissue.

The situation prevailing with cross-linked systems where only two insoluble, macroscopic phases may be observed is somewhat different from that which may be observed in the case of soluble collagen or uncross-linked systems. In fact, when no chemical constraints (native or added) are present in the native fibrous arrays, only one insoluble phase may be observed: the fibrous, swollen one. Melting in the presence of a diluent results in dissolution of individually dispersed macromolecules which may or may not possess intramolecular order, that is, the triple-helix tropocollagen unit [2] or the random coiled conformation. The two soluble forms may, in turn, participate in an equilibrium of the helix random coil type. For a description of transformations involving soluble forms of collagen, see the recent works of Veis [2] and von Hippel [4]. A unified description, in terms of phase diagrams, of the role of variables such as pH, temperature, and solvent composition on the three possible transformations involving the insoluble crystalline, dispersed helical, and dispersed random coiled form of collagen, has been recently presented by Bianchi et al. [5].

Swelling and phase transition in cross-linked tendons, which are the sole consideration here, may be investigated with a variety of approaches which include studies of birefringence, x-ray diffraction [6], dimensional changes, membrane properties, and elasticity [7].

A brief discussion of the significance of the techniques and of various theories describing the process of swelling and melting is presented in the next section. This discussion is limited to the background necessary for the presentation of the results of swelling, selective absorption of one of the solvent components, and shrinkage which form the subjects of the ensuing sections.

3.1   TECHNIQUES AND THEORIES USED IN CONNECTION WITH SWELLING AND SHRINKAGE OF COLLAGEN

3.1.1   Techniques

The cross-linked systems which are the main concern in this chapter were obtained by water-washing rat tail tendons removed from mature animals and immersing them in a large excess of 0.1% p-benzoquinone solution for 1 hr [7]. A higher degree of cross-linking could be obtained by increasing the p-benzoquinone concentration or the time of exposure of the tendons to the 0.1% solution. In the terminology of Veis [3], the system may be described as "native collagen" nonpurified from its polysaccharide component.

The behavior of the crystalline and amorphous phases of cross-linked collagen may be analyzed by the various techniques which are described below.

Birefringence

The study of the anisotropy of collagen fibers by means of birefringence reveals that usually the birefringence is positive in the direction of the fiber axis, indicating the occurrence of fibrils aligned parallel to this direction. The value of birefringence $\Delta\eta$ is calculated from the retardation measured in the presence of a diluent and the actual thickness of the sample [7]. The $\Delta\eta$ is usually divided by v, the volume fraction of polymer, in order to eliminate the effect of swelling per se on the birefringence [7]. Upon melting, the value of the birefringence exhibits a sharp decrease and approaches zero at sufficiently high temperatures.

X-Ray Diffraction

The study of the x-ray diffraction patterns of collagen tendons is usually performed at room temperature for tendons in excess of diluent using thin, lead-free glass capillaries which may be filled with tendons and diluent [7]. In the wide-angle pattern of collagen below the shrinkage temperature, the prominent features are [8] the meridional arc corresponding to 2.86 Å, the equatorial halo at $\approx$4.5 Å, and the 11 Å equatorial spot. The 2.8 Å spacing represents the repeat distance along the axis of the triple-helix tropocollagen unit; the 4.5 Å reflection is attributed to an average spacing between the three minor helices which form the major helix, and the 11 Å equatorial spot is attributed to the spacing between adjacent triple helices. The 11 Å spacing is known to be sensitive to hydration increasing from about 10.3 Å in perfectly dry materials to about 15–16 Å in wet, uncross-linked materials. In addition, a large axial repeat distance ($\sim$650 Å) can be revealed from small-angle x-ray diffraction patterns [2]. In contrast, the x-ray diffraction pattern of collagen above the shrinkage temperature exhibits only a diffuse halo, typical of amorphous polymers [7].

Dimensional Changes

Variations of the degree of swelling and shrinkage transitions are usually investigated following dimensional changes of tendons [7]. Variations in the length of swollen tendons with temperature, pH, or salt concentrations are generally measured with a cathetometer while the tendon, immersed in an excess of water or salt solution, is maintained in a water-controlled bath. Mean diameters may be similarly determined with a microscope, equipped with a hot stage, using short pieces of tendons. A fixed, slow rate of temperature increase ($\sim$5°C hr^{-1}), or of pH and salt concentration changes, is often used, and the tendons are carried through temperature, pH, or concentration cycles in order to assess the reproducibility of the results. The equilibrium degree of swelling, v^{-1} (inverse of the volume fraction of polymer in the swollen gel) is the volume of swollen tendons referred to the volume of dry polymer.

Elasticity

Elasticity measurements also serve to characterize differences among crystalline and amorphous tendons [7]. In the crystalline state the collagen has high modulus and exhibits limited deformability in contrast to the amorphous state where low modulus and long-range elasticity are exhibited. Stress-strain isotherms in the crystalline state may be described by simple phenomenological equations such as $\tau = M(\alpha - 1)$ where the modulus M is of the order of 5×10^5 kg cm^{-2} and the maximum extension ratio α (stretched length/rest length) is of the order of 1.1. In the amorphous state the stress-strain equation of the rubber elasticity theory applies; the modulus is of the order of 5 kg cm^{-2} and α may be as high as 3. Thus a large change in the rigidity and deformability of the material accompanies the shrinkage transition. An additional difference is that while the modulus of the crystalline tendon decreases with increasing temperature, the modulus of an amorphous network is often directly proportional to temperature. The detailed stress-strain equation for an amorphous rubber in swelling equilibrium with a diluent is [9], in fact

$$\tau v^{\frac{1}{3}} = \frac{RT\rho}{M_c} \frac{\overline{r_i^2}}{r_0^2} (\alpha - \alpha^{-\frac{3}{2}}) \tag{1}$$

where τ is the stress (force per unit, dry cross-sectional area), T the absolute temperature, R the gas constant, ρ the polymer density, M_c the molecular weight between cross-links, v the volume fraction of polymer, and the parameter $\overline{r_i^2}/r_0^2$ the ratio between the mean square end-to-end distance of a chain constrained by the cross-links and free, respectively.

Membrane Properties

Transport properties of collagen membrane [10] are characterized by the filtration coefficient L_p defined by the relationship for volume flow J_v across the membrane given by irreversible thermodynamics treatment

$$J_v = L_p \, \Delta P + L_{pE} \, \Delta V + L_{pD} \, \Delta \pi \tag{2}$$

where ΔP is the hydrostatic pressure difference across the membrane and L_{pE} and L_{pD} are the phenomenological cross-coefficients which connect the volume flux to the electrical potential gradient ΔV and to the osmotic pressure gradient $\Delta \pi$, respectively. For the experimental determination of L_p, the collagen membrane may be clamped between two half-cells filled with a salt solution of a given pH (the salt concentration being identical on the two sides). The net flux of solution is measured when a hydrostatic pressure gradient ΔP is applied across the membrane, following the movement of the meniscus in a horizontal capillary connected with one of the half-cells [10]. Under the experimental conditions usually adopted $\Delta V = 0$ and $\Delta \pi = 0$. Thus the filtration coefficient L_p can be simply obtained by dividing J_v (the volume flow per unit area and unit time) by ΔP.

3.1.2   Theories

Swelling

No theory is available for describing the swelling of a crystalline polymer. For an amorphous network, however, the Flory-Huggins theory of polymer solutions and the rubber elasticity theory lead to the following equation for the equilibrium volume fraction of polymer in the swollen gel [11, 12]

$$\left(\frac{RT\rho}{M_c}\frac{\overline{r_i^2}}{r_0^2}\right)V_1\left[v^{1/3} - v\frac{\overline{r_0^2}}{r_i^2}\right] = -[\ln(1-v) + v + \chi_1 v^2] \qquad (3)$$

where, in addition to parameters defined in connection with the stress-strain equation (1), V_1 is the molar volume of diluents and χ_1, the free-energy parameter, may be defined as [11]

$$\chi_1 = \frac{\Delta F_m^*}{kTn_1\xi} \qquad (4)$$

where ΔF_m^* is an excess free energy of mixing, k the Boltzmann's constant, n_1 the number of diluent molecules, and ξ the volume fraction of polymer. (Of the two symbols v and ξ used to denote the volume fraction of polymer, only v refers to equilibrium conditions for a swollen gel in an excess diluent.) A corresponding enthalpy parameter k_1 may be defined as [11]

$$k_1 = \frac{\Delta \bar{h}_1}{RT\xi^2} \qquad (5)$$

and it may be easily shown from Equation 3 that

$$k_1 = -T\left(\frac{\partial \chi_1}{\partial T}\right) \qquad (6)$$

Thus the measure of v and its temperature coefficient along with the knowledge of the rubber-elasticity theory modulus (determined by ordinary stress-strain measurements for the same amorphous network) permit, according to Equations 3 and 6, an evaluation of the thermodynamic parameter of dilution χ_1 and its enthalpy component k_1. Relative differences in solvent power from solvent to solvent for a given polymer network are probably more reliable than absolute values of χ_1 in view of general theoretical limitations [11, 12] which affect Equations 3 and 1.

Equation 3 is based on a theory which is strictly valid for a polymer network in the presence of a one-component diluent. The extensions to pluricomponent diluent may be rigorously made by introducing the several interaction parameters, χ_{ij}, describing the interaction between the polymer with the various diluent components [11]. A simpler alternative is often used, particularly for solvent mixtures containing a component which interacts strongly with the polymer. This interaction should involve attractive forces strong enough to justify classification of the preferences of the polymer for these media as binding. The remaining, much weaker interaction of the bound polymer with the diluent is then described by considering the entire solvent environment as a single component from the point of view of the latter secondary interaction. In applying such a simplifying assumption to a water-salt-polymer system, χ_1 in Equation 3 should be regarded as a parameter characterizing the interaction of the polymer (modified by bound water and salt) with the remaining salt and water solution regarded as a one-component diluent [12].

Melting

In the case of binary polymer-diluent systems, the following equation [11] describes the dependence of the melting temperature T_m upon the volume fraction of diluent ξ_1 and the previously defined χ_1 parameter:

$$\frac{1}{T_m} - \frac{1}{T_m{}^0} = \frac{R}{\Delta H_u} \frac{V_u}{V_1} (\xi_1 - \chi_1 \xi^2) \tag{7}$$

where $T_m{}^0$ is the melting point of the undiluted polymer, ΔH_u the melting enthalpy, and V_u the molar volume of the polymer repeating unit. According to Equation 7, as well as in classical melting point depression theory, the *diluent effect* in depressing $T_m{}^0$ depends on both the quantity of diluent, expressed by ξ_1, and its quality (diluent power), expressed by the χ_1 parameter [11]. This equation is valid for a closed system, and its application to collagen has been discussed by Flory and Garrett [13] and Witnauer and Fee [14]. In the case of an open system such as that of a cross-linked collagen fiber melting into an amorphous network in equilibrium swelling with an excess diluent, a term should be added to Equation 7 accounting for the increase of T_m due to the dilation of the network brought about by swelling. This term [15] is, however, generally small and thus the character of the dependence of T_m on diluent content may be approximated by Equation 7 even for an open system.

Equation 7 cannot, however, be easily applied to pluricomponent diluents unless a proper account of selective interaction is made. Two ways in which this can be done for collagen have been considered. One approach consists of modifying Equation 7 by introducing a term involving a binding constant [16]. This approach is coherent with a separation of the polymer-diluent interaction in two terms: a specific effect which may be described as binding of a low molecular weight component to the polymer, and a nonspecific polymer-solvent interaction in which the mixture of low molecular weight species is treated as a single component diluent [16]. The approach is the same as that considered for interpreting the swelling behavior of a polymer network in the presence of a two-component solvent. With the alternative approach, given by Katchalsky and Oplatka [17], no distinction is made between a component which may be partially bound to the polymer and partially present in the diluent. The depression of the melting temperature is attributed simply to an enrichment of that component within the polymer domain.

In terms of the first approach, and in the particular case in which binding only occurs in the amorphous state and there is no competition between the solvent components for binding to the same site, one obtains [16]

$$\frac{1}{T_m} - \frac{1}{T_m{}^0} = \left(\frac{R}{\Delta H_u} \frac{V_u}{V_1}\right) (\xi_1 - \chi_1 \xi_1{}^2) + \frac{R}{\Delta H_u} p \ln (1 + Ka) \qquad (8)$$

where p is the number of reactable sites per repeating unit and K is the binding constant between the polymer and a solvent component with activity a. In Equation 8 the first term on the right-hand side, similar to that appearing in Equation 7, describes the activity of the bound polymer [16] and represents the nonspecific or diluent effect on the melting point depression. The second term on the right-hand side of Equation 8 describes the additional depression resulting from the formation of the bound polymer. The separation is to a large extent arbitrary, but it has the advantage that in the absence of binding it yields the expression valid for a one-component solvent.

The Effect of Stress

The application of a tensile force f on the collagen fiber will influence the crystal-amorphous transition temperature in accordance with general thermodynamic considerations valid for systems where a dimensional change occurs as a result of a phase transition [18]. Flory [18] uses the function

$$d(F - fL) = -S \, dT + V \, dp - L \, df$$

where F, S, V, and L are the Gibbs free energy, entropy, volume, and length of the sample, respectively, to obtain a force-temperature relationship analog of the Clausius-Clapeyron equation. If c and a denote the crystalline and amorphous phases, respectively, at equilibrium melting and constant pressure

$$d(F_c - fL_c) = d(F_a - fL_a)$$

and

$$\left(\frac{df}{dT}\right)_p = -\frac{(S_a - S_c)}{(L_a - L_c)} = -\frac{\Delta S}{\Delta L} \qquad (9)$$

or, alternatively,

$$\left[\frac{\partial(f/T)}{\partial(1/T)}\right]_p = \frac{\Delta H}{\Delta L} \tag{10}$$

where ΔH is the heat of melting. The application of a tensile force has, generally, a small effect on L_c while L_a (the length of the shrunken amorphous sample) depends on f according to Equation 1. As long as the length of the stretched amorphous fiber does not exceed L_c, the melting temperature will increase with an increase of applied stress since, in Equation 9, ΔS is positive and ΔL is negative. Moreover, according to the phase rule for a one-component, two-phase system which is univariant at constant pressure, the force remains constant during the isothermal transformation. The latter condition applies even if the fiber is in equilibrium with a liquid phase composed of a one-component diluent, in which case ΔH will contain a contribution due to alteration in dilution of one form [18]. Only in the case where the fiber is in equilibrium with a liquid phase composed of a two-component diluent, is the system bivariant and the force is not expected to remain constant during an isothermal transformation. In the latter case, particularly when the two-component diluent is a salt solution, there is the possibility of triggering the phase transition by alteration of solvent composition for constant values of the tensile force and temperature. Thus, in general, three state variables (i.e., T, f, and μ_s, the chemical potential of one of the solvent components) may affect the crystal-amorphous equilibrium and these correspond to the possibilities of a thermal melting (f and μ_s constant), a mechanical melting (T and μ_s constant), and a chemical melting (T and f constant).

Katchalsky and Oplatka [17] have derived analogous Clausius-Clapeyron equations relating the change of any two variables for a constant value of the third. They select a model which allows both the crystalline and amorphous phases to be composed of three components: polymer, solvent, and solute. These phases are in equilibrium with a supernatant solute-solvent solution. At constant temperature and pressure the Gibbs free energy of a gel is

$$dF = f\, dL + \mu_s\, dN_s + \mu_w\, dN_w + \mu_p\, dN_p$$

where μ is the chemical potential and N represents the number of moles. The subscripts s, w, and p represent solute, solvent, and polymer, respectively. It follows that an analogous Gibbs-Duhem relationship holds:

$$L\, df + N_s\, d\mu_s + N_w\, d\mu_w + N_p\, d\mu_p = 0$$

Therefore, at equilibrium between the crystalline and amorphous fiber the following relationships hold:

$$L^c \, df + N_s{}^c \, d\mu_s + N_w{}^c \, d\mu_w + N_p{}^c \, d\mu_p = 0 \tag{11}$$

$$L^a \, df + N_s{}^a \, d\mu_s + N_w{}^a \, d\mu_w + N_p{}^a \, d\mu_p = 0 \tag{12}$$

Dividing Equation 11 by $N_p{}^c$ and Equation 12 by $N_p{}^a$ and subtracting one from the other, we have

$$(\bar{L}^c - \bar{L}^a) \, df + (\bar{N}_s{}^c - \bar{N}_s{}^a) \, d\mu_s + (\bar{N}_w{}^c - \bar{N}_w{}^a) \, d\mu_w = 0$$

where $\bar{L}$ and $\bar{N}$ denote length and number of moles per mole of polymer. Furthermore, the bath components (outside the gel) must obey the Gibbs-Duhem relationship:

$$N_w{}^0 \, d\mu_w + N_s{}^0 \, d\mu_s = 0$$

Therefore, since $\mu_p{}^c = \mu_p{}^a$ and μ_w and μ_s are equal in all three phases

$$(\bar{L}^c - \bar{L}^a) \, df + \left[(\bar{N}_s{}^c - \bar{N}_s{}^a) - \frac{N_s{}^0}{N_w{}^0} (\bar{N}_w{}^c - \bar{N}_w{}^a) \right] d\mu_s = 0$$

Katchalsky and Oplatka define the *chemical enrichment*, ϵ, as

$$\epsilon = N_s - \frac{N_s{}^0}{N_w{}^0} N_w$$

Hence

$$\left(\frac{\partial \mu_s}{\partial f} \right)_{pT} = - \frac{\Delta \bar{L}}{\Delta \bar{\epsilon}} \tag{13}$$

which is the analog of the Clausius-Clapeyron equation for mechanochemical melting. If the change in chemical enrichment upon melting $\Delta \bar{\epsilon}$ is positive (i.e., $\epsilon_a > \epsilon_c$), $(\partial \mu_s/\partial f)_{pT} > 0$ since $\Delta L < 0$. Thus the chemical potential of the solute (or the solute concentration) necessary to trigger the melting will increase with f.

An alternative relationship can be obtained from the thermodynamic potential ψ defined as

$$\psi = F - N_s\mu_s - N_w\mu_w - fL$$

or

$$d\psi = dF - N_s \, d\mu_s - \mu_s \, dN_s - N_w \, d\mu_w - \mu_w \, dN_w - f \, dL - L \, df$$

Because $dF = v \, dp - s \, dT + f \, dL + \mu_s \, dN_s + \mu_w \, dN_w$, we have

$$d\psi = V \, dp - S \, dT - L \, df - N_s \, d\mu_s - N_w \, d\mu_w$$

at constant p, and f phase equilibrium is maintained when

$$- (S_a - S_c) \, dT - (\epsilon_a - \epsilon_c) \, d\mu_s = 0$$

where the subscripts a and c refer to the amorphous and crystalline phases, respectively. Therefore

$$\left(\frac{\partial \mu_s}{\partial T}\right)_{pf} = -\frac{\Delta S}{\Delta \epsilon} \tag{14}$$

According to Equation 14 when $\Delta S > 0$ and $\Delta \epsilon > 0$ the solute concentration necessary to trigger the melting process will decrease with increasing temperature. This theoretical result is equivalent to that expressed by Equation 8 indicating the role of binding in depressing the melting temperature.

3.2   SWELLING

3.2.1.   Osmotic Swelling [1]

This type of swelling is brought about by alteration of pH at low and constant ionic strength and temperature. Typical data [19] obtained for cross-linked tendons at 25°C are reported in Fig. 3.1. In the intermediate pH region from pH $\sim$4 to pH $\sim$8 no sensible alterations of either length or cross-section is exhibited. However, when the pH is lowered below $\sim$4 or increased above $\sim$8, a decrease of length and an increase of cross-sectional area are observed, leading to an almost tenfold increase of the total volume of the swollen tendon. At the low end of the pH scale, a deswelling may be observed on decreasing pH below $\sim$2. It is to be noticed that the degree of swelling (relative to the value observed at neutral pH) is greatly reduced by an increase of ionic strength. In fact, for salt concentration, C_s, of the order of 0.5 M NaCl, the degree of swelling is largely independent of pH. The pH variation of the degree of swelling of uncross-linked tendons, amorphous tendons, skin and gelatin follows a trend similar to that reported in Fig. 3.1, although the actual values of degree of swelling may vary. The overall behavior can be justified in terms of the Donnan effect arising from an increase of the net fixed charge on the protein upon changing pH below or above the isoelectric value. In terms of Donnan's theory, the occurrence of fixed charges causes an excess of mobile counter-ions in the interior of the gel, hence the osmotic forces.

While the Donnan effect offers a suitable thermodynamic framework for the description of the pH variation of the degree of swelling, the problem of the detailed mechanism of solvent uptake deserves further consideration. Of particular interest here is the question of possible modi-

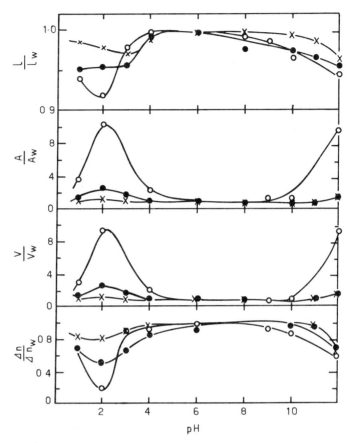

Figure 3.1. The relative length, cross-sectional area, volume, and birefringence of cross-linked rat-tail tendons swollen for 30 min at 25°C in solutions at different pH values. The reference state in each case is the tendon in water or salt at neutral pH; ○, No added electrolyte; ●, 0.1 M NaCl; ×, 0.5 M NaCl. (Reproduced from Ref. 19)

fications of the crystal structure of the tendon brought about by the large swelling occurring at pH 2.

In order to answer this question, it is appropriate to consider the results of studies of elasticity, x-ray diffraction, and membrane properties. In Fig. 3.2 stress-strain isotherms [17] at 25°C for tendons in HCl solutions of varying pH in absence of added salt are reported. The results indicate a progressive reduction of the modulus which appears to reach a minimum at pH 2 and to increase again at still lower pH. Comparison with the swelling behavior illustrated in Fig. 3.1 indicates that the reduction of the modulus is well correlated with an increase of swelling. This behavior may be ascribed to a reduction of the crystalline order of the tendon. However, even at pH 2 when the degree of swelling is at maximum, a complete melting out of the structure has not occurred. This is indicated by the fact that the stress-strain isotherm at pH 2 and T = 40°C exhibits a modulus still lower than that observed at 25°C. The shrinkage behavior (cf. Fig. 3.15) also indicates that the tendon is still crystalline at pH 2 when T = 40°C.

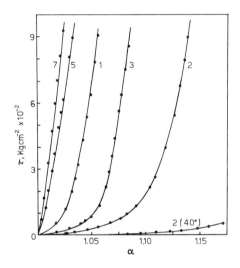

Figure 3.2.   Stress-strain curves for crystalline rat-tail tendons in acid solution of the indicated pH; $T = 25°C$, except for the lower curve. (Reproduced from Ref. 7).

Turning to the x-ray evidence, Burge et al. [20] found an increase of the intertropocollagen spacing from about 13.5 Å at neutral pH to about 15 Å at pH 2 in the absence of salt. This is a very small increase especially if compared to the extremely large osmotic swelling which occurred at pH 2 for the uncross-linked tendons they used. More recent results by Puett et al. [7] indicate that for lightly cross-linked tendons the intertropocollagen spacings measured in the dry state, at neutral pH, and at pH 2 are, respectively 10.72 Å, 14.31 Å, and 14.28 Å. Similarly, no effect was found on the 2.86 Å spacing.

It thus appears that in spite of the positive charges on the protein, the large swelling, the decrease in length and of the modulus, and the low birefringence, the tendon is not only still crystalline at 25°C but the crystalline structure of the component which remains crystalline has not been altered.

The suggestion [7] is that after the initial lattice adjustment brought about by water, additional water uptake is associated with an alteration of a component which is relatively less stable rather than to an alteration of the crystalline structure responsible for the scattering. Moreover, these results suggest that the stability of the crystalline structure is not pri-

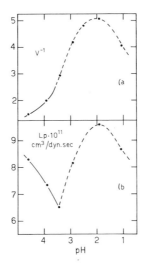

Figure 3.3. (a) Degree of swelling (ratio of swollen volume to dry volume) at different pH in KCl 10^{-2} M; (b) The filtration coefficient L_p as a function of pH in KCl 10^{-2} M. Data obtained at 52°C for a cross-linked collagen membrane. (Reproduced from Ref. 21)

marily due to electrostatic forces but rather to interactions within less polar sections of the chain. The permanence of the latter interaction assures the stability of the architectural framework of the tendon until its collapse occurs at the melting temperature.

The study of membrane properties serves to put in evidence some additional details. The pH variations of the degree of swelling and of the filtration coefficient L_p measured for cross-linked collagen films at 52°C and in a 0.01 M KCl solution are reported in Fig. 3.3 [21]. The films were prepared by casting a dispersion of fibrils obtained from steer tendons [10]. Independent optical and elasticity studies indicate that at 52°C the melting transition occurs between pH 3.2 and 2.2. Thus the large increase of swelling observed between pH 3.5 and 2.0 includes, besides the Donnan effect, the effect associated with the complete transition to the amorphous state. In the pH range where the tendon is still essentially crystalline (i.e., from pH 5 to pH 3.5), an increase of swelling is accompanied by a *decrease* of L_p, whereas when the structure is disorganized (i.e., pH < 3.5) an increase of swelling is accompanied by an *increase* of L_p. The behavior of the filtration coefficient thus reveals that significant differences exist between swelling in the crystalline and in the amorphous state. In terms of the pore model [21], which is often used for interpreting membrane properties, it can be said that the reduction of the permeability coefficient with increasing swelling in the crystalline state is equivalent to a reduction of pore size. In the amorphous state, instead, when the permeability increases with increasing swelling, the pore size increases with swelling. As will be discussed later, this behavior is common to both osmotic and lyotropic swelling. The behavior in the crystalline state seems to suggest the occurrence of pores, among the interfibrillar spaces, which may be closed up when an increase of absorbed water causes an expansion of adjacent less organized regions. An instructive analogy for describing the behavior in the amorphous state may be that of a sponge where pore size increases by swelling and decreases by deswelling.

3.2.2   Lyotropic Swelling

Lyotropic swelling is the swelling observed in salt solutions where Donnan's osmotic forces are negligible. As a rule it can be observed at any pH provided salt concentration is high enough (i.e., > 0.5 M) or in the neutral pH range (6–8) even at relatively low salt concentration. In contrast to osmotic swelling which produces translucent fibers, no alteration in the naturally opaque aspect of tendons is manifested in lyotropic swelling. A characteristic of lyotropic swelling is that, for a given collagen sample, the degree of swelling is considerably less than for osmotic swelling. Length changes during lyotropic swelling are negligible and cross-sectional swelling is also considerably smaller than in osmotic swelling. Figure 3.4 represents a quantitative description of the effect of salt concentration on length, cross-sectional area, volume and birefringence of cross-linked tendons. The changes observed are fully reversible.

Additional data [19] describing the role of salt type, salt concentration, and temperature on the lyotropic swelling of cross-linked collagen tendons are collected in Fig. 3.5. The occurrence of a rather abrupt

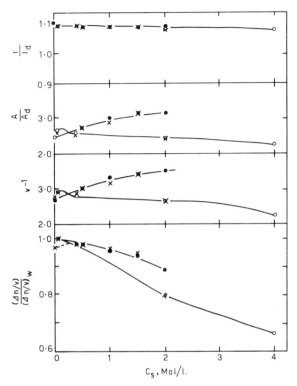

Figure 3.4. The relative length, cross-sectional area, degree of swelling, and birefringence of cross-linked rat-tail tendons as a function of salt concentration; ●, KSCN; ○, KCl; circles, salt concentration increasing; ✕, salt concentration decreasing. The reference state in each case is the dry tendon except for the birefringence data. (Reproduced from Ref. 19).

increase of swelling at intermediate salt concentration is associated with the shrinkage or melting transition (cf. Section 3.4). Thus the dashed line characterizes the behavior in the amorphous state while the continuous line indicates the behavior in the crystalline state. A general feature is that the degree of swelling at first increases and then decreases on increasing salt concentration. This behavior may be referred to [12] as a salting-in followed by a salting-out of the protein. The viscosity of soluble gelatin in salt solution reveals a similar behavior [12] and, in fact, the results obtained from swelling and viscosity measurements may be used for obtaining similar kinds of quantitative information concerning the interaction between the protein and the salt solution [12, 23].

From data such as those reported in Fig. 3.5, viscosity data [12, 23], and from swelling data for soluble gelatin at low temperature [24] it is possible to establish a well-defined order from both anions and cations for favoring salting-in or salting-out. Considering data in 1 M salt solu-

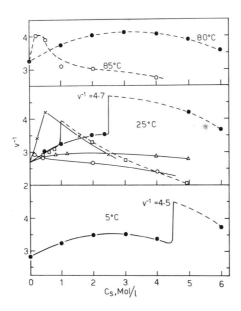

Figure 3.5. Degree of swelling of cross-linked rat-tail tendon collagen at 25°C as a function of salt concentration. Solid lines represent data taken on native fibers, dashed lines on denatured fibers; ○, KCl; △, NaCl; ●, KSCN; □, Ca(SCN)₂; ✕, AlCl₃. (Reproduced from Ref. 19).

tion, the deduced order for univalent ions is (swelling or salting-in increasing from left to right):

$$F^- < Cl^- < NO_3^- < Br^- < SCN^- \qquad (15)$$

$$K^+ < Na^+ < Cs^+ < Li^+ \qquad (16)$$

The swelling behavior of amorphous tendons may be analyzed in terms of Equation 3 with the limitations which have been discussed in Section 3.1. Results obtained [12, 23] for the volume fraction of polymer, v, its temperature coefficient and the thermodynamic parameters χ_1 and k_1 for several salts are collected in Table 3.1. The data have been obtained in the temperature interval where the shrunken tendon was com-

Table 3.1   Swelling Data for Amorphous Cross-Linked Collagen (Refs. [12, 23])

C_s, M	v	$\dfrac{dv}{dT} \times 10^3$	χ_1	$-k_1$
		H_2O (80°C)		
0	0.303	1.02	0.624	0.220
		KCl (80°C)		
0.2	0.238	0.95	0.589	0.187
1.0	0.333	0.83	0.634	0.151
4.0	0.370	—	0.666	—
		KSCN (80°C)		
1.0	0.267	0.95	0.611	0.166
2.0	0.248	0.68	0.588	0.154
3.0	0.244	0.51	0.594	0.088
4.0	0.248	0.40	0.590	0.081
5.0	0.259	0.35	0.597	0.067
6.0	0.279	0.14	0.608	0.021
		NaBr (80°C)		
1.0	0.281	1.55	0.612	0.322
2.0	0.315	0.98	0.632	0.209
3.0	0.330	0.73	0.642	0.156
		LiCl (80°C)		
1.0	0.300	1.31	0.623	0.275
2.0	0.300	0.91	0.623	0.189
3.0	0.309	0.82	0.628	0.172
4.0	0.328	0.82	0.640	0.176
		KF (86°C)		
1.0	0.334	0.17	0.644	0.031
2.0	0.408	—	0.695	—
		$MgSO_4$ (86°C)		
0.2	0.220	—	0.576	—
0.4	0.225	0.11	0.579	0.016
1.0	0.333	—	0.634	—

pletely istropic (cf. Section 3.4) and the experimental stress-strain curve was satisfactorily represented [7] by Equation 1 of the rubber elasticity theory (cf. Fig. 3.22). The data in Table 3.1 indicate that the enthalpy of dilution parameter k_1 is negative at low C_s and its absolute value continuously decreases on increasing salt concentration. This continuous decrease of the exothermicity of dilution (also observed by Flory and Spurr [25]) contrasts with the trend of χ_1 (which reflects the excess chemical potential of the diluent) generally going through a minimum on increasing C_s. The complete thermodynamic analysis of these data and those obtained from intrinsic viscosity measurements [12, 23] indicate that the initial increase of v^{-1} with C_s (cf. Fig. 3.5) results from the balance of an enthalpy component which, on increasing C_s, becomes less favorable to dilution and an entropy component which, conversely, becomes more favorable. The subsequent decrease of v^{-1} with C_s is then due to the prevailing of the adverse enthalpy component.

A definite molecular interpretation of these effects has not been given and the limitations due to the use of an approach strictly valid for one-component diluents probably forbid the attachment of more than a qualitative significance to the results. The reduced exothermicity of dilution with increasing C_s might suggest that the polar character of the chain is decreased on increasing C_s. This could result from increased ion immobilization at the polar sites of the chain. The increase of the entropy component with C_s can be associated with an increased conformational freedom of the macromolecules arising from ion binding and/or with an increased liquid character of the diluent, particularly in solutions of those salts which are known as "breakers" of the water structure. A fuller discussion of these effects has been presented by Rajagh et al., [12] and by Puett and Rajagh [23].

A detailed analysis of the data in Fig. 3.5 reveals that the variation of swelling with salt concentration when the tendon is crystalline, is qualitatively similar to that observed when the tendon is amorphous. Considering that no theory is available for interpreting the swelling of a crystalline system, the simplest interpretation of this observation is that amorphous regions coexist within the crystalline tendon. However, this possibility appears to be ruled out by the high degree of crystallinity of collagen [8]. Other authors [25] have preferred the view that the majority of the diluent is retained among major helices and structural voids; however, the observed variation of the degree of swelling with C_s raises significant doubt as to the acceptability of this view since this variation indicates that the space available to the diluent is not fixed but depends upon the nature of the diluent. The observed swelling-deswelling could, alternatively, be attributed to the possible ability of the diluent to sever the intertropocollagen bonds at low C_s and re-establish them in some manner at high C_s [26]. In this case, one would expect corresponding variations in the meridional 14 Å spacing; however, the results of a detailed analysis [7] of the effect of salt solutions on the lattice spacing of cross-linked collagen tendons (cf. Table 3.2) reveals that no alteration of the spacing is exhibited when the tendon is in equilibrium with KSCN and KCl solutions of different concentrations,

Table 3.2   Effect of Diluents on Lattice
Spacings of Cross-Linked Collagen [7]

	Reflection, Å	
Medium	a	b
Dry	2.86	10.72
H_2O	2.86	14.31
KSCN, 0.1 M	2.86	14.25
KSCN, 0.5 M	2.86	14.27
KSCN, 1 M	2.86	14.23
KCl, 0.2 M	–	14.26
H_2O + HCl, pH 2	2.86	14.28

in spite of the large alterations in the degree of swelling illustrated in Fig. 3.5.

The behavior of the amorphous and the crystalline swelling is similar enough to support the occurrence of the same effects. These results may then be interpreted as indicating that, in the presence of strong salting-in agents, such as KSCN, the degree of ordering is reduced and less-ordered regions are able to interact with the diluent in the amorphous-like manner regardless of the high degree of crystallinity of collagen in water. The interpretation is thus similar to that advanced in the case of osmotic swelling. The postulated regions of reduced order and stability may be associated with the occurrence of particular sequences along the tropocollagen unit and their proper juxtaposition in the crystalline lattice. Such regions may coincide with the bands and interbands observed through high-resolution electron microscopy [8] within the axial pattern repeat of about 650 Å. It was suggested [8] that the band represents regions of relative disorder due to a concentration of long polar side chains. The regions where the different tropocollagen units meet and where the poorly organized chain ends are concentrated, or the telopeptide regions [27], may represent additional loci of reduced order. Complete disorganization in these regions can be expected with small salt concentrations or pH variations. As long as the main crystalline framework is stable, the swelling will be anisotropic. The most perfect crystalline regions which are responsible for the x-ray diagram (and may have dimensions of perhaps only 50 Å as the diffusiveness of the spots suggest) may not be essentially altered by the reagent below the shrinkage temperature.

Elasticity measurements of crystalline tendons in equilibrium swelling with different salt solutions [7], reported in Fig. 3.6, support the above conclusions. In fact, a progressive softening (i.e., a reduction of the modulus) is seen on increasing KSCN concentration in line with the noticeable effect of this salt on increasing the degree of swelling in the crystalline state (cf. Fig. 3.5).

The birefringence of crystalline tendons in salt solutions reveals, however, a behavior which is somewhat puzzling. As the data in Fig. 3.4 indicate, the birefringence is continuously depressed by increasing KSCN and KCl concentration in spite of the fact that of the two salts considered one promotes swelling and the other deswelling.

A somewhat more detailed insight into the situation caused by swelling and deswelling of the crystalline tendons in KSCN and KCl solutions is afforded by the study of membrane properties of cross-linked collagen films [10]. The variation of the filtration coefficient with KSCN and KCl concentration is represented in Fig. 3.7 and 3.8, respectively. The upper part of the figure represents the variation of the cross-sectional swelling of the membrane and reveals a trend similar to that exhibited in Fig. 3.4 and 3.5. The discontinuity of L_p at ~ 3 M KSCN can be attributed [10] to the melting transition, as confirmed by independent optical studies. Thus, the solid line and the dashed line characterize the behavior of the crystalline and of the amorphous membrane, respectively. It is seen that while in the amorphous state an increase (or a decrease) of swelling corresponds to an increase (or a decrease) of the filtration coefficient, in the crystalline state an increase of swelling (KSCN) brings about a decrease of L_p and a decrease of swelling (KCl) causes an increase of L_p. While the behavior in the amorphous state is typical of homogeneous structures (cf. also the similar behavior ex-

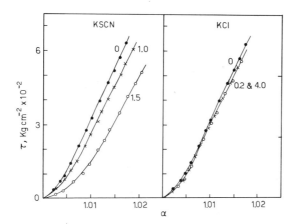

Figure 3.6. Stress-strain curves for crystalline rat-tail tendons in salt solution of the indicated molarity, $T = 30°C$. (Reproduced from Ref. 7).

hibited by the data in Fig. 3.3), the behavior in the crystalline state suggests that swelling improves the homogeneity of the structure, perhaps by closing up structural voids, whereas deswelling makes the structure somewhat more porous [10].

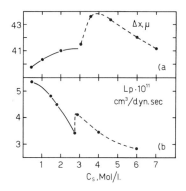

Figure 3.7.   (*a*) Thickness Δx, (*b*) filtration coefficient L_p plotted against KSCN concentration for a cross-linked collagen membrane, $T = 26°C$. (Data from Ref. 10).

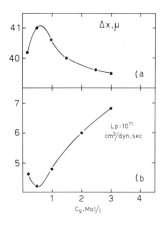

Figure 3.8.   (*a*) Thickness Δx, (*b*) filtration coefficient L_p plotted against KCl concentration for a cross-linked collagen membrane, $T = 26°C$. (Data from Ref. 10).

3.2.3   Swelling in Alcohol Solutions

Gustavson [1] has described and discussed the role of urea, phenols, and nonelectrolytes such as sucrose and glucose on the swelling of collagen. These substances generally increase the degree of swelling of col-

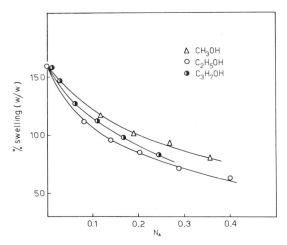

Figure 3.9. Variation of the equilibrium degree of swelling of a cross-linked collagen membrane with the molar fraction N_A of several alcohols; $T = 20°C$, pH ~ 6. (Reproduced from Ref. 28).

lagen. Aliphatic alcohols, instead, invariably cause a reduction of the degree of swelling relative to the value measured in pure water. The effect is illustrated in Fig. 3.9 in the case of collagen films obtained by casting a dispersion of steer tendons and cross-linking with p-benzo-quinone [28]. The order for increasing deswelling deduced from Fig. 3.9 is $CH_3OH > C_3H_7OH > C_2H_5OH$. However, there is a crossover of the curves for the latter two alcohols in concentrated alcohol solutions since the degree of swelling (w/w) of the same membrane in the pure alcohols in 60% in CH_3OH, 15% in C_2H_5OH and 3% in C_3H_7OH. This indicates that the affinity of pure alcohol for collagen follows the order $CH_3OH > C_2H_5OH > C_3H_7OH$.

3.3   SELECTIVE INTERACTION OF COLLAGEN WITH ONE OF THE SOLVENT COMPONENTS

3.3.1   Ion Binding

In the preceding section the overall degree of swelling of collagen in equilibrium with two-component solutions (water-salt or water-alcohol) was discussed. Under consideration in this section is the occurrence of solvent disproportion, leading to an enrichment of one of the solvent components within the collagen gel.

Most common methods for measuring solvent disproportion rely upon the determination of solvent composition outside the domain occupied by the polymer molecules. For instance, Docking and Heymann [24] equilibrated dry, insoluble gelatin in a salt solution of known initial concentration $C_s{}^i$ and, using conventional analytic techniques, determined the final concentration, $C_s{}^f$, of the excess solution in equilibrium with the gel. A positive value of the difference $C_s{}^i - C_s{}^f$ indicates an enrichment [17] of salt in the solution within the gel (with respect to the outside solution) due to a preferential collagen-salt interaction. A determination of this type of enrichment is often, and somewhat arbitrarily, referred to as a determination of salt binding [29]. For instance, if the ratios of "free" (i.e. unbound) water to salt molecules outside and inside the gel are taken to be equal, then the $C_s{}^i - C_s{}^f$ difference represent the variation due to selective binding of salt and water molecules to the polymer molecules. The underlying model is that of a polymer-salt-water complex swollen by a salt solution which can be regarded as a one-component diluent [16] (cf. Section 3.1). In terms of this model it becomes reasonable to calculate binding constants using enrichment data.

Selected data from Docking and Heymann are reproduced in Fig. 3.10. High positive values of $C_s{}^i - C_s{}^f$ mean, of course, that a large adsorption of salt overshadows the normal adsorption of water by the initially dry gelatin while high negative values indicate that the salt adsorption is small or negligible. In fact, the decrease of $C_s{}^i - C_s{}^f$ with increasing C_s which is observed in the case of the strongest salting-out agent (K_2SO_4, $MgSO_4$) can be attributed to the adsorption of about three water molecules for each peptide residue by the initially dry gelatin [29]. Such a figure is in line with the data of Sponsler et al. [30], who calculated that one residue should have a maximum binding capability corresponding to four water molecules although they did point out that due to chain interactions and space restrictions a reasonable value should be about two. The order for increasing salt adsorption deduced from the data in Fig. 3.10 is

$$SO_4{}^{2-} < \text{acetate} < Cl^- < NO_3{}^- < Br^- < SCN^- \qquad (17)$$

$$K^+ < Mg^{2+} < Na < Cs^+ < Li^+ < Ca^{2+} \qquad (18)$$

The data of Docking and Heymann may be used for calculating binding constants of salts to gelatin. The evaluation of Ciferri et al. [29], is based on the assumption of no competition between salt and water for binding to the same site and of a fixed hydration value of two water molecules per residue. The equilibrium constant K for the reaction

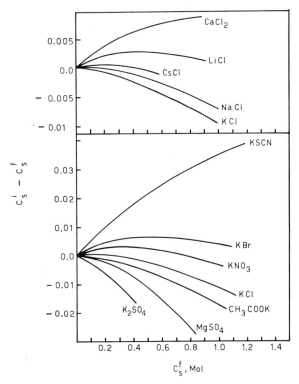

Figure 3.10. Apparent adsorption of salts on gelatin plotted as a function of the concentration of the (outside) solution in equilibrium with the gel. (Data from Ref. 24).

$P + S \rightleftharpoons PS$, where P denotes a protein hydrate, S the salt, and PS the hydrated protein-salt complex, may be written as [31].

$$Ka = \frac{\alpha}{(1 - \alpha)} = \left(\frac{\bar{\nu}}{n}\right)\left(1 - \frac{\bar{\nu}}{n}\right) \qquad (19)$$

where a is the salt activity, α is the mole fraction of reactable groups occupied, and n is the total number of binding sites per mole of protein (not necessarily either the number of residues or the number of amide or carbonyl groups). The $\bar{\nu}$ is the number of moles of salt bound per mole of protein which may be obtained from experimentally measured quantities as

$$\bar{\nu} = \frac{(C_s{}^i - C_s{}^f)}{C_P} \qquad (20)$$

where C_P is the molar concentration of polymer after proper account is taken [29] of the protein hydration. Rearrangement of Equation 19 gives the following equation:

$$\frac{\bar{\nu}}{a} = K(n - \bar{\nu}) \tag{21}$$

Thus a plot of $\bar{\nu}/a$ versus $\bar{\nu}$ permits calculation of both K and n. If $\bar{\nu}/a$ is linearly dependent upon $\bar{\nu}$, a single type of noninteracting site is in-

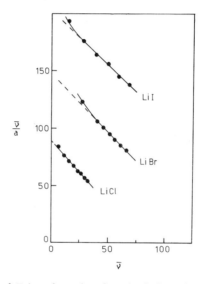

Figure 3.11.   Ratio of $\bar{\nu}$ (number of moles of salt bound per mole of protein) to the molar salt activity versus $\bar{\nu}$ for gelatin. Calculated from the data of Docking and Heymann [24] using a hydration of 2 water molecules per residue. (Reproduced from Ref. 29)

volved [31]. Data reported in Fig. 3.11 indicates that this linear relationship is, in fact, verified from about 0.2 to about 2 M. In Table 3.3 are collected values of the parameter $p \ln (1 + Ka)$ where p is the number of reactable sites per repeating unit (equal to $n/1000$ assuming 1000 residues per α chain) obtained from Docking and Heymann's data [29].

The question of the ion-binding site on collagen was considered in detail by Veis [2]. In general, ion binding should occur at the polar sites of the macromolecule, that is, basic hydroxyl and carboxyl side-chain groups and main-chain peptide bonds. In the case of charged poly-

Table 3.3   Values of $p \ln (1 + Ka)$ for the Absorption of Salts to Gelatin at 0°C in 1 M Salt Solutions. A Hydration of Two Water Molecules/ Residue Was Assumed [29]. Calculated Using the Data of Docking and Heymann [24]

K^+	$p \ln (1 + Ka)$	Cl^-	$p \ln (1 + Ka)$	Li^+	$p \ln (1 + Ka)$
SCN^-	0.101	Ca^{2+}	0.072	I^-	0.132
I^-	0.090	NH_4^+	0.038	Br^-	0.087
Br^-	0.055	Cs^+	0.032	Cl^-	0.050
NO_3^-	0.042	Na^+	0.031		
Cl^-	0.021	Rb^+	0.026		
CH_3COO^-	0.013				

peptides [32], such as poly-L-lysine and poly-L-glutamic acid, evidence based on the relative stability of helical versus random coiled conformation indicates that ion binding occurs preferentially at the charged side chain. However, the evidence quoted by Veis suggests that a direct interaction of the ions with the peptide bonds is prevailing in the case of near-isoelectric collagen. A convincing point was the similarity of the melting point depression caused by several salts in acelylated, nitrated, and original gelatins.

Another determination of salt binding to gelatin (in a 1% solution) was recently performed by Threlkeld et al. [33] using high-speed ultracentrifugation techniques. The technique is based on the principle that one can sediment a protein toward the bottom of the centrifuge cell leaving an area at the meniscus free of polymer. If salt or water are preferentially absorbed by the protein, the absorbed ions or molecules are no longer free to diffuse but must sediment with the protein. The amount of preferential absorption that has taken place may be determined by measuring the change in salt concentration above the sedimentation boundary as compared to the salt concentration in absence of polymer. No account of the hydration of the polymer is necessary using this technique. Results obtained for four different salt solutions, including some tetraalkylammonium salts, are listed in Table 3.4. The binding values found for KSCN and KCl are in good agreement with those which can be calculated from the Docking and Heymann data reported in Table 3.3. The latter are 0.044 and 0.011 for KSCN and KCl, respectively [33].

The question as to whether the preferential salt absorption by collagen depends upon the physical state (i.e., crystalline or amorphous) of the protein cannot be answered using data from Docking and Heymann or Threlkeld et al. [33], since the situation prevailing in the case of gelatin is that of a bulk sample stabilized by a small and probably very imperfect degree of crystallinity. The data of Ciferri et al. [29] allow, however, one to establish that ion binding is greater in the amorphous than in the crystalline state and that there is an increase of ion binding at the denaturation temperature. Using ^{14}C-labeled KSCN and [36]Cl-labeled KCl and a radioisotope comparison technique, Ciferri et al. [29] determined the difference $C_s{}^i - C_s{}^f$ both below and above the denaturation temperature of cross-linked collagen tendons. Their results, reported in Fig. 3.12, exhibit the variation of $C_s{}^i - C_s{}^f$ with temperature for several values of $C_s{}^i$. Rather sudden variations of $C_s{}^i - C_s{}^f$ occur at temperatures which correspond to the shrinkage temperature. Values of n,K and the parameter $p\ln(1 + Ka)$ calculated

Table 3.4   Salt Adsorption to Gelatin at 25°C [33]

Salt (0.4 M)	Moles Salt Bound/ Mole Monomer
KSCN	0.042
(C$_4$H$_9$)$_4$NBr	0.040
(CH$_3$)$_4$NBr	0.023
KCl	0.012

from the $C_s{}^i - C_s{}^f$ values in the amorphous state are collected in Table 3.5 for various hydration values. Also included are the values of the intrinsic thermodynamic parameters of the binding process calculated from the temperature dependence of K for the case corresponding to two water molecules for residue. The discrepancy in the binding values reported in Table 3.5 and those obtained from the Docking and Heymann data (cf. Table 3.3) is not unexpected since the temperature is not the same and the structure of cross-linked denatured collagen is somewhat different from that of commercial gelatin. The increase of ion binding at the denaturation temperature reflects the greater exposure of binding sites to the solvent in the amorphous than in the crystalline state. The fact that $C_s{}^i - C_s{}^f$ is greater than zero below the denaturation temperature was attributed to the occurrence of regions of reduced organization in native collagen, such as that discussed in Section 3.2.

Among additional determinations of ion binding to collagen and gela-

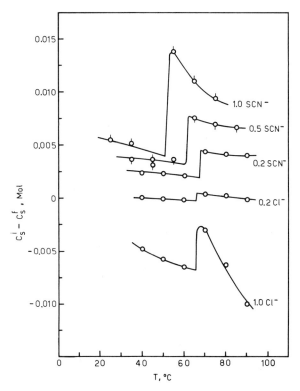

Figure 3.12. Apparent adsorption of KSCN and KCl by cross-linked collagen tendons as a function of temperature in solutions of different salt molarity. Collagen content increases from about 25 mg ml^{-1} at the lowest temperature to about 33 mg ml^{-1} at the highest temperature for each curve. (Reproduced from Ref. 29).

Table 3.5 Binding Parameters for Amorphous, Cross-Linked Collagen [29]

Salt	Temperature, °C	Water, moles/mole residue	n	K, M^{-1}	$p \ln (1 + Ka)$ at 1 M
KSCN	75	0	50	2.54	0.044
KSCN	75	1	85	1.67	0.056
KSCN	75	2[a]	160	0.95	0.069
KSCN	75	3	214	0.81	0.081
KCl	80	2	10	10.1	0.0098

[a] $\Delta F°$, 36 cal mole^{-1}; $\Delta H°$, -2800 cal mole^{-1}; $\Delta S°$, -8.1 eu

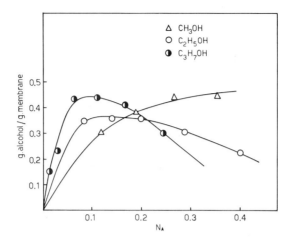

Figure 3.13. Selective absorption of several alcohols by a cross-linked collagen membrane as a function of the molar fraction of alcohol, $T = 20°C$, pH $\sim$ 6. (Reproduced from Ref. 28).

tin, results based on isoionic pH shifts have been reported [2, 29]. These results are often considered in order to assess unequal ion binding of anions and cations. However, the validity of this method for determining ion binding appears to be questionable on both experimental and theoretical grounds [29].

3.3.2 Alcohol Enrichment

As discussed in Section 3.2 the overall degree of swelling of collagen decreases on increasing alcohol content in binary water-alcohol mixtures of simple aliphatic alcohols.

Simultaneous with this decrease of swelling, however, there is a selective increase of the amount of alcohol absorbed and, necessarily, a decrease of absorbed water. Results for the water-alcohol disproportion obtained by Bianchi et al. [28] are collected in Fig. 3.13. The collagen sample was in the form of a cross-linked membrane obtained by casting a dispersion of steer tendons [10] and the composition of external solution in equilibrium with the swollen membrane was determined by gas chromatography. On increasing the molar fraction of alcohol, the apparent amount of alcohol absorbed by the membrane goes through a maximum in the case of C_2H_5OH and C_3H_7OH. For composition less than that corresponding to the maximum the order for increasing absorption is: $C_3H_7OH > C_2H_5OH > CH_3OH$ (which is not the same as the order for increasing affinity of pure alcohol toward collagen, cf. Section 3.2).

In the case of binary water-alcohol mixtures, the activity of the alcohols follows the order [28] $C_3H_7OH > C_2H_5OH > CH_3OH$, over the whole compositional range. However, the difference between the activities of these alcohols is abnormally large for $N_A \sim 0.1$–0.2. This is a possible correlation with the effects illustrated in Fig. 3.13. Note also, that the absorption of alcohols by collagen may be, in principle, described as a binding. Recently Strassmair et al. [34] have demonstrated the binding of alcohols to the peptide CO-group of poly-L-proline in the I and II conformation by infrared spectroscopy and optical rotatory dispersion.

3.4 SHRINKAGE AND MELTING OF TENDONS

3.4.1 Characteristics of the Shrinkage of Tendons

Typical length-temperature (at constant C_s), length-C_s (at constant temperature) and length-temperature (at constant pH) curves [7, 19] are reproduced in Figs. 3.14 and 3.15. The midpoint of the transformation is usually taken as the shrinkage temperature T_s or the critical pH or salt concentration for isothermal shrinkage. The transition from crystalline to amorphous tendon is generally rather abrupt although it is particularly broad in the case of the curve at pH 2 in the absence

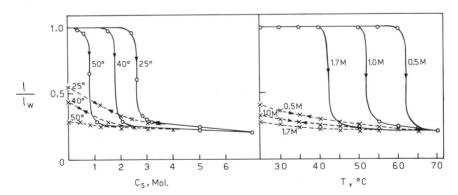

Figure 3.14. Length-concentration and length-temperature curves for cross-linked collagen tendons at the indicated molarities of KSCN, $f = 0$. A reversible cycle can be performed after the first shrinkage, as indicated by the dashed lines. (Reproduced from Ref. 7).

of salt (Fig. 3.15), when the occurrence of large osmotic forces tends to oppose full shrinkage. Moreover, one generally observes the occurrence of a tail which appears to protract the transformation at much higher temperatures and salt concentrations than those corresponding to the midpoint of the transformation. This effect is shown in more detail in Fig. 3.16 which reproduces only the region after the shrinkage and where the critical concentration for shrinkage is represented by an arrow. A very slow rate was used for these experiments and the results (i.e., the variations of birefringence with C_s) clearly demonstrates that true iso-

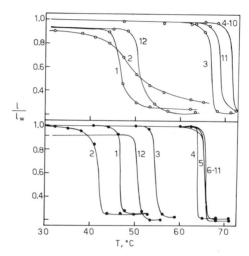

Figure 3.15.   Length-temperature curves for cross-linked tendons at the indicated pH: (○) no added salt, (●) 0.1 M KSCN. The reference state is the tendon in water at room temperature. (Reproduced from Ref. 19).

tropy is reached only after C_s is several molar higher than the value corresponding to the shrinkage. That this behavior might be interpreted as a nonequilibrium effect is excluded by the perfect reversibility in this region [7]. A similar trend was exhibited at other temperatures. It would seem that in spite of the high degree of swelling and of the disorganization of the matrix, the presence of a stable network restricts the disordered dispersion of residual helical regions thus assuring a kind of "memory" of the original oriented state.

Further inspection of Fig. 3.14 reveals that a reversible length change, which may be as high as 300% of the shrunken length, can be obtained when shrunken samples are carried through a cyclic process of heating

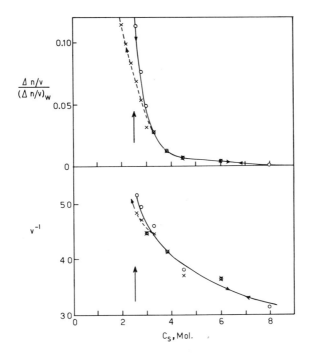

Figure 3.16. Variation of birefringence (relative to the value measured in water) and degree of swelling with KSCN concentration for a shrunken cross-linked tendon, $T = 25°C$ and the critical concentration for shrinkage = 2.5 M: ($\bigcirc$) increasing and ($\times$) decreasing salt concentration, 24 hr between successive determinations. (Reproduced from Ref. 7).

and cooling (or of varying the salt concentration). Depending upon the conditions adopted, including the rate of temperature and concentration change, the amount of recovery differs. However, the amount of recovery remains substantially the same at the end of each cycle when a sufficient period is allowed, indicating the slowness of recrystallization. Even after long periods of standing (and the use of a high degree of cross-linking) the original length, which amounts to about 500% of the shrunken length, is not recovered. The failure of the original structure to regenerate is noted in all cases where complete shrinkage occurs [7, 28]. However, in the case of the tendon immersed in an acid solution at pH 2 there is, at 25°C, a reduction of length (cf. Fig. 3.1) of about 10% which, as discussed in Section 3.2, may be regarded as a selective melting. When the tendon is reimmersed in pure water this kind of dimensional change is completely reversible, although the transformation is still somewhat slow. Clearly then, recovery of the original length, after full shrinkage, cannot be secured by the simple insertion of cross-linkages in the oriented state. Although by using this method one can secure a reversible contractible system following the first shrinkage, in order to obtain a contractile system with full recovery of the original length a more complex pattern of the original organization must be maintained.

Occurrence of time effects not only affects the recovery of length, once shrinkage has occurred, but also the value of the shrinkage temperature (or of the critical salt concentration for shrinkage) which may be slightly decreased by increasing the time scale of experiment [19]. In fact, Weir [35] was able to describe the shrinkage as a rate process and concluded that a true shrinkage temperature did not exist.

The difficulty of eliminating time effects and, especially, the recognition that a component of the material may be disordered before shrinkage and another component ordered after shrinkage, should not, however, be regarded as evidence that the process underlying shrinkage is not a melting or first-order phase transition. As discussed by Flory and Garrett [13], a large body of experimental facts do indicate the validity of the latter description which was earlier suggested by Wöhlish [36] The fact that a crystalline and an amorphous phase are involved in the process is amply documented by measurements of x-ray diffraction, birefringence, and elasticity, such as those presented in Section 3.2. Reversibility, though incomplete, is nevertheless observed as the data in Fig. 3.14 illustrates. The effect of increasing diluent content is invariably that of reducing the melting temperature, as predicted by Equation 7. This conclusion holds even in the case of open systems (i.e., swollen tendons in equilibrium with an excess of diluent) and it is reflected in the increase of the shrinkage temperature observed [14, 19] on increasing cross-linking density. In fact, an increase of the latter is known to decrease the amount of diluent available to the molten network [1]. Ciferri et al. [19] point out that an additional contribution to the increase of T_s with degree of cross-linking may be ascribed to a decreased conformational entropy in the amorphous state, as theoretically predicted [18] when the cross-linking reaction occurs in the oriented fibrous state.

Occurrence of volume changes is evident from the data in Fig. 3.5 and latent heat effects have been directly measured [37]. Moreover, Witnauer and Fee [14], as well as Flory and Garrett [13], were able to successfully apply melting-point depression theory to the collagen-gelatin transition. Witnauer and Fee measured shrinkage temperatures for bovine corium collagen-glycol systems as a function of the volume fraction of solvent and, using Equation 7, calculated ΔH to be 17 cal

g^{-1}. Flory and Garrett used dilatometric measurements for collagen tendon-glycol systems obtaining ΔH equal to 24 cal g^{-1}. The value of T_m^0 (cf. Equation 7) was found to be 145°C. Considering the fact (cf. Section 3.2) that a certain amount of firmly bound diluent may be retained by collagen even in the crystalline state, Flory and Garrett proposed that the observed T_m^0 should refer to the melting point of the pure collagen-diluent complex (assuming its composition to remain constant with ξ_1). Melting temperatures determined by dilatometry were found to be the same for the first and second melting of a given collagen sample [13]. With regard to differences between the shrinkage and the melting temperature, Oth [38], as well as Flory and Spurr [25], were able to demonstrate that the measured shrinkage temperature T_s is usually some 4–7°C above the true thermodynamic melting temperature T_m, (i.e., shrinkage corresponding to the melting of a superheated crystal). This observation justifies the finding that the shrinkage temperature may be reduced by increasing the time scale of the experiment.

An additional feature which is in line with the description of the collagen-gelatin transformation as a first-order phase transition is the variation of the shrinkage temperature of cross-linked tendons with the applied stress to be described in detail next.

Before closing this subsection it seems appropriate to call attention to an additional transition, which may be observed upon heating collagen tendons. Careful determinations by Flory and Garrett [13] and by Mason and Ribgy [39] indicates that at about 40°C, that is, below both T_s or T_m, there is a change of slope of the specific volume-temperature dependence for swollen collagen, as is commonly observed for glass transitions. Ribgy [40] analyzed the effect of this transition on the stress-relaxation of stretched tendons and found that above 40°C large stress-relaxation and irreversible deformation of the fiber occur. The nature of this transition is not entirely clear (cf. Mason [41]).

3.4.2   The Role of pH

The variation of the shrinkage temperature with pH is illustrated in Fig. 3.17. These data were obtained from length-temperature curves at constant pH such as those reported in Fig. 3.15.

On the basis of the titration data of Kenchington and Ward [42] for gelatin and those of Bowes and Kenten [42] for intact bovine corium collagen, the pH ranges for titration of the significant carboxyl, α-amino + imidazole and ϵ-amino groups are, respectively, 1.5–6.5, 6.0–8.5, and 8.0–11.5. Thus the data in Fig. 3.17 suggest that a certain amount of net cationic charge can exist within the tropocollagen units

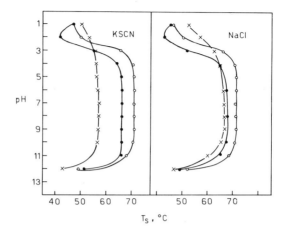

Figure 3.17. Variation of the shrinkage temperature (midpoints of the transition data in Fig. 3.15) for cross-linked collagen tendons with pH in (○) solutions containing no added salt: (●) 0.1 M and 0.5 M (×) NaCl or KSCN. (Reproduced from Ref. 19).

without altering the stability of the crystalline tendon. However, at pH <4 the number of cationic charges begin to be appreciable, and the resulting destabilization of the tendon, evidenced by the reduction of the shrinkage temperature, may be attributed to the electrostatic repulsion of the positive charges and associated Donnan osmotic effect. The same consideration can be extended to the case of a net anionic charge on the alkaline side of the pH scale when only at pH >10 a depression of the shrinkage temperature with pH is observed. Comparison of the shrinkage data in Fig. 3.17 with the swelling data reported in Fig. 3.1 reveals an excellent correlation between the two effects.

3.4.3   The Role of Salts

Isoelectric or Near-Isoelectric Conditions

Gustavson [1] as well as Theis and Steinhardt [26] have reviewed some of the earlier studies on the dependence of the shrinkage temperature T_s of collagen upon salt type and salt concentration under isoelectric conditions. The latter authors, in an extensive investigation of the effect of both acids and mono- and divalent salts, pointed out the differences in the behavior of some salts for which the shrinkage temperature in an excess of pure water, T_s^w, is continuously depressed on increasing C_s, and other salts for which T_s^w, is reduced at low C_s and increased at high C_s. Typical C_s versus T_s curves [23, 35] are collected in Fig. 3.18. Above $C_s = 1\ M$ all data admit the following order of ions for increasing depression of the shrinkage temperature (generally, salting-in) from left to right (note that the order can be altered at lower C_s).

$$F^- < SO_4^{2-} < OAc^- < Cl^- < NO_3^- < Br^- < SCN^- \qquad (22)$$

$$K^+ < Mg^{2+} < Na^+ < Cs^+ < Li^+ < Ca^{2+} \qquad (23)$$

The effects of various ions for a given salt are largely additive.

Comparison of series (22) and (23) with series (15) and (16) and with series (17) and (18) immediately reveals full agreement between the order of salting-in deduced from swelling, ion binding, and shrinkage data. This suggests the possibility of describing the role of salt on the shrinkage temperature in terms of swelling and/or ion binding. The en-

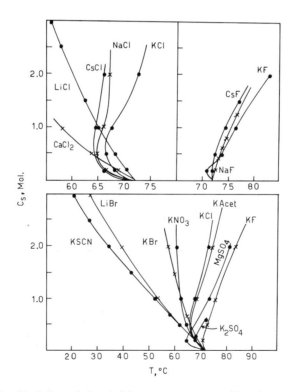

Figure 3.18.   Variation of the shrinkage temperature with salt concentration for cross-linked rat-tail tendons in equilibrium with several salt solutions. (Reproduced from Ref. 23)

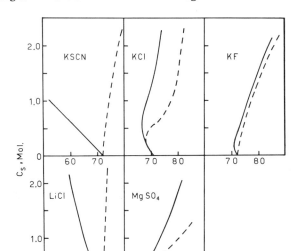

Figure 3.19. The solid lines represent experimental shrinkage curves similar to those reproduced in Fig. 3.18 for cross-linked tendons in several salt solutions. The dashed lines represent theoretical curves obtained from Equation 7 and the equilibrium swelling data, extrapolated at the shrinkage temperature, collected in Table 3.1. (Reproduced from Ref. 23).

suing discussion indicates that both effects are necessary for a proper description of the role of salts.

To be considered first is the correlation between shrinkage and swelling in neutral salt solutions. Examination of Fig. 3.18 and Fig. 3.5 reveals that there is a difference in the two sets of results in the dependence of the effect considered upon C_s. For salts such as KCl and $MgSO_4$ there is an apparent correlation between the shape of the T_s versus C_s curves and the shape of the isothermal swelling versus C_s curves in the sense that in the range of the salt concentration where swelling increases T_s is depressed, and when v^{-1} decreases T_s is raised. The correlations, however, becomes less apparent with increasing salting-in power, an observation which was also made by Gustavson [1]. Figure 3.19 illustrates a more quantitative correlation between the degree of swelling and shrinkage temperature for KSCN, KCl, KF, LiCl, and $MgSO_4$. Equation 7 was used to calculate the theoretical melting curves (dashed lines) using values of χ_1 and ξ_1 corresponding to the equilibrium degree of swelling extrapolated to the shrinkage temperature using the data collected in Table 3.1. Values of ΔH_u and T_m^0 were chosen to fit the experimental shrinkage curves at $C_s = 0$. Figure 3.19 clearly reveals that in the case of salting-out agents there exists a satisfactory correlation between the shapes of experimental and theoretical curves. However, as salting-in becomes more pronounced, a large and continuous depression is experimentally observed, although the theoretical curve, which reflects the variation of v^{-1} and χ_1, would predict a small increase of T_m with C_s.

Thus while the swelling behavior and the simple equation 7 are adequate for describing the role of salting-out agents, an additional effect must be introduced for describing the role of salting-in agents. There is little doubt that this additional effect is ion binding which, as evident from series (17) and (18), is larger for the strongest salting-in agents. As discussed in Section 3.1, the overall polymer-salt-water interaction may be described in terms of (1) a strong specific interaction described as binding, and (2) a remaining weaker interaction described as a generic diluent effect [16]. This division is thermodynamically represented by Equation 8 which indicates that when ion binding occurs to the denatured form of the protein (as experimentally was found to be the case, cf. Fig. 3.12) a larger depression of the melting temperature than predicted from Equation 7 should occur. One can actually evaluate from Equation 8 the parameter $pRT \ln (1 + Ka)$ (i.e., the free energy of binding $-\Delta F_b/RT$) from the experimentally determined shrinkage temperature in various salt solutions. For this evaluation the diluent term in Equation 8, that is, $(1/T_m^0) + (R/\Delta H_u) (V_v/V_1) (\xi_1 - \chi_1\xi_1^2)$, may be treated as constant (this term, cf. Fig. 3.19, is relatively insensitive to salt concentration) and detemined by measuring the shrinkage temperature for tendons in pure water. The results of this determination [29] are collected in Table 3.6 which includes data from Tables 3.3 and 3.5. Comparison of the free energy of binding obtained from direct measurements of salt binding and from melting point depression (cf. Table 3.6) reveals that not only is the ranking of salts for their salting-in behavior similar for the two methods but also that reasonable agreement is obtained. Virtually complete agreement between the two methods could be obtained using $\Delta H_u = 1.35$ kcal mole^{-1} [25] or a somewhat larger hydration value. Mandelkern and Stewart [43] also used Equation 8 to evaluate binding constants (assuming $p = 1$) from the helix-coil transition data of von Hippel and Wong [44] for soluble gelatin and their results are in satisfactory agreement with those reported in Table 3.6. The limited effect of binding for salting-out agents such as KCl support the contention [19, 23] that the corresponding salt solution can be approximated as

Table 3.6   Free Energy of Binding, $-\Delta F_b =$ $pRT \ln (1 + Ka)$, for 1 M Salts [29]

Salt	$-\Delta F_b$, cal mole^{-1}		
	Binding		
	From Table 3.3	From Table 3.5[b]	Melting[a]
K$^+$			
SCN$^-$	55.2	48.0	115.7
I$^-$	49.1	—	—
Br$^-$	30.0	—	55.0
NO$_3^-$	22.9	—	51.7
Cl$^-$	11.5	6.9	23.2
CH$_3$COO$^-$	7.1	—	17.1
Li$^+$			
I$^-$	72.1		—
Br$^-$	47.5		110.8
Cl$^-$	27.3		41.2
Cl$^-$			
Ca^{2+}	39.3		92.8
Li$^+$	27.3		41.2
NH$_4^+$	20.8		
Cs$^+$	17.5		40.6
Na$^+$	16.9		33.2
Rb$^+$	14.2		—
K$^+$	11.5		23.2

[a] Determined from shrinkage data [16, 23] by using Equation 8 with $\Delta H_u = 2$ kcal mole^{-1} and $T_m = T_s$.
[b] Calculated from the binding data of Table 3.5 for two water molecules per residue.

a one-component diluent. The fact that binding constants are quite small for the salting-in agents justifies some of the observations [44], such as the additive effects of various ions and the lack of site saturation even at high molarites.

Puett and Rajagh [23] have critically analysed the role of other effects which have been suggested for describing the interaction of proteins in water-salt solutions. They concluded that the large depression of melting temperature caused by salting-in agents was not adequately explained by any of the following: Donnan effects (arising from unequal anion and cation binding), ion hydration of water activity, water structure, internal pressure of the solutions and electrostatic properties of the solutions.

While thermodynamic binding of salts to the randomly coiled form explains the large melting point depression, the detailed molecular description of the binding process is somewhat obscure. It is plausible, as suggested by Mandelkern et al., [45], that a local alteration of the electronic configuration of the peptide group at which binding takes place destabilizes the tropocollagen helix. The generality of series (22) on depressing the denaturation temperature of such diverse polymers as collagen, DNA [46], and ribonuclease [44] suggests that anion binding is primarily controlled by factors which pertain to the hydration of ions and to the structure of the solutions, at least, for the relatively loose ionic complexes which are generally involved. Robinson and Jencks [47] stated that binding reflects more the poor interaction of the anions with water than a specific preference of the ions for the solute. In fact, the order for decreasing exclusion of anions from a water-air interface is in close agreement with the order for increasing salting-in of collagen and of an uncharged peptide [47]. The foregoing interpretation fails to explain the large salting-in by cations such as Li^+ and Ca^{2+} which are strongly hydrated and net-structure-former. For these, it is possible [2, 47] that more definite classes of compounds are formed involving a more specific role of the polymer structure and of the hydration layer of the ions.

Nonisoelectric Behavior

In the preceding section it was indicated that polyelectrolyte or Donnan effects resulting from unequal ion absorption cannot be regarded as responsible for the large melting point depression caused by salting-in agents. One simple observation which substantiates this finding is that the depression caused by salts where both anions and cations are absorbed, such as $Ca(SCN)_2$, is larger than for a salt where only one ion is preferentially absorbed, such as $CaCl_2$ and $KSCN$ [cf. series (12) and (18)]. Very likely any polyelectrolyte or Donnan effect resulting from unequal ion absorption plays a negligible role at the relatively high salt concentration considered in the preceding section due to the screening effect of couter-ions and co-ions in proximity to the polymer.

The situation may be, however, quite different at low pH or low salt concentration [5]. Data reported in Fig. 3.20 illustrate the role of salt on the shrinkage temperature at pH 2 when extreme nonisoelectric conditions exist. The data clearly indicate that the role of salts is similar to that observed under isoelectric conditions only for salt concentrations $> \approx 0.8\ M$. The typical polyelectrolyte effect exhibited in salt concentration $< \approx 0.8\ M$ can be described (cf. Fig. 3.20) as a competition of two effects: a tendency for decreasing the shrinkage temperature prevailing at very low salt concentration and a tendency for reincreasing the shrinkage temperature prevailing at somewhat higher salt concentration [5]. The former effect is probably associated with the effect of salts on the apparent pK values of the ionizable groups of the protein [48, 32]. The latter effect can be associated [49] with a decrease of the electrostatic free energy of the polyelectrolyte which may result

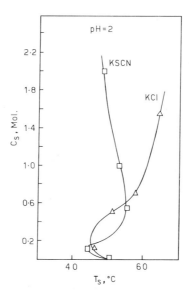

Figure 3.20.   Variation of the shrinkage temperature with salt concentration at pH = 2 for cross-linked collagen tendons. (Data from Ref. 5).

from both anion binding and from screening of the fixed charges by the mobile ions. Detailed inspection of the data in Fig. 3.20 indicates that KSCN is more effective than KCl in causing a prevailing of the latter over the former effect. In fact, for KSCN we find a $\sim 10°$ higher denaturation temperature in 0.4 M solutions than in the case of KCl. This observation is interpreted [5] as additional support for the view discussed in the preceding section that SCN$^-$ possesses a stronger ability than Cl$^-$ to bind to polar groups of the protein. Binding of SCN$^-$ under such conditions may preferentially occur to the ϵ-amino groups of lysine and hydroxylisine residues rather than at the peptide bonds [32].

Cross-linking Salts

The effect of neutral salts on native collagen is not, generally, a permanent one and after washing out the salt solutions, the original value of the shrinkage temperature $T_s{}^w$ measured in pure water may be observed a second time.

A different situation is exhibited in the presence of some particular salts such as $AlCl_3$ and, particularly, $KCr(SO_4)_2$ which have a cross-linking power toward collagen [1]. T_s versus C_s curves for collagen in $KCr(SO_4)$ solutions are exhibited in Fig. 3.21. The upper curve corresponds to unbuffered solutions, the actual pH of the solutions being indicated on the insert. Under these conditions, particularly at low salt concentrations, the cross-linking effect is overshadowed by the polyelectrolite effect which was discussed in the preceding section. The occurrence

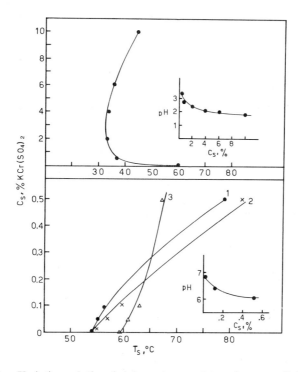

Figure 3.21. Variation of the shrinkage temperature of uncross-linked collagen tendons with $KCr(SO_4)_2$ concentration. The data for the upper curve correspond to unbuffered solutions (1) 30 min and (2) 24-hr immersions in each solution at 25°C before the determination of T_s in chrome alum solution buffered with CH_3COONH_4; (3) same conditions as for curve 2 but shrinkage measured in pure water. (Reproduced from Ref. 19).

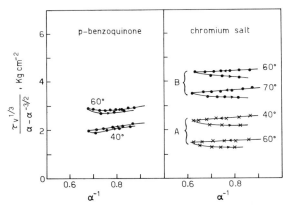

Figure 3.22. Stress-strain isotherms at different temperatures and in 6 M KSCN solutions for tendons cross-linked with chromium salt (samples A and B) as compared with tendons cross-linked with p-benzoquinone. (Reproduced from Ref. 7).

of a cross-linking reaction may be, however, revealed by eliminating the latter effect using $KCr(SO_4)_2$ solutions buffered with 0.15 M ammonium acetate (pH 6–7), as was done in the case of curves 1 and 2 reported in the lower part of Fig. 3.21, (the point at $C_s = 0$ refers to the tendon in excess 0.15 M CH_3COONH_4 solution). Each curve represents a different time of immersion in the $KCr(SO_4)_2 + CH_3COONH_4$ solution prior to the measurement of shrinkage. It is seen that in contrast to all cases so far considered (cf. Fig. 3.18), the shrinkage temperature is continuously raised upon increasing C_s. Independent measurements [19] reveal a simultaneous decrease of the degree of swelling of the tendons. That stable cross-links are indeed involved is demonstrated by measuring the shrinkage temperature of tendons after they had been immersed in $KCr(SO_4)_2 + CH_3COONH_4$ solutions of different C_s for 24 hours and then carefully washed. The shrinkage temperature was measured in pure water and the results are illustrated in curve 3 of Fig. 3.21. In contrast to the case of salts such as NaCl, $Ca(SCN)_2$, and KSCN which, after washing, did not leave any permanent effect on the tendons, chromium salts are effectively strongly bound to the protein.

The occurrence of a cross-linking reaction in the presence of chromium salts may be also evidenced by elasticity measurements [7], from dilute solutions studies [50], and other effects [1]. Figure 3.22 represents the elastic characteristics of amorphous tendons treated with chromium salts. Stress-strain curves were obtained in a 6 M KSCN solution. The occurrence of a rubbery network can be deduced from the good reversibility, the relatively high modulus and from the fact that the theoretical Equation 1 satisfactorily represents the data. In contrast to the case of quinone cross-linking, however, the thermal stability of chromium networks is rather poor, and the expected increase of the modulus with temperature (cf. Equation 1) which is observed for the former networks fails to be evident in the latter.

Some of the elastic characteristics of chromium cross-linked tendons are similar to those exhibited by collagen tendons obtained from old rats [51]. This led to the suggestion [7] that the accumulation of polyvalent ions within cells and connective tissue could have been associated with the natural aging process of collagen. However, according to recent results [52], there is no evidence to substantiate this possibility.

3.4.4   The Role of Nonelectrolytes

Gustavson [1] has reviewed earlier data concerning the role of various nonelectrolytes on the shrinkage temperature. He points out that there is not a simple relation between the effect on T_s and the dielectric constant of the solvent. Moreover, comparing the effect of sucrose and glucose on T_s and on the degree of swelling, Gustavson concludes that other factors besides swelling must be involved in controlling T_s.

Recent data [28] for soluble collagen in the presence of simple aliphatic alcohols are reported in Fig. 3.23. It is seen that on increasing

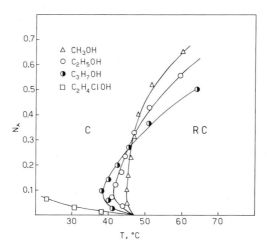

Figure 3.23. Variation of the melting temperature of soluble collagen with the molar fraction N_A of several alcohols. pH = 6. The field of stability of each phase is indicated. (Reproduced from Ref. 28).

alcohol concentration the melting temperature is initially depressed. The order for increasing depression is

$$C_2H_4ClOH > C_3H_7OH > C_2H_3OH > CH_3OH \qquad (24)$$

Upon further increasing of the alcohol concentration a subsequent re-increase of T_m is observed and, in this region, the order for increasing depression is

$$CH_3OH > C_2H_5OH > C_3H_7OH \qquad (25)$$

Similar results were obtained by Schnell and Zahn [53] using rat tail tendons. Comparison of the data in Fig. 3.23 with the data in Fig. 3.9 reveals that also in the case of collagen-alcohol systems there is no correlation between the melting and swelling behavior. The measurement of the selective absorption of alcohols by collagen (cf. Fig. 3.13) reveals, however, an effect which can be correlated to the melting behavior. In fact, the absorption goes through a maximum on increasing alcohol content and the order for increasing absorption coincides with series (24) below the maximum and with series (25) above the maximum. Thus, similar to the case of neutral salts, the effect of aliphatic alcohols on the melting temperature may be thermodynamically interpreted in terms of the selective enrichment of one of the solvent components within the polymer domain. A quantitative analysis in terms of Equations 8 or 14 has not, however, been attempted. Bianchi et al., [28] who compared the role of alcohols on the conformational stability of synthetic polypeptides and collagen, suggested that the depressing effect on T_m observed in diluted alcohol solutions should be attributed to a solvation of the side chain apolar groups of collagen which become exposed during the melting transition.

3.4.5   The Effect of Stress

Experimental examples of crystal $\rightarrow$ amorphous transitions for collagen tendons subjected to an external tensile force were considered by Oth [38]), Spurr and Flory [25], and Yonath et al. [54].

Flory and Spurr, and Oth used an elaborate technique for determining the stress-strain behavior at the melting temperature for cross-linked collagen tendons in excess of water. If full shrinkage of the crystalline fiber is prevented by holding the sample between clamps and if the temperature is held in the proximity of the shrinkage temperature, co-existing amorphous and crystalline phases can be established and visually observed along a well-constructed and well-behaved fiber. The force which can be measured under this situation is the force for phase equilib-

rium at a given temperature and it should be independent of sample
length as a consequence of the monovariance of the systems (cf. Section
3.1). This was verified by performing small alterations in length within
the range L_c–L_a. After a transient alteration of the force, the equilibrium
value was eventually recovered. Results obtained with this procedure
[38] for cross-linked collagen in excess of water are represented in Fig.
3.24. A region of constant f between the stress-strain curves for the
fully amorphous and fully crystalline fiber is quite evident. The value
of the equilibrium force corresponding to the plateau for different tem-

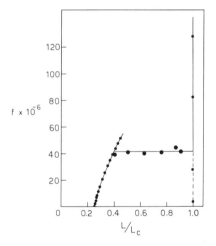

Figure 3.24. Experimental stress-length isotherm at 75°C for a cross-linked
collagen tendon in water. (Reproduced from Ref. 38).

peratures is reported in Fig. 3.25. The curve indicates that the melting
temperature increases with increasing applied stress and the intercept
at $f = 0$ denotes that value of the "isotropic melting temperature" [25,
38]. In accordance with Equation 9, the curvature of the plot reflects
the decrease of the difference $\Delta L = L_a - L_c$ on increasing f due to the
relatively higher deformability of the fiber in the amorphous than in
the crystalline state.

Regarding ΔS and ΔH as temperature independent and using the experimentally determined ΔL value, it is possible, according to Equations
9 and 10, to obtain the values of the latent entropy and enthalpy changes
on melting. Following this approach Oth found a value of $\Delta H_u = 2$ kcal
mole^{-1} of average peptide residue in case of dry collagen (correction

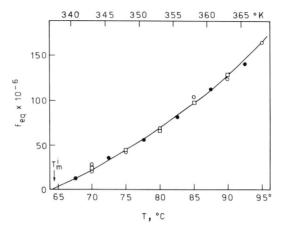

Figure 3.25. Variation of the stress for solid → melt equilibrium with temperature for a cross-linked collagen tendon in water. (Reproduced from Ref. 38).

for the contribution due to the heat of dilution was asserted using samples with different cross-linking degree and extrapolating the overall heat of transformation to unit volume fraction of polymer). This value compares favorably with the result of a similar investigation by Spurr and Flory [25] yielding $\Delta H_u = 1.3$ kcal mole^{-1}.

Flory and Spurr [25], Yonath et al. [54], and Rubin et al. [55] have investigated the melting of collagen under stress in the presence of salt solutions. Typical length-C_s isotherms for different values of the applied stress obtained by Yonath et al. for collagen fibers in KSCN solutions are reported in Fig. 3.26. The shrinkage is markedly unsharp (note that the system is not monovariant, cf. Section 3.1), particularly when the applied load is large and, thus, it is impossible to define a simple f versus C_s diagram for phase equilibrium, as was done using f and T as state variables, in the case of data in Fig. 3.25. It is seen that the critical salt concentration increases with the stretching force indicating, according to Equation 13, a positive change in chemical enrichment upon melting. This was, in fact, verified by Oplatka and Yonath [54] by direct measurements of KSCN and water uptake. Enrichment values measured by the latter authors were found to be in satisfactory agreement with the binding constant measured by Ciferri et al. [29].

Rubin et al. [55] have recently analysed the variation of fiber length with LiBr activity and with tensile force using reconstituted collagen which had undergone several contraction-expansion cycles. They analysed the result in terms of the two-state model proposed by Hill [56] which they found to be a satisfactory framework for the characterization of the mechanochemical transition. The measured enrichment decreased linearly with fiber length; in 5 M LiBr the molar ratio of excess LiBr/amino acid residue varied from 1:4 in relaxed fibers to 1:7 in fully stretched ones.

One interesting application of the chemical melting of collagen was reported by Steinberg et al. [57]. Using the forces developing during the melting process, they were able to construct an engine based on a cross-linked collagen belt with one extreme immersed in a concentrated

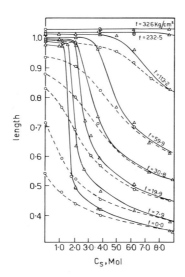

Figure 3.26. Length versus KSCN concentration at constant load for collagen tendons at 32°C:∆ increasing concentration (first run), ○ decreasing concentration (second run). (Reproduced from Ref. 54).

LiBr solution and the other in water. Mechanical work resulted from the conversion of the chemical free energy associated with the transfer of LiBr from the concentrated solution to water.

REFERENCES

1. K. H. Gustavson, *The Chemistry and Reactivity of Collagen,* Academic Press, New York, 1956.
2. A. Veis, *The Macromolecular Chemistry of Gelatin,* Academic Press, New York, 1964.

3. A. Veis, *Treatise on Collagen*, G. N. Ramachandran, Ed., Academic Press, London, 1967.

4. P. H. von Hippel, *Treatise on Collagen*, G. N. Ramachandran, Ed. Academic Press, London, 1967.

5. E. Bianchi, G. Conio, A. Ciferri, D. Puett, and L. Rajagh, *J. Biol. Chem.*, **242**, 1361 (1967).

6. W. F. Harrington and P. H. von Hippel, *Advan. Protein Chem.*, **16**, 1 (1961).

7. D. Puett, A. Ciferri, and L. V. Rajagh, *Biopolymers*, **3**, 439 (1965).

8. R. S. Bear, *Advan. Protein Chem.*, **7**, 149 (1952).

9. J. Bashaw and K. J. Smith, *J. Polymer Sci.*, **6**, 1041 (1968).

10. A. Gliozzi, R. Morchio, and A. Ciferri, *J. Phys. Chem.*, **73**, 3063 (1969).

11. P. J. Flory, *Principles of Polymer Chemistry*, Cornell University Press, Ithaca, N.Y., 1953.

12. L. V. Rajagh, D. Puett, and A. Ciferri, *Biopolymers*, **3**, 421 (1965).

13. P. J. Flory and R. R. Garett, *J. Amer. Chem. Soc.*, **80**, 4836 (1958).

14. L. P. Witnauer and J. G. Fee, *J. Polymer Sci.*, **26**, 141 (1957).

15. K. J. Smith, A. Greene, and A. Ciferri, *Kolloid-Z.*, **194**, 49 (1964).

16. T. A. Orofino, A. Ciferri, and J. J. Hermans, *Biopolymers*, **5**, 773 (1967).

17. A. Katchalsky and A. Oplatka, *Procedings of the 4th International Congress on Rheology*, E. H. Lee and A. L. Copley, Eds., Interscience, New York, 1965.

18. P. J. Flory, *J. Amer. Chem. Soc.*, **78**, 5222 (1956).

19. A. Ciferri, L. V. Rajagh, and D. Puett, *Biopolymers*, **3**, 461 (1965).

20. R. E. Burge, P. M. Cowan, and S. McGavin, *Recent Advances in Gelatin and Glue Research*, Pergamon Press, London, 1958.

21. A. Gliozzi, R. Morchio, and A. Ciferri, *The Chemistry and Molecular Biology of the Intercellular Matrix*, E. A. Balazs, Ed., Academic Press, New York, 1970.

22. G. Thau, R. Bloch, and O. Kedem, *Desalination*, **1**, 129 (1966).

23. D. Puett and L. V. Rajagh, *J. Macromol. Chem.*, **A2**, 111 (1968).

24. A. R. Docking and E. Heymann, *J. Phys. Chem.*, **43**, 513 (1939).

25. P. J. Flory and O. K. Spurr, Jr., *J. Amer. Chem. Soc.*, **83**, 1308 (1961).

26. E. R. Theis and R. G. Steinhardt, Jr., *J. Amer. Leather Chemists' Assoc.*, **37**, 433 (1942).

27. A. L. Rubin, M. P. Drake, P. F. Davison, D. Pfahl, P. T. Speakman, and F. O. Shmitt, *Biochemistry*, **4**, 181 (1965).

28. E. Bianchi, R. Rampone, A. Tealdi, and A. Ciferri, *J. Biol. Chem.*, **245**, 3341 (1970).

29. A. Ciferri, R. Garmon, and D. Puett, *Biopolymers*, **5**, 439 (1967).

30. O. L. Sponsler, J. D. Bath, and J. W. Ellis, *J. Phys. Chem.*, **35**, 2053 (1940).

31. C. Tanford, *Physical Chemistry of Macromolecules*, Wiley, New York, 1961.

32. A. Ciferri, D. Puett, L. Rajagh, and J. Hermans, Jr., *Biopolymers*, **6**, 1019 (1968).

33. J. O. Threlkeld, J. J. Burke, D. Puett, and A. Ciferri, *Biopolymers*, **6**, 767 (1968).

34. H. Strassmair, J. Engel, and G. Zundel, *Biopolymers,* **8,** 237 (1969).
35. C. E. Weir, *J. Res. Nat. Bur. Stand.,* **42,** 17 (1949).
36. E. Wöhlish, *Biochem. Z.,* **247,** 329 (1932); *Kolloid Z.,* **89,** 239 (1939).
37. E. Wöhlish and R. de Rochemont, *Z. Biol.,* **85,** 406 (1927); A. Küntzel and K. Doehner, *Angew. Chem.,* **52,** 175 (1939).
38. J. M. F. Oth, *Kolloid-Z.,* **164,** 114, 124 (1959); ibid., **171,** 1 (1960).
39. P. Mason and B. J. Ribgy, *Biochem. Biophys. Acta,* **66,** 448 (1963).
40. B. J. Ribgy, N. Hirai, J. D. Spikes, and H. Eyring, *J. Gen. Physiol.,* **43,** 265 (1959).
41. P. Mason and B. J. Ribgy, *Polymer,* **6,** 90 (1965).
42. A. W. Kenchington and A. G. Ward, *Biochem. J.,* **58,** 202 (1954); J. H. Bowes and R. H. Kenten, *ibid.,* **43,** 358 (1948).
43. L. Mandelkern and W. E. Steward, *Biochemistry,* **3,** 1135 (1964).
44. P. H. von Hippel and K. Y. Wong, *Biochemistry,* **1,** 664 (1962); *J. Biol. Chem.,* **240,** 3909 (1965).
45. L. Mandelkern, J. C. Halpin, A. F. Diorio, and A. S. Posner, *J. Amer. Chem. Soc.,* **84,** 1383 (1962).
46. K. Hamaguchi and E. P. Geiduschek, *J. Amer. Chem. Soc.,* **84,** 1329 (1962).
47. D. R. Robinson and W. P. Jencks, *J. Amer. Chem. Soc.,* **87,** 2402 (1965).
48. A. Wada, *Mol. Phys.,* **3,** 409 (1960).
49. C. Schildkraut and S. Lifson, *Biopolymers,* **3,** 195 (1965).
50. J. Purradier, J. Roman, A. Venet, H. Chateau, and A. Accary, *Bull. Soc. Chim. France,* **19,** 928 (1952).
51. A. Ciferri and Rajagh, *J. Gerontol.,* **19,** 220 (1964).
52. R. Morchio and A. Ciferri, *Biophysik.* **5,** 327 (1969).
53. J. Schnell and H. Zahn, *Makromol. Chem.,* **84,** 192 (1965).
54. A. Oplatka and J. Yonath, *Biopolymers,* **6,** 1147 (1968).
55. M. M. Rubin, K. A. Piez, and A. Katchalsky, *Biochemistry,* **8,** 3628 (1969).
56. T. L. Hill, *J. Chem. Phys.,* **20,** 1259 (1952).
57. I. Z. Steinberg, A. Oplatka, and A. Katchalsky, *Nature,* **210,** 568 (1966).

4

The Optical Properties of Skin and its Biochemical Substituents

KIRK C. HOERMAN

Chief, Biophysics Division, Naval Dental Research Institute, Great Lakes, Illinois

Skin possesses the optical property of self-luminescence. The major forms of this luminescence, fluorescence and phosphorescence, are consequences of the absorption of incident light cast upon the skin from artificial sources or the sun. The radiation capable of causing self-luminescence in skin must be of such energy that, when absorbed, it produces a molecular distortion of the chromophores in the tissue. This distortion is rapidly minimized by dissipation of absorbed energy as heat and/or luminescence. Prolonged or intensified radiation and excitation of tissue chromophores may bring about pathologic conditions, such as sunburn, erythema, and, in the worst case possible, neoplastic lesions.

The light which produces chromophoric excitation in skin is invisible to the human eye. This radiation is nonionizing and falls in the ultraviolet range of the electromagnetic spectrum, that is, less than 390 nanometers (nm) in wavelength (λ). Merely 5.7% of the sun's incident light on the earth's atmosphere is composed of wavelengths in the ultraviolet region from 250 to 350 nm. The lower end of this spectral interval, from 250 to 265 nm, is known to critically damage nucleic acids in cells. Fortunately, very little of the sun's energy below 300 nm in wavelength reaches the surface of the earth. Atmospheric ozone absorbs this energy and thus forms a shield which prevents the penetration of these biologically dangerous photons onto the earth's surface. The absorption spectrum of atmospheric ozone and that of ribonucleic acid (RNA) are compared in Fig. 4.1. The umbrella effect of ozone is clearly demonstrated [1].

There is among scientists a fair understanding of the absorbance and transmission of light in skin and its strata. On the other hand, room temperature fluorescence of skin, teeth, finger and toe nails, eyes, and other integumental tissues exposed to ultraviolet light, as often dramatically displayed in nightclubs and other darkened settings, is imperfectly understood. Notwithstanding, there is an increasing knowledge of the low-temperature ultraviolet fluorescence and phosphorescence of skin, cartilage, bone, tooth, and their biochemical substituents such as collagen and glycoprotein.

In all, the property of self-luminescence in skin, and its substituents, constitutes a means to probe and assess the structure of connective tissue at the molecular level adjunctive to what is already known from chemical analyses.

4.1. BIOLOGICAL FLUOROPHORES

4.1.1 General

Luminescence of skin provided the first clue to the fact that protein was capable of attaining excited states. It started with the work of Stübel in 1911 when he published a remarkable account of luminescence of skin after ultraviolet light radiation [2]. In the years that followed, especially in the 1930s, the scientific literature was filled with descriptions of luminescence of skin, other connective tissues, and proteinaceous materials [3–7]. Unfortunately, many of these authors observed bluish-white and yellowish-blue fluorescence present in some proteins and absent

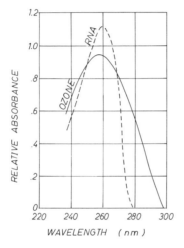

Figure 4.1. The absorption spectra of ozone compared to that of ribonucleic acid (RNA) showing the "umbrella" effect of ozone against solar critical radiation between $\sim \lambda = 200$ and 300 nm.

in others. They also noted that heat and the state of aggregation correlated directly with intensity of luminescence. These effects were later shown to be associated with excited states and quantum laws not ordinarily ascribed to proteins [8].

The first observation of significance related to fluorescence of skin and other connective tissue resulted from the work of Reeder and Nelson in 1940 [9]. Actually, these authors, rather than discovering the authentic protein fluorophore, that is the ring-membered amino acid, found a bluish-white fluorescence in solid proteins, hair, wool keratin, and gelatin. This luminescence arose after excitation at $\lambda = 325$ nm, a wavelength significantly red-shifted away from the absorption band of proteins.

Surprisingly, the resulting bluish-white fluorescence, whose emission maximum was $\lambda = 405$ nm, has been noted many times over in solid tissues such as skin, bone, and tooth and remains a mystery—indeed the darkened room curiosity—even to this day. A subsequent section of this Chapter will attempt to bring the reader up to date on the understanding of this elusive, yet fascinating, emissivity.

In 1952, Debye and Edwards [10] studied protein and amino acid luminescence at liquid nitrogen temperature ($-196°C$). This supercooled state of the fluorophore environment produced long-lived, low energy— relative to fluorescence—emissions, or phosphorescence. These workers noted that in all of the 18 amino acids studied, none exhibited visible fluorescence, including the ring-membered molecules, tryptophan, tyrosine, and phenylalanine. However, a visible emission, phosphorescence, was noted in these amino acids as well as in most proteins studied. Thus the stage was set for the subsequent pioneering work of Duggan and Udenfriend [11] in which ultraviolet fluorescence of proteins was first described. At this time in 1956, other laboratories were recording the existence of ultraviolet fluorescence of proteins and definitively relating them to fluorophores consisting of ring-membered amino acid residues in polypeptide chains [12–14]. The origin and nature of protein fluorescence was finally clarified by Teale in 1960 [15]. He noted that, at room temperature, protein solutions displayed fluorescent spectra and maxima in the ultraviolet range. These emissions were characteristic of the dominant residual aromatic amino acid. For example, when tryptophan was present it was found that the peak emission always occurred at $\lambda \simeq 353$ nm, even if tyrosine $\lambda \simeq 303$ nm, was in disproportionately high concentration. This predominant emissivity of tryptophan in polypeptide chains implied migration of energy from tyrosine to tryptophan in the molecule.

4.1.2   Energy Migration

The fact that tyrosine and phenylalanine could not be found in the luminescent state in proteins in the presence of authentic tryptophan residues convinced Teale [16] and others working with the phenomenon that this quenching was due, in the large measure, to donor-acceptor mechanisms and resonance transfer of energy between the three aromatic amino acids [17–20].

The physical principles and working formulation of the events of inductive resonance between two molecules have been worked out by Förster [21]. His theory and application of the principles involved were based on earlier work by J. Perrin and Choucroun [22] and F. Perrin

[23]. They described the transfer of energy by electrodynamical inter-action from an excited oscillator to an oscillator in resonance with it and so close that their distance was small compared with the wavelength of the vibrating electromagnetic field emitted by the excited oscillator. From these tenets, Förster derived equations which yielded the number of intermolecular transitions per second between the donor and acceptor, and more importantly, provided the basis for measurement of the critical distances between them.

Briefly, the probability of energy migration is known to be directly proportional to the square of the interaction energy. The efficiency of the migration emerges to be inversely proportional to the sixth power of the intermolecular distance. In a practical matter, the following data are needed to calculate intermolecular transitions and critical distances, (1) the life-time of the excited state of the fluorescent molecule, (2) the average of the wave numbers of the peak of the fluorescent and of the longest wavelength peak of the absorption spectrum of the fluores-cent substance and (3) the overlap integral. Figure 4.2 shows an example of these interactions displayed as plotted spectra in absorption and fluorescent modes.

It is highly probable that critical distances are of such orders in skin and its molecular substituents that energy migration occurs between

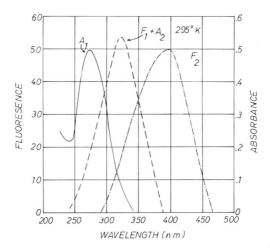

Figure 4.2. Spectral curve displays of "overlap" principles in energy migration. A_1 (————) is the absorption spectrum of the photon-acceptor; $F_1 + A_2$ (- - - -) is the fluorescence spectrum of the photon-donor which has an "overlap" integral with A_1; F_2 (-·-·-·) is the fluorescent spectrum of the photoacceptor.

such resonant molecules as tryptophan, tyrosine, and phenylalanine. Therefore, the existence of inductive resonance must be considered when critical interpretations are made of the emissivities of connective tissues. It is important then to offer a useful and practical experimental example of the mathematical means to be applied to assessment of energy migration between donors and acceptors in polypeptide chains.

The critical distance, or the last intermolecular distance at which energy migration will take place, may be calculated by the equation proposed by Karreman and Steele [24]. In our example, let us consider the resonance of transfer of energy between phenylalanine as the donor and tyrosine as the acceptor, as would be the case in most collagens where tryptophan is not an authentic residue. The following simplified formula may be used:

$$R_0 = \sqrt[6]{0.95 \times 10^{-33} \frac{\tau J\bar{\nu}}{\bar{\nu}_0^2}} \tag{1}$$

where τ is the lifetime of the lowest singlet state of the donor, phenylalanine, $(\tau = 1.1 \times 10^{-8}$ sec), $J\bar{\nu}$ is the integral of overlap of the fluorescence spectrum of the donor and the absorption spectrum of the acceptor, tyrosine $(J\bar{\nu} = 4.1 \times 10^8$ cm$^3)$, and where $\bar{\nu}_0$ is the mean wave number between the fluorescence and absorption spectra of the donor $(\bar{\nu}_0 = 37{,}100$ cm$^{-1})$. The calculation of R_0, the critical distance in Ångstrom units proceeds by substitution as follows:

$$R_0 = \sqrt[6]{0.95 \times 10^{-33} \times \left(\frac{1.1 \times 4.1}{1.38 \times 10^9}\right)}$$

$$= \sqrt[6]{\frac{4.2 \times 10^{-33}}{1.38 \times 10^9}}$$

$$= \sqrt[6]{3.02 \times 10^{-42}}$$

$$\log 3.02 \times 10^{-42} = -42.4820$$

$$-42.4820 \div 6 = -7.0803$$

$$\text{antilog } -7.0803 = 1.2 \times 10^{-7}$$

$$= 12 \times 10^{-8} \text{ cm}$$

$$R_0 = 12 \text{ Å}$$

Figure 4.3 presents the absorption spectrum of tyrosine, the fluorescence spectrum of the donor, phenylalanine, and its overlap interval with the former, and the fluorescence spectrum of the acceptor, tyrosine.

4.1.3   Classification of Proteins as Fluorophores

As noted previously, the luminescent centers in proteins are formed by the aromatic amino acids, tyrosine and tryptophan. Phenylalanine does not, apparently, contribute to emissivity [25]. On this basis, Weber [26] has divided proteins into two classes; class A containing tyrosine exclusive of tryptophan and class B possessing both residues. In the latter case, the dominant emission is because of tryptophan even when this residue is sparse compared to tyrosine. Hoerman and co-workers [27, 28] have suggested that the monomeric polypeptide chains of col-

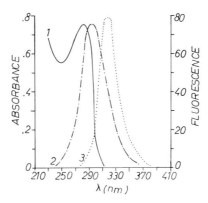

Figure 4.3.   Spectral curves showing the Förster mechanism in donor phenylalanine (curve 2, fluorescent spectrum) "overlapped" with the absorption spectrum of acceptor tyrosine (curve 1) resulting in fluorescence due to tyrosine (curve 3). Excitation was at $\lambda_{max} = 258$ nm.

lagen displayed a low-temperature luminescent spectra which qualified this fibrous protein as neither a class A nor a class B molecule. It could easily be assumed, however, that these authors were, in fact, dealing with a class A protein since the observed excitation maximum was $\lambda = 275$ nm and the emission maximum was $\lambda = 395$ nm. These data were not unlike those derived from such class A proteins as ribonuclease and insulin [29]. Additionally, the lifetime of the phosphorescent state, $\tau = 2.00$ sec, was quite near to that noted by Longworth in class A proteins [30]. Nonetheless, the possibility that collagen may constitute a third class of protein emissivity may not be totally discounted since its tyrosine content is low, 2 residues per 1000 residues, and the spacing along the polypeptide chain is unique [31]. These factors could support a case against inductive resonance between phenylalanine and tyrosine and, in turn, encourage a view toward a strict phenylalanine emissivity

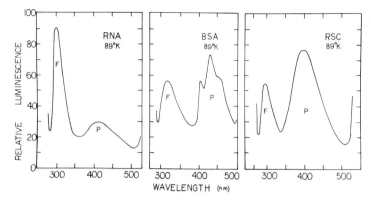

Figure 4.4.   Low-temperature total emission curves of Class A and B proteins. Fluorescence F and phosphorescence P. Emission bands and peaks are characteristic of the predominant emitting center; in Class A proteins, ribonuclease (RNA), and rat-skin collagen (RSC) the chromophore is tyrosine, and in Class B protein, bovine serum albumin (BSA) the emitting center is tryptophan, irrespective of the presence of tyrosine in the structure.

in collagen. Indeed this possibility has been set forth by Burshtein [32] who found a low-temperature emission (phosphorescence) at a maximum, $\lambda = 412$ nm, in tryptophan-free mixtures of polypeptides, collagen and gelatin.

Figure 4.4 presents for consideration the low-temperature total emission spectra for ribonuclease (class A protein), bovine serum albumin (class B protein), and rat skin collagen, α chains. It may be readily noted that the fluorescent and phosphorescent peak positions are nearly the same, but that the ratio of fluorescence total area to that of phosphorescence is markedly different, the singlet state (fluorescence) being virtually nil.

4.1.4   Other Biological Fluorophores

Skin contains, as substituents, molecules which possess potential for optical activity. Generally these molecules exhibit ring-membered structures, such as certain of the polynucleotides and biogenic amines, and have ultraviolet light absorbancies. One of the most obvious fluorophores in this category would be the ring-structured purine and pyrimidine bases of nucleic acids. However, there is some doubt that these molecules function as fluorophores in viable cells. *In vitro*, nonetheless, luminescence of the purine bases, guanine and adenine, obtains when environmental conditions are severe, for example at pH 2.0 or when supercooled

[32–36]. On the other hand, certain polynucleotides do possess emissivities. For instance, Velick [37] and Chance et al. [38] have demonstrated the authenticity of fluorescence of cellular nicotinamide adenine dinucleotide in the reduced form (NADH). The peak emission of NADH occurs at $\lambda \simeq 460$ nm after excitation at $\lambda \simeq 340$ nm and the intensity of fluorescence relates directly to the state of oxidation of the excited system [39]. It is doubtful, however, that under normal conditions NAD plays a significant role in luminescence of skin or its substituents, since the metabolic activity of epidermal strata is relatively low. Thus the absolute quantities of NADH at any point in time in normal skin would be insignificant.

Epidermis has been shown to contain the strongly ultraviolet light absorbing chemical urocanic acid. The molecule, a nonoxidative deaminated product of histidine, has been shown by Schwartz and Spier [40] to be present in skin and callus. Its ultraviolet absorption spectrum, peaking in the region from $\lambda = 260$ to 275 nm, strongly suggests a potentially fluorophoric molecule. This was not confirmed, however.

According to Adams-Ray, Bloom, and Ritzen [41] cells with autofluorescent pigment granules are common in the connective tissue of human dermis. Using a microspectrograph with fluorescence measuring capabilities, as devised by Caspersson, Lomakka, and Rigler [42], the spectrum of these autofluorescent pigments, *in situ*, displayed a maximum of emission at about $\lambda = 500$ nm, a wavelength significantly shifted to the red from the emission bands of protein or many of the polynucleotides. The intensity of emission in this pigment in connective tissue cells was low, detectable only by exquisite microfluorimetric techniques. Its origin according to Bloom and Ritzen [43] could be from one or both of melanin granules or lipo-pigments in the dermal autofluorescent (DAF) cells. Macroscopically, however, an emission of these DAF cells must be inconsequential compared to the total fluorescence of skin arising from such fluorophores as ring-membered amino acids in collagen and glycoproteins, other indole derivatives such as 5-hydroxytryptamine or the catecholamines.

With specific regard to the presence of 5-hydroxytryptamine in skin, Welsh and Zipf found levels of 5-HT in dorsal frog skin (*R. pipiens*) as high as 370 μg per gram of fresh tissue [44]. These authors related the ecology of ranids to the content of 5-HT in the dorsal skin. For example, the exclusively aquatic, *R. catesbeiana*, showed less than 0.09 μg per gram of fresh tissue as opposed to *R. pipiens*, a semiterrestrial ranid, in which 5-HT was 3 to 4 orders of magnitude greater. The question arises as to what function 5-HT possesses in skin. Water conservation was considered for a period of time then ruled out by experimentation. However, studies of Welsh and Zipf clearly pointed out that, because the accumulation of 5-HT occurred inordinately in venom glands, the role must be one of protection against predators.

It should be pointed out most clearly here that the fluorescence of 5-HT and of catecholamines in tissue sections is an induced emissivity (yellowish) obtaining after treatment with paraformaldehyde [45]. The natural fluorescence of indole derivatives usually peaks at from $\lambda = 320$–430 [46], the long-wavelength tails of which could be faintly visible to the human eye. Thus the natural fluorescence of these chemicals in skin would not contribute greatly to the visible noninduced fluorescence. Nonetheless, the fluorescent analysis of biogenic amines in tissues has provided a sensitive tool for the study of such important metabolic processes as the decrease in tissue 5-HT and catecholamines as a result of reserpine administration [47].

4.2 PRINCIPLES OF LUMINESCENCE

4.2.1 General

Fluorescence and phosphorescence are potentially the most exact analytical methods available in chemistry and biology today. Indeed their limits of precision are fixed mainly by instrumental constraints, namely, (1) attenuation and fluctuation of light sources, (2) absorptive qualities of monochromators, (3) variation in the effective solid angle viewed by the photodetector, and (4) the variation in the quantum conversion factor of the photomultiplier tube as a function of wavelength. The methods of the experimenter are eminently important. For example, the purity and/or homogeneity of specimens are firm requirements. Also of great importance are the concentration of the fluorophore, its molar extinction coefficient and the light-path length on the axis of irradiation. According to the Stark-Einstein law of photochemical equivalency, if these constraints were tacitly controlled, one could measure exactly a single quantum of energy, or photon, its precise vibrational frequency and the luminescent efficiency of the reaction in which it derived. A thorough treatment of the limitations imposed by measurement devices and sample characteristics may be obtained reading a recent article by Hercules [48] .

An extensive perusal of the current literature dealing with luminescence in chemistry and biology revealed that many attempts have been made to assess and fully compensate for instrumental inadequacies. Regrettably, there are more instances where authors have not as much as mentioned the make of photomultipliers, nor their response curve characteristics, thus making reproducing of their experiments in other laboratories impossible. Notwithstanding, there appeared to be no single instance where all affecting variables on the fluorescence and phosphorescence signals were definitively controlled or compensated.

4.2.2 Excited States

The excited state in a molecule occurs after the absorption of quanta of light and the concomitant promotion of electrons into energy bands

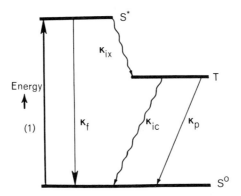

Figure 4.5. Electronic state diagram for a typical molecule. Ground state (S_o); lowest excited singlet state (S^+); lowest excited triplet state (T); absorption (1); fluorescence (κ_f); intersystem crossing, (κ_{ix}); phosphorescence (κ_p); internal conversion (triplet to ground) (κ_{ic}). [48]

above that of the ground-state level. An extended discussion of these events and the quantum mechanical principles capable of producing, in the excited state, conditions favoring fluorescence and phosphorescence is beyond the scope of this chapter. The reader is most vigorously recommended, if interested in a very comprehensive and understandable treatise on the excitation of molecules by light, to read Chapter 2 in Seliger and McElroy, *Light, Physical and Biological Action* [49]. For an understanding of luminescence and the excited state for our present purposes, look at Fig. 4.5 which is an energy diagram of a molecule in an excited state. The ground state is represented by S_0. The lowest singlet state is shown as S^*. The electron transition from S_0 to S^* is accompanied by the absorption of a photon of light, $h\nu$, and the return to S_0 may occur from S^* with the expulsion of a photon of lower energy, or fluorescence. Ground state may be reached also from the lowest triplet excited state, T^* with the expulsion of a photon of yet a lower energy level as phosphorescence. In order for this triplet-state transition to occur, it is required that the molecular environment favor it, for example when the environment of a biological macromolecule is supercooled to about liquid nitrogen temperatures. In Fig. 4.5, the κ values are rate constants for each of the processes in the excited state. Table 4.1 lists these electronic state processes and their rate constants.

The usual luminescent experiment proceeds as follows. The specimen is irradiated with monochromated light having a wavelength at which maximum photon absorption occurs. This process is always at a greater rate than any of the subsequent electronic excited state events. As

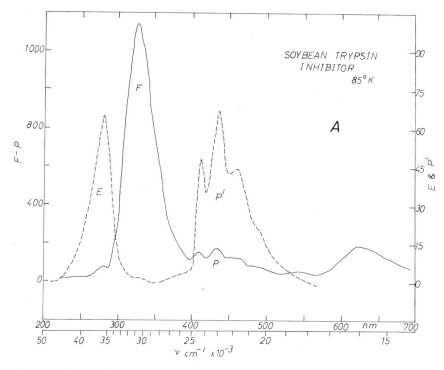

Figure 4.6. (*a*) Total emission spectra for 0.1% crystalline soybean trypsin inhibitor (*STI*) in 50% aqueous propylene glycol frozen solution, pH 7.0. Fluorescence (*F*), Phosphorescence (*P*)-(*P'*), Excitation spectra with λ_{em} = 437 nm (*E*). RCA 1P28 photomultiplier detector used. Spectra plotted on energy and wavelength bases. *STI* is a Class B protein. (*b*) Total emission spectra for crystals of *STI*. Note the exalted triplet state emission due to altered physical environment of the fluorophore.

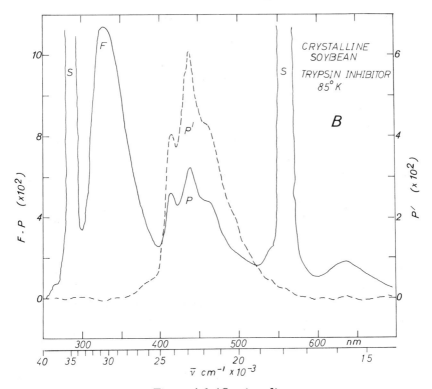

CRYSTALLINE
SOYBEAN
TRYPSIN INHIBITOR
85° K

B

Figure 4.6 (*Continued*)

shown in Fig. 4.5 and Table 4.1, the rates are related as follows: (1) Absorption $\gg \kappa_f, \kappa_{ix}, \kappa_p, \kappa_{ic}$. After about 10^{-8} sec the excited state commences a rapid deactivation provided no further excitation energy is available. The fluorescence produced during the deactivation decays in

Table 4.1   Electronic State Processes and Rates for Fluorescence and Phosphorescence

Process	Rate	Description
$S^0 + h\nu \to S^*$	1	Absorption
$S^* \to S^0 + h\nu_f$	$\kappa_f(S)^*$	Fluorescence
$S^* \to T^*$	$\kappa_{ix}(S^*)$	Intersystem crossing
$T \to S^0 + h\nu_p$	$\kappa_p(T^*)$	Phosphorescence
$T \to S^0$	$\kappa_{ic}(T^*)$	Radiationless energy loss

a fashion similar to the discharge of a condenser, that is,

$$A = A_0 e^{-\lambda t} \tag{2}$$

where A is the charge intensity and λ is the rate constant at time t. The lifetime of the excited state is $1/\lambda$, or the time at which,

$$A = A_0 e^{-1} \tag{3}$$

Because of the very short lifetimes of the singlet state, 10^{-8} sec, it is technically difficult to secure data adequate enough for calculation. Recently, the work of Weber, however, has made the measurement of fluorescent lifetimes feasible. Naturally, the lifetimes of phosphorescence, being orders of magnitude longer than the singlet-state lifetime, are easier to calculate [50].

The maximum peak or λ of the fluorescence spectrum will correspond to the lowest singlet excited state level. If the molecular environment is rigid, for example as it would be in a frozen solution at liquid nitrogen temperature ($-196°C$), the electronic excited state becomes metastable due to characteristic changes in spin and momenta of the electron. As a consequence a transition, or the intersystem crossover (κ_{ix}) occurs to the lowest triplet-state level and the transition from this energy level to ground state produces phosphorescence (κ_p). In skin, this series of quantum events may produce excited state lifetimes (triplet) of seconds up to minutes.

In summary, two modes of analysis of luminescence are available to the experimenter. The first deals with the spectral characteristics of the specimen, or the distribution of light energies in the excited state. The second mode involves the lifetime of the excited state. Figure 4.6 shows a spectral distribution in the singlet and triplet excited states of purified soybean trypsin inhibitor. Additionally, the excitation spectrum is shown. The luminescent intensities are plotted as functions of λ and vibrational frequencies showing the correspondence between the two optical energy scales. Spectra of frozen glasses and solid specimens are shown.

4.3   INSTRUMENTATION

4.3.1   General

There are several instrumental modes capable of inducing excited states in fluorophoric material [51]. However, the most usual equipment arrangement employs a 90° geometry between the light source and the detector systems, as shown in Figure 4.7.

The principal elements of a spectrofluorophotometer are the light source, the primary monochromator, the specimen compartment, the secondary monochromator, and the photomultiplier tube with an accompanying signal amplifier or processing system. There are commercially available instruments offering various combinations of these system elements including temperature ranges providing for experimentation from room to liquid nitrogen temperatures. The ultimate instrument has not been developed, however, and work in various laboratories continues to attempt to improve geometries and increase sensitivities through optimization of luminescent signals in the presence of electronic and other

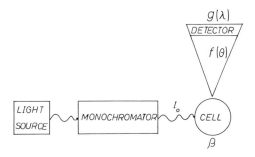

Figure 4.7.   Geometrical arrangement for luminescence measurements; $f(\theta) =$ geometry factor depending upon the effective solid angle viewed by the detector, $g(\lambda) =$ quantum conversion factor for detector, variable as a function of wavelength, $I_0 =$ intensity of exciting radiation, $a =$ molar extinction coefficient, $b =$ path length along axis of irradiation, and $c =$ concentration (moles/liter) of fluorescent material. [48]

system noise. Some of these advances will be discussed later in Section 4.3.

4.3.2   Light Sources

Generally the excitation light source for biological material must provide ultraviolet light energies. The light source and primary monochromator constitute a part of the overall system which may vary widely according to the desires of the experimenter. Currently the widest range of monochromated wavelengths with intensities at useful levels may be derived from pressurized gas lamps such as the electrically ionized xenon lamp. The wavelength distribution and relative output intensities of a typical 150-watt xenon lamp are shown in Fig. 4.8a. Other light sources are restricted to, or are especially effective in, certain intervals

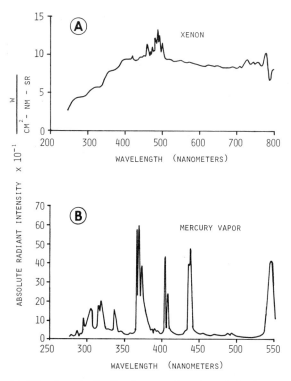

Figure 4.8. (*a*) Wavelength distribution as a function of absolute radiant intensity for a 150-W Xenon lamp. (*b*) Wavelength distributions as a function of absolute radiant intensity for a 500-W mercury vapor lamp.

of the electromagnetic spectrum. For example, the classical mercury vapor lamp provides a series of high-intensity emission bands which may provide excellent excitation sources in the ultraviolet range when the experiment specifically calls for these energies. The mercury vapor emission lines are shown in Fig. 4.8b.

Recently ionized gas and frequency divided crystal lasers have produced emission bands in the ultraviolet range. In these cases a fine advance has been accomplished in that the primary monochromator could be discarded on the basis that the laser was tunable within a desirable spectral range or that the emission lines of the gas satisfied the experiment. For example, an argon laser has been produced [52] which provides 1 watt peaks on precise emission lines at 2912.92 and 2926.24 Å. Obviously protein excitation at ~280 nm can be obtained. Also a recent attempt to lase oxygen has succeeded and a band at 298.4 Å was emitted.

In the use of high voltage lamps as light sources, that is, the xenon device, the salient operating problem lay in attenuation and fluctuation of intensity because of slight voltage changes, arc shifting, aging of the pressurized gas, and inherent absorptive characteristics of the glass envelope. These constraints obviously could have deleterious effects on final output at the photomultiplier. Actually the prime perplexity in spectroscopy today involves light sources and acquisition of an uniform energy output, especially through the ultraviolet range from a xenon lamp. To date, no single compensating system, such as feedback circuits designed to maintain constant lamp intensities [53] or corrective photon counters [54] have been absolute in producing light source homogeneity. Without doubt, the solution to the problem lay in successful development of a totally tunable laser, the ultimate light source.

4.3.3   Specimen Compartment

The presentation of biological specimens for luminescent studies has been done primarily in a 90° geometry between the source and detector with the sample in solution in a square cuvette. This mode of fluorescent analysis is not without constraints, however. According to Hercules [55] the main problems to consider are the effects of solute concentration (fluorophore), the molar extinction of the solute and the light path length along the axis of irradiation. Certain geometric considerations come into play as well as the luminescent efficiency of the fluorophore. The fluorescent or phosphorescent signal may be represented by,

$$(S)_{f,p} = f(\theta)g(\lambda)I_0\phi_{f,p}(1 - e^{-abc}) \tag{4}$$

and the definition of terms may be found in the caption of Fig. 4.7. There are two main precautions to be taken in the use of fluorescence as a quantifying tool. First, it must be assured that the relationship of concentration of the fluorophore to luminescent intensity is linear within the range of values anticipated in the experiment. Also it must be kept in mind that the nature of the linearity, in terms of concentration, is highly dependent on the extinction coefficient of the fluorophore and too that there is a strong relationship between the light path length and the luminescent intensity. These factors are demonstrated graphically in Fig. 4.9 and 4.10. In the case of light path effects, the problem develops because of a variance in fluorescence along the light path due to changes in absorbancy from the excitation face of the cell through to the center where most detectors view. In effect, the geometry of the system, factor $f(\theta)$ in Equation 4, becomes variable (see Fig. 4.7). The errors introduced by this nonuniformity of luminescent intensity along

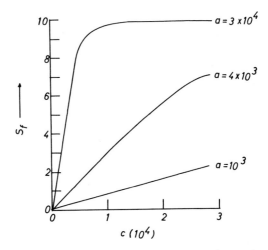

Figure 4.9. Relationship between fluorescence intensity and concentration for various values of a, assuming a 1-cm-cell path length. [48]

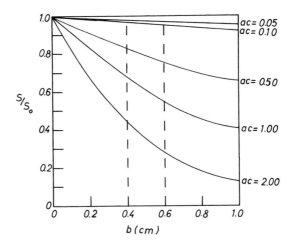

Figure 4.10. Relationship between fluorescence intensity and excitation path length. S = fluorescence intensity at b, S_o = fluorescence intensity at $b = 0$, b = path length along direction of excitation (excitation direction is from left to right), a = molar extinction, and c = concentration. Vertical dotted lines refer to estimated portion of cell seen by detector for Equation 4. [48]

the light path may be best controlled by arranging the product of the extinction coefficient and concentration of the fluorophore to be around 0.10 or less (see Fig. 4.9).

In the final analysis these constraints on luminescent measurements may be brought to a minimum by careful planning of the experiment. That is to say that the investigator who understands the limits of his instrument, with special regard to signal to noise characteristics, and knows the chemical and physical properties of the fluorophore can adjust all parameters so that precise, useful information may be obtained in the system.

Finally it should be noted that frontface or reflectance specimen presentation (solid specimens) is, in theory, free of many of the affecting variables relating to light-path length and concentration. However, in actual experiment, the problems of light scattering, unknown depth of penetration of exciting light (absorbancy), and discontinuities of concentration of fluorophore in the dispersing medium may be overwhelming and produce spurious results. Van Durren and Bardi [56] and Hoerman and Mancewicz [57] have studied luminescence derived from the frontface mode using solid specimens dispersed in potassium bromide discs. The latter authors induced the triplet-state in calcified tissues by supercooling and eliminated light scatter and fluorescence by mechanical chopping of the front-face emission. Similar studies have been performed on amino acids [58], proteins and other biological materials [59] in which the excited state distortions brought about by viewing the condensed system are rigorously discussed (see Fig. 4-6 a & b for demonstrated effects).

4.3.4 Photodetectors, Photomultipliers

Two properties of light, or the photon, make possible a direct relationship between the wave function (s) it possesses and its quantum energy. For example, when a photon strikes the photosensitive cathode of a photomultiplier, it is always absorbed as a whole quantum. Upon striking a diffraction grating, the photon behaves according to the laws of interference of continuous waves. Accordingly, the following relationship holds:

$$\frac{1 \text{ quantum}}{\text{sec}^{-1}} = \frac{1987}{\lambda \text{ (Å)}} \times 10^{-18} \text{ watt}^* \tag{6}$$

---

* The term 1987×10^{-18} is derived from the constant, hc, where h = Planck's constant, 6.624×10^{-27} erg-sec, and c = the speed of light, 3.0×10^{10} cm sec^{-1}.

From this relationship the basis for the development of instruments of great precision has been formed. Notwithstanding, one very serious limitation always arises, and that is, so far as could be determined at this writing, there is no photosensitive metal surface to be placed in a photomultiplier which responds uniformly with respect to changing wavelength. Thus, the photomultiplier must be chosen to fit the experiment, or the particular wavelength range where the emissivity is predicted to occur, and where the response curve of the photosensitive surface is flat, or at least functionally suitable and defined. Where the experiment demands spectra to be taken, there is a constant desire to correct the photodetector so that the emissivity will be a true quantum representation of the energy distribution in the fluorphore. Many techniques are available for this procedure, none of which taken alone are totally adequate. The reader is again referred to Ref. 49, if he desires to learn the details of photomultiplier function, correction and application to experiment.

4.4   LUMINESCENCE OF UNALTERED SKIN AND CONNECTIVE TISSUE

4.4.1   General

The property of fluorescence and phosphorescence of unaltered skin and other connective tissues is not precisely understood. Attempts to isolate and characterize tissue substituents which appear to be prime loci of ambient temperature fluorescence have generally led to some confusion and unrewarding results. As a consequence, little advance has been made in establishing an a priori relationship between fluorescent emissions and either health or disease of skin or other connective tissues. Nor have these electronic excited states yielded outstanding information about molecular structure in connective tissues. Undoubtedly the fact that nearly all matter interacts in some manner with radiant energy, with production of luminescence as frequent sequela, opens the distinct possibility that tissue fluorescence may be spuriously attributed to authentic substituents, like aromatic amino acids, peptide bonds, or polynucleotides, when indeed the origin may be environmental contaminants or impurities possessing relatively high quantum efficiencies. Such a condition may prevail in the case of room temperature fluorescence of skin, cartilage, bone, tooth, collagen, and elastin which betrays the usual emissivity attributable to aromatic compounds in globular proteins where the fluorescence is exclusively in the ultraviolet region of the spectrum.

4.4.2   Total Transmission of Light in Skin

The penetration of light into skin is of considerable importance, physiologically, for the conversion of 7-dehydrocholesterol into vitamin D_3. And of more dubious importance is production of sunburn erythema and its esthetic consequences—be there truly any—plus solar carcinogenesis. Some discussion has transpired regarding the location of these events in skin—exclusively epidermal thus inferring the lack of penetration of u. v. light into the dermis, cornium, and capillary blood vessels. Everett, Yeagers, Sayre, and Olson [60] have addressed themselves to this problem in a very precise and careful study. They hold that there is a physiologically significant quantity of ultraviolet light which may penetrate the epidermis into dermis. The notion that erythema in dermis layers is brought about by photoreaction material extending from the epidermis is questionable. Their contention is supported by the findings of Van der Leun [61] who noted that there is very little lateral extension of sunburn beyond areas exposed to light, as well as the pronounced basophilic degeneration of collagen associated with actinic exposure. Everett and co-workers managed to successfully separate epidermis from dermis of black and white volunteer persons and at autopsy. The precision of their work is exemplified by the fact that of the fourteen specimens collected, the mean thickness was 15 microns with little variation. The samples were mounted on quartz slides for subsequent spectral studies using a modified Cary 15 spectrophotometer. Measurements were made of the fraction of light transmitted directly through the specimen, the light scattered backwards, and the total light forward consisting of light directly transmitted plus that scattered forward. From these data the authors calculated the light actually absorbed and the total transmission. The shortcomings of the method, such as possible underestimation of total transmitted light due to 2π light scattering and the inability of the phototube to see all of this light, were accounted for. The light energy required to produce minimal preceptible erythema (MPE) was determined by administration of measured quantities of monochromated ultraviolet light (280 nm) through a section of intact epidermis onto the abdominal skin of a volunteer subject. With this system, it was found that 4.8% of the total light was transmitted and it required 12,000 μW-sec cm^{-2} to cause erythema when no epidermal filter was used. When the filter was used, 240,000 μW-sec cm^{-2} were required. Obviously, epidermal layers possess great absorptive powers. Figure 4.11 shows the total transmission spectrum of stratum corneum in which the absorbancy is depicted. Notwithstanding, it seems clear now, according to Evert and co-workers, that the significant consequences of incident ultraviolet irradiation on human skin—erythema and solar carcinogenesis—are not primary epidermal events, but that ultraviolet light does transverse the epidermis in the concentration of about 10^{15} photons cm^{-2} in the subjacent dermis. The strong absorbance of light in skin at about 280 nm (see Fig. 4.11) firmly suggests the role of protein as a protective agent and certainly attests to the fact that electronic excited states exist and luminescent sequela surely follow in terms of dissipation of absorbed energy.

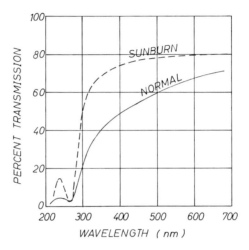

Figure 4.11. Total emission characteristics of human skin (stratum corneum) showing comparison of normal and sunburned tissue. Note the coincidence of the absorptive characteristics at $\lambda \simeq 280$ nm, but the greater transmission of sunburned stratum corneum at longer wavelengths. [60]

4.4.3   Ambient Temperature Fluorescence

Undoubtedly the most interesting and provocative issue in the study of luminescence in connective tissues is the visible ambient temperature fluorescence at $\lambda \simeq 415$ nm which, by it's apparent high efficiency and excitation maximum ($\lambda \simeq 320$ nm), denies an origin in primary protein structure. The scientific literature reaching as far back as 1911 is replete with reports dealing with this fluorescence [2]. The source of the phenomenon has been variously ascribed to a range of substances from the arcane, through lipids, nucleotides, to a recent popular source, the poly-L-tyrosine molecules. The author will attempt to synthesize the current understanding of this fluorescence in connective tissue.

It would be of no great moment to commence the synthesis earlier than 1953 when Hartles and Leaver [62] removed a visible fluorescent (bluish-white) material from dentin using alkaline alcohol for the extraction. These workers suggested that the fluorescence could be derived from pyridinium compounds in the organic matrix of the tissue. Later in 1955, these same investigators found fluorescent pyrimidine thymine in the tooth cementum of the sperm whale and suggested that nucleoproteins could contribute principally to connective tissue luminescence. The evidence presented was based on absorption data alone; fluorescent emission data lacking. We know now, however, that natural fluorescence of nuceoproteins *in vivo* is remote, unless the environmental conditions are rendered somewhat severe. Fluorescence from polynucleotides, on the other hand, must not be totally discounted as a contributor to overall emissivity from connective tissue [32–38].

Subsequently in 1962, Armstrong [63], and Mancewicz and Hoerman [64] measured the fluorescent spectra and characteristics of relatively insoluble fractions and peptides of human dentin and enamel. Both in gelatinized (autoclaved) and decalcified organic material, a fluorescent substance was found emitting a maximum at $\lambda \simeq 405$ nm with an excitation maximum at $\lambda \simeq 320$ nm. It was of interest also that Hoerman and Mancewicz were able to demonstrate fluorescent emission and absorption spectra in alkaline hydrolyzates of dentin collagen (human) which indicated the presence of approximately one authentic residue of tryptophan per mole of collagen [65]. Tyrosine emissivities were noted also while the fluorescence at $\lambda \simeq 405$ nm was absent.

At about the same time, Andersen [66] liberated, by prolonged hydrolysis, two visible fluorescent compounds from native resilin, a component of the elastic ligaments of insects. These compounds were shown to be associated with the cross-linking structures between molecules of resilin. It was striking that in native resilin, and the two isolates, a fluorescent emission maximum of 415 nm was noted. The absorption maxima of compound I and II in acid were 286 and 283 nm, respectively. In alkali, the absorption maxima shifted to the red by 36 and 34 nm. The excitation spectra in alkaline solution revealed maxima for compound I at 254 and 325 nm and for compound II at 254 and 315 nm. These compounds were later isolated by Andersen in highly pure form [67] and it was quite clear that both were aromatic amino acids containing phenolic groups. There was no indole configuration present and tests for diphenols were negative. A biphenyl linkage was found, however. Thus it was concluded the compounds were essentially dityrosines with biphenyl linkages. Lehrer and Fasman [68] provided considerable evidence for the authenticity of this visible fluorescent molecule. They observed the same blue fluorescence as that noted by Andersen in compounds isolated from resilin when poly-L-tyrosine, copolymers of tyrosine and L-tyrosine monomers were irradiated with ultraviolet light at 280 and 295 nm. These investigators are to be complimented for their careful use of spectrophotofluorometric equipment. The interested reader should heed the precision and care given to the accurate collection of data going into the confirmation and identification of a bityrosine photoproduct having properties similar to those found naturally in resilin. It seems most probable that a fluorescence at $\lambda_{max} = 405$ nm with excitation at $\lambda \simeq 320$ nm found in biological material, especially connective tissues, must be carefully analyzed for a possible origin in structures of the following form:

Bityrosine

One slight dichotomy remains for discussion here. It is known that irradiation of tyrosine in air at room temperature results in the formation of dihydroxyphenylalanine (DOPA) [69]. Leherer and Fasman did not, apparently, take this possibility into account in all experimental cases. Vladimirov and co-workers [70] did consider this possible photoproduct (DOPA) in similar experiments aimed at learning something of the effects of low temperature (77°K) on photoproduct formation. In matter of fact, DOPA does not absorb at 313 nm, where Vladimirov was exciting specimens, and these authors attributed the observed fluorescence at 400 nm to formation of tyrosine dimers similar to those formed upon ultraviolet irradiation of phenol [71]. Thus the photoproduct, bityrosine, does seem authentic, but the question remains to be answered; how could the photoproduct be formed *in situ* during the synthesis of such structures as the cross-link of resilin when the likelihood of irradiation of magnitude great enough to bring about formation is virtually nil?

LaBella and co-investigators have attempted to provide some explanations through studies on the formation of insoluble gels and dityrosine by the action of peroxidase on soluble collagens [72]. The enzyme peroxidase has been shown capable of producing dityrosine from free tyrosine and in a few isolated cases from protein substrates [73, 74]. LaBella sets forth the proposition that dityrosine formation through the action of ubiquitous peroxidases may represent one type of cross-linking process concerned with polymerization and maturation of collagen. His data to support that idea are based solely on fluorescent emissivity of isolates from the chromatographic separation of acid hydrolyzates of peroxidase treated and untreated rat skin collagen. The fluorescent experimental data supporting the contention that dityrosine is naturally present in acid or neutral salt extracted rat skin collagen were not convincing since the fluorescent intensities at $\lambda \simeq 410$ nm were very weak and in some instances not present at all. Additionally, in the peroxidase-treated collagens, and in the dityrosine control chromatogram, no positive ninhydrin reactions occurred corresponding to fluorescent peaks. Also, these authors recognized that their data could be artifactual and in some cases dependent upon values well within the experimental error of the methods. In all likelihood the role of dityrosine in formation of collagen cross-links remains obscure. With further regard to the intramolecular cross-linkage in rat skin collagen, Bornstein and Piez et al. [75, 76] appear to have identified an authentic cross-link structure in the monomeric polypeptide chains of collagen. Through cleavage of $\alpha1$ and $\alpha2$ chains with cyanogen bromide, it was shown that a lysyl residue in each chain was converted to the δ-semialdehyde of α-aminoadipic acid in peptide linkage, thus setting the chemical stage for aldol-type condensations of aldehydes on adjacent chains. Piez, Martin, Kang, and Bornstein [77] have presented strong evidence to directly support this idea. These investigators have shown that chromatographic heterogeneity of $\alpha1$ chains exists and is due to a lysyl residue, $\alpha1^{Lys}$, in one species and an aldehyde residue, $\alpha2^{Ald}$, in the other. The same species of residues were found in $\alpha2$ chains. The essential factor in bringing about the aldol-type condensation and formation of the lysine to aldehyde conversion—and the cross-linkage— was not identified, a catalyst. Siegel and Martin [78] have provided that precise information. These investigators have extracted an enzyme, lysyl oxidase, from embryonic chick cartilage. The enzyme was responsible for the production of cross-linked collagen and the lysine-derived cross-link precursor allysine (α aminoadipic-δ-semialdehyde). Additionally, the location was found on the α chains where the first step in cross-linking occurs. It was residue 9, the site of action of lysyl oxidase.

4.4.4 Low-Temperature Luminescence

Hoerman, Balekjian and Boyne [79] had investigated the low-temperature luminescence of collagen and its substituents as provided by Piez and co-workers. The total emission spectra as well as spectra of

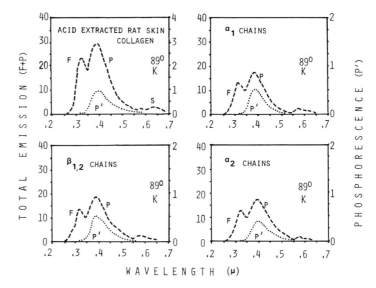

Figure 4.12. Low-temperature (89°K) total emission spectra of rat-skin collagen and its subunits: (———) total emission, F (fluorescence), P (phosphorescence) and P' (phosphorescence alone). $\lambda_{\max}$ excitation = 277 nm. Emissivity is due to authentic tyrosyl residues in polypeptide chains.

phosphorescence alone are shown in Fig. 4.12. Studies were conducted on acid extracted rat skin collagen, $\beta12$, $\alpha1$, and $\alpha2$ purified chains. None of the emission spectra taken at 89°K showed the presence of fluorescence at $\lambda \simeq 405$ nm. Rather the emission spectral contours and peaks were consistent with tyrosine (free) emissions or a class A protein. Excitation was accomplished at $\lambda_{\max} = 277$ nm. Excitation at 320 nm did not give rise to fluorescence at $\lambda_{\max} \simeq 405$ nm. Thus it was apparent that dityrosine compounds, similar to those identified in resilin, were not present in rat skin collagen and that this finding was consistent with the fact that the cross-link between molecules was not formed by a luminescent substance. The presence of an excited triplet-state in collagen was of interest. The data presented by Hoerman, Balekjian, and Boyne [79], and shown here in Table 4.2, revealed mean lifetimes of the triplet of about 2.00 sec in all collagen preparations. This value was consistent with a tyrosine emitting center. It was of further interest to note that the transition from singlet to triplet states (κ_{ix}) in collagen was of high efficiency as delineated by F/P ratios of less than 1.00. This fact renders the study of luminescence at low temperatures very attractive since the authentic emissivity is efficient, relatively, and the contaminating

Table 4.2   Phosphorescence spectral maxima and
lifetimes at 89°Kelvin for aromatic amino acids,
rat skin collagen and its molecular subunits

Specimen	λ Maximum (nm) Excitation	Emission	Phosphorescent Life-time (τ)* (sec)
Rat skin collagen	277	395	2.1
β12 chains	277	395	1.8
α1 chains	277	395	2.2
α2 chains	277	395	2.4
Tyrosine†	277	404	1.7
Tryptophan	292	436	4.8

* Derived from $P = P_o e^{-at}$, where $a = \tau^{-1}$
† Data obtained in 50% ethelyene glycol, pH 7.4

light scatter and fluorescence (low efficiency) may be mechanically chopped out. In this case the phosphorescence becomes somewhat more reliable for critical study of structural status.

Using low-temperature luminescence (phosphorescence alone) of monkey cartilage and bone, Hoerman, Balekjian, and Boyne [79] were able to resolve, both spectrally and in terms of lifetimes of excited triplet-states, collagen emissivity from that of globular proteins in tissue slices. The combined spectra of phosphorescence arising from the tyrosine center in collagen (class A protein) and globular protein—glycoprotein—(class B protein) with a triplet-state emissivity owing to tryptophan are shown in Fig. 4.13. Employing these methods, these investigators noted that collagen phosphorescence in cartilage remained constant with respect to intensity, as a function of age of the monkey, while globular protein intensities diminished markedly, especially after age 11 years (corresponding to human age $\simeq$ 45 years). Additionally, it was noted that bone phosphorescence arose from the same centers as that in cartilage and that newly established bone, 35 days after transplantation in defect sites, was not typical, showing instead of the normal combined spectrum, one which was predominantly owing to globular protein material. After 95 days of regeneration, the transplanted bone returned to normal emissivity. The proposition set forth appears quite tenable, to wit: that luminescent changes in connective tissue, at least bone and cartilage of monkeys due to advancing age, are detectable as decreased phosphorescent intensities arising from other than collagen structures. That the observed changes are due to diminished quantities of globular protein in cartilage and bone, as a function of age, may be supported by the observation of Eastoe that chrondroitin sulfate levels in older age groups are lowered [80]. The risk in this line of reasoning lies in the fact that contaminating substances in the tissues accumulating with age could act as quenchers of the triplet state. There was some evidence to support such an idea [79].

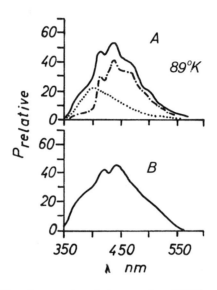

Figure 4.13. (*a*) Phosphorescent emission spectra (89°K) of rat-skin collagen: (··········) and human glycoprotein (-·-·-·) showing additive result (————). (*b*) Phosphorescent emission spectrum of cartilage from the ear tragus of a 6-month-old monkey. Note similarity between the combine spectra in A and the emissivity in B. Excitation at λ = 277 nm.

Using similar methods, Hoerman and Hughes [81] studied the total emission characteristics of sliced rat tail skin, and tendon in a series of five litter mates, and submitted to experiment the skin and tendon dissected at the tenth tail joint and exhaustively washed in Ringers solution. An example of the differences noted in the two connective tissues, with special regard to the relative detectable quantities of collagen and globular protein in each, is depicted in Fig. 4.14. Before discussion of the Figure, the reader is asked to note Fig. 4.15, in which is shown, diagrammatically, the interface of fibrous and globular protein in tendon. It is the selective singlet and triplet state emissivities of these two tissues which

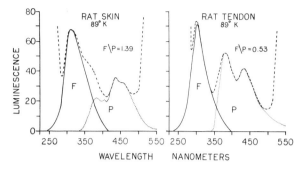

Figure 4.14. Low-temperature total emission spectra of tissue slices of rat-tail skin and tendon: (-----) total emission; (———) fluorescence; (······) phosphorescence. Sepctral contour and F/P differences due to relative concentration of collagen and globular protein. Excitation maximum at $\lambda = 277$ nm.

form the basis of the spectral presentations in Fig. 4.14. Additionally, these data allow some observations to be made concerning the existence of a dityrosine cross-linkage in collagen of rat skin and tendon. The data shown in Fig. 4.14 were collected using an excitation maximum of 277 nm. This irradiation favored the phosphorescence of collagen, the excitation maximum for globular protein emissions being at 288 nm. In the case of rat tail tendon, if one assumes an authentic dityrosine cross-link with absorption maxima, and corresponding excitation

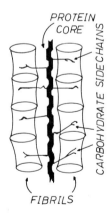

Figure 4.15. Drawing of the two-component protein system occurring in tendon. Each component, collagen and glycoprotein, functions independently with respect to interaction with radiant energy. See Fig. 4.14 for low-temperature emission spectra.

maxima, at $\lambda \simeq 254$ and 315 nm and fluorescence peaking at $\lambda \simeq 405$ nm, then the Förster mechanism must come into play. That is, energy migration must occur when the fluorescence spectrum of the energy donor, in this case authentic tyrosyl residues in tendon collagen, overlaps the absorption spectrum of the energy acceptor, in this case dityrosine covalently linked to the collagen polypeptide chain. Referring again to Fig. 4.14, it was noted that the fluorescent emission maximum in rat tail tendon occurred at $\lambda \simeq 310$ nm (tyrosine). This energy most certainly overlapped the absorption spectrum of dityrosine, if present within critical distances, and the result would be a dominant fluorescence at $\lambda \simeq 405$ nm. Quite obviously this situation did not obtain. The conclusion reached is that the data do not tacitly rule out the presence of a substance in connective tissues which possesses a fluorescence similar to that of dityrosine, only that the fluorophore, whatever it may be, is independent of the physiology of development and maturation of collagen. It is gratifying to note that in the case of resilin, the tenets of the Förster mechanism held, that is, irrespective of the excitation wavelength, the fluorescence of the molecule (compound I and II or native material) always appeared to be due to dityrosine, even though other authentic fluorophores occurred in the tissues.

4.4.5   Isolation of the $\lambda_{max} \simeq 405$ nm Fluorophore

Among the various attempts to isolate the visible fluorophore in connective tissues, excluding resilin, the work of Armstrong and Horsley [82] seems nearest success. Using a Sephadex ion-exchange column, these investigators separated a fluorescent material from alkaline hydrolyzates of bone (oxen), human dentin, and gelatin. The substance displayed ultraviolet absorption spectra with maxima at 264 and 325 nm. The fluorescent excitation maximum was at 330 nm and the emission peaked at 400 nm. These optical characteristics were identical to those derived from native and solubilized dentin and bone [63, 64]. Armstrong and Horsley postulated from their data that the fluorescent material was not intrinsic to the collagen structure but rather was a substance bound to matrix, being separable by alkaline hydrolysis as per their methods. They roughly estimated a molecular weight of 700 or less. These findings are not in controversy with the existence of a nonfluorescent intra- and intermolecular cross-link as delineated by Piez et al. [77, 78] and as revealed by Hoerman and Balekjian [79, 81]. It is unlikely too that these data support the contention of LaBella [72] that dityrosine could form as an intrinsic portion of the collagen molecule to make up the cross-link. Undoubtedly a fluorescent component of connective tissue exists which is not like the cross-link of resilin but, coincidentally, possesses very similar optical properties. The important matter is whether this luminescent material has any physiological importance such as the new enzyme, lysyl oxidase, isolated and characterized by Siegel and Martin [78].

4.4.6   Elastin and Aging

According to Partridge [83] elastin is essentially a cross-linked gel. And analysis of the stress and strain curves and other physical properties of moist elastin shows it to be composed of random coils which are kinetically free throughout the greater part of their length but are cross-linked by firm chemical bonds. This kind of structure is ideally suited for the walls of arteries and veins, and occurs almost uniformly to some degree in all connective tissues, with the possible exception of densely calcified tissues. Partridge, Elsden, and Thomas [84] have identified and characterized the cross-link in elastin. It emerges to be a pyridinium ring formed by the condensation of four lysine residues. The molecule of elastin is composed of ten lysine residues which are arranged on the outside of two polypeptide chains. Eight of these would condense with adjacent lysine pairs on the neighboring molecules. This then, according to Partridge [83] would bring about a functional structure in which each globular molecule is combined with its neighbor at four points directed toward the corners of a tetrahedron. The cross-link is synthesized, *in situ*, with great dependence upon copper [85]. Recently, an intermediate, tropoelastin has been identified [86]. Partridge and co-workers have called the cross-link desmosine (isodesmosine) and have not found the structure in any other biological material other than elastin.

LaBella, Keeley, Vivian, and Thornhill [87] using tyrosine-C^{14} have presented evidence of conversion of tyrosine into dityrosine in chick aortic elastin. The dityrosine was located and assessed using fluorescence at 405 nm and by chromatographic characteristics. Since the authentic cross-link in elastin, desmosine, has been precisely identified, it would seem presumptive to ascribe the cross-link in elastin to the same structures—di- and trityrosine—as found in resilin. Notwithstanding, Blomfield and Farrar [88] have suggested, on the basis of fluorescence and excitation peak shifts, that human pulmonary artery changes with advancing age could be accounted for by increasing cross-linking as in the conversion of dityrosine to polytyrosines. A far more attractive explanation of the fluorescence of elastin (405 nm) is presented by LaBella et al. [89] in which the proposition is set forth that the desmosines are fixed in concentration at about age 11 and that it is the accumulation of oxidized derivatives of constituent aromatic acid residues which account for the visible fluorescence. This idea may be harmonized with the yet unanswered question of whether these visibly fluorescent substances in connective tissues are physiologically important. As best as could be determined in this review, this question remains unanswered. The fluorophore, $\lambda_{max} \simeq 405$ nm, is there awaiting precise identification following isolation directly from the tissue providing the emissivity.

REFERENCES

1. Smithsonian Physical Tables, Table 808, 1959.
2. P. Stübel *Arch. Ges. Physiol.,* **1,** 142 (1911).
3. P. Nels, *Pflügers Arch.,* **219,** 738 (1928).
4. H. Pringsheim and O. Gerngrass, *Ber. Deutsch. Chem. Ges.,* **61,** 2009 (1928).
5. A. C. Giese and P. A. Leighton, *J. Gen. Physiol.,* **18,** 557 (1935).
6. W. G. Leighton and P. A. Leighton, *Can. J. Chem.,* **12,** 139 (1935).
7. S. Hoshijima, *Sci. Papers Inst. Phys. Chem. Res. (Tokyo),* **20,** 109 (1933).
8. H. W. Leverenz, *An Introduction of Luminescence of Solids,* Wiley, New York, 1950.
9. W. Reeder and V. E. Nelson, *Proc. Soc. Exp. Biol. Med.,* **45,** 792 (1940).
10. P. Debye and I. O. Edwards, *Science,* **116,** 143 (1952).
11. D. Duggan and S. Undenfriend, *J. Biol. Chem.,* **223,** 313 (1956).
12. F. W. J. Teale and G. Weber, *Biochem. J.,* **68,** 476 (1957).
13. S. V. Konev, *Dokl. Akad. Nauk SSSR,* **116,** 594 (1951).
14. R. H. Steele and A. Szent-Györgi, *Proc. Nat. Acad. Sci.,* **43,** 477 (1957).
15. F. W. J. Teale, *Biochem. J.,* **76,** 381 (1960).
16. G. Weber, *Biochem. J.,* **73,** 335 (1960).
17. S. V. Konev and M. A. Katibnikov, *Biofizika,* **6,** 638 (1961).
18. L. Stryer, *Radiation Res. Suppl.,* **2,** 432 (1960).
19. Yu A. Vladimirov, *Dokl. Akad. Nauk SSSR,* **136,** 960 (1961).
20. F. W. J. Teale, *Photoelec. Spectrometry Group Bull.,* **13,** 346 (1961).
21. Th. Förster, *Discussions Faraday Soc.,* **27,** 7 (1959).
22. J. Perrin and F. Choucroun, *Compt. Rend. Acad. Sci.,* **189,** 1213 (1929).
23. F. Perrin, *Ann. Chim. Phys.,* **17,** 283 (1932).
24. G. Karreman, R. H. Steele, and A. Szent-Györgyi, *Proc. Nat. Acad. Sci., U.S.,* **44,** 140 (1958).
25. R. H. Steele and A. Szent-Györgyi, *Proc. Nat. Acad. Sci.,* **44,** 540 (1958).
26. G. Weber, in *Light and Life* (W. McElroy and B. Glass, Eds.), John Hopkins Press, Baltimore, 1960, p. 82.
27. K. C. Hoerman and A. Y. Balekjian, *Fed. Proc.,* **25,** 1016 (1966).

28. K. C. Hoerman, S. A. Manceiwiez, and A. Y. Bakekjian, *J. Dent. Res.,* **45,** 216 (1966).

29. S. V. Konev, in *Fluorescence and Phosphorescence of Proteins and Nucleic Acids,* Plenum Press, New York, 1967, p. 100.

30. J. N. Longworth, *Biochem. J.,* **81,** 23P (1961).

31. P. Bornstein, A. H. Kang, and K. A. Piez, *Biochemistry,* **5,** 3803 (1966).

32. E. A. Burshtein, *Disertation: Functional States of Proteins,* Moscow, 1964.

33. D. Duggan, R. Bowman, B. B. Brodie, and S. Udenfriend, *Arch. Biochem. Biophys.,* **68,** 1 (1957).

34. J. W. Longworth, *Biochem. J.,* **84,** 104P (1962).

35. R. Bersohn and I. Isenberg, *J. Chem. Phys.,* **40,** 3175 (1964).

36. P. Dauzou, J. C. Fraucq, M. Hauss, and M. Ptak, *J. Chim. Phys.,* **58,** 926 (1961).

37. S. F. Velick, in *Light and Life* (W. McElroy and B. Glass, Eds.), Johns Hopkins Press, Baltimore, 1960.

38. B. Chance, P. Cohen, F. Jobsis and B. Schoener, *Science,* **137,** 499 (1962).

39. E. E. Harrison and B. Chance, *Appl. Microbiol.,* **19,** 446 (1970).

40. E. Schwarz and H. W. Spier, *J. Invest. Derm.,* **45,** 319 (1965)

41. J. Adams-Ray, G. Bloom, and E. M. Ritzen, *Acta Morphol. Neerl.-Scand.,* **3,** 131 (1960).

42. T. Casperson, G. Lomakka, and R. Rigler, Jr., *Acta Histochem. Suppl.,* 6 (1965).

43. G. Bloom and E. M. Ritzen, *Z. Zellforschung,* **67,** 319 (1965).

44. J. H. Welsh and J. B. Zipf, *J. Cell. Physiol,* **68,** 25 (1966).

45. B. Falck, N. A. Hillarp, G. Thieme, and A. Torp, *J. Histochem. Cytochem.,* **10,** 348 (1962).

46. H. Sprince, G. R. Rowley, and D. Jameson, *Science,* **125,** 442 (1956).

47. L. S. Van Orden, III, I. Vugman, K. G. Bensch, and N. J. Giarman, *J. Pharm. Exp. Ther.,* **158,** 195 (1967).

48. D. M. Hercules, *Anal. Chem.,* **39,** 29A (1966).

49. H. H. Seliger and W. D. McElroy, in *Light: Physical and Biological Action,* Academic Press, New York, 1965.

50. G. Weber, *Biophys. J.,* **9,** A-23 (1969).

51. D. M. Hercules (ed.), *Fluorescence and Phosphorescence Analysis,* Interscience, New York, 1966.

52. P. K. Cheo and H. L. Cooper, *J. Appl. Phys.,* **36,** 1862 (1965).

53. C. A. Parker, *Nature,* **182,** 1002 (1958).

54. J. D. S. Hamilton, *J. Sci. Instrum.,* **43,** 49 (1966).

55. D. M. Hercules (ed.), *idem.,* chap. 1.

56. B. L. Van Duuren and C. E. Bardi, *Anal. Chem.,* **35,** 2198 (1963).

57. K. C. Hoerman and S. A. Mancewicz, *Arch. Oral Biol.,* **9,** 517 (1964).

58. Y. A. Vladimirov, *Izvest Akad. Nauk. SSSR,* **23,** 86 (1959).

59. J. Nag-Chaudhuri and L. Augenstein, *Biopolymers,* Symposium No. 1, 441 (1964).

60. M. A. Everett, E. Yeagers, R. M. Layre, and R. L. Olson, *Photochem. Photobiol.,* **5,** 533 (1966).

61. J. C. Vander Leun, *Photochem. Photobiol.,* **4,** 447 (1965).

62. R. L. Hartles and A. G. Leaver, *Biochem. J.,* **54,** 632 (1953).

63. W. G. Armstrong, *Arch. Oral Biol.,* **5,** 115 (1961).

64. S. A. Mancewicz and K. C. Hoerman, *Arch. Oral Biol.,* **9,** 535 (1964).

65. K. C. Hoerman and S. A. Mancewicz, *J. Dent. Res.,* **40,** 1293 (1964).

66. S. O. Andersen, *Biochem. Biophys. Acta,* **69,** 249 (1963).

67. S. O. Andersen, *Acta Physiol. Scand. 66,* Suppl., 263 (1966).

68. S. S. Lehrer and G. G. Fasman, *Biochemistry,* **6,** 757 (1967).

69. L. E. Arnow, *J. Biol. Chem.,* **120,** 151 (1937).

70. Y. A. Vladimirov, *Biofizika,* **11,** 237 (1966).

71. E. V. Land and G. Porter, *Trans. Faraday Soc.,* **59,** 2016 (1963).

72. F. S. La Bella, W. Prabhaker, and C. Queen, *Biochem. Biophys. Res. Commun.,* **30,** 333 (1968).

73. A. J. Gross and I. W. Sizer, *J. Biol. Chem.,* **234,** 1611 (1959).

74. S. O. Andersen, *Biochem. Biophys. Acta,* **93,** 213 (1964).

75. P. Bornstein, A. H. Kang, and K. A. Piez, *Proc. Natl. Acad. Sci., U.S.,* **55,** 417 (1966).

76. P. Bornstein, A. H. Kang, and K. A. Piez, *Biochemistry,* **5,** 3803 (1966).

77. K. A. Piez, G. R. Martin, A. H. Kang, and P. Bornstein, *Biochemistry,* **5,** 3813 (1966).

78. R. C. Siegel and G. R. Martin, *J. Biol. Chem.,* **245,** 1653 (1970).

79. K. C. Hoerman, A. Y. Balekjian, and P. J. Boyne, *J. Dent. Res.,* **48,** 661 (1969).

80. J. E. Eastoe, in *Biochemists Handbook, Chemical Composition of Bone Teeth and Cartilage* (Cyril Long, ed.), Von Nostrand, Princeton, N.J., p. 715, (1961).

81. K. C. Hoerman and F. L. Hughes, *Biophysical J.,* **9,** A-273 (1969).

82. W. G. Armstrong and H. J. Harsley, *Nature,* **211,** 981 (1966).

83. S. M. Partridge, *Fed. Proc.,* **25,** 1023 (1966).

84. S. M. Partridge, D. F. Elsden, and J. Thomas, *Nature,* **197,** 1297 (1963).

85. L. B. Sandberg, N. Weissman, and D. W. Smith, *Biochemistry,* **8,** 2940 (1969).

86. E. J. Miller, G. R. Martin, C. E. Mecca, and K. A. Piez, *J. Biol. Chem.,* **240,** 3623 (1965).

87. F. S. La Bella, F. Keeley, S. Vivian, and D. Thornhill, *Biochem. Biophys. Res. Commun.,* **26,** 748 (1967).

88. J. Blomfield and J. F. Farrar, *Biochem. Biophys. Res. Commun.,* **28,** 346 (1967).

89. F. S. La Bella, S. Vivian, and D. P. Thornhill, *J. Gerontol.,* **21,** 550 (1966).

5

The Structure of Elastin Fibers

DAVID A. HALL

Department of Medicine, University of Leeds, England

Knowledge of the structure, chemistry, and function of the elastic fiber has developed considerably since the present author commenced work in this field in 1951 [1]. A number of excellent review articles [2–8] have been written dealing with elastin and the pancreatic and bacterial enzymes which attack it. Because of these it will not be necessary to consider, at length, the earlier work in this field, and emphasis will be placed on recent observations from which it may soon be possible

187

to explain, on a biochemical basis, the physical properties reported fully in Chapter 6.

One of the difficulties in writing a chapter on elastic fibers for inclusion in a book dealing with skin is the fact that only a small proportion of the research carried out on elastic tissue has been based on material derived from this source. The reason for this will become apparent as this chapter proceeds; suffice it to say at this stage that it will be necessary to refer repeatedly to work which has been carried out on elastic tissues from ligamentum nuchae, aorta, and lung in addition to that from skin in order that an overall picture may be obtained.

5.1   ELASTIC FIBERS AND LAMELLAE

5.1.1   Gross Structure

Elastic fibers can be observed in a variety of tissues of the human and animal body where they appear as yellow wavy elements intermeshed with collagen bundles. Such fibers are, however, not the only elastica staining elements in the body, elastica staining sheets being apparent in the large arteries and ribbonlike fibers of considerably greater thickness occurring in the ligaments. In these ligaments and more especially in the nuchal ligaments of grazing animals, where up to 80% of the fibrous material consists of elastin, the fibers are broad and lie parallel to one another. If this tissue is teased out, it can be seen that even these structures branch and anastomose with one another. The lamella structures which lie as concentric cylinders around the lumen of the large blood vessels have fibrillar appendages protruding from their inner and outer surfaces. These cross the spaces between adjacent lamellae interweaving among the collagen bundles which lie between them [4]. The lung demonstrates a truly isotropic three-dimensional structure consisting of a network on fine fibers [9], whereas the skin presents a mixture of these various forms [10]. Fibrils are condensed into flattened bands deep in the corium whereas free and fibrillar elements exist in the papillary layer. Elements from the deeper ribbons and the upper fibrillar network are interconnected to form a three-dimensional network which enmeshes the collagen bundles. Except where the fibers are cut during the preparation of a section for examination, there is no evidence that they have free ends, and they appear to anastomose with one another throughout the whole depth of the dermis.

In early papers on elastic tissue, the elastic fibers are referred to as yellow connective tissue fibers, and in unstained tissue they are recognizable by this appearance. When examined by polarized light, elastic fibers only demonstrate a slight degree of birefringence in the unstretched state being easily distinguishable in this respect from collagen fibers which are very anisotropic. However, when stretched, they assume a high degree of anisotropy which can be further enhanced by immersing the fibers in toluene [11].

Estimates of the amount of elastin present in a tissue based solely on visual appraisal may provide completely erroneous results. In the dermis, especially where the elastic fibers are arranged in a rather sparse three-dimensional network in between the collagen bundles, it is possible to cut sections which dissect the majority of elastic fibers either at right angles to their length or mainly in a longitudinal direction (Fig. 5.1 and 5.2). The former presents a situation in which it is extremely difficult to assess the elastin quantitatively in view of the relatively small areas of the cross-sections of the fibers, whereas the latter may, in contrast, induce an overestimation of the amount of elastin present.

Chemical analysis of the amount of elastin present in the skin may be equally ambiguous, since the values obtained depend to such a marked

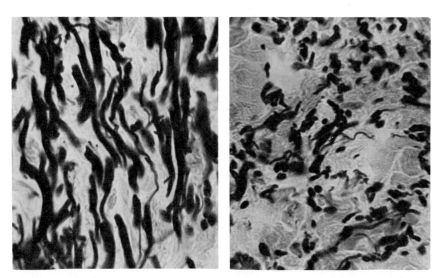

Figures 5.1 and 5.2. Difficulties in the assessment of elastin content in the dermis by visual appraisal of stained sections. Both sections were from the same block but were cut from planes at right angles to one another; otherwise staining and magnification are identical.

extent on the method employed for its estimation. A comparison of the various methods of analysis has been made in a number of earlier reviews [5, 8, 12]. At the present time four main methods are in general use, differing from one another in the way in which the extraneous protein is cleared from the preparation [12–17]. Once a relatively pure preparation of elastin is obtained it is possible to make a quantitative estimation of the amount of elastin present either gravimetrically [18] or following the dissolution of the elastin by elastase using one of the methods devised to study the elastolytic process [19, 20].

Partridge and his group [14] advocate the use of neutral extraction carried out by autoclaving with distilled water, whereas other workers have suggested the use of boiling dilute alkali [15, 18] or autoclaving with dilute acetic acid [13]. The acid extraction of collagen is complete, but this method does not remove as large a proportion of the associated polysaccharide as the neutral method. It is still not clear whether this polysaccharide represents the remains of the ground substance [21] which it is not possible to remove from the elastin under acid conditions or whether on the other hand it is a true component of the physiological entity, which suffers a small but finite degree of degradation during purification with hot water at neutral pH. Alkaline treatment is recognized as providing the most likely method for the production of a perfectly pure protein preparation [15, 22], but it has been shown [23, 24] that prolonged treatment with boiling alkali can result in the total solution of an elastin preparation. It is therefore quite possible that even the limited period of treatment used for the removal of the associated collagen and ground substance will be adequate to initiate a small amount of degradation. Loeven [25] has demonstrated marked differences in the relative degrees of susceptibility of acid and alkali treated elastin preparations to attack by elastase.

Recently more gentle methods of purification have been described [16, 17] in which the collagen is removed by treatment with collagenase at pH values close to neutrality, and the ground substance is removed by prolonged extraction with neutral salt solutions. An appreciable amount of material is left behind after this type of treatment; more polysaccharide and in certain instances, especially in the case of foetal tissue and that from "middle-aged" subjects, more nonelastin, noncollageneous protein (see below).

Normal human knee skin [26] has 3.1% elastin expressed in terms of the dry weight of tissue after purification with alkali, and similar values have also been obtained for neck and abdomen skin [27]. Thus it is possible that there may be a uniform proportion of elastin in all nonexposed skin areas of the body.

Exposed areas of skin apparently show markedly increased concentrations of elastin when studied by histological methods [28–30] and this is apparent whatever the angle from which the observation is made. It will be demonstrated in a Section 5.2.3 that this is most probably due to the simultaneous existence in these sites of another protein, the so-called pseudoelastin [31], which among its other properties differs from true elastin in being soluble in alkali. It is not therefore estimated together with the elastin when alkali is employed for purification, but may be so to a greater or lesser extent, if one or other of the methods of purification is employed [22].

5.1.2   Histological Characteristics of Elastic Tissue

Apart from their differences in gross structure by which it is often possible to distinguish between collagen and elastin, these two components of connective tissue also differ quite markedly in their staining properties. It is therefore relatively easy to differentiate between them when they are present in their normal undegraded state. The two principal stains for elastic tissue are Unna's acid orcein [32], and Weigart's resorcinol-fushin in one or other of its many variations [33, 34]. It would appear likely that the actual mode of attachment of these two types of dye, both based as they are on the presence of a phenolic group, is dependent on the availability of sites for hydrogen bonding along the backbone of the molecule [35]. However, the selectivity of these stains for elastin as opposed to collagen would appear to be associated with the differing numbers of basic and acidic residues which are present in the two proteins. As is shown in a later section elastin differs in its amino acid analysis from collagen in being relatively devoid of basic and acidic amino acids and hence is not able to take up acidic or basic dyes to any marked extent. Nor, however, is there any marked repulsion of the phenolic dyes. The presence of such groups in the collagen molecules on the other hand prevents the uptake of dyes such as orcein and resorcinol-fuchsin. That this is in fact the case has been demonstrated by blocking carboxyl groups by esterification [36] when collagen can be shown to take up elastica stains as easily as elastin. The opposite would also appear to be true since it has been shown [37] that partially degraded elastin after short periods of treatment with elastase, although retaining its structure, is completely devoid of staining ability. During the early stages of elastolysis [14, 38] new α-amino and α-carboxyl groups are liberated thus creating a charge pattern which in many ways resembles that appertaining in collagen.

A number of other stains can be used to identify elastin, but these are in the main less specific than those based on phenols. For instance Mallory's aniline blue stain [39] stains collagen blue and elastin red, and a similar differentiation occurs under ideal conditions with Masson's trichrome stain [40]. However, the slightest degree of pathological degeneration results in less clearly defined staining of the two proteins. Verhoeff's haematoxylin [41], Nile Blue sulphate, basic fuchsin, osmic acid, and Sudan Black [42] all attach themselves to elastin, as does the specific stain for reducing structures, the McManus periodic acid-Schiff reagent, although their reaction appears in many instances to be restricted to the periphery of the fiber and may be due to closely associated components of the ground substance rather than to integral components of the elastic fiber itself.

Gillman [43] examined a number of elastica stains as a means of differentiating not only collagen and elastin but also the normal and degenerate forms of these two proteins. This had first been accomplished by Unna [44] who coined the terms collastin, collacin and elacin to identify the degradation products of collagen and elastin respectively which he observed in degenerate skin. Gillman discarded Unna's staining technique as being insufficiently selective, and also arrived at the same conclusion with respect to most of the other commonly used stains, but derived a variety of stain mixtures which in his hands were capable of distinguishing between true elastica staining elements and the material which he referred to as "elastotically degenerate collagen."

Braun Falco [45] studied the attachment of those elastica stains which were dependent on the presence of phenolic groups and showed that the adsorption of the dye molecule on to the fiber is dependent on the setting up of a dipole between basic centers on the dye molecule and the main protein chains of the fiber. Electron microscopy [46, 47] has made it possible to demonstrate that the dye molecules are in the main associated with the amorphous region of the elastic fiber. Suggestions [37] that the digestion of this matrix by elastase results in a failure to attract the stain were at an earlier stage taken as indicating that it was to this material only that the dye became attached. However, as was mentioned it is more likely that failure to stain following partial elastolysis is due to the appearance in the molecules of increasing numbers of polar groups consequent on main-chain degradation, and that these groups prevent the approach of the dye molecules. It has been shown that stained elastin can be used as a suitable substrate for elastase [48, 49] but that whole tissue stained with one of the resorcinol fuchsin stains is resistant to elastolysis [50]. It appears, therefore, that although the markedly polar basic and acid groups are not required for, and indeed are antagonistic to, the adsorption of the dye molecules on to the fibers some other center which is necessary for the formation of an active enzyme substrate complex plays a part in the attachment of the dye molecule. In view of the fact that both carboxyl and hydroxyl groups are required for the formation of the complex between enzyme and substrate [5] it would appear likely that hydroxyl groups may be involved in dye attachment. As yet little is known as to the distribution of active groups on the surface and in the body of the elastic fiber. If this hypothesis regarding the relationship between the attachment of dye and enzyme to the substrate is correct, it would appear that active centers within the body of the fiber uncovered by mechanical degradation must consist of sites in which hydroxyl and carboxyl groups are relatively close together. These will not only provide adequate centers for the formation of active enzyme-substrate complexes, but also situations in which free carboxyl groups can prevent the approach and attachment of dye molecules which would otherwise block these active sites and so prevent elastolysis.

5.1.3   Microstructure of Elastic Fibers

When the electron microscope was first used to examine connective tissue components [51] the methods available were by no means as sophisticated as those available today. To obtain a preparation suitable for study it was necessary to tease the sample, discard the majority of the material as being too gross for examination and shadow the small amount which could be deposited on the grid from one drop of fluid, to intensify the contrast, and to give some indication of the surface irregularities. Examined in this way small pieces of elastic tissue from skin, aorta, and ligament showed a considerable variety of structures [52–55]. In the aorta two forms of elastica were apparent, fine fibrils which branched and anastomosed with one another and large sheets of material from the edges of which short lengths of fiber could be seen protruding. The exact relationship of these two forms was difficult to assess but it was suggested that the sheets consisted of networks of the fine fibrils coated with masses of amorphous substance. Following observations on the effect of elastase on these structures [53] the fibers themselves were shown to be dual in nature with fine fibrils embedded in an amorphous mass, which itself formed aggregates with other such structures to form the sheetlike elements present in certain tissues [54].

When more elegant methods of electron microscopy became available, instead of the picture becoming clearer, other difficulties arose [55, 56]. The majority of workers [57–59] reported that cross-sections through elastic fibers showed that they were without internal structure consisting of electron-lucent material surrounded by an electron-dense membrane. However certain other workers [60, 61] observed signs of fibrillar patterns within such structures, especially if the fibers were cut longitudinally [62]. Later it became apparent that internal structure was mainly apparent in very young and aging elastic fibers [63]. The suggestion has now been made [61] that the fine fibrils which represent the first stage in the laying down of elastic fibers coalesce to form relatively structureless elements and that the mature elastic fibers consists of an amorphous core surrounded by an array of fibrils which have not become absorbed into the main structure. Because of this, the outer surface of the fiber presents a rough appearance due to these semiabsorbed elements on its surface [61].

It would appear that the early and later forms of the elastic tissue demonstrate different degrees of susceptibility to elastase. The studies which were made of the effects of elastase on elastic fibers when teased preparations were used showed that the relatively cylindrical fibers (demonstrated by the length of the shadow cast during the preparation of samples for electron microscope examination) collapsed during elastolysis [53] and it was at this collapsed stage that signs of a fibrillar inner structure became apparent. At that time the author and his collaborators suggested [64] that the elastic fiber consisted of a bunch of fibrils surrounded by amorphous material. It was therefore suggested that the first stage of elastolysis consisted in the dissolution of the surrounding material to reveal the underlying fibrils. It would appear that although this concept is still fundamentally true, newer observations on the structure of the molecule would indicate that the original model should in fact be turned inside out leaving the only partially absorbed fibrils on the surface. The collapse of the structure following the early stages of elastolysis would then be due to the removal of the more susceptible amorphous inner portion of the fiber.

Biochemical observations on the structure of the elastic fiber which will be dealt with in detail in a later section are also in agreement with this concept, since if the central more susceptible part of the elastic fiber consists of material which is derived in the first instance from intact young elastic fibrils, it would be expected that total solution of the elastic material would result in the production of substances which might differ from one another in their degree of physical aggregation, but would be identical or nearly so from the point of view of their chemical composition. That this is indeed the case, was demonstrated as long ago as 1951 by Partridge and his collaborators [65] in their studies on the high and low molecular weight preparations obtained from elastin following treatment with boiling dilute oxalic acid. They found no difference between the amino acid composition of the so called α-elastin with a molecular weight of 80,000 and the β-elastin with a molecular weight of 6,000. The author of this chapter suggested [21] that the high molecular weight species of the α-elastin might represent material which consisted of direct polymers of a fundamental protein unit whereas the β-elastin might be derived from the amorphous material which he suggested might consist of the same elastin subunits linked together by polysaccharide and possibly also by lipid.

5.2   CHEMISTRY OF ELASTIN

5.2.1   Amino Acid Analysis

The first amino acid analyses of elastin to provide more than a partial picture of the overall pattern were those of Stein and Miller [66]. They employed boiling 40% urea solution to remove collagen from the crude elastic tissue. Although Hall later showed [67] that this reagent, if present in a high enough liquor/solid ratio, was capable of taking elastin completely into solution, he also demonstrated that before it did so it dissolved not only the collagen which was present in the crude elastic tissue, but also another protein species to which the name *pseudoelastin* has been given [22]. This species of protein which is not soluble in boiling acetic acid, and hence is retained with elastin preparations purified in this fashion, renders amino acid analyses of elastin preparations from elastic tissues of aging subjects completely different from those of classical youthful elastins.

Stein and Miller's results, although still relatively crude, paved the way for subsequent analyses which have since been carried out using either microbiological assay methods [68] or ion-exchange resin chromatography [69–77] for the estimation of the individual constituents.

Elastin resembles collagen in that approximately one-third of the amino acid residues are glycine (Table 5.1). It also has a relatively high proline content but here its formal similarity to collagen ceases. The numbers of basic and acidic amino acid residues are appreciably smaller than those present in collagen (152 as opposed to 250 residues per 1000). The long-chain monoamino monocarboxylic amino acids, especially valine are however markedly more abundant (135 valine residues in elastin as compared to 22 valine residues in collagen).

Fractionation on DEAE-Sephadex of the high molecular weight material resulting from the digestion of elastin by pancreatic elastase [78] results in the separation of a number of peptides which can be distinguished from one another in that they differ in their amino acid analysis.

The first fraction from the column, which is essentially nonpolar, had on average 47 amino acid residues of which 87% were the three nonpolar ones—glycine, proline and valine—in relative molar ratios of 2:1:2. The glycine content is roughly similar to that of intact elastin, and the proline level is only slightly raised. The valine content on the other hand is 2.5 times larger than that in the intact molecule. The only other residue present in this peptide, at a level appreciably higher

Table 5.1   Amino Acid Composition of Elastin from the Skin of a Normal Subject

g amino Acid/100 g Protein	
Aspartic acid	0.4
Threonine	0.6
Serine	0.6
Glutamic acid	2.4
Proline	18.0
Glycine	23.4
Alanine	23.0
Valine	13.0
Isoleucine	2.8
Leucine	7.6
Tyrosine	3.4
Phenylalanine	3.7
Quarter desmosine	0.7
Quarter isodesmosine	0.9
Lysine	0.6
Histidine	Trace
Arginine	0.7
Hydroxyproline	0.9

than 1%, is hydroxyproline. These results are of fundamental importance in indicating firstly that, in common with collagen, elastin contains large nonpolar regions, and secondly that a high proportion of the valine, which is a significant component of elastin that differentiates it from other connective tissue proteins, is present in the nonpolar section of the molecule. Finally, the enrichment of the hydroxyproline content of this fraction supports the belief, which has been strengthening of recent years [77], that the small levels of this amino acid which have been observed in all samples of elastin so far analysed are not, as was first believed to be the case, the result of incomplete removal of collagen from the preparation, but represent an integral part of the molecule. This highly nonpolar fraction does not account for more than 6.3% of the total elastin digest, the largest fraction being one containing between ten and twenty times more basic and acidic residues and accounting for some 30% of the total nondialysable portion of the molecule. Another fraction although only accounting for 11.5% of the total was of considerable interest not only because it was the major fraction with antigenic activity, but also in view of the fact that it contained about 7% carbohydrate and about 50% of chloroform-extractable lipids. The presence of high concentrations of basic and acidic amino acids and aromatic residues is in conformity with observations on collagen where fractions rich in these amino acids have been shown to demonstrate a similar degree of antigenicity [79]. The desmosine and isodesmosine contents of both the polar and the slightly polar peptides are between three and four times higher than those in intact elastin, whereas the nonpolar peptide contains less than a third as much. It would appear that the inner chain linkages provided by these polydentate amino acids are in the main restricted to the polar regions. This is as would be expected if the hypothesis that the biosynthetic pathway whereby these linkages are formed entails the interaction of intact and oxidatively deaminated lysine residues is in fact correct. The presence of lipid in such large amounts in the most polar fraction is rather unexpected since it might be thought likely that at least some of the lipid would be associated through van der Waal's forces with the more nonpolar regions of the molecule [80]. It is always possible that whereas the main attachment site for the lipid, be it phospholipid or free fatty acid, is through its lyophillic center and the polar groups in the protein, the other lipophyllic end of the molecule may associate with the nonpolar regions, thus providing a semipermanent cross-linkage which may be completely resistant to polar solvents, but can be broken by molecules with paraffinoid residues of increasing chain length. Robert [81] has shown that the alkaline hydrolysis of elastin may be enhanced considerably by the addition of alcohols of increasing chain length.

5.2.2   Secondary and Tertiary Structure

In view of the fact that so little is as yet known regarding the way in which the molecules of elastin are arranged in relationship to one another to form physiologically intact entities, it is not surprising that it is difficult to differentiate between secondary structures in the elastic fibers and those more highly organised structures which verge on the fibrillar.

Partridge was the first to provide evidence [14] for the existence of a complex molecule with numerous parallel chains. From end-group determinations on soluble elastin derived from the intact ligament protein by prolonged treatment with boiling 0.25 M oxalic acid he deduced that at least seventeen chains must exist, joined presumably by covalent linkages. More recent studies by Mandl and her co-workers have shown [78] that this highly branched structure is retained even after dissolution by elastase. The nondialysable fraction in an elastolysate must have a molecular weight of more than 10,000 to be retained by the dialysis membrane, but the longest polypeptide recovered from elastolysates only contained 47 residues, based on the concentration of the least frequent residue; some fractions had as low as 8.8 residues. Even the largest peptide must therefore consist of two or more chains, and the smaller ones of up to ten or twelve chains. The numbers of desmosine, isodesmosine and lysinonorleucine residues in these fractions increase with increasing complexity, but not in a directly proportional fashion. Thus the partially polar fraction which represents the major portion of the molecule as a whole has the highest concentration of cross-links (0.923%). The other fractions for which Dr. Mandl and her co-workers give analytical data containing only 0.143 and 0.647 moles% must have come from regions of the molecule which are appreciably less cross-linked. In view of the suggested biosynthetic pathway whereby these cross-linkages are formed [82], necessitating the juxtaposition of aldehydes derived from lysine residues and intact lysine molecules, it is interesting to note from these figures that there are portions of the elastin molecule which are apparently aligned in such a fashion that four lysine residues can react with one another with the production of one or other of the desmosines, whereas in other regions of the molecule only two lysines react to produce lysinonorleucine. The recent discovery [83] by Partridge and his colleagues of yet a third condensation product of residues and lysine, so-called merodesmosine, in which three amino acid residues are combined to form an open chain compound, may indicate either an intermediate in the production of the quaternary pyridinium molecules of desmosine or isodesmosine, or on the other hand it may represent a situation in which the spacial alignment of the chains is such that it is impossible for the four required for desmosine production to lie in the correct relationship to one another with the result that only three residues enter into combination. Of the cross-linkages in the nonpolar regions of the molecule 47.5% are the simplest lysinonorleucine structures whereas in the two more polar fractions only between 19.4 and 20.0% are of this type.

The tertiary structure of elastin has been discussed by a number of groups of workers, but with certain notable exceptions such discussion has been based in the main on hypothetical considerations rather than on experimental fact. It has been suggested [21] on the basis of evidence for the rates of production of high and low molecular weight material following the treatment of elastin with boiling oxalic acid solution [14], that elastin may consist of protein units of constant composition joined either directly to others 'of similar type, or indirectly to similar units through carbohydrate. At the state in the elucidation of the structure of elastin when this hypothetical scheme was propounded, little account was taken of the lipid present in the molecule. Later observations that free fatty acids could be observed in elastolysates necessitated an alteration to be made to this hypothesis [84] to include this third component, and it was then suggested [5] that the elastin units are linked to one another through lipid, but that this part of the molecule bears a carbohydrate moiety. The lipid is released into solution in an intact state together with the carbohydrate when the protein is attacked by the proteolytic enzyme elastase alone, but may appear as free fatty acid when this enzyme is contaminated by the presence of other enzymes, also present in the pancreas, which have lipolytic activity [84]. Considerable confusion has arisen over this question of the macromolecular structure of elastin during the past 20 years, since it has been variously reported [81, 85] that elastin contains either carbohydrate or lipid or both as an integral part of the molecule.

As an example of this, an alternative structure has been proposed which is different from that mentioned previously in that the various subunits of elastin are united through carbohydrate rather than lipid [86] and that this part of the molecule carries the lipid. It is not yet possible to discriminate between these two theories, and both may be applicable in different parts of the molecule, or conversely a lipopolysaccharide may link the elastin subunits, with the effective linkage being from lipid to protein at one end and from carbohydrate to protein at the other.

The theory in which these two hypotheses are embedded was initially devised to explain among other things the fact that digestion with elastase causes elastin fibers to collapse from their original cylindrical structure to flattened arrays of microfibrils [53] (see above). It was therefore suggested that the pure protein aggregate occupies the center of the fiber whereas the polysaccharide-protein complex (and later the lipopolysaccharide-protein complex) covers the array of microfibrils formed by this association of protein subunits. On the basis of more refined observations on the biogenesis of elastin in foetal tissues [62] and of the ratios of nondialysable to dialysable products of elastolysis

[87] it has been suggested that the structure proposed on the basis of this earlier concept should be turned inside out, with the amorphous carbohydrate-rich fraction in the interior of the fiber and pure elastin protein on the outside.

5.2.3   Age Changes

Lansing and his colleagues [88–91] were the first to suggest that the amino acid composition of elastin varies with age. They noticed that there are marked increases in the amounts of polar amino acids; for instance aspartic and glutamic acids provide only 1.8% of the total nitrogen of the protein in elastin from samples of aorta from the 15 to 20 year age group as apposed to 3.55% in the age group 55 to 75. They were able to demonstrate that the elastin preparations from the aorta could be separated into two fractions depending on their differential centrifugation in sucrose solution (sp. gr. 1.30). The major part of the material in preparations of aorta from young subjects floated in this solution, whereas the reverse was the case for elastin from old subjects. These elastin preparations had been obtained following the removal of the associated collagen and ground substance by treatment with alkali [90]. This method of purification was apparently incapable of removing calcium from the tissue. Thus the calcium content of the young aortas was on average 0.35% whereas that of the elastin from old tissue was 5.93% a difference which is reflected in the relative amount of "light" and "heavy" forms of the protein.

It was later suggested that the changes in amino acid analysis which are apparent in elastin with increasing age [2] are due to the simultaneous presence in the elastic tissue of a third protein with an amino acid analysis midway between that of collagen and elastin, in that its polar amino acid and hydroxyproline content is considerably greater, whereas its valine content is considerably lower than that of young elastin.

In cattle aorta, it has been demonstrated [22] that these changes in amino acid composition are most pronounced, not, as might be expected, in the oldest samples examined, but in samples from mature but "middle-aged" animals. Thus there are changes in the amino acid pattern in an upward direction (Table 5.2) in the case of seven amino acids and in a downward direction in five. The levels of proline and glycine, (not recorded in the table) remained essentially constant, thus indicating that the contaminating protein is in all probability derived either from collagen or elastin, since no other proteins have such high levels of both these acids. Studies on human aortic tissue [72] have

Table 5.2 Amino Acid Analyses of Elastin Preparations[a]

Amino Acids with Mixed Concentration		Amino Acids with Lowered Concentration	
Hydroxyproline	4	Alanine	0.8
Aspartic acid	4	Isoleucine	0.5
Threonine	3	Leucine	0.9
Serine	2	Lysine	0.1
Tyrosine	2	Valine	0.9
Arginine	5		
Histidine	5		

Changes in the other amino acids were not significant.

[a] From the aortae of 4-year-old cattle and those of older and younger animals (2 and 7 years). The figures indicate the numbers of times greater the concentrations of individual amino acids are than those of the same amino acids in the other preparation.

also demonstrated that normal methods of purification of elastin leave behind a fraction of similar type with the elastin from tissues of subjects in the 51 to 60 age group, and again this material is either not present or is more easily removed from both older and younger tissues. Treatment of aortic elastin fom elderly subjects with boiling 40% urea solution [22, 92] ultimately results in the total dissolution of the elastin if the liquor/solid ratio is sufficiently high. Before the elastin passes into solution, however, two other components of the tissue are dissolved. Firstly the collagen passes into solution leaving behind an elastin preparation with the abnormal analysis observed when elderly elastin is freed from collagen by treatment with boiling acetic acid, and then the intermediate protein, pseudoelastin, passes into solution. The residue at this stage is elastin with a classical amino acid analysis; this is the third and last fraction to be dissolved.

Pseudoelastin of this type has been extracted from old skin as well as aorta and would appear to account, at least in part, for the abnormal elastica staining material which appears with age in exposed dermis [29, 31]. The amino acid analysis of the pseudoelastin fraction demonstrating as it does, a high level of basic and acidic amino acids and hydroxyproline, together with a valine level which is appreciably less than that present in elastin, would appear to indicate that this protein fraction is derived from collagen.

Elastin from foetal tissue also exhibits an amino acid analysis which differs considerably from that of classical adult elastin [22, 74]. Under normal circumstances it is impossible to separate a fraction from such foetal elastins which is comparable to the pseudoelastin of old tissues. It has recently been demonstrated, however, that pretreatment of the elastin preparation with α-amylase [77] removes a fraction from the elastin which has a different amino acid analysis from that of the classical substance, leaving a preparation behind which has the same amino acid analysis as elastin from adult tissue.

There are two possible ways in which these two extra proteins—pseudoelastin and the foetal protein—may remain in close association with elastin so as to be segregated with it during the less complicated purification procedures. The proteins may have a physical make-up which is so similar to that of elastin that they are insoluble in the same reagents, or they may actually be combined with the elastin by relatively stable bonds. If this is the case, they would be regarded as integral parts of the elastin molecule, but the fact that they can be removed by treatment with urea and α-amylase would indicate that they are less permanent structural components than the integral chains of the elastin molecule.

5.3   ENZYMOLOGICAL STUDIES OF ELASTIC STRUCTURE

5.3.1   The Reaction Between Elastase and Elastin

The interaction between elastase and its insoluble substrate elastin poses a number of problems which have not been fully investigated. Under normal enzymic circumstances in which a high molecular weight protein, the enzyme, interacts with either a low molecular weight substance, the substrate or in the case of proteolytic enzymes in general, with another high molecular weight substance which is also soluble, the reaction can be assumed to follow the normal kinetic pathways. In the present instance, however, the enzyme apparently has a molecular weight of between 10,000 and 25,000 and is soluble, whereas the substrate is of virtually infinite molecular weight and is completely insoluble. It is therefore of importance how the two proteins approach one another and whether reactive sites on the substrate are available for attachment to active sites on the enzyme molecule.

It has been shown that both carboxyl and hydroxyl groups are essential on the surface of the substrate for the close association of enzyme and substrate [93] and similar requirements have been reported for the enzyme [94]. The presence of the same type of reactive group on both enzyme and substrate limits the number of possible ways in which the two can become united to one another. Either the pair of reactive groups can form a couple of ester linkages, or they can both react with some intermediate group which is capable, because it is bidentate, of reacting equally with enzyme and substrate. Based on the observation that chelating agents such as citrate [95] ethylenediamine tetraacetic acid [95, 27] uramil diacetic acid, nitrolotriacetic acid, methylene diacetic acid, and aminodiacetic acid [96] and certain metal EDTA complexes are capable of inhibiting elastolysis, whereas calcium EDTA can activate the system [97], it has been suggested that calcium atoms may provide this intermediate group to which both sets of carboxyl and hydroxyl groups attach themselves.

Any likelihood of the former suggestion being correct would appear to be slight in view of the alterations which can be observed in the rate of elastolysis when either carboxyl or hydroxyl groups are blocked [93]. Esterification of the hydroxyl groups results in a greater amount of enzyme being absorbed on to the substrate, but completely inhibits elastolysis. Such a differential effect on adsorption and elastolysis respectively could not occur if the linkage between enzyme and substrate were to occur directly between carboxyl and hydroxyl groups since the blockage of either would result in a reduction in both adsorption and activity.

The suggestion has been made that the enzyme-substrate complex might result from the formation of a coordination shell around the calcium atom [27, 95], the electrons being supplied in part by the enzyme and in part by the substrate. Although EDTA inhibits elastolysis when present in the elastolysis mixture, no effect can be observed when either substrate or enzyme are pretreated with the chelating agent; excess of which is subsequently removed by thorough washing or dialysis prior to the two components of the system being brought together [27]. This phenomenon may be explained in either of two ways. Either sufficient calcium is derivable from the glassware or from the reagents to permit the formation of the necessary complex even after the removal of all endogenous calcium by chelation, or calcium is so firmly bound either to the substrate, to the enzyme or to both, as to be completely resistant to extraction by EDTA. Yu and Blumenthal [98] have demonstrated that there are two forms of calcium in elastic tissue, an EDTA-extractable form and one which is resistant to extraction with this reagent. It would appear therefore that the second supposition advanced is the more likely to be correct.

The strength of the bonds binding calcium to both enzyme and substrate can be demonstrated by measuring the amount of EDTA which is picked up by an elastolytic system when enzyme substrate and chelating agent are incubated together. Table 5.3 shows that the amount of EDTA adsorbed by a given amount of elastase and elastin is directly

Table 5.3   The Effect of Variations in the Concentration of EDTA, Elastin, and Elastase on the Amount of the Former Reagent Absorbed on to the Solid Phase of an Elastolytic System Containing All Three Components

Changing EDTA Concentration (1.0 mg Elastase, 1 µg Elastin)

EDTA Added, µmoles	EDTA Removed from Supernatant
1	0.105
2	0.225
5	0.605
10	1.247

Changing Elastin and Elastase (2 µmoles EDTA Added to Each System)

Elastase Concentration, µg ml^{-1}	µmoles of EDTA Removed from Supernatant. Elastin Concentration, mg ml^{-1}			
	0	1	2	3
0	0	0	0	0
0.5	0	0.105	0.385	0.667
1.0	0	0.225	0.667	0.842
2.0	0	0.281	0.821	0.947
3.0	0	0.316	0.918	1.02

proportional to its initial concentration in the elastolytic system whereas for a fixed EDTA concentration the uptake of the latter is dependent on the relative concentrations of the other two components (i.e., enzyme and substrate).

The amount of EDTA taken up by the protein in the elastolysis system is not only proportional to the amount of enzyme and substrate present but also to the amount of calcium present in these two components of the system. Values for the amount of EDTA taken up by systems in which both enzyme and substrate differ in their calcium content from standard preparations are given in Table 5.4. Since EDTA is not taken up by either the substrate or the enzyme when either is incubated with the chelating agent in the absence of the other, it would appear that the linkages binding calcium to each of the two proteins are too strong to be broken by EDTA. However the uptake of EDTA from a complete elastolytic system must imply that during the formation of the enzyme/substrate complex these coordinate calcium linkages are broken. It has, therefore, been suggested that both enzyme and substrate exist in monomeric and polymeric forms [5], the latter consisting of at least a dimer; the individual monomeric subunits of this species of enzyme being joined together by coordinately bound calcium atoms. The approach of a monomeric form of one of the components to the dimeric form of the other may then be supposed to result in the fission of the coordination shell followed by its reformation employing electrons from the other component.

$$E-Ca-E + S = E-Ca-S + E \qquad (1)$$

$$S-Ca-S + E = S-Ca-E + S \qquad (2)$$

The net result of both these two postulated reactions will be the production of identical enzyme/substrate complexes and monomeric forms of the opposite component from that present as the monomeric form at the beginning of the reaction. If one can assume that both enzyme and substrate consist of a mixture of both forms these two reactions will be self-perpetuating.

The involvement of a bidentate chelating agent in either Equation 1 or 2 may result in a variety of subsidiary reactions which can produce either active or inactive complexes.

$$2(E-Ca-E) + 2S + V = E-Ca-V-Ca-S + 3E + S \qquad (3)$$

$$2(E-Ca-E) + 2S + V = E-Ca-V-Ca-E + 2S + 2E \qquad (4)$$

Table 5.4   The Uptake of EDTA by Elastolytic Systems in Which the Calcium Content of Both Enzyme and Substrate Differ (Elastin 2.0 mg ml^{-1}; Elastase 1.0 μg ml^{-1})

Substrate Calcium Concentration, %	EDTA Uptake from 2 μmoles, μmoles
0.012	0.667
0.020	0.91
0.060	1.4
Calcium content of elastase 0.032%	

Enzyme Substrate Concentration, %	EDTA Uptake from 2 μmoles, μmoles
0.02	0.48
0.032	0.667
0.052	0.915
0.064	1.170
0.141	1.690
Calcium content of elastin 0.012%	

where V represents the chelating agent. Equation 3 represents a system in which an active enzyme/substrate complex is formed, Equation 4 is a system in which an inactive complex resulting in the sequestering not only of the calcium but also of half of the available enzyme. There are of course other equations which can be written for conditions in which the dimeric form of the substrate is involved. The complex formed in the system referred to in Equation 3 in which the enzyme and substrate are separated not only by a pair of calcium atoms, but also by

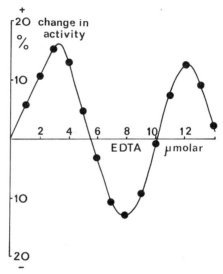

Figure 5.3. One activation and inhibition cycle in an elastolysis system brought about by the introduction of between 1 and 14 μ molar EDTA to a system containing 5 mg elastin ml^{-1} and 4 ug elastase ml^{-1}. Activity was determined in the usual way after 3 hr incubation.

an EDTA molecule represents the condition in which EDTA is picked up by the insoluble component of the elastolysis system. It has been shown that variations in the amount of EDTA added to an elastolysis system can result in alterations in the effect which it produces [27; 97]. At low concentrations of EDTA, activation may occur followed by inhibition as the amount of EDTA present increases (Fig. 5.3). The activation may be due to the fact that the insertion of an EDTA molecule between enzyme and substrate provides a more mobile linkage between the two. When the enzyme attaches itself directly to the surface of the elastin molecule it is possible that there is a marked steric hinderence due to the fact, mentioned previously, that both are large molecules, at least one of which is highly immobile due to its insoluble nature. A longer linkage between the enzyme and its substrate may permit interaction between the two to be much more easily attained.

Because of the changing uptake of EDTA which results from changes in the amount of calcium bound to the substrate and the enzyme it may be deduced that there will be associated changes in the rate of elastolysis depending on the amount of calcium. This is in fact true as can be seen from Fig. 5.4, where the amount of elastin taken into solution is plotted against the calcium content of the substrate. Calcium

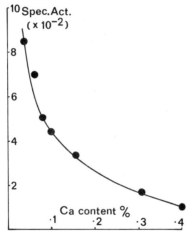

Figure 5.4. The effect of endogenous calcium in the substrate on the specific activity of an elastase preparation itself containing 0.012% calcium.

can be taken up by elastic tissue in either of two ways [98] providing calcified products which differ in their resistance to decalcification with chelating agents. It is possible to deposit calcium which is resistant to extraction by EDTA by treating the solid substrate with the calcium salt of EDTA (Fig. 5.5). This modified substrate also demonstrates a varied susceptibility to elastase (Fig. 5.6).

Lansing [91] and his co-workers demonstrated that there is an increase in the calcium content of elastic tissue on aging, but their figures included an appreciable amount of calcium which was not necessarily bound to the elastin by coordinate linkages and would represent both the forms of calcium reported in elastic tissue by Yu and Blumenthal [98]. Cattle

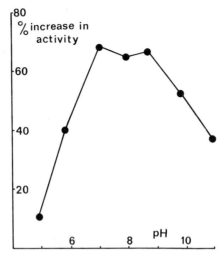

Figure 5.5. Change in susceptibility of a standard preparation of elastin, pre-incubated for 3 hr at a liquid/solid ratio of 50–1 with 0.005 mM Ca-EDTA complex in veronal/phosphate buffers over the pH range 4.8–10.4. Susceptibility is expressed in terms of the percentage increase in the activity of a standard elastase preparation (Ca content 0.032%) incubated under standard conditions with each pretreated sample over its activity when an untreated substrate is employed.

aorta also shows a marked increase in calcium content with age (Table 5.5). The figures reported here represent only the EDTA-resistant form of bound calcium. If the hypotheses outlined above are correct, it should be possible to isolate a monomeric and a dimeric form of elastase and to show that the latter is more active against young elastin in which

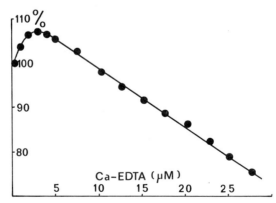

Figure 5.6. The effect of treatment with increasing concentrations of Ca-EDTA at pH 7.9 on the susceptibility of elastin to standard elastase (Ca content 0.032).

Table 5.5   The Calcium Content of Elastin
Preparations Obtained by Various
Purification Techniques from the
Aortae of Cattle of Differing Ages

Method of Purification	Age of Animal, years Calcium Content, %		
	2	4	7
Acid extraction	0.49	0.82	0.5
Alkali extraction	0.52	0.55	0.71
Enzyme extraction	0.12	0.25	0.37

a larger number of carboxyl and hydroxyl groups are not linked through calcium, whereas the opposite will be the case in elastin from old animals in which the amount of coordinately bound calcium is greatly increased.

Elastase is normally extracted from pancreas powder by buffers of pH 4.7 and the majority of the material can be extracted in the first and second extracts (1:10 w/v). If however buffers of other pH value are used for the extraction it can be seen that there are two separate species of enzyme extractable (Fig. 5.7); one being optimally extracted at pH 5 and coming out predominantely in the first extract, and the other at pH 1.5 and being more readily extracted in the second and third serial extracts. The normal extract at pH 4.7 consists of a mixture of the two species. Studies on the gel filtration properties of these two enzymes indicates that the one extracted at the more alkaline pH has a higher molecular weight than the other and when both enzymes are tested against elastin preparations of increasing age and hence increasing calcium content, it can be seen that the ratio of the susceptibilities to the two enzymes changes with age in conformity with the suggestion that elastin becomes increasingly cross-linked by coordinately bound calcium with increasing age (Fig. 5.8).

A further indication of the existance of free and coordinately bound carboxyl and hydroxyl groups in elastic fibers can be obtained from a study of the effect of elastase on the physical properties. Elastic tissue from ox ligamentum nuchae, purified from collagen by treatment with boiling 2% acetic acid can be stretched by the application of weights with a resulting linear-load extension curve. Being linear there is no hysteresis factor to consider when the load is removed, and repeated extension cycles are absolutely reproducible. It is therefore possible for any individual strip of elastic tissue to be used as its own control in experiments in which successive treatments are carried out. Using apparatus devised by Ridge and Wright [99] for their study of the tensile properties of skin, it was possible to surround the strip of elastic tissue by a solution of elastase maintained at a constant temperature of 37°C by circulating liquid from a thermostat. Young's modulus can be calcu-

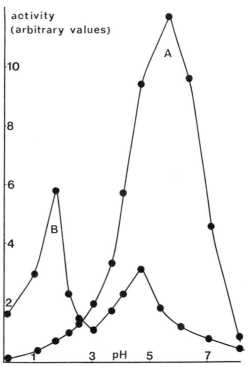

Figure 5.7. The yields of elastolytic activity (in terms of arbitrary activity values) following the extraction of defatted pancreas powder at various pH values. (a) Activity in the euglobulin fraction from the first serial extracts. (b) activity in the albuminon fraction from the second serial extracts.

lated for the system after each extension cycle, and the reduction in this parameter plotted against time of treatment with elastase (Fig. 5.9). Within a relatively short period, the value for Young's modulus falls by 20% [104]. If samples of the enzyme solution are removed at intervals during treatment it can be seen that the amount of elastin passing into solution during the period in which this large change in Young's modulus occurs is only 5%. From this it may be inferred that the change in Young's modulus occurs during the formation of the enzyme-substrate complex and before the dissolution of the substrate which results from the fission of this complex. The reduction in stability [100] of the molecule which is consonant with the fission of half of the linkages so as to lengthen the interlinkage distance from a residue weight of 2,000 to 11,000, can only be accomplished by the monoeric form of the enzyme. It may thus be deduced that the formation of the enzyme-substrate complex necessitates the fission of stabilising linkages in the molecule, and the enzymic requirements for this to happen point to these linkages being the coordinately bound calcium atoms already referred to.

5.3.2   Nonprotein Constituents of Elastin

It has been suggested that elastin may contain both carbohydrate and lipid components and there is a certain amount of evidence from enzyme studies as to the role which these particular constituents may play in the stabilisation of the fiber.

The addition of other fractions of pancreatic extract to the proteolytic

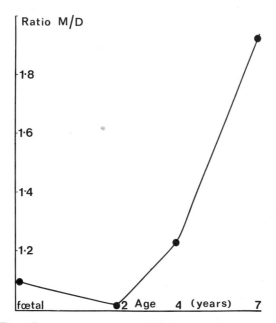

Figure 5.8.   The effect of age on the relative susceptibility of ligament elastin to attack by the two forms of elastase. The curve represents the ratio of the susceptibilities to "monomeric" (euglobulin) form of the enzyme and the "dimeric" (albuminoid) form of ox aorta elastin from a calf foetus and from 2-, 4-, and 7-year-old cattle.

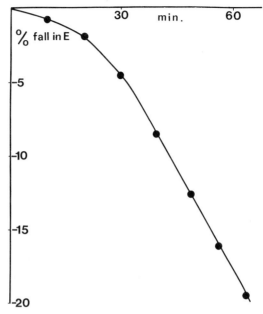

Figure 5.9. The fall in Young's Modulus E of strips of elastic tissue from the ligamentien nuchae of an Ox during 60 min treatment at 37°C with elastase (a preparation from the euglobulin fraction, see Fig. 5.7).

enzyme enhances the activity in its role as a solubilizer of elastin [101]. This was first observed in 1953 when the suggestion was first advanced that there was more than one enzyme responsible for total elastolysis. When sections of whole tissue are employed [102] it is apparent that the presence of these secondary factors is increasingly important as the age of the subject from which the elastic tissue is obtained increases. Since it has more recently become apparent that these ancillary enzymes are either mucolytic [103] or lipolytic [84, 104] there are only two ways in which they can act. Firstly, it is possible for them to potentiate the solubilizing action of elastase itself, by breaking cross-linkages (see above) thus rendering the elastin more easily soluble when a limited number of main chain-linkages are broken by elastase, or secondly, it may provide an increasing number of sites at which elastase can attack the elastin molecule by liberating carboxyl and/or hydroxyl groups which were previously blocked either by carbohydrate or lipid. There is some evidence [105] for the former possibility in Banga's observations regarding the changes which occur in the tensile properties of elastic tissue after it has been treated with the so-called elastimucase, one of the ancillary enzyme preparations obtained from pancreas. Since this enzyme has never been completely purified, however, it might be that the preparation used contains a small but adequate amount of the monomeric form of elastase which would of course, on the basis of the observations reported above, be capable of bringing about these changes in the physical properties of the elastin molecule. The liberation of active groups is not easy to assess but would appear to be the more likely of the two hypotheses to explain enhanced elastolysis, although this does not invalidate the possibility that the groups which block these centers are themselves part of a cross-linking moiety in the molecule as a whole.

The other and most highly documented form of cross-linkage—that deriving from the metabolism of lysine—cannot be studied directly by the use of the elastolytic enzymes since structures containing these cross-links are completely refractory to attack by elastase. The regions of the molecule which are not cross-linked in this fashion are degraded into peptides containing five or six residues [38]. This can be demonstrated by a comparison of the rate of appearance of terminal amino groups and the tricarboxylic acid precipitability of the soluble protein. If the molecule is split into two and then two again, the amount of soluble, nonprecipitable protein would not mirror the amino group production, but would remain relatively constant, until a threshold level of molecular size was reached after which there would be a rapid increase in the amount of nonprecipitable material.

5.4   CONCLUSION

Elastin consists of a protein which resembles collagen to a certain extent in so far as it contains a high concentration of glycine and proline. The small amount of hydroxyproline which can be observed in all preparations, is an integral part of the molecule and is not due to contamination by small amounts of collagen which cannot be removed during purification. The further analysis of elastin shows marked differences from collagen being relatively devoid of polar amino acid residues and containing an extremely high level of valine. There is little evidence now in favor of the concept which was apparently well-founded in the 1950s to the effect that elastin suffered a change in amino acid composition with increasing age. It would now appear to be far more likely that these apparent changes in composition are due to the retention with apparently purified elastin of a third protein, pseudoelastin, probably derived from collagen. This abnormal protein, which has an amino acid analysis part way between that of collagen and elastin, has physical properties which render it easily confusable with true elastin, especially in tissues such as skin in which in elderly exposed sites there is appreciably more of it present than there is of true elastin.

There appear to be at least three cross-links which have different roles to play in the stabilization of elastin fibers. The transformation from foetal elastin to the adult form which is associated with the formation of the isodesmosine type of cross-linkage is accompanied by the disappearance from close association with the elastin of a protein fraction which has little or no direct analytical relationship with elastin. It appears likely that this material holds the elastin molecules in the desired spatial arrangement for the interaction of the modified lysine residues with some of the remaining intact examples of this amino acid during the formation of these polydentate amino acids.

The second form of cross-linkage which is most prevalent in aging tissue is the coordinately bound calcium atom. This introduction of an inorganic focus into the elastin molecule may explain why the elastic fibers act as centers of calcification in tissues such as the aortic wall. The third type of cross-linkage, for which there is less evidence is the hypothetical lipopolysaccharide one. Here, again, the provision of lipid molecules within the elastic fiber may explain why these components of connective tissue act as centers for lipid deposition. Again, the major example of this is in the connective tissue of the aortic wall but it is also possible that the bound lipid which is present in the dermis may also be associated with the integral lipid of the elastic components of this tissue.

At a higher level of organization, the molecules of elastin, together with their associated calcium, lipid, and polysaccharide combine to form fibrils. In certain sites these combine further to form either fibers or membranes, and in aging tissues become associated with pseudoelastin which appears to be a degradation product of collagen.

The physical properties of the elastic fiber which impart typical structural properties to the tissues of which it forms a part would appear to be dependent on the close association of the paraffinoid portions of the molecule together with the cross-linkages which impart a rubberlike consistency to the fiber as a whole. In tissues such as the skin the innate nature of the elastin fibers themselves combines with the properties of the tissue as a whole (the weave of the collagen bundles) to provide exactly the right degree of elasticity and tone required for a containing membrane. When the relative amounts of elastin and collagen are altered in aging and exposed dermis, the tensile properties of the tissue, as a whole, change with the resulting sagging and wrinkling associated with aged skin.

REFERENCES

1. D. A. Hall, *Nature,* **168,** 513 (1951).
2. S. M. Partridge, *Advan. Protein Chem.,* **17,** 227 (1962).
3. G. M. Hass, *Arch. Pathol.,* **27,** 334 (1939).
4. J. P. Ayer, *Intern. Rev. Conn. Tissue Res.,* **2,** 33 (1964).
5. D. A. Hall, *Elastolysis and Ageing,* Charles C Thomas, Springfield, 1964.
6. W. A. Loeven, *Intern. Rev. Conn. Tissue Res.,* **1,** 184 (1963).
7. I. Mandl, *Advan. Enzymol.,* **23,** 163 (1961).
8. I. Banga, *Structure and Function of Elastin and Collagen,* Akademiai Kaido, Budapest, 1966.
9. R. W. Carton, J. Dainauskas, B. Tews, and G. M. Hass, *Amer. Rev. Respirat. Diseases,* **82,** 186 (1960).
10. M. K. Keech, *Ann. Rheum. Diseases,* **17,** 23 (1958).
11. G. Romhanyi, *Acta. Morphol. Acad. Sci. Hung.,* **5,** 311 (1955).
12. D. A. Hall, *Intern. Rev. Cytol.,* **8,** 211 (1959).
13. D. A. Hall and J. E. Gardiner, *Biochem. J.,* **59,** 465 (1955).
14. S. M. Partridge and H. F. Davis, *Biochem. J.,* **61,** 21 (1955).
15. A. I. Lansing, *Symposium on Atherosclerosis,* National Academy of Sciences-National Research Council, 1954 p. 50.
16. M. J. Fitzpatrick and V. D. Hospelhorn, *J. Lab. Clin. Med.,* **56,** 812 (1960).
17. J. W. Czerkawski, *Nature,* **194,** 869 (1962).
18. J. Balo and I. Banga, *Biochem. J.,* **46,** 384 (1950).
19. D. A. Hall and J. W. Czerkawski, *Biochem. J.,* **73,** 356 (1959).
20. L. A. Sachar, K. K. Winter, N. Sicher, and S. Frankel, *Proc. Soc. Exptl. Biol. Med.,* **90,** 323 (1955).
21. D. A. Hall, *Connective Tissue,* R. E. Tunbridge, Ed. Blackwell, London, 1957 p. 238.
22. D. A. Hall, *Exptl. Gerontol.,* **3,** 77 (1969).
23. G. C. Wood, *Biochem. Biophys. Acta,* **15,** 311 (1954).
24. D. A. Hall, *Biochem. J.,* **59,** 459 (1955).
25. W. A. Loeven, *Acta Physiol. Pharmacol. Neerl.,* **9,** 473 (1960).
26. D. P. Varadi and D. A. Hall, *Nature,* **208,** 1224 (1965).
27. D. A. Hall, *Abstr. of Eighth Internat. Cong. Gerontology,* Vol. 1, 113, 1969.
28. R. E. Tunbridge, R. N. Tattersall, D. A. Hall, W. T. Astbury, and R. Reed, *Clin. Sci.,* **11,** 315 (1952).
29. J. G. Smith Jr., E. A. Davidson, and R. D. Clark, *Nature,* **195,** 716 (1962).
30. J. G. Smith Jr., A. E. Davidson, and R. L. Hill, *Nature,* **197,** 1108 (1963).
31. D. A. Hall, Progress in the Biological Sciences in Relation to Dermatology, 2, A. Rook & R. H. Champion, Eds., Cambridge, 1964 p. 77.
32. P. G. Unna, *Histopathology of the Diseases of the Skin* (trans. by N. Walker), Macmillan, New York, 1896.

33. C. Weigert, *Zentr. Allgem. Pathol. Pathol. Anat.,* **9,** 287, (1898).

34. K. Hart, *Zentr. Allgem. Pathol. Pathol. Anat.,* **19,** 1 (1958).

35. R. L. Engle Jr. and E. W. Dempsey, *J. Histochem. Cytochem.,* **2,** 9 (1954).

36. H. M. Fullmer and R. D. Lillie, *J. Histochem. Cytochem.,* **4,** 64 (1956).

37. H. Saxl, *Gerontologia,* **1,** 141 (1957).

38. D. A. Hall and J. W. Czerkawski, *Collagen,* N. Ramanathan, Ed., Interscience, New York, 1962, p. 419.

39. F. B. Mallory, *Stain Technol.,* **11,** 101 (1936).

40. P. Masson, *J. Tech. Methods,* **12,** 75 (1929).

41. F. H. Verhoeff, *J. Amer. Med. Assoc.,* **50,** 876 (1908).

42. A. I. Lansing, 2nd Conf. on Connective Tissues, C. Ragan, Ed., Josiah Macy Foundation, 1951, p. 45.

43. T. Gillman, J. Penn, D. Bronks, and M. Roux, *A.M.A. Arch. Pathol.* **59,** 733 (1955).

44. P. G. Unna, *Monatschr. Prakt. Dermatol.,* **11,** 365 (1890).

45. O. Braun-Falco, *Arch. Klin. Exptl. Dermatol.* **203,** 256, (1956).

46. W. Schwatz and N. Dettmer, *Arch. Pathol. Anat. Physiol. Virchow's,* **323,** 243 (1953).

47. N. Dettmer, *Z. Zellforsch. Mikroskop. Anat.,* **37,** 89 (1952).

48. S. Chao, J. J. Sciarra, and C. J. Vosburgh, *Proc. Soc. Exptl. Biol. Med.,* **109,** 342 (1967).

49. D. A. Hall, *Biochem. J.,* **101,** 29 (1966).

50. G. H. Findley, *Brit. J. Dermatol.,* **66,** 16 (1954).

51. J. Gross, *J. Exptl. Med.,* **89,** 699 (1949).

52. C. Wolpers, *Klin. Wochshchr.,* **23,** 169 (1944).

53. D. A. Hall, R. Reed, and R. E. Tunbridge, *Exptl. Cell Res.,* **8,** 35 (1955).

54. O. Kawase, *Bull. Res. Inst. Diathetic Med.,* Kukakoto University, **9,** 1 (1959).

55. A. Charles, *Brit. J. Dermatol.,* **73,** 57 (1961).

56. J. Rhodin and T. Dahlamn, *Exptl. Cell. Res.,* **9,** 371 (1955).

57. M. K. Keech, *J. Biophys. Biochem. Cytol.,* **7,** 533 (1960).

58. D. C. Pease and W. J. Paule, *J. Ultrastruct. Res.,* **3,** 469 (1960).

59. J. G. Jensen, *Acta Pathol. Microbiol. Scand.,* **56,** 388 (1962).

60. M. D. Haust, R. H. More, S. A. Bencosme, and J. U. Balis, *Exptl. Molec. Pathol.,* **4,** 508 (1965).

61. T. K. Greenlee Jr., R. Rose, and J. L. Hartmann, *J. Cell. Biol.,* **30,** 59 (1966).

62. W. H. L. B. Sandberg and E. G. Cleary, *Anat. Record,* **155,** 563 (1966).

63. R. Ross, *Treatise on Collagen,* Vol. 2, Biology, B. S. Gould, Ed., Academic Press, New York, 1968, p. 1.

64. D. A. Hall, R. Reed, and R. E. Tunbridge, *Nature,* **170,** 264 (1952).

65. G. S. Adair, H. F. Davies, and S. M. Partridge, *Nature,* **167,** 605, (1951).

66. W. H. Stein and E. G. Miller Jr., *J. Biol. Chem.,* **125,** 599 (1938).

67. D. A. Hall, *Nature,* **168,** 513 (1951).

68. R. E. Newman and M. A. Logan, *J. Biol. Chem.*, **186,** 549 (1950).

69. M. Fitzpatrick and V. D. Hospelhorn, *Amer. Heart J.*, **69,** 211 (1965).

70. L. Gotte, V. Meneghelli, and A. Castellani, *Structure and Function of Connective and Skeletal Tissue*, Butterworth, London, 1965.

71. R. A. Grant, *Brit. J. Exptl. Pathol.*, **47,** 163 (1966).

72. F. S. Labella, S. Vivian, and D. P. Thornhill, *J. Gerontol.*, **21,** 550 (1966).

73. A. Serafini-Fracassini and G. R. Tristram, *Proc. Roy. Soc. B.*, **59,** 334 (1966).

74. E. G. Cleary, L. B. Sandberg, and D. S. Jackson, *J. Cell. Biol.*, **33,** 469 (1967).

75. F. S. Labella and S. Vivian, *Biochem. Biophys. Acta*, **133,** 189 (1967).

76. J. A. Petruska and L. B. Sandberg, *Biochem. Biophys. Res. Commun.*, **33,** 222 (1968).

77. F. S. Steven and D. S. Jackson, *Biochem. Biophys. Acta,* **168,** 334 (1968).

78. S. Keller, M. M. Levi, and I. Mandl, *Arch. Biochem. Biophys.*, **132,** 565 (1969).

79. S. Seifter and P. M. Gallop, *Abstr. Int. Collagen Symp., Velka Karlovice Czechoslovakia, Collagen Currents*, **4,** 40 (1963).

80. H. Saxl and D. A. Hall, *Cowdry's Atherosclerosis,* H. T. Blumenthal, Ed., Charles C Thomas, Springfield, 1968, p. 141.

81. N. Kornfeld-Poullain and L. Robert, *Bull. Soc. Chim. Biol.*, **50,** 759 (1968).

82. S. M. Partridge, D. F. Elsden, J. Thomas, A. Dorfman, and A. Telser, *Biochem. J.*, **93,** 30c (1964).

83. B. C. Starcher, S. M. Partridge, and S. F. Elsden, *Biochem. J.*, **6,** 2425 (1967).

84. D. A. Hall, *J. Atherosclerosis Res.*, **1,** 173 (1961).

85. A. I. Lansing, T. B. Rosenthal, M. Alex, and E. W. Dempsey, *Anat. Record,* **114,** 555 (1952).

86. I. Banga, W. A. Loeven, and G. Romhanyi, *Acta Morphol. Acad. Sci. Hung.,* **13,** 385 (1965).

87. R. L. Walford, D. L. Mayer, and R. B. Schneider, *Arch. Pathol.,* **72,** 158 (1961).

88. A. I. Lansing, M. Alex, and T. B. Rosenthal, *J. Gerontol.,* **5,** 112 (1950).

89. A. I. Lansing, T. B. Rosenthal, and M. Alex, *J. Gerontol.,* **5,** 211 (1950).

90. A. I. Lansing, M. Alex, and T. B. Rosenthal, *J. Gerontol.,* **5,** 314 (1950).

91. A. I. Lansing, E. Roberts, G. B. Ramasarma, T. B. Rosenthal, and M. Alex, *Proc. Soc. Expt. Biol. Med.,* **76,** 717 (1951).

92. T. J. Bowen, *Biochem. J.,* **55,** 766 (1953).

93. D. A. Hall and J. W. Czerkawski, *Biochem. J.,* **80,** 128 (1961).

94. D. Bagdy, P. Tolnay, J. Borsy, and K. Kovacs, *Magy. Tud. Akad. Biol. Orvosi. Tud. Oszt. Kozlemeni,* **11,** 277 (1960).

95. D. A. Hall, *Old Age in the Modern World,* R. E. Tunbridge, Ed., Livingstone, Edinburgh, 1954, p. 165.

96. G. N. Graham, Thesis, Leeds University (1958).

97. E. Cacciola, R. Cristaldi, and R. Giustolisi, *Arch. Ricmabio.,* **27,** 681 (1963).

98. S. Y. Yu and H. T. Blumenthal, *Federation Proc.*, **19,** 19 (1960).

99. M. D. Ridge and V. Wright, *Brit. J. Dermatol.*, **77,** 639 (1965).

100. J. W. Czerkawski, Ph.D. Thesis, Leeds University (1960).

101. D. A. Hall, *Arch. Biochem. Biophys.*, **67,** 366 (1957).

102. H. Saxl, *Proc. Fourth Internal. Cong. Gerontol.*, 67, (1957).

103. W. A. Loeven, *Acta Physiol. Pharmacol. Neerl.*, **9,** 44 (1960).

104. W. A. Loeven, *Acta Physiol. Pharmacol. Neerl.*, **14,** 475 (1967).

105. I. Banga and J. Balo, *Biochem. Biophys. Acta,* **40,** 367 (1960).

6

Physical and Mechanical Properties of Elastin

DEBI P. MUKHERJEE* and ALLAN S. HOFFMAN†

Chemical Engineering Department, Massachusetts Institute of Technology, Cambridge, Massachusetts

Elastin, a fibrillar protein present in the connective tissues and blood vessels, is responsible for carrying out the elastic functions of tissue systems. The loss of elasticity, due to the different tissue diseases and normal aging, has motivated researchers from diverse areas to investigate

* Presently with the Research Division, The Goodyear Tire and Rubber Company, Akron, Ohio.
† Now at the Department of Chemical Engineering and Bioengineering Program, University of Washington, Seattle, Washington.

the structure of elastin. The sources of elastin primarily are ligamentum nuchae and aorta (blood vessel) from humans and animals with elastin contents of 60–70% (wt.) and 30–40% (wt.) respectively. The methods of purification are:

1. Autoclaving at 15 psig for 45 min [1].
2. NaOH (0.1 M) treatment at 95°C for 45 min [1].
3. Treatment with the enzyme collagenase [2].
4. Treatment with 90% formic acid at 45°C for 72 hours [3, 4].

There are considerable variations in physical properties and nature of the surfaces of elastin obtained from various sources [5, 6], even though their amino acid analyses are the same. Elastin contains 90% nonpolar amino acids and 10% polar amino acids. Purified elastin in water exhibits the physical properties of cross-linked rubber in contrast to its brittle glasslike state when dried. It is this rubberlike property of elastin that makes it so interesting for polymer physicists to examine the applicability of the kinetic theory of rubber elasticity.

6.1   PRINCIPLES OF RUBBER ELASTICITY

6.1.1   Closed Systems

If one takes any material (e.g., protein, plastic, rubber, glass, metal) which is at equilibrium with its surroundings and applies a force such that there is a differential change in length, one may write the first law of thermodynamics for the specimen as the system, describing this differential disturbance from equilibrium as

$$dE = dQ - dW$$
$$= T \, dS - \left(P \, dV - f \, dL - \sum_i \mu_i \, dn_i - \gamma \, dA \right) \qquad (1)$$

(where the terms have their usual meanings). If the system is closed, that is, if there is no exchange of mass with the surroundings, all dn terms will be zero. One may also assume that the $\gamma \, dA$ term is negligible and, neglecting gravitational, kinetic, magnetic, and electrical effects, the expression simplifies to

$$dE = T \, dS - P \, dV + f \, dL \qquad (2)$$

Applying the definition of Helmholtz free energy,

$$F \equiv E - TS$$

$$dF = dE - T\,dS - S\,dT$$

$$= -S\,dT - P\,dV + f\,dL \tag{3}$$

from which

$$f = \left(\frac{\partial F}{\partial L}\right)_{T,V,n} = \left(\frac{\partial E}{\partial L}\right)_{T,V,n} - T\left(\frac{\partial S}{\partial L}\right)_{T,V,n} \tag{4}$$

Thus the force of retraction may be broken up into two major contributions, one due to internal energy changes and representing the changes in inter- and intramolecular energies on stretching and the other due to entropy changes, representing the change in the order or degree of randomness of the molecules. It is desirable to measure each of these terms separately in order to interpret the effects of an applied force on the molecular structure of the material. Then from (3) it may be seen that

$$\left(\frac{\partial S}{\partial L}\right)_{T,V,n} = -\left(\frac{\partial f}{\partial T}\right)_{L,V,n} \tag{5}$$

so that

$$\left(\frac{\partial E}{\partial L}\right)_{T,V,n} = f - T\left(\frac{\partial f}{\partial T}\right)_{L,V,n} \tag{6}$$

Thus if a series of experiments is run in which the force required to keep a specimen at fixed length is measured as a function of temperature, if the specimen volume is kept constant, and if there is no exchange of mass with the surroundings, one may, derive $(\partial S/\partial L)_{T,V,n}$ from the slope of the force-temperature (or $f - T$) curve and $(\partial E/\partial L)_{T,V,n}$ from the intercept at $T = 0°K$. In order to keep the specimen at constant volume it would be necessary to test under pressure, and since this is inconvenient, the question is raised as to whether measurement of $f - T$ curves at constant pressure (e.g., 1 atm) would be as useful. It may be similarly shown that under constant pressure

$$f = \left(\frac{\partial G}{\partial L}\right)_{T,P,n} = \left(\frac{\partial E}{\partial L}\right)_{T,P,n} + P\left(\frac{\partial V}{\partial L}\right)_{T,P,n} - T\left(\frac{\partial S}{\partial L}\right)_{T,P,n}$$

$$\cong \left(\frac{\partial E}{\partial L}\right)_{T,P,n} - T\left(\frac{\partial S}{\partial L}\right)_{T,P,n} \tag{7}$$

and

$$\left(\frac{\partial S}{\partial L}\right)_{T,P,n} = -\left(\frac{\partial f}{\partial T}\right)_{L,P,n} \tag{8}$$

$$\left(\frac{\partial E}{\partial L}\right)_{T,P,n} = f - T\left(\frac{\partial f}{\partial T}\right)_{L,P,n} \tag{9}$$

where the same assumptions are made for the constant volume system and where $P(\partial V/\partial L)_{T,P,n}$ is assumed to be small relative to the other terms in (7).

The terms that are desired, $(\partial E/\partial L)_{T,V,n}$ and $(\partial S/\partial L)_{T,V,n}$, are related to the experimentally derived quantities, $(\partial E/\partial L)_{T,P,n}$ (intercept of $f - T$ curve at constant L, P, n) and $(\partial S/\partial L)_{T,P,n}$ (slope of this same curve) as follows:

$$\left(\frac{\partial S}{\partial L}\right)_{T,V,n} = \left(\frac{\partial S}{\partial L}\right)_{T,P,n} - \left(\frac{\partial S}{\partial V}\right)_{T,L,n}\left(\frac{\partial V}{\partial L}\right)_{T,P,n} \tag{10}$$

$$\left(\frac{\partial E}{\partial L}\right)_{T,V,n} = \left(\frac{\partial E}{\partial L}\right)_{T,P,n} - \left(\frac{\partial E}{\partial V}\right)_{T,P,n}\left(\frac{\partial V}{\partial L}\right)_{T,P,n} \tag{11}$$

It may be shown that for a rubbery material $(\partial V/\partial L)_{T,P,n}$ is very small relative to the other terms. However, $(\partial S/\partial V)_{T,L,n}$ and $(\partial E/\partial V)_{T,L,n}$ represent the changes in degree of molecular randomness and in intra- or intermolecular energies as the volume is, say, increased slightly while the sample is maintained at constant length, temperature, and composition. The resultant small increases in local "free volume" may permit large changes in the conformational entropy of network chains and in the intermolecular interaction energies where, for example, the latter is inversely proportional to the sixth power of distance for Van der Waals' interactions. Thus

$$\left(\frac{\partial f}{\partial T}\right)_{L,V,n} \neq \left(\frac{\partial f}{\partial T}\right)_{L,P,n}$$

Fortunately, it has been shown (Equation 7) that if the $f - T$ experiment for a closed system is run at constant pressure and constant extension ratio, $\alpha(= L/L_0$, unstretched length at any temperature/stretched length at that same temperature), then

$$\left(\frac{\partial f}{\partial T}\right)_{L,V,n} \cong \left(\frac{\partial f}{\partial T}\right)_{\alpha,P,n} \tag{12}$$

Based on these principles it has been found that for many typical rubbers extended to moderate elongations

$$T \left(\frac{\partial S}{\partial L}\right)_{T,V,n} \gg \left(\frac{\partial E}{\partial L}\right)_{T,V,n}$$

Thus the force of retraction is mainly entropic in nature or

$$f \cong -T \left(\frac{\partial S}{\partial L}\right)_{T,V,n}$$

Statistical mechanics have been used (Equation 7) to calculate the entropy decrease in an idealized network of chains under stress, and the following stress-strain relationship for an "ideal rubber" has been derived:

$$\frac{F}{A_0} = \frac{\rho RT}{M_c} \left(\alpha - \frac{1}{\alpha^2}\right) \tag{13}$$

where A_0 = unstretched cross-sectional area
ρ = dry density of rubber
R = gas constant
M_c = average molecular weight between cross-links

If the rubber is swollen with a solvent but there is still no exchange of matter with the surroundings when the sample is stretched, this becomes

$$\frac{f}{A_{01}} = \frac{\rho RT}{M_c} v_2^{-1/3} \left(\alpha - \frac{1}{\alpha^2}\right) \tag{14}$$

where A_{01} = unswollen, unstretched cross-sectional area
v_2 = volume fraction of rubber in the swollen specimen

Thus measurement of the extent of swelling and of the elongation for any particular applied force will permit calculation of M_c, a useful and interesting molecular parameter of the network.

6.1.2   Open Systems

When a force is applied to a swollen rubber specimen, it is possible that there will be an exchange of mass with the surroundings, such that the $\sum_i \mu_i \, dn_i$ terms in Equation 1 can no longer be neglected. This problem has been recognized in the literature [8, 9, 10] and Oplatka, Michaeli, and Katchalsky [9] have derived the equations for an open system at constant pressure where the solvent and specimen together were taken as the system (thus reducing the open system to a "closed" system, which now includes the surroundings). However, if we continue to take the specimen as our system then the following modified equations for the constant volume condition may be derived [11].

$$\left(\frac{\partial F}{\partial L}\right)_{T,V,\text{open}} - \sum_i \mu_i \left(\frac{\partial n_i}{\partial L}\right)_{T,V,\text{open}}$$

$$= \left(\frac{\partial E}{\partial L}\right)_{T,V,\text{open}} - T\left(\frac{\partial S}{\partial L}\right)_{T,V,\text{open}} - \sum_i \mu_i \left(\frac{\partial n_i}{\partial L}\right)_{T,V,\text{open}} \qquad (15)$$

where it can be shown that

$$\left(\frac{\partial E}{\partial L}\right)_{T,V,n} = \left(\frac{\partial E}{\partial L}\right)_{T,V,\text{open}} - \sum_i \left(\frac{\partial E}{\partial n_i}\right)_{T,V,L} \left(\frac{\partial n_i}{\partial L}\right)_{T,V,\text{open}} \qquad (16)$$

and

$$\left(\frac{\partial S}{\partial L}\right)_{T,V,n} = \left(\frac{\partial S}{\partial L}\right)_{T,V,\text{open}} - \sum_i \left(\frac{\partial S}{\partial n_i}\right)_{T,V,L} \left(\frac{\partial n_i}{\partial L}\right)_{T,V,\text{open}} \qquad (17)$$

Recognizing that for each solvent component (superscript s here) in the surrounding medium

$$\mu_i \equiv \left(\frac{\partial F^s}{\partial n_i}\right)_{T,V,n} = \left(\frac{\partial E^s}{\partial n_i}\right)_{T,V,n} - T\left(\frac{\partial S^s}{\partial n_i}\right)_{T,V,n} \qquad (18)$$

Combining Equations 16, 17, and 18 with Equations 5 and 6 we obtain

$$\left(\frac{\partial E}{\partial L}\right)_{T,V,n} = f - T\left(\frac{\partial f}{\partial T}\right)_{T,V,\text{open}} - \sum_i \Delta \bar{E}_i \left(\frac{\partial n_i}{\partial L}\right)_{T,V,\text{open}} \qquad (19)$$

and

$$\left(\frac{\partial S}{\partial L}\right)_{T,V,n} = \left(\frac{\partial f}{\partial T}\right)_{L,V,\text{open}} - \sum_i \Delta \bar{S}_i \left(\frac{\partial n_i}{\partial L}\right)_{T,V,\text{open}} \qquad (20)$$

where

$$\Delta \bar{E}_i = \left[\left(\frac{\partial E}{\partial n_i}\right) - \left(\frac{\partial E^s}{\partial n_i}\right)\right]_{T,V,L,n_j\ldots} \qquad (21)$$

= the "partial molar isometric internal energy of rubber dilution" [9]

and

$$\Delta \bar{S}_i = \left[\left(\frac{\partial S}{\partial n_i}\right) - \left(\frac{\partial S^s}{\partial n_i}\right)\right]_{T,V,L,n_j\ldots} \qquad (22)$$

= the "partial molar isometric entropy of rubber dilution" [9]

Once again, as for the closed system, the constant pressure (1 atm) experiment is easier to perform, and Oplatka et al. [9] have derived the similar equations for this case

$$\left(\frac{\partial H}{\partial L}\right)_{T,P,n} = f - T\left(\frac{\partial f}{\partial T}\right)_{T,P,\text{open}} - \sum_i \Delta\bar{H}_i \left(\frac{\partial n_i}{\partial L}\right)_{T,P,\text{open}} \tag{23}$$

and

$$\left(\frac{\partial S}{\partial L}\right)_{T,P,n} = -\left(\frac{\partial f}{\partial T}\right)_{T,P,\text{open}} - \sum_i \Delta\bar{S}_i \left(\frac{\partial n_i}{\partial L}\right)_{T,P,\text{open}} \tag{24}$$

It can be seen that there are two new terms in Equations 19, 20, 23, or 24 which were not present in the closed system analysis. These must be evaluated (or eliminated) in order to obtain the desired $(\partial E/\partial L)_{T,V,n}$ and $(\partial S/\partial L)_{T,V,n}$ terms.

Hoeve and Flory [8] studied the elastic properties of ligamentum nuchae and showed that in a 30% glycol/70% water mixture $(\partial V/\partial T)_{L,P,\text{open}} \cong 0$ (as temperature rises, thermal expansion is counterbalanced by deswelling) and since

$$\left(\frac{\partial V}{\partial T}\right)_{L,P,\text{open}} = \left(\frac{\partial V}{\partial L}\right)_{T,P,\text{open}} \left(\frac{\partial L}{\partial T}\right)_{V,P,\text{open}}$$

where $(\partial L/\partial T)_{V,P,\text{open}}$ must be finite, they noted that $(\partial V/\partial L)_{T,P,\text{open}} \cong 0$. On the basis of this they have evidently assumed that the $(\partial n_i/\partial L)_{T,P,\text{open}}$ terms will be very small, since $(\partial V/\partial L)_{T,P,n}$ is very small for a rubbery material and

$$\left(\frac{\partial V}{\partial L}\right)_{T,P,\text{open}} = \left(\frac{\partial V}{\partial L}\right)_{T,P,n} + \sum_i \left(\frac{\partial V}{\partial n_i}\right)_{T,P,\text{open}} \left(\frac{\partial n_i}{\partial L}\right)_{T,P,\text{open}} \tag{25}$$

where the partial molar volume terms must be finite. They then arrive at the following approximation:

$$\left(\frac{\partial E}{\partial L}\right)_{T,V} \cong \left(\frac{\partial E}{\partial L}\right)_{T,P} = f - T\left(\frac{\partial f}{\partial T}\right)_{T,P}$$

where E refers to the sample phase plus solvent phase and f, P, V, and L refer only to the sample phase, an unusual choice of system in which the $(\partial E/\partial L)$ terms denote essentially a "closed" system while any $(\partial V/\partial L)$ terms denote an open system. It is not clear whether they have overlooked the possibility of glycol and water exchange with the surroundings (e.g., as suggested by Oplatka et al. [9] where the sum of the individual $\mu_i(\partial n_i/\partial L)_{T,P,\text{open}}$ terms could be finite) or whether they conclude that their choice of system plus the fact that the sum of the $(\partial n_i/\partial L)_{T,P,\text{open}}$ terms will be very small eliminates this consideration. They do state explicitly that "possible disproportionation of the two components between the two phases is of no consequence provided only that the diluent phase is present in large excess." In any case, it is not clear what part would be played by the collagen or mucopolysaccharide components in native ligamentum nuchae, with respect to the soption of glycol and water and in the resultant $\mu_i(\partial n_i/\partial L)_{T,P,\text{open}}$ terms. They are able to estimate $(\partial E/\partial L)_{T,V}$ from the approximation above, based on $f - T$ measurements at 1 atm. They conclude from tests that $(\partial E/\partial L)_{T,V}$ does not deviate from zero by more than 1% of the total force, for extensions up to 50% and for the temperature range between 0°C to 50.5°C. (See Fig. 6.2.)

However, it is desirable to work with the purified protein as the system, if at all possible, since the results would be easier to interpret. This is true when the material is elastin, resilin, keratin, collagen, and so on.

Indeed, if solvent systems were found for which the *individual* $(\partial n_i/\partial L)_{T,P,\text{open}}$ terms were each measured to be zero or very small, then the approximations of Hoeve and Flory would apply (as long as $(\partial V/\partial L)_{T,P,n}$ also remained small, which would be the case for elastic materials). If it can be shown that the force of retraction of a rubberlike protein is all entropic in nature, then one may use Equation 14 to calculate M_c for the particular protein immersed in the particular solvent system. In order to do this, one must measure the actual unswollen, unstretched cross-section (A_0) of the elastic fibers which sustain the stress, as well as the actual volumetric swelling of these fibers in the solvent environment (to obtain v_2). It should be mentioned that Equation 14 is really simplified and does not include the effect of temperature on the r.m.s. end-to-end distance of the random chain coils between crosslinks (i.e., the "front factor") or chain end corrections (e.g., see [12] for a discussion of these effects).

6.2   SWELLING BEHAVIOR OF ELASTIN

Elastin swells in various solvents without going into solution. The swelling behavior of elastin (purified from ligamentum nuchae) is shown

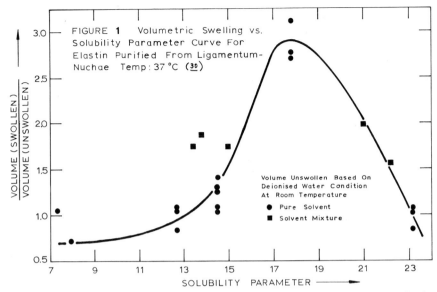

Figure 6.1. Volumetric swelling versus solubility parameter curve for elastin purified from ligamentum-nuchae; $T = 37°C$. (From Ref. 30).

in Fig. 6.1, where the degree of volumetric swelling in various solvents (e.g., formamide, formamide-water solutions, methanol, ethanol, butanol) was plotted against solubility parameter, λ. The extent of swelling increases with the solubility parameter of the solvent and reaches maximum at a particular solubility parameter value. The solubility parameter, defined as the square root of the molal heat of vaporization, measures the nature of interactions present in the solvent molecules. The maximum in the swelling curve of a cross-linked polymer represents the maximum compatibility with the solvent. Hence the solubility parameter of the polymer is presumed to be identical with that of the solvent showing such maximum [13]. Hence the solubility parameter of elastin from the swelling data is approximately 18 corresponding to the value for the solvent formamide. This solubility parameter, however, has contributions due to the polar, dispersion, and hydrogen-bonding forces.

The studies of Lloyd [14] and Partridge [15] have indicated qualitatively that elastin also swells in formic acid, lactic acid, thioglycollic acid, and aqueous solutions of sodium salicylate, thiourea, zinc chloride, and potassium iodide. Although elastin swells in these reagents, it is not soluble in any reagent without considerable degradation accompanying dissolution.

6.3   MECHANICAL BEHAVIOR OF ELASTIN

6.3.1   Stress-Strain Behavior of Impure Elastin

The study of the mechanical properties of elastin was first initiated by Meyer and Ferri [16] and Wohlisch [17], who attempted to measure the thermoelastic behavior of impure ligamentum nuchae. They found that above a certain threshold elongation the stress-strain curve rose steeply. They attributed this phenomenon to crystallization of elastin at higher elongation. However, the x-ray diffraction pattern of the stretched elastin did not show any sign of crystallinity [18]. So there remained contradictions between the results from thermoelastic behavior

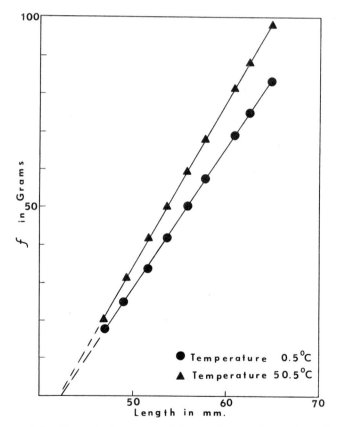

Figure 6.2.   Stress-strain curves of ligamentum nuchae. (From Ref. 8).

of elastin and x-ray results for a long time, until Hoeve and Flory [8] made a careful study of the stress-strain behavior of impure ligamentum nuchae in glycol-water mixture of glycol concentration of 30% (vol.). Their data, shown in Fig. 6.2, were measured at 0.5 and 50.5°C. They made a thermodynamic analysis of these stress-strain data by the method described in Section 6.1. They concluded from the analysis of their data that behavior of elastin fibers is very similar to an ideal rubber and the elasticity is essentially entropic in nature. They also indicated that the steep portion of stress-strain behavior at higher elongation is due to the elongation of collagen fibers.

6.3.2   Mechanical Properties of Blood Vessels

Since elastin is a major constituent of blood vessels, the study of mechanical behaviors of intact aorta or arteries has helped in gaining a great deal of information regarding the relative contributions of collagen, elastin, and smooth muscles. Some of the recent observations on the viscoelastic properties of intact blood vessels have been summarized in Table 6.1.

The relation of structure to function of the tissue of the walls of blood vessels has been very extensively reported by Burton et al. [27–29]. Models have also been suggested incorporating the contributions of each individual component (e.g. elastin, collagen, and smooth muscle) on the overall behavior of the arterial wall or aorta. However, the exactness of these models needs to be verified from a similar study of purified elastin or collagen or smooth muscle. The mechanical properties of purified elastin are little studied; a recent study by the authors will be considered here [30].

6.3.3   Stress-Strain Behaviors of Purified Elastin

Deionized Water

The equilibrium stress-strain behavior of elastin purified from ligamentum nuchae by a repeated autoclaving technique is shown in Fig. 6.3. The stress (based on original unstretched area) is plotted against $(\alpha - 1/\alpha^2)$. Although the plot is linear, as expected from the theory (see Section 6.1), there is a positive intercept, which is not expected from the relation shown in Equation 14. Therefore, the stress-strain behaviors at lower load levels are necessary to clarify the point, and the plot in Fig. 6.4 shows that indeed there are two regions in the stress-strain behavior of elastin. At the lower load region extensibility is high,

**Table 6.1 Viscoelastic Properties of Intact Blood Vessels
(A Selective Review of the Literature)**

Study	Material	Conclusions
Stress-relaxation behavior by application of step function of stretch [19]	Aorta and pulmonary artery of dogs	A mathematical model consistent with the stress relaxation curve was developed to show how to use the tension curves to measure a viscous, a series-elastic, and parallel-elastic constant unique for a given curve. The viscous and series-elastic constants were higher where muscle content was high and increased markedly when the muscle was contracted. The parallel-elastic constant was high when elastin was high and in the presence of contracted muscle, but independent of collagen content at moderate tension levels.
Stress relaxation by the application of circumferential stretch at various temperatures 0–70°C [20]	Aorta, pulmonary artery, as well as isolated collagen, elastin, and smooth muscle	Two crystalline polymers, collagen and smooth muscle have a negative force-temperature relationship and elastin has a positive relationship. Collagen differed from smooth muscle in its inertness to autonomic drugs and its elastic modulus. Intact arteries stretched slightly (2–20%) in the presence of phenylphrine behaved like smooth muscle, arteries stretched more (20–70%) behaved like elastin. At both strain levels, the tensions developed were compatible with *in vivo* pressure. Arteries stretched even more (>100%) comparable to 300 mm Hg, behaved like collagen.
Sinusoidal Loadings at low and at resonance frequencies [21]	Aorta of dogs	At frequencies below 1 Hz, the force registered was sinusodial with the same frequency as the stretch and lagged behind the strain at frequencies below 0.05 Hz. As frequencies rose above 1

Table 6.1 (*Continued*)

Study	Material	Conclusions
		Hz, the force amplitude rose to a maximum value, resonating at a frequency which was higher at higher initial strains. From the study it was shown under what condition there is negligible viscous loss, that is, collagenlike behavior and condition at which there is high viscous losses representing elastinlike or smooth musclelike behavior. Smooth muscle or elastin may be distinguished by the response to drugs or temperature.
Dynamic study [22]	Aorta of dog	Measurements in 14 aortic regions demonstrated a smooth transition from one aortic region to another and provided numerical values for parameters suitable for use in mathematical models of aorta. Moduli and viscous losses were functions of mean tension level, of location along the aorta, and of direction (longitudinal versus circumferential). Absolute dynamic moduli were generally higher and viscous losses lower in the longitudinal than in the circumferential direction. Anisotropy was minimal near the aortic valve and increased down the aorta, reaching a maximum near the abdominal aorta. In addition, in the less anisotropic regions near the heart, the moduli increased only slightly with increasing mean tension level, thereby resembling elastin which is in high concentration. In the more highly anisotropic regions lower down the aorta, the moduli increased with increasing tension level,

Table 6.1 (*Continued*)

Study	Material	Conclusions
		thereby resembling the anisotropic collagen which is in high concentration. Moreover, the positive temperature—modulus relationship of elastin was characteristic of isotropic aorta, while the negative temperature-modulus relationship of collagen was found in anisotropic aorta.
Light and electron microscopic study followed by relationship of pressure with wall thickness [23]	Abdominal aorta	The mechanical properties and organization of the collagen and elastic components of the aortic media indicate that the wall normally functions as a "two phase" material. At and above physiological pressures, circumferentially aligned collagen fibers of high tensile strength and relatively high modulus of elasticity, bear most of the stressing force. Elastin lamella and fibrile of relatively low modulus of elasticity distribute stressing forces uniformly.
Static and dynamic tests to correlate pressure, radius, and wall thickness [24]	Thoracic aorta, abdominal aorta, femoral and carotid artery	The increase in modulus with increase in pressure depends both on the elastic properties of collagen, elastin and muscle within the arterial wall and on their arrangement and linkage. The study supports the view that the collagen and elastin in arterial wall function in parallel. It is claimed that the difference between thoracic aorta and other vessels between 60 and 100 mm Hg pressure is due to the great preponderance of elastin over collagen (2:1) that has been found in thoracic aorta and to a relatively loose collagen network. Thus elastin, collagen, and smooth muscle in arteria wall carry some load at all internal pressures.

Table 6.1 (*Continued*)

Study	Material	Conclusions
Dynamic testing [25]	Dog arteries	The dynamic elastic modulus abruptly increases between 0 and 2 Hz and then the dynamic modulus remains essentially constant. The phase angle between pressure and dilation is very small and alters with frequency in a manner different from that predicted by the use of simple mechanical model containing elastic and viscous elements.
Histological examination [26]	Thoracic aorta of dogs and cats	The number of lamellar units in the media of mammalian aorta is very nearly proportional to aortic radius regardless of species or variations in measured wall thickness. The findings suggest that elastin lamella and the contents of its adjacent interlamellar zone represent the unit of structure and function of the mammalian aortic wall.

hence modulus value is low (i.e., the slope of the plot in Fig. 6.4).

This region is presumed to represent the initial "slack" present in the nonwoven fabriclike structure of elastin. Beyond this low load region at the intermediate load level the load is carried by the peptide chains of elastin, and in this region the theory of rubber elasticity is applicable. The situation is, however, complicated by the void spaces in elastin produced during purification process; consequently the area of cross-section needs to be corrected for this void content. An estimate of void spaces was obtained from the study of diffusion of NaCl, from presoaked samples of elastin in NaCl solution, when transferred to deionized water. The data from such diffusion study are shown in Fig. 6.5.

The breaks in the curve in the case of purified elastin are assumed to be due to the presence of two types of void regions; (a) macrovoid and (b) microvoid. The absence of any break in the impure sample (ligamentum nuchae) confirms the view that the breaks are due to the

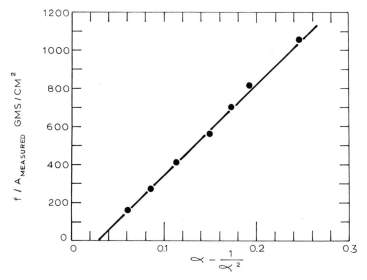

Figure 6.3. Elastic deformation of purified elastin (sample 112) E2YB at 37°C in deionized water. (From Ref. 30).

presence of voids. The void volumes are estimated as (a) macro-void = 28% (vol.) and (b) microvoid = 19% (vol.). Partridge [31] in his studies of diffusion of the sugar molecule through the elastin fiber preparation (which did not have macrovoids) has indicated the void content of 17–20% which agrees with the value of microvoids estimated from this salt diffusion study.

Finally, the value of M_c (molecular weight between cross-links) was calculated using Equation 14, with corrected area of cross-section. The M_c has an average value of 4,000. There is considerable variations in the M_c values (at 95% confidence limit the variation is $\pm 12\%$) even though the samples were obtained from the animals of the same age (2 years). This variation probably represents variability in the biological specimens.

Different Nonaqueous Solvents and Their Aqueous Solutions

The equilibrium stress-strain behaviors of purified elastin in different nondegrading solvent media are summarized by presenting the calculated M_c values in Table 6.2. Corresponding values of degree of swelling are also shown. The values of M_c were also obtained by measuring the stress-strain behavior of elastin after the solvents were leached out by deionized water. The data in Table 6.2 clearly show that M_c values after pretreatment with solvents are different from the value of M_c

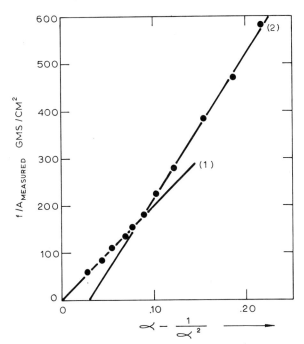

Figure 6.4. Elastic deformation of elastin in low and intermediate load regions. (From Ref. 30).

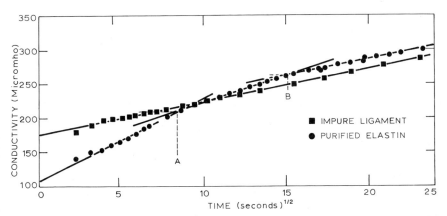

Figure 6.5. Leaching of NaCl from elastin into deionized water. (From Ref. 30).

235

for untreated elastin in deionized water measured as 4000. The degree of reversibility is defined as the closeness of the value of M_c in deionized water after leaching out the solvent to the value of M_c in the untreated condition in deionized water. Thus different degrees of irreversibility are seen in the values reported in Table 6.2. The reasons for this kind of irreversible change have not been clearly understood. However, the controlled experiments showed that stress effects, sudden change in swelling pressure during leaching operation, and the time effect in this relaxation process of the chains to come back to the original native state, do not initiate this kind of irreversible change in elastin. The uv absorption of the solvent media in which samples of elastin were equilibrated does not show any sign of elastin being dissolved, but the possibility remains that these solvents might cause scission to the network without producing

Table 6.2 M_c **Values in Different Solvents**

| | | | M_c **Value** | |
| | | | In Solvent Media | In Deionized Water After Leaching Out Solvent |
Solvent Media	Concentration, vol. %	Volumetric Swelling $\left[\dfrac{\text{Swollen Volume}}{\text{Unswollen Volume}}\right]$		
Formamide and its	100	2.7	5350	4150
aqueous solution	65	2.1	5700	4150
	44	2.0	7200	7100
	5	1.2	5900	5000
Methanol and its	100	1.2	4550	5650
aqueous solution	88.0	1.2	4550	—
	64.0	1.2	3900	4250
	32.0	1.2	5000	—
	9.0	1.2	5400	—
Ethanol and its	100	1.0	830	3700
aqueous solution	79.0	1.0	2800	—
	64.0	1.0	2800	—
	32.0	1.0	3900	—
	9.0	1.0	3600	—
Butanol and its	100	1.0	<830	7300
aqueous solution	8.0	1.0	6200	—
	6.0	1.0	6200	—
Water	100	1.0	4000	(4000)

any appreciable amount of dissolved products. It is possible, however, that a new equilibrium arrangement of the peptide chains different from the native one has been imposed by these solvents, hence the peptide chains in elastin are unable to come back to the same native state even when the solvents are leached out.

The swelling behavior reported in Table 6.2 is interesting, since the solvents may be divided into two categories based on their swelling effect on elastin: (1) good swelling agent and (2) poor swelling agent. However, in each group of solvents the M_c values increase, indicating that these solvent systems have a loosening effect on the structure of elastin. To gain some insight into the nature of secondary forces of interactions which are disrupted by these solvents, M_c values were correlated with the solubility parameter. Instead of using the overall solubility parameter, the individual solubility parameter value due to polar, δ_p, dispersion, δ_d, and hydrogen bonding, δ_H, are used. A technique has been suggested by Hansen [32] to calculate these individual solubility parameter values of pure solvents. The values for solvent mixtures were calculated using the following relationship (where ϕ = volume fraction and V = molar volume):

$$\delta_{\text{mixture}} = \sum_i \frac{\delta_i \phi_i V_i}{\phi_i V_i} \qquad \text{for} \quad \delta_p, \delta_d, \text{ or } \delta_H \text{ of the mixture}$$

Plots of M_c versus δ_p, δ_d, and δ_H show that maximum value of M_c for each solvent group lies between 6000 and 7000 and the overall solubility parameter value between 18 and 19, as reported from swelling data. (See Section 6.2.) These values indicate that once they meet certain contributions of polar, dispersion, and hydrogen-bonding forces which are probably the reflections of the nature of interactions in elastin, these solvent systems are able to increase the M_c values. The role of hydrophobic bond in the secondary forces in elastin has been well demonstrated in the studies of alkaline hydrolysis of elastin powder exposed to different alcohol systems [33]. The system consisted of the mixture of aqueous solution—of $1M$ KOH and methanol plus higher alcohols keeping $H_2O/MeOH + ROH = 8/2$, where ROH represents the higher alcohols. The data in Fig. 6.6 showed an increase in weight percent dissolved with increase of nonpolar chains in the alcohol, that is, the effectivity of dissolution is in order of isoamyl > alcohol > n-butanol > n-propanol > ethanol. Based on the correlation of rate of degradation with increasing chain length of aliphatic alcohol, it was suggested that the three-dimensional conformation of the peptide chains of elastin is such that the hydrophobic amino acid residues interact with each other in

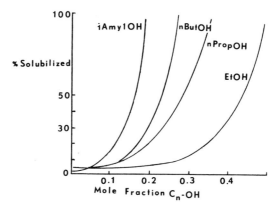

Figure 6.6.   The effect of alcohols at different chain lengths on the rate of alkaline hydrolysis of elastin. (From Ref. 33).

turtleshell-like structure which makes the peptide bonds inaccessible to other molecules or other ions. They also suggested that the hydrophobic forces are responsible for the strong chemical resistance of elastin; the hydrophobic forces cause the water molecules to arrange around the aliphatic chains in clusters. This reorganization of the solvent in the vicinity of the fibers accompanied the considerable high negative entropy and they suggest that this is the basis of the entropic elasticity as shown by the fibers of elastin.

6.4   PHYSICAL MODEL OF ELASTIN

Partridge [34, 35] has suggested a model of elastin in which he assumes a globular structure connected by the demosine cross-linkages. It was shown experimentally that four lysine groups condense to give desmosines, *in vitro* studies. During the biosynthesis of desmosine cross-linkages *in vivo*, the situation requires four lysine containing chains to come close together in such an orientation so as to produce one desmosine cross-linkage. Partridge has suggested that this requires an exact geometrical arrangement similar to a globular protein. He has examined his model by studying the diffusion of different sized sugar molecules and glycols and concluded from this study that elastin fibers are like gels containing pores of about 32 Å in diameter or a structure consisting of rods of about 16 Å in diameter which carry hydration water to the extent of 0.2–0.25 g water per g of dry protein. The swelling and stress-strain behavior of elastin suggest the peptide chains are present in an associated form showing rubberlike elastic behavior. This would require the peptide chains having a conformation similar to random coil as expected for an elastomer. In fact, Piez [36] in his review pointed out the possibility that elastin fibers were initially composed of identical units in a regular order, but that during or after cross-linking a process similar to denaturation converted the structure to the randomly coiled cross-linked network of chains similar to an elastomer. The x-ray data also suggest that there is no apparent order in the structure similar to globular unit. The study of differential thermal analysis of elastin powder shows also an absence of ordered structure of elastin [30]. The isotropic swelling of elastin in different solvents is consistent with this view. However, the highly hydrophobic nonpolar amino acids compel the peptide chains to exist in an associated form in order to expose minimum nonpolar surface area in contact with external polar water. These water molecules around the hydrophobic part of the peptide chains are more structured compared to bulk water molecules. The hydrophilic groups are partially buried inside the associations of peptide chains. This association of peptide chains exerts both inter- and intrachain interactions, and these interactions affect the cross-linking structure [30]. In addition to these, the covalent cross-linkages are present and some of the compounds responsible in cross-linking of elastin have been isolated. These cross-linking compounds are demosine, isodesmosine, and lysinonorleucine. It has been shown that the synthesis of these compounds occur in following steps [37–39]:

1. Deamination of ϵ-amino group of specific lysine residue along the polypeptide chain leading to the formation of adipic semialdehyde.

2. Three aldehyde residues either on different chains or on the same chain together with a fourth intact lysine condense to form the carbon and nitrogen skeleton of desmosines. In the case of lysinonorleucine after the first step of deamination the adipic semialdehyde reacts with ϵ-amino group of lysine of the same chain or other chain forming an intermediate base which is finally reduced to lysinonorleucine.

Thus the possibility cannot be ruled out that the compounds as aldols or Schiff bases or their condensation products might act as cross-linkages in elastin in addition to the compounds already isolated. Franzblau and Lent [40] recently have been able to isolate some of the decomposable intermediates by reducing the elastin with sodium borohydride prior to hydrolysis. They have found evidences for the presence of Schiff-base intermediate and α-amino adipic semialdehyde in elastin. The possibility of the presence of additional compounds derived from lysine acting as cross-linkages, has been emphasized by a recent study by Smith and his co-workers [41] who isolated from Cu-deficient pigs a soluble protein resembling matured elastin in amino acid compositions without the desmosines. This protein is supposed to be the precursor of the matured elastin or soluble elastin in uncross-linked form. The soluble form of elastin contains about 42 lysine residues as opposed to 18 equivalent residues per 1000 residues in matured elastin in cross-linked form. This difference of 24 lysines could not be accounted for in the process of biosynthesis of cross-links. Hence there is strong possibility of presence of other types of cross-linkages in elastin. In addition to these covalent cross-linkages, there are effects due to hydrogen bonding and hydrophobic interactions. Once these secondary forces of interactions are reduced to minimum, the value of M_c is around 7000 which is probably due to covalent cross-links [30].

ACKNOWLEDGMENTS

The authors wish to thank Mr. R. M. Pierson of Research Division, The Goodyear Tire and Rubber Company, for his assistance in preparing the manuscript.

REFERENCES

1. S. M. Partridge, et al., *Biochem. J.* **61,** 21 (1955).
2. E. J. Miller, et al., *J. Exptl. Med.,* **123,** 1097–1108 (1966).
3. A. L. Lewis and R. S. Jones, *Stain Technol.,* **26,** 85 (1951).
4. G. M. Haas, *AMA Arch. Pathol.,* **34,** 807 (1939).
5. F. S. Labella, *Arch. Biochem. Biophys.,* **93,** 72 (1961).
6. F. G. Lemox, *Biochem. Biophys. Acta,* **3,** 170 (1949).
7. P. J. Flory, *Principles of Polymer Chemistry,* Cornell University Press, Ithaca, N.Y., 1953.
8. C. A. J. Hoeve and P. J. Flory, *J. Amer. Chem. Soc.,* **80,** 6523 (1958).
9. A. Oplatka, I. Michaeli, and A. Katchalsky, *J. Polymer Sci.,* **46,** 365 (1960).
10. A. Oplatka and A. Katchalsky, *Makromol. Chem.,* **92,** 251 (1966).
11. A. S. Hoffman, *A Critical Evaluation of the Applicability of Rubber Elasticity Principles to Structural Proteins such as Elastin,* (to be published in 1970 as part of a book based on the Battelle University of Washington Biomaterials Conference at Battelle Memorial Institute, Seattle, Wash., November 1969).
12. P. Meares, *Polymers, Structure and Bulk Properties,* Van Nostrand, London, 1965.

13. L. R. G. Treolar, *The Physics of Rubber Elasticity*, 2d ed., Oxford University Press, 1958.
14. D. J. Lloyd, et al., *Trans. Faraday Soc.*, **44**, 441 (1948).
15. S. M. Partridge, et al., *Biochem. J.*, **61**, 21 (1955).
16. K. H. Meyer and E. Farri, *Arch. Ges. Physiol. Pfugers*, **238**, 78 (1936).
17. T. Wohlisch, et al., *Kolloid-Z.*, **104**, 14 (1943).
18. W. T. Astbury, *J. Internat. Soc. Leather Trades' Chemists*, **24**, 69 (1960).
19. J. T. Apter, *Circulation Res.*, **19**, 104 (1966).
20. J. T. Apter, *Circulation Res.*, **21**, 901 (1967).
21. J. T. Apter, *Circulation Res.*, **22**, 393 (1968).
22. J. T. Apter, Paper presented at 21st ACEMB at Houston, Texas, November 18–21, 1968.
23. H. Wolinsky, *Circulation Res.*, **15**, 400 (1964).
24. D. H. Bergel, *J. Physiol.*, **156**, 445 (1961).
25. D. H. Bergel, *J. Physiol.*, **156**, 458 (1961).
26. H. Wolinsky, S. Glagov, *Circulation Res.*, **20**, 99 (1967).
27. A. C. Burton, *Physiol. Rev.*, **34**, 619 (1954).
28. M. R. Roach and A. C. Burton, *Can. J. Biochem. Physiol.*, **35**, 618 (1957).
29. A. C. Burton and R. H. Stinson, *J. Physiol.*, **153**, 290 (1960).
30. D. P. Mukherjee, *The Viscoelastic Properties of Elastin*, Sc.D. Thesis in Chemical Engineering, M.I.T., January 13, 1969.
31. S. M. Partridge, *Biochem. Biophys. Acta*, **140**, 132 (1967).
32. C. M. Hansen, *J. Paint Technol.*, **39**, No. 511, 104 (1967).
33. L. Robert, et al. *Bull. Soc. Chim. Biolog. Extrait du Tome*, **4**, 759 (1968).
34. S. M. Partridge, D. F. Elsden, and J. Thomas, *Nature*, **197**, 1297 (1963).
35. S. M. Partridge, *Biochem. Biophys. Acta*, **140**, 132 (1967).
36. K. A. Piez, *Ann. Rev. Biochem.*, **37**, 557 (1968).
37. C. Franzblau, F. M. Sinex et al., *Biochem. Biophys. Res. Commo.*, **21**, 575 (1965).
38. E. J. Miller, G. R. Martin, and K. A. Piez, *Biochem. Biophys. Res. Commun.*, **17**, 248 (1964).
39. S. M. Partridge, D. F. Elsden, and J. Thomas, *Nature*, **197**, 1297 (1963).
40. C. Franzblau and R. Lent, *Symposium on Structure, Function, and Development of Proteins*, Brookhaven National Laboratory Symposium No. 20, 1968 (in press).
41. D. W. Smith, N. Weissman, and W. H. Coranes, *Biochem. Biophys. Res. Commun.*, **31** (3), 309 (1968).

7

Cross-links in Elastin and Collagen*‡

FRANK S. LABELLA, Ph.D.†

*Professor of Pharmacology and Therapeutics, University of Manitoba,
Faculty of Medicine, Winnipeg, Manitoba, Canada*

Collagen and elastin are the two major fibrous proteins of connective (supporting) tissues and each serves a distinctive mechanical function.

* Investigations by the author were supported by the Medical Research Council of Canada, the Canadian Arthritis and Rheumatism Society, the Manitoba Heart Association, and the American Heart Association.
‡ Literature review completed in December, 1969.
† Medical Research Associate, MRC of Canada.

Collagen fibers are almost inextensible but possess high mechanical strength. Elastin, in most areas of the body, contributes little to mechanical support and stability of a tissue but permits its reversible deformation. It is present in greatest amount in those tissues subjected to regular, periodic deformation, such as in arteries, lung, and skin. The molecular structure and the supramolecular organization of the fibrous proteins both constitute the basis for their characteristic participation in tissue construction and function. Collagen exists as bundles of parallel fibers each composed of linear aggregates of polypeptide chains; covalent and noncovalent bonds result in marked cohesion between the triple-helical polypeptide chains which comprise the collagen monomeric unit, and between the triple-chain molecules. These interchain bonds prevent any significant longitudinal displacement between adjacent chains. Elastin is generally believed to be a true elastomer, composed of aggregates of randomly coiled, linear peptide chains laterally connected by covalent links; when hydrated the molecule may be stretched to two or three times its resting length but then returns to its original configuration, by virtue of the strategically placed cross-links and relatively weak interchain hydrogen bonds.

The presence of cross-links between the peptide strands in collagen and elastin molecules results in fibrous proteins which are relatively insoluble, resistant to enzymic degradation and, therefore, removed from the utilizable metabolic pool of the body. Cross-linked, mature collagen and elastin are permanent structural elements, the bulk being metabolically inert. As a consequence, they exhibit cumulative degenerative changes produced by constant physical and chemical insult. Control of cross-linking reactions in these proteins determines the rate, duration and extent of their deposition in tissues. Mechanisms for inhibition of cross-link formation appear to be required during those phases of tissue growth and development in which tissue remodelling and reorganization occurs with extensive resorption of collagen and elastin. Furthermore, the formation or scission of cross-links is implicated in a number of physiological and pathological processes involving the fibrous proteins. Thus, elucidation and possible control of mechanisms for the deposition and removal of collagen and elastin hinges on a knowledge of the chemical types, molecular dimensions, and number of cross-links.

7.1   STRUCTURE AND CHEMICAL COMPOSITION OF ELASTIN AND COLLAGEN

7.1.1   Defining Elastin and Collagen

One cannot describe with much confidence the chemical composition, including the cross-links, of elastin or collagen without indicating the tissue source and methods of purification of the proteins. One fraction of collagen, the so-called soluble collagen, can be isolated, purified, and its chemical composition reproducibly determined. Indeed, amino acid sequence studies are in progress on the individual peptide chains which constitute the fundamental unit, the triple-helical collagen molecule [1, 2]. It is for this easily prepared fraction that relatively well-established cross-links (see Section 7.2) have been described for collagen; these links are covalent *intramolecular* cross-links (those within a triple helix). It appears that *intermolecular* cross-links (those covalently joining peptide chains of one triple-helix to another) are the more significant from the aspect of collagen fiber stability, accumulation, maturation, and deterioration. It is this highly cross-linked molecular network referred to as "insoluble" collagen that resists attempts to characterize it, because it is often covalently associated with other substances, including proteins, and solubilization procedures tend to degrade its primary structure.

Elastin has been generally defined in large part on the basis of its relative insolubility. It represents the tissue residue following the extraction, hopefully, of all other proteins and nonproteins. A reasonably reproducible protein component with rubberlike properties can be prepared from many tissues by this procedure. Elastin, then, defines this protein preparation which can be characterized chemically, physically, and morphologically. However, even with elastin prepared from the same tissue and from animals of the same species, sex, and age, controversy exists among laboratories on several issues. Disagreement exists on the exact amino acid composition, whether or not hydroxyproline is a component of the protein itself, and whether or not nonprotein elements, such as lipids, carbohydrates, and noncharacterized fluorescent and pigmented materials, are covalently linked to the protein. The controversy becomes magnified when dealing with very young, very old, or unfamiliar tissues. For example, conventional purifications, indeed, apparently any extractive procedure, fails to provide from aortas of individuals over 80 years of age a protein fraction corresponding to purified elastin prepared from younger individuals [3]. One interpretation for this observation is that surrounding proteins and other substances gradually become covalently joined to elastin, and by age 80 essentially no part of the elastic fiber is unaffected. Conversely, embryonic or fetal elastin-rich tissues are completely dissolved when purified in a manner similar to that from adult aortas [4, 5].

Ideally, the types and number of cross-links in a protein are ascertained from the amino acid composition, the amino acid sequence, amino acid functional groups, and the characterization of atypical amino acids or other unknown components in the pure, soluble protein. In the case of the connective tissue proteins, this ideal has been reasonably achieved only for soluble collagen. Of course, for elastin prepared from a source such as beef ligamentum nuchae or from aortas of animals and non-senescent humans, certain components can be characterized and reasonably assigned to the primary structure of the protein, as in the case of the desmosine cross-links (see Section 7.2.1). However, even with elastin preparations of consistent composition, some uncertainty exists as to the possible extraction of substances which are essential to the functional integrity of the elastin molecule. Conceivably, certain aspects of the primary structure of elastin, including cross-links, may be altered or destroyed during purification procedures which are known to be too severe for proteins in general.

Thus, confusion about the chemistry and physical properties of collagen and elastin, and of collagenous or elastic structures, has often come about because of the failure to recognize that a single purification procedure is inadequate for the isolation of the proteins from all tissues. In the discussion that follows, attempts will be made to point out the problem of purity where applicable.

7.1.2   Some Features of the Chemistry of Elastin and Collagen

The chemistry of collagen and elastin has been extensively considered in a number of books, review articles and symposia (see References). Only a summary of some important characteristics of these two proteins, pertinent to the present discussion, will be presented here.

Amino Acid Composition in Relation to Tertiary Structure and Fiber Formation

The fundamental feature of structural supporting proteins is their relative chemical inertness. The mature, weight-bearing and/or stressed connective tissue fibers must be highly resistant to circulating enzymes and reactive metabolites. Therefore, the evolution of structural proteins of animals has resulted in molecules with an extremely high proportion of amino acids with aliphatic side chains. These amino acids in the peptide backbone of proteins tend to be generally unreactive. The high proportion of nonpolar amino and imino acids also contribute to formation of certain peptide bonds, relatively rare in nonstructural proteins, which are not attacked by most proteases but rather by specific enzymes, designated collagenases and elastases in the case of the proteins under present consideration. Thus, glycine, alanine, proline, valine, leucine, and isoleucine, constitute about 90% of the amino acids in elastin; nonreactivity of amino side chains is essential in this protein in which peptide chains must be free to slide past one another during extension and relaxation.

However, it should be pointed out that the rubberlike properties of elastin are evident only when the protein is hydrated. Dried elastin from ligamentum nuchae or rat aorta is brittle and cannot be stretched. Hydrophilic groups apparently play some role in the physiological elasticity of elastin. In collagen, where the polypeptide chains are fixed relative to one another, these same amino acids make up a lower proportion of the total, amounting to about 60%, still an unusually high proportion relative to nonstructural proteins. Glycine in collagen from all sources is invariably present as one-third of the total amino acid residues, because of the essential role of this amino acid in establishing the helical structure of the native polypeptide chains.

LaBella and Vivian [4] found for human aortic elastin that there was considerable variation in the absolute amounts of glycine, alanine, or proline from individual to individual. However, these three amino acids always totalled exactly two-thirds of the amino acids in elastin from a given aorta; the amount of each of the other amino acids was constant for all individuals. This finding indicates that the requirements for the primary structure of elastin are quite rigorous; functional integrity of the molecule is maintained only when genetic alterations are limited to a few substitutions among three amino acids with nonpolar side-chains.

Collagen and elastin are unique among animal proteins in that they contain a hydroxylated form of proline, hydroxylation taking place after the amino acid has been incorporated into a large peptide precursor. Although the hydroxyproline in elastin has been considered by some to reflect contamination with collagen, several studies on highly purified elastin [4, 6] leave little doubt that this amino acid is an inherent part of the elastin molecule. The hydroxyproline content of collagen varies widely from species to species and is correlated with certain physical properties of the molecule, such as thermal stability [7]; others [8], however, have suggested that the total imino acid content (proline plus hydroxyproline) is a better correlate. The content of hydroxyproline in elastin from various species is only one-fifth to less than one-tenth that in the collagens, and constitutes about 7, 10, and 20 residues per 1000 total residues in elastin from human aorta [4], bovine ligamentum nuchae [5], and chick aorta [5], respectively. Whereas this amino acid is known to play a significant role in the helical structure of collagen through hydrogen bond formation, its role in elastin is uncertain. Because the denaturation temperature of fibrous proteins is well correlated with the total imino acid content, Harrington and Rao [9] concluded that a collagen species with less than 130 to 140 pyrollidine residues per 1000 total amino acid residues would be expected to be unstable and transform from a helix to a random coil about $0°$. Elastin, then, exists as a random coil, because it may be regarded as a collagen species, with glycine as every third residue and a low content of pyrollidine residues [10].

Hydroxylysine is another unique amino acid found in collagen but not elastin and is concerned with glycosylation and interchain covalent cross-linking; hydroxylation of lysine appears to render the amino acid more susceptible to enzymic conversion to aldehyde precursors of certain cross-links (see Section 7.2.1).

Collagen exists in a given tissue in two forms: that fraction which can be extracted in a native form by nonhydrolytic methods such as extraction with cold neutral salt solution or dilute acid buffers, and another fraction which is dissolved only by procedures which break down its primary structure and/or interchain cross-links. Presumably, collagen in the native solid phase exists as an aggregate of triple-helical molecules and as a continuous spectrum of molecules with varying degrees of both intramolecular and intermolecular cross-links. Veis and co-workers [11] and Piez and his group [12, 13] believe that cross-linking reactions within and between collagen molecules are simultaneous and continuous processes, involving the same functional groups. This hypothesis is supported by the work of Gross [14], who found that lathyrogen administration (see Section 7.3.1) to animals inhibited formation of intra- and intermolecular cross-links. Cold neutral salt or acid buffers solubilize the apparently least cross-linked components. Procedures which disrupt noncovalent linkages, that is, denaturation, result in only single chain, α, or double chain, β, components; the neutral salt extract (see Fig. 7.1) tends to contain a higher proportion of α chains than does acid extracts. The amount of "soluble" collagen obtained depends upon the tissue concerned, and is in greatest abundance in young animals.

Veis [15] uses the term "intact collagen" to refer to the fraction, freed of polysaccharide and other noncollagen constituents of the ground substance, containing the native array of polymerized (cross-linked) tropocollagen (triple-helix monomer) units plus noncross-linked, "soluble," tropocollagen monomers. Removal of the "soluble", nonincorporated collagen by nonhydrolytic and nondenaturing procedures yields "matrix collagen" [15], consisting of the network of tropocollagen units covalently linked to each other and to noncollagen components (Fig. 7.1). The high stability of matrix collagen is probably due to the fact that each tropocollagen unit is linked to adjoining units by several covalent links. In gelatin derived from matrix collagen, all possible combinations of covalently linked components have been obtained; however, γ111 and γ222 are present in larger amounts than would be predicted

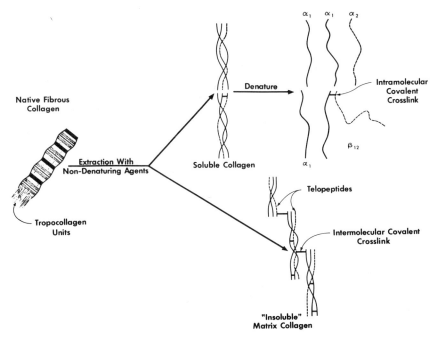

Figure 7.1.

by random intramolecular and intermolecular cross-linking. From renaturation studies, Veis concluded that γ111 arose largely from intermolecular cross-linking of molecules with their ends aligned and γ222
from cross-links formed between staggered molecules [16]. He proposes
a model for the packing of tropocollagen monomers into fibrils and suggests that the molecular alignment favors α1 to α2 and α2 to α2 linkages.

Veis [15] postulates that collagen from two different tissues may have
the same number of cross-links, but in one case the collagen may be
almost entirely extracted with dilute acid and in the other be present
entirely as matrix collagen. The acid soluble collagen would contain
only intramolecular cross-links, thereby preventing the same reactive
groups from forming the intermolecular links characteristic of relatively
insoluble matrix collagen. He also suggests that selective conversion of
the noncross-linked collagen precursors to acid soluble collagen or to
matrix collagen may depend upon removal from potential cross-linking
sites on the protein of tissue-specific "protecting" moieties, or by the
incorporation of tissue-specific "bridging" moieties.

Schmitt and co-workers [17–19] reported that treatment of purified collagen with proteases cleaved peptides which protruded from the triple-helix body of the molecule. These peptides are rich in polar amino acids, including tyrosine, and constitute an estimated 1 to 5% by weight of the soluble collagen. They believed that one or more of the peptides were located at the ends of each polypeptide chain and referred to these nonhelical regions as "telopeptides" (Fig. 7.1). These workers [20, 21] believed that there were numerous telopeptides branching from along the length of the helical portion of the molecule as well as at the end. Piez [22] criticized this work and cited Bornstein and Piez [23] who found only one protease-susceptible region per α chain. Bornstein et al. [24] provided good evidence that the aldol condensation, intramolecular cross-link (see Section 7.2.1) is located at the amino terminal, nonhelical portion of the molecule. Rubin et al. [18, 19] showed that after treatment of soluble collagen with pepsin, the number of single chains increased and of double chains decreased, indicating removal of the cross-linking regions of the chains. They put forth the attractive hypothesis that telopeptides in collagen, which participate in intramolecular cross-linking, may modulate fiber deposition, stabilization, and removal. Alteration of load-extension curves (see Section 7.1.2) of tendon fibers following treatment with trypsin has been attributed to degradation of a noncollagen stabilizing matrix [25]; in retrospect, it seems more likely that the cross-linked telopeptides were removed by the enzyme, leading to a loss of intermolecular associations. The action of endogenous proteases in removing telopeptides before or after cross-link formation would appear to be a very efficient mechanism for controlling collagen deposition and resorption. Rubin et al. [18, 19] suggest that telopeptides may also participate in pathological, immunological, and aging processes involving collagen.

Staining of native collagen fibrils with heavy metals reveals a characteristic banding, with a repeating period of about 640 Å, when viewed electronmicroscopically. It has been proposed that the light bands in native collagen correspond to regions where the aligned macromolecular chains are bonded together, since the introduction of artificial cross-links with glutaraldehyde, benzoquinone, or tetrazobenzidine increased the size of these bands [26].

Just as the tropocollagen monomer units constitute the fundamental building blocks for collagen fibrils which aggregate to form massive tendons, filmy organ coverings, or dense fibrous mattings, so do fine elastin fibrils serve as the basic units for a variety of elastic structures. Fine, undulating, relatively sparse elastic fibers occur in skin; some ligaments are composed of large, densely packed elastic fibers in parallel, and even the concentric sheets of elastin found in arterial walls are apparently the result of networks of fibrils in close apposition. Ayer [27] believes that the apparent amorphous matrix of aortic lamellae and of large fibers is an artifact of nonresolution of submicroscopic, closely applied fibrils. The factors which determine the degree of fibril deposition and packing, presumably through intermolecular cross-linking reactions, understood to some extent for collagen, are completely unknown for elastin.

Cross-linking Density Estimated by Physical Parameters

Wiederhorn et al. [28, 29] developed an equation based on the stress-strain behavior of thermally denatured collagen (kangaroo tail tendon), whereby the average molecular weight of the polymer chain between junction points may be calculated:

$$F = \left(\frac{RTpv_2^{1/3}}{M_c}\right)\left(\alpha - \frac{1}{\alpha^2}\right) \tag{1}$$

where f is the retractive force per unit area, T the absolute temperature, R the gas constant, α is the ratio of stretched length to initial length, p the density of the dry elastomer, v_2 the volume fraction of the elastomer in the composition which is being stretched, and M_c the average molecular weight between cross-links. It is pointed out that the equation assumes no change in internal energy with length, that is, there are no intramolecular attractive or repulsive forces between the various groups on the chains, hence, the basis for carrying out measurements above denaturation temperature. Under the conditions defined by Wiederhorn et al., M_c is apparently a measure of covalent bonds rather than of hydrogen bonds or salt linkages.

M_c, determined for three different batches of tail tendons, believed to be an almost pure preparation of collagen, was estimated to be about 55,000 ± 5,000, or about 594 amino acid residues [28]. The calculated value was little influenced by media with different dielectric constants or by different temperatures, indicating the covalent nature of the cross-links. Gotte et al. [30] examined strips of alkali-purified ligamentum nuchae, presumably pure elastin, and obtained a value of 3,000, or about 30 residues between cross-links. It is of interest that Andersen [31], using the same technique, arrived at values of between 2,800 and 3,800 for various preparations of resilin, a rubberlike protein from the wing hinges of the locust.

A modified form of Equation 1 was put forth by Flory [32] for extension under load. Bowes and Cater [33] estimated M_c for kangaroo tail tendon to lie between 190,000 and 375,000, or 0.4 to 0.8 cross-links per triple helix. The method is assumed to measure only the cross-links in excess of those necessary to give a continuous polymer network, a minimum of 2 intramolecular and 1 intermolecular cross-links. Therefore, it was estimated that there are between 3.4 and 3.8 cross-links per three chains of the tropocollagen unit of 300,000 molecular weight. Cater [34] cross-linked kangaroo tendon collagen with a variety of aldehydes and obtained values for M_c as low as 4,000, indicating a maximum potential number of cross-links of 10 to 12 per tropocollagen molecule. The data of Bowes and Cater are at variance with those of Wiederhorn and Reardon [28] for the same type of material, although the discrepancies may be due to differences in pre-test histories of the kangaroo tail tendons. The estimates of Bowes and Cater for M_c of artificially imposed cross-links were similar by the physical method and by direct chemical estimation of the cross-linking material.

Mohr and Bendall [35] estimated M_c for purified collagen from tail tendon and skeletal muscle of the rat, using extension under load. Skeletal muscle collagen was much less soluble than tendon collagen, and estimates of 8,000 to 24,000 for the former and 100,000 to 300,000 for the latter were obtained. The higher degree of cross-linking for muscle collagen was supported by estimates obtained from other physical parameters. These workers pointed out that the covalent links are thermostable and probably not of the aldimine-type (Schiff base) (see Section 7.2.1) which are thermolabile. Also, tendon collagen fuses with muscle collagen and a drastic increase in cross-links in the continuous collagenous structure takes place over just a few millimeters. In another study [36] M_c for rat tail tendon gave a constant value of about 50,000 in animals aged 3 to 24 months. On the other hand, defatted, salt-extracted skin strips gave values of about 200,000 at 3 months of age, progressively decreasing to about 40,000 at 24 months. These results suggest that the rate of apparent aging of collagen varies from tissue to tissue in the same animal. However, these findings are at apparent variance with those of others which indicate changes in tail tendon with age to be compatible with increased cross-linking of the constituent proteins (see Section 7.3.2).

Another commonly used procedure considered to reflect the degree of cross-linking in collagen and elastin is thermal contraction (expressed generally in terms of the "shrinkage temperature"). Contraction of a fiber occurs at that temperature at which the crystallinity or ordered cohesive forces break down, that is, the melting point. Covalent bonds in general are not affected by temperatures required for contraction, although Schiff bases may be degraded (see Section 7.2.1). Gustavson [37] showed that thermal contraction of collagen fibers is related to the number of cross-links present in the protein, but is also influenced by many other factors, such as the weave of the fibril network and the structure of the fiber which includes noncollagen components. There is little doubt that artificial cross-linking, such as "tanning", elevates the shrinkage temperature for purified collagenous tissues [34, 38, 39], and is due to covalent cross-link formation. However, Jackson [40] points out that, considering the variations in thermal contraction of tissues from the same individual and the multiplicity of factors influencing the reaction, the one or two degree changes observed with aging must be interpreted cautiously. There is uncertainty as to whether these changes occur in the collagen molecule itself. Mohr and Bendall [35] measured the tension produced during thermal contraction of rat tail tendon and skeletal muscle collagen; the latter developed a higher tension and maintained it at a temperature above 100°, whereas the tension of tail tendon decreased at temperatures above 80°. This study indicated the presence of more cross-links in muscle collagen, as did extension under load studies referred to previously.

Measurement of tensile strength, defined as the maximum load the fiber can bear without rupturing, is another frequently used technique for assessing the degree of cross-linking. Generally, tanning and aging of collagenous and elastic tissues result in increased tensile strength, compatible with increased covalent cross-linking. However, this physical parameter, is also influenced by a variety of factors due to the inherent complexity of strips of tissue.

For a more detailed consideration of the physical properties of macroscopic collagen fibers, interpreted in relation to the molecular structure of collagen, see Elden [41].

Fluorescence and Pigmentation

Elastin.   Elastic fibers, sheets, or lamellae have long been noted by histologists to be autofluorescent when illuminated with ultraviolet light. Highly purified elastin is also visibly brilliantly fluorescent [3, 42, 43]. Elastin is yellow, and an easily oxidized pigmented material can be separated from acid hydrolysates of the protein [44,45]. A fatty aldehyde has been reported to be associated with elastin [46, 47] and has been considered to contribute to the fluorescence of the protein. Recent studies (Thornhill, unpublished), however, indicate that extraction of alkali-purified elastin with hot pyridine removes the fluorescent lipid and the extracted elastin is still brilliantly fluorescent. The pronounced swelling of elastin that occurs in pyridine may permit removal of lipid confined within the fiber. Dityrosine (see Section 7.2.2), although intensely fluorescent, is present in elastin in amounts too small to account for the fluorescence of the protein [48, 49]. Neither the desmosines nor the typical amino acids found in proteins can account for the intense fluorescence of elastin, which is characterized by a maximum emission and activation near 405 and 340 nm, respectively.

Chromatography of acid hydrolysates of elastin resolves several unknown yellow, fluorescent fractions [44, 45]; whether the several components represent a family of chemically related compounds or are degradative products of one parent substance remains to be determined.

LaBella [50] and Walford et al. [51] found that most of the fluorescence and color of elastin remained associated with the undigested, nondialyzable fraction after prolonged incubation with elastase. Thornhill (personal communication) reports similar findings with the use of elastase followed by pronase. LaBella postulated that the large unattacked fragment is extensively cross-linked and resembles enzyme resistant, artificially cross-linked, or "tanned", proteins. Partridge et al. [52, 53] digested elastin sequentially with elastase, papain, aminopeptidase, and carboxypeptidase and attempted to isolate the cross-linked portions of the protein; by molecular sieve techniques, large yellow, fluorescent peptides were isolated. These observations suggest that the fluorescent component(s) is a cross-linking species in elastin.

The yellow, fluorescent components isolated from hydrolysates of elastin darken with exposure to air, adhere tenaciously to Dowex-50 ion-exchange resin, and are adsorbed on charcoal, properties highly indicative of aromatic compounds. LaBella [3, 42, 43] suggested that tyrosine and phenylalanine-derived quinones would have the spectral characteristics and chemical reactivity exhibited by the unknown compounds in elastin. He also pointed out similarities to the cuticle-hardening substances in certain invertebrates. Tanning of cuticle proteins appears to take place by polyphenols and quinones secreted by specialized gland cells. A cross-linked protein fragment has not been isolated and covalently-linked peptide chains identified. However, detection of circulating polyphenolic compounds and their deposition and subsequent "toughening" of the cuticular protein are convincing circumstantial evidence for the presence of cross-linking aromatic compounds. Furthermore, tanning by quinones is an effective, widely-used procedure in the leather industry [55]. Quinones, produced from aromatic compounds by oxidative processes, are extremely reactive and could easily combine with a number of functional groups protruding from the surface of the protein. The products formed from the reaction of quinones with amino acids or proteins *in vitro* have been characterized [56, 57].

Evidence for the formation of the pigment in elastin (and in another apparently fibrous connective tissue, an alkali-soluble protein) from tyrosine was obtained by LaBella and co-workers [48, 49]. They labelled elastin in chick embryo aortic cultures with tyrosine-C^{14} and examined the distribution of C^{14} among components separated during amino acid analysis of acid hydrolysates. In addition to C^{14} in tyrosine, a small amount of label was found in dityrosine and much more in the NaOH wash used to regenerate the Dowex 50 column. Among several protein fractions labelled with tyrosine-C^{14} in tissue culture, hydrolysates of only elastin and the alkali-soluble protein, presumably derived from microfibrils (see Section 7.1.2) yielded significant radioactivity in the column-wash fraction. It is of significance that only these two proteins were found to contain dityrosine. These workers suggested that dityrosine is an intermediate, because it disappears from maturing elastin. Support for this suggestion was the tentative identification of traces of trityrosine in elastin and the alkali-soluble protein [58].

These observations are compatible with the hypothesis that tyrosine residues in elastin (and perhaps free tyrosine derived from circulating tissue fluid) are polymerized to a reactive cross-linking species. LaBella et al. [43] made additional observations which agree with this concept: for example, ultraviolet irradiation of purified elastin caused a loss of tyrosine, a corresponding increase in fluorescence at wavelengths identical to those of the native protein, and an increase in yellow pigmentation. Irradiation of tyrosine solutions produces identical effects. Also, elastin was labeled with I^{131} under conditions in which only tyrosine rings are expected to be iodinated, the protein was irradiated with ultraviolet light and I^{131} labeled fluorescent products isolated.

Thornhill (unpublished results) hydrolyzed bovine ligamental elastin and fractionated the products, both under reducing conditions. Three yellow, fluorescent ampholytes were resolved, and neither the hydrolysate nor the isolated components had darkened. On the basis of the properties of the isolated compounds, Thornhill considers that quinonelike complexes with amino acids might be involved.

Collagen.   Collagen in tissues or in purified form has long been noted to be fluorescent under ultraviolet light. Brown et al. [59] examined several human tissues and reported that fluorescence was absent from collagen in fetuses or stillborn, at one year of age was extremely weak, but beyond age four years was very intense. Uterine collagen, on the other hand, showed weak or no fluorescence in individuals under 45 years, but was intensely fluorescent in older women. These findings may be related to the observations that dry, purified soluble collagen is not visibly fluorescent, in contrast to gelatin derived from highly cross-linked matrix collagen in rat skin [60]. Consden and Kirrane [61] reported that freshly purified acid soluble and neutral salt soluble collagen were very weakly fluorescent as determined fluorometrically, but, became highly fluorescent upon standing for a few days. Furthermore, fibers formed from the aggregated soluble collagen showed increased thermal stability with time, indicative of enhanced interchain interactions.

All of these observations suggest correlations among the extent of cross-linking, fiber and gel stability, and intensity of fluorescence.

Evidence for Carbonyl Compounds as a Source of Fluorescence and Cross-links.   LaBella (unpublished observations) believes that carbonyls are the major source of fluorescence in elastin and collagen. All carbonyl compounds examined, aliphatic or aromatic, aldehydes and ketones, showed activation/emission near 340/405 nm; furthermore, a progressive bathochromic shift occurs with these compounds. This spectral shift, absent in all fluorescent non-carbonyl compounds examined, is characteristic of solutions of elastin or collagen or their hydrolysates [43]. Aldehydes have been detected in both collagen and elastin, but it seems unlikely that the brilliant fluorescence of elastin is due to any large extent to the lysine-derived aldehydes which represent only one or two residues per 1000 total amino acids (see Section 7.2.1). As discussed previously, aromatic polymers may contribute significantly to the flourescence of elastin. Thus, the fluorescence characteristics of elastin and its isolated compounds are entirely compatible with the presence of carbonyl and quinonelike compounds referred to earlier.

Aldehyde groups were first detected in collagen by Landucci [62], and several aldehydic compounds have been isolated and characterized from soluble collagen. A cross-linking function has been demonstrated for certain aldehydes derived from lysine (see Section 7.2.1). Rosmus and Deyl [63] reported that each molecule of purified soluble collagen contains 2 moles of aldehyde and 2 to 3 moles of α-keto acids. Insoluble collagen was reported to contain 2 to 3 moles of aldehyde groups and 4 to 5 moles of keto acids. Ayad et al. [64], however, have denied the presence of α-keto acids in collagen and criticized previous reports on the basis of experimental technique.

Assuming that fluorescence in collagen is due to aldehydes and other carbonyl compounds, one can reasonably explain the differences in fluorescence intensity observed in different collagen preparations. Oxidation of ϵ-amino groups to aldehydes is the first step in cross-link formation involving lysine residues (see Section 7.2.1). Thus, soluble collagen which is very weakly fluorescent, might contain only a few chains having lysine-derived aldehydes. On the other hand, insoluble collagen is brilliantly fluorescent and highly cross-linked with aldehyde-containing intramolecular and intermolecular bonds. In addition, insoluble collagen may be covalently linked with quinones, aldehydes, and other carbonyl compounds in tissues.

Uterine collagen is unusual in that it is reported to be nonfluorescent until the menopause [59], and remains in a labile form for the relatively prolonged period of pregnancy. Woessner [65] has reviewed the literature on uterine collagen, and points out that the protein is unique in its rapid degradation and reabsorption in the postpartum period. Although it is not unusually soluble, the relatively low-thermal shrinkage temperature and elevated metabolic turnover indicate that uterine collagen contains fewer covalent cross-links than does collagen from other tissues of the same individual or older individuals.

Furthermore, decreased solubility and increased stability that occur with time in gels and aggregates of soluble collagen are correlated with increased fluorescence of the protein [61], perhaps due to nonenzymic oxidation of tyrosine, lysine ε-amino groups, or other reactive amino acid sidechains. Ultraviolet irradiation increases the stability of collagen and the characteristic carbonyl fluorescence [61, 66], and appears to promote the formation of covalent cross-links [66, 67]. Ultraviolet irradiation or *in situ* aging is accompanied by modification of tyrosine residues in collagen [43, 66, 68].

Increased fluorescence of purified human aortic elastin with age [3, 42, 69] or after ultraviolet irradiation [43] is associated with loss of tyrosine. Quinones produced from phenolic residues may account for the increased fluorescence produced artificially or during natural aging of collagen and elastin. The unusually high degree of fluorescence in elastin from the human neonate [69] may be due to extensive conversion of lysine ε-amino groups to aldehyde cross-link precursors. These cross-links are known to be formed for the most part in newly synthesized elastin.

Evidence for Elastin-Precursor Role of an Alkali-Soluble Protein

Keeley et al. [49] extracted from chick aorta and bovine ligamentum nuchae a protein which contained more dityrosine than did elastin, the only other mammalian protein known to contain this apparent cross-link. The tissues were freed of collagen by autoclaving in water and the dityrosine-containing protein fraction extracted with hot 0.1 N NaOH, the final step in the purification of insoluble elastin. The alkali-soluble protein was rich in polar amino acids, including cysteine and methionine (Table 7.1) and contained dityrosine in about 2 and 10 residues per 100,000 total amino acids from ligamentum and aorta, respectively.

Table 7.1   Amino Acid Composition of Alkali-soluble
Protein and Apparent Soluble Elastin[a]

| | Alkali Soluble Protein[b] | | Copper Deficiency[c] |
	Bovine Ligament	Chick Aorta	Soluble Elastin
Hypro	0	0	11.8
Asp	102	103	8.2
Thr	35	37	10.8
Ser	51	60	6.0
Glu	139	125	22.2
Pro	87	61	113
Gly	103	115	321
Ala	75	85	212
Val	73	69	127
Cys[d]	8	12	—
Met[d]	13	12	1.7
Ileu	38	43	16.8
Leu	81	93	48.2
Tyr	31	29	17.0
Phe	42	39	28.9
Lys	62	54	45.2
His	17	16	1.0
Arg	37	40	8.6
Des	0	0	0
Isodes	0	0	0

[a] Residues/1000 total residues.
[b] From Keeley et al. [49].
[c] From Smith et al. [77].
[d] Probably underestimates in these acid hydrolysates.

Keeley et al. [49, 58] showed, using tyrosine-C^{14} in aortic tissue culture, that dityrosine, as well as the apparent aromatic polymer previously described for elastin, were derived from tyrosine.

Ross and Bornstein [70] reported that dithioerythritol in 5 M guanidine extracted a protein from fetal bovine ligamentum nuchae which appeared to be derived from a microfibrillar component, observed electron microscopically at the periphery of an amorphous component of elastic fibers. These workers cite others who proposed that the microfibrils probably play a primary role in the morphogenesis of the elastic fiber, since their appearance always precedes elastin formation. The microfibrils extracted by Ross and Bornstein showed an amino acid composition very similar to that of the alkali-soluble protein of Keeley et al. [49]. The former workers reported that conventionally purified, that is, alkali-extracted elastin, lacks the peripherally oriented microfibrils as determined electron microscopically. Haust [71] and Karrer [72] believe that the microfibril forms a continuum with the elastic fiber and is, in fact, an integral part of morphologically defined elastin. Ross and Bornstein suggest that microfibrillar protein may form an ionic association with elastin, because of the apparent differences of charge resulting from their dissimilar amino acid compositions.

Keeley [5] purified elastin from aortas of chick embryos as young as six days and chicks as old as several months by treatment with 0.1 N NaOH at 98°C. Elastin prepared in this manner from chicks only a few days old and older showed the typical amino acid composition, except for small increases in the content of desmosines with increasing age. In animals less than five days old, however, the presumed elastin showed an increase in the content of polar amino acids with decreasing age (Table 7.2). In attempts to remove possible contaminating proteins in the elastin preparations from young and embryonic animals, repeated extraction with alkali was performed, but failed to yield a "typical" elastin substrate. Keeley concluded that elastin is formed from a pre-

Table 7.2 Amino Acid Composition of Elastin in the Developing Chick Aorta[a]

	10-Day Embryo	17-Day Embryo	80-Day Chick
Hypro	25	23	19
Asp	13	7.8	4.2
Thr	11	8.7	6.7
Ser	11	7.7	5.7
Glu	23	18	13
Pro	116	121	127
Gly	324	349	355
Ala	162	164	182
Val	161	171	172
Cys	tr.	0	0
Met	2.3	0.7	0
Ileu	22	20	19
Leu	64	55	51
Tyr	14	13	12
Phe	24	21	20
Lys	11	6.8	2.7
His	2.7	1.4	0.8
Arg	9	6.9	4.9

From Keeley [5].
[a] Residues/1000 total residues. Desmosine and isodesmosine were not resolved from ammonia in these nondeaminated hydrolysates.

cursor protein, the latter composed of a segment with an amino acid composition typical of mature elastin, in covalent linkage with a highly polar microfibrillar protein (Fig. 7.2). Presumably, the polar-protein portion is subsequently removed, perhaps by enzyme hydrolysis, having served to align the polypeptide chains of the immature elastin moiety for the subsequent imposition of stabilizing cross-links (Fig. 7.2). The liberated polar portion of the microfibril, thus, represents the alkali-soluble protein, which occurs in highest concentration in the youngest aortas.

According to this concept, elastin from very young embryos would be present largely as precursor protein, and when isolated in the conventional manner from these animals, would exhibit the most atypical amino

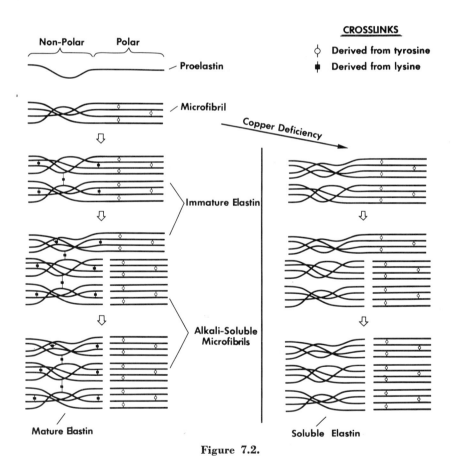

Figure 7.2.

acid composition. The amino acid composition of very young elastin is, in fact, an apparent composite of typical, mature elastin and the alkali-soluble protein. Thus, elastin from the ten-day old embryo is calculated to contain about 15% alkali-soluble protein, which is present as proelastin. The proportion of alkali-soluble protein in elastin diminishes to about 2% in the day-old chick. Several laboratories [73, 74] reported that isolation of elastin by extraction with alkali fails to yield a protein with the expected amino acid composition from fetal ligamentum nuchae. The atypical composition was attributed to contamination by a noncollagen protein rich in polar amino acids.

Apparent Soluble, Cross-link-Deficient Elastin from Copper-Deficient Animals

Keeley [5] proposes that elastin originates as part of a larger microfibrillar protein which is cross-linked by dityrosine and possibly higher tyrosine polymers as well. The polar portion of the precursor molecule is ultimately divorced from the rest of the molecule, presumably through the action of enzymic hydrolysis, and an immature form of elastin is produced, having the typical amino acid composition but being less extensively cross-linked. The polypeptide chains of this newly-formed elastin lack lysine-derived cross-links but may be stabilized and oriented by other types of cross-links, such as those formed from tyrosine residues. Subsequently, the desmosines are gradually formed in this immature elastin. In normal, developing animals hot 0.1 N NaOH fails to solubilize detectable amounts of protein with an amino acid composition characteristic of elastin. This observation indicates either that immature elastin, even prior to desmosine formation, is relatively insoluble, or that, at any given time, the pool of incompletely cross-linked, soluble elastin is extremely small. Or, the immature protein may have been removed during extraction with salt and by autoclaving.

Studies on copper-deficient or lathyrogen-treated (see Section 7.3.1) animals might help to elucidate some of these areas of uncertainty in elastin fibrogenesis. The formation of the desmosines appears to involve an amine oxidase which deaminates the side chains of lysine residues in the elastin molecule (see Section 7.2.1). The enzyme is inhibited by lathyrogenic agents or by the lack of copper, this trace metal apparently serving as a cofactor [75, 76].

Smith et al. [77] isolated a soluble protein from the aortas of copper-deficient pigs by extraction in the cold with phosphate buffer containing sodium chloride; upon standing at 23° the protein formed a coacervate. The amino acid composition of the purified soluble protein was remarkably similar to that typical of elastin, except that it contained no desmosines and had a much higher lysine content. In contrast to normal mature elastin which contains about five to eight residues of lysine per 1,000 residues, the soluble component in aortic elastin from copper-deficient pigs contains over 40 residues (Table 7.1).

From these observations, it appears that newly formed, that is, immature, elastin is deposited in the tissues in a readily extracted form and that achievement of its ultimate insoluble state depends upon the formation of desmosine cross-links. These particular cross-links must be formed soon after immature elastin has been laid down, because normal developing animals, in which there is active elastic fiber formation, yield no extractable elastinlike protein. The model of elastin formation (Fig. 7.2) proposes the stage at which copper deficiency interferes.

7.2 NATURE OF THE CROSS-LINKS IN ELASTIN AND COLLAGEN

To unequivocally establish the existence and chemical identity of an interchain cross-link, certain criteria should be satisfied. Ideally, an "H-peptide" should be isolated and shown to consist of segments of two chains joined by a covalent link. This task is a formidable one but appears to have been satisfied in the case of the aldol condensation product (see Section 7.2.1), isolated from the purified β component of soluble collagen. It should be established, also, whether a given cross-link is formed by interaction between side chains of amino acid residues in the protein or by incorporation of exogenous substances. Studies using radioactive lysine have demonstrated that the continual loss of labelled lysine per se from collagen and elastin parallels the appearance of label in lysine derivatives, the apparent cross-links. In the case of elastin, it is uncertain what proportion of the tyrosine residues preexisting in the protein contributes to formation of dityrosine and to the presumed aromatic polymers referred to earlier. A functional role for a putative cross-link is strongly indicated in experiments where the administration of agents known to prevent biosynthesis of the compound leads to significant changes in the stability and molecular size of the protein or its aggregates. Experiments of this type have been carried out for the lysine-derived cross-links which require prior enzymic conversion of side-chain amino groups. As for proof of chemical identity of isolated potential cross-links, in several instances this appears to have been achieved brilliantly by means of a variety of powerful physical and chemical techniques and, in some cases, biosynthesis and chemical synthesis of the compounds. Rapid advances over the span of a few years in the characterization of individual potential cross-links in connective tissue proteins and other proteins, has in many instances, been the product of investigations carried out in a single laboratory. It would be desirable, ultimately, to have independent confirmation of structure and function for each of the apparent cross-links.

7.2.1   Cross-links Involving Lysine Residues

Desmosine and Isodesmosine

A most fascinating chapter in the area of fibrous protein chemistry, and indeed in the field of protein chemistry, unfolded with the isolation by Partridge and his group [78] of two unique compounds from acid hydrolysates of purified elastin. It is apparent from their structures that they could be formed by the condensation of side chains of four lysine residues in elastin; each of three lysine residues reacting as an aldehyde derivative, that is, α-aminoadipic acid semialdehyde, and the fourth residue incorporated unaltered. Because these two isomeric components appear to be logical candidates for cross-links, joining as many

$$\begin{array}{ccc}
\text{N}_2\text{H} & & \text{N}_2\text{H} \\
\diagdown & \text{oxidative} & \diagdown \\
\diagdown \text{CH---(CH}_2)_4\text{---NH}_2 \xrightarrow{\text{deamination}} & \diagdown \text{CH---(CH}_2)_3\text{---CHO} \\
\diagup & & \diagup \\
\text{HOOC} & & \text{HOOC} \\
\text{Lysine} & & \alpha\text{-Aminoadipic acid semialdehyde}
\end{array}$$

as four different polypeptide chains, Partridge and his co-workers named them desmosine and isodesmosine (Fig. 7.3 and Fig. 7.4).

Verification that the desmosines are formed within the elastin molecule by condensation of four lysine residues was obtained from experiments in which ^{14}C-labelled lysine was supplied to tissues actively synthesizing elastin. The loss with time of ^{14}C-lysine per se corresponded to a progressive increase in ^{14}C-labeled desmosines [79–82]. Also, the total amount of lysine in newly formed elastin decreases while that of the desmosines increases in the chick [80], the human [4] and the ox [81] (see also Table 7.3). Mature elastin from all species thus far examined contains about three residues of desmosine plus isodesmosine (equivalent to twelve residues of lysine) per 1000 total amino acid residues. Intermediates, including the expected aldehyde derivatives of lysine, in the reactions leading to desmosine formation can be identified in elastin [75, 84, 85, 90].

Partridge and co-workers [75, 90] isolated from reduced elastin an apparent desmosine precursor, merodesmosine, consisting of the condensation of three lysine residues. They outlined the possible pathways

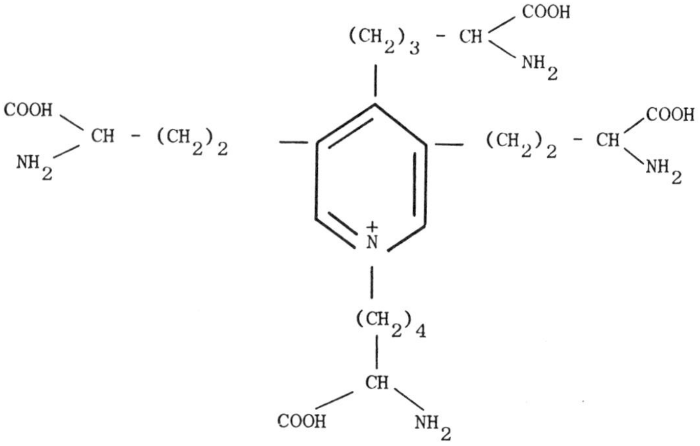

$(CH_2)_3 - CH \begin{smallmatrix} COOH \\ NH_2 \end{smallmatrix}$

$\begin{smallmatrix} COOH \\ NH_2 \end{smallmatrix} CH - (CH_2)_2$ —   — $(CH_2)_2 - CH \begin{smallmatrix} COOH \\ NH_2 \end{smallmatrix}$

$\overset{+}{N}$

$(CH_2)_4$

$CH \begin{smallmatrix} COOH \\ NH_2 \end{smallmatrix}$

DESMOSINE

Figure 7.3.

in the synthesis of this compound; it is an apparently slow process and involves several steps. Partridge points out that aldols and Schiff bases are first stages in cross-link formation in both collagen and elastin, and these early bonds are labile and reversible by a number of agents. He suggests that these nonpermanent bonds permit remodelling of con-

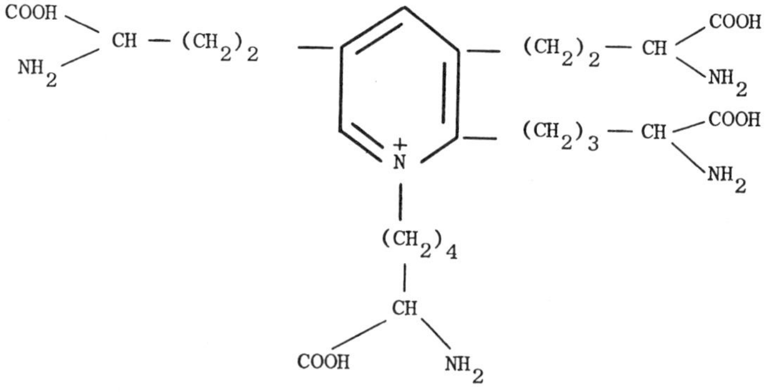

$\begin{smallmatrix} COOH \\ NH_2 \end{smallmatrix} CH - (CH_2)_2$ —   — $(CH_2)_2 - CH \begin{smallmatrix} COOH \\ NH_2 \end{smallmatrix}$

$(CH_2)_3 - CH \begin{smallmatrix} COOH \\ NH_2 \end{smallmatrix}$

$\overset{+}{N}$

$(CH_2)_4$

$CH \begin{smallmatrix} COOH \\ NH_2 \end{smallmatrix}$

ISODESMOSINE

Figure 7.4.

Table 7.3 Amino Acid Composition of Human Aortic Elastin from Fetuses and Individuals of Various Ages*

	14-Week Fetus	23-Week Fetus	33-Week Fetus	5-Month Infant	1 Year	5 Years	10 Years	51 Years
Hydroxyproline }	24[a]	9.0	11	9.3	6.7	6.6	4.9	5.8
Aspartic acid		3.7	2.5	2.5	3.4	3.9	3.5	4.3
Threonine		8.2	7.4	7.9	10	11	9.8	5.3
Serine		8.4	6.8	4.6	4.8	5.9	5.2	3.1
Glutamic acid	16	17	15	16	18	18	15	19
Proline	127	132	145	113	93	89	94	114
Glycine	293	330	297	323	321	318	325	314
Alanine	249	212	223	233	250	242	248	251
Valine	142	123	135	134	144	136	139	135
Isoleucine	24	27	25	25	24	28	23	23
Leucine	57	54	54	58	58	65	60	58
Tyrosine	7.2	11	19	20	18	23	20	19
Phenylalanine	27	27	26	25	23	25	24	22
Arginine	5.0 (9.5)[b]	4.2 (7.4)	1.2 (7.2)	1.4 (6.0)	4.8 (7.5)	4.1 (7.0)	3.8 (6.5)	3.8 (7.6)
Ornithine	4.5	3.2	6.0	4.6	2.7	2.9	2.7	3.8
Lysine	7.8	9.7	9.6	6.5	6.3	4.9	5.0	4.8
Desmosine[c]	3.2 (6.6)[g]	6.1 (10.4)	6.6 (12.3)	7.0 (12.4)	6.5 (11.2)	7.7 (13.3)	7.0 (12.2)	7.6 (14.4)
Isodesmosine[c]	3.4	4.3	5.7	5.4	4.7	5.6	5.2	6.8
U1[d]	3.1	0.7	1.6	0.7	1.9	2.4	3.2	
U2[e]								
U3[d]	0.4	0.9	1.0	1.2	1.4	1.6	1.4	1.1
U4[d,f]	9.6	8.3	2.5	0.7	0.3	0.4	0.2	0.2
U5[d,f]								
Recovery of nitrogen (%)	86	89	97	96	97	97	98	94

From LaBella and Vivian [4].

* Residues/1000 total residues.
[a] These amino acids were not resolved due to technical difficulty and are expressed as leucine equivalents.
[b] Arginine plus ornithine.
[c] Quarter residues, expressed as leucine equivalents × 1.09.
[d] Expressed as leucine equivalents.
[e] Not resolved in all preparations.
[f] U4 and U5 determined together.
[g] Desmosine plus isodesmosine.

265

nective tissue structures. Immature elastin from chick aorta contains about 4 residues of the semialdehyde of α-aminoadipic acid per 1000

$$
\begin{array}{c}
\text{NH}_2 \\
| \\
\text{COOH} \qquad\qquad \text{CH}_2\text{—CH}_2\text{—CH—COOH} \\
| \qquad\qquad\qquad\qquad\qquad\qquad\qquad\qquad\quad \\
\text{CH—(CH}_2)_4\text{—NH—CH}_2\text{—CH—CH=CH—(CH}_2)_2\text{—CH—COOH} \\
| \qquad\qquad\qquad\qquad\qquad\qquad\qquad\qquad\qquad\quad | \\
\text{NH}_2 \qquad\qquad\qquad\qquad\qquad\qquad\qquad\qquad\quad \text{NH}_2
\end{array}
$$

Merodesmosine

total amino acid residues [85]. Because desmosine formation is still incomplete in newly formed elastin, the aldehyde precursor is probably at its highest level here.

Although it appears highly unlikely that four lysine residues on a single polypeptide chain could achieve the necessary steric configuration for condensation into the desmosines, unequivocal proof that different chains are involved is not available. Fragmentation of desmosine and isodesmosine, without cleavage of peptide bonds, was achieved by reduction of the pyridinium rings with borohydride followed by treatment with permanganate-periodate [86]. This technique offers promise of providing information concerned with the number of peptide chains involved in desmosines formation. Partridge [75] expressed the view that, in order for the four lysine side chains to be brought into accurate apposition for the formation of the desmosine cross-links, the tertiary structure of the immature elastin must be globular. He also experimented with water-swollen elastin fibers packed in columns and showed that the column behaved as a molecular exclusion system when sugars and glycols were used as solutes [87]. The results suggested a structure which could be represented as short rods 16 Å in diameter and cylindrical pores about 30 Å in diameter [88]. However, the compatibility of the proposed globular components of elastin with the concept of randomly coiled aggregates of long chain polypeptide chains remains to be shown. Piez [22] has criticized this concept, and pointed out that the proposed model is self-contradictory, since globular proteins are believed to have rigid structures held together by interactions between chain segments, and elasticity requires the absence of interactions. Piez points out a possible compromise implied by Partridge [88], whereby the repeating globular units in immature elastin become denatured and linearly oriented following the insertion of cross-links. The desmosines have not been found in collagen and are apparently unique to elastin.

Lysinonorlecucine

Franzblau et al. [89, 91] identified in elastin another amino acid which is apparently derived from condensation of two lysine side chains, via reactions that probably also lead to desmosine formation. These workers established the structure of this compound by means of several techniques, including nuclear magnetic resonance, infrared and mass spectroscopy, and by its chemical synthesis.

$$
\begin{array}{ccc}
HOOC & & COOH \\
\diagdown & & \diagup \\
CH-(CH_2)_3-CH_2-NH-(CH_2)_4-CH & \\
\diagup & & \diagdown \\
HN_2 & & NH_2
\end{array}
$$

Lysinonorleucine

The lysine-derived aldehyde and postulated Schiff-base precursor of lysinonorleucine was subsequently identified in elastin by this same laboratory [92, 93]. Lysinonorleucine and its precursor are present in beef elastin in 1 residue per 1,000 and 1 residue per 4,000 total amino acid residues, respectively. Lysinonorleucine also appears to be unique to elastin, although other apparent cross-links formed by the union of two lysine side chains have been reported in collagen (Section 7.2.1).

Aldol Condensation Product

The structure of an apparent intramolecular cross-link in highly purified, mammalian soluble collagen was deduced by Bornstein and Piez [23] to be an aldol condensation product of two moles of α-aminoadipic acid semialdehyde. That the compound is derived from lysine was indi-

$$
\begin{array}{ccc}
HOOC & & COOH \\
\diagdown & & \diagup \\
CH-(CH_2)_2-C=CH-(CH_2)_3-CH & \\
\diagup & | & \diagdown \\
H_2N & CHO & NH_2
\end{array}
$$

Aldol Condensation Product

cated from experiments in which rats were given ^{14}C-lysine; the compound contained label, but not lysine per se. Reaction with aldehyde reagents resulted in products with the absorption-spectra characteristic of α, β-unsaturated aldehydes. Although Tanzer et al. [94] concluded that production of α, β-unsaturated aldehydes may be unrelated to cross-linking, Piez [22] rejected this notion. Piez bases his conclusion of a cross-linking function for the aldehyde on analysis of peptides produced from collagen β components (pairs of α chains linked covalently) by cyanogen bromide which cleaves peptide bonds involving methionine. Rojkind et al. [95, 96] supported the conclusion that the aldol product is formed from two residues of α-aminoadipic acid semialdehyde. They carried out experiments using [14]C- and ^{3}H-lysine in conjunction with the isolated, cross-linked peptide studies also by Bornstein and Piez [23]. Purified $\alpha 1$ and $\alpha 2$ chains of chick collagen did not contain the aldol condensate. The covalently-linked dimer, β12, contained one equivalent, thus supporting the intramolecular cross-linking role of the compound [97]. Piez [22] points out that, although lysine-derived aldehyde precursors of cross-links are localized to the N-terminal region of the individual collagen chains, other intermolecular cross-links must exist which involve a region, at least on one of the joined chains, remote from N-terminal. This assumption is based on the fact that collagen fibrils are formed, in part, from regularly staggered molecules.

Lent et al. [93] reported the presence of this same aldol condensation product in elastin, as determined by studies with ^{14}C-lysine in chick embryo cultures. They propose that this compound may serve a dual role in elastin: as an independent cross-link (4–5 residues/1000 amino acids) and as a precursor of the desmosine cross-links. They also identified 2–3 residues of α-aminoadipic acid semialdehyde per 1000 amino acids in elastin and demonstrated its formation from lysine and its rapid conversion to the aldol compound [84]. Citing Smith et al. [77] who isolated an apparent soluble elastin from copper deficient pigs containing a reported 42–45 residues, Lent et al. [92, 93] calculated that desmosine, isodesmosine, aldol condensate, lysinonorleucine, α-aminoadipic acid semialdehyde, plus four unaltered lysine residues account for 38–41 of the lysine residues in the apparent precursor protein.

Hydroxylysino-norleucine, Syndesine, and Schiff Bases

The aldol condensation product derived from lysine in collagen (see Section 7.2.1) is well established as an *intramolecular* cross-link. Tanzer [99] and Bailey et al. [100, 101] have presented evidence for the presence of chemically and thermally labile bonds which are apparently covalent *intermolecular* cross-links in collagen. Reduction of reconstituted native-type collagen fibrils with sodium borohydride produced a firmly cross-linked polymer as determined by solubility, thermal shrinkage and dissolution, ultracentrifugation, and other techniques [99]. Reduction of collagen in solution did not result in formation of cross-links, and reduction of collagen which was polymerized into other than native-type fibrils resulted in only partial cross-linking. Apparently, the collagen molecules must be properly aligned, as occurs in the native-type fibrils formed *in vitro*, before cross-linking can occur. With sodium borotritide an estimated 1 mole ^{3}H was incorporated per mole of collagen. Reduction stabilizes the intermolecular bonds. Blocking aldehyde groups with thiosemicarbazide precluded the formation of labile covalent bonds and prevented the subsequent production of insoluble fibrils by borohydride. Lathyritic collagen, known to contain less aldehyde than normal collagen [102, 103], failed to form insoluble fibrils. Tanzer [99] interprets these results as indicative of the initial formation of aldimines (Schiff bases), these bonds being stabilized by reduction.

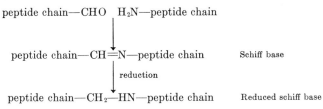

peptide chain—CHO   H₂N—peptide chain

peptide chain—CH=N—peptide chain   Schiff base

reduction

peptide chain—CH₂—HN—peptide chain   Reduced schiff base

Bailey and co-workers [104–106] extracted collagen from chick bones and teeth and reduced the protein with borohydride. By means of lysine-H³ incorporation, elemental analysis, mass spectroscopy, as well as biosynthesis and chemical synthesis, they proposed the following structures for two compounds isolated from hydrolysates of reduced collagen:

$$\begin{array}{c} \text{HOOC} \\ \diagdown \\ \text{N}_2\text{H} \diagup \end{array} \text{CH—(CH}_2)_4\text{—NH—CH}_2\text{—CH—(CH}_2)_2\text{—CH} \begin{array}{c} \diagup \text{COOH} \\ \\ \diagdown \text{NH}_2 \end{array}$$

Hydroxylysino-norleucine

$$\begin{array}{c} \text{HOOC} \\ \diagdown \\ \text{N}_2\text{H} \diagup \end{array} \text{CH—CH}_2\text{—CH}_2\text{—CH—CH—CH—CH}_2\text{—CH}_2\text{—CH} \begin{array}{c} \diagup \text{NH}_2 \\ \\ \diagdown \text{COOH} \end{array}$$

Syndesine

Hydroxylysino-norleucine was found in tendon collagen, also. Administration to chick embryos of compounds known to inhibit intermolecular cross-linking in collagen resulted in a dose-related decrease in the content of these two compounds. These workers estimated that one aldol bond is present for every two collagen molecules from chick bone and may be the major stabilizing bond. They also feel that the fact that hydroxylysine is a component of both presumed cross-links establishes a role in collagen for this unique amino acid. They suggest that hydroxylysine formation in the telopeptides may control the extent of cross-link synthesis, the amino acid being preferentially converted by enzyme action to the aldehyde precursor of the cross-link. Page et al. [107] reported that a certain few of the side chains of lysine and hydroxylysine in collagen specifically react with pyridoxal phosphate to form Schiff bases, and suggested that these residues may be concerned with molecular aggregation and fibril maturation, that is, with cross-linking. They estimated that only one lysyl and two hydroxylysyl residues per chain (1,000 amino acids) react; Bornstein and Piez [23] had reported that one lysine per alpha chain was converted to the corresponding aldehyde. In the developing chick, the extent of hydroxylation of lysine in newly synthesized collagen was greater in the youngest animals studied and decreased with age [108]. Presumably, tissue factors modulate lysine hydroxylase activity which in turn appears to determine those lysine residues which are to be converted to cross-link precursors.

Enzymes Involved in Lysine Conversion

The available evidence indicates that enzymic mediation is involved in the conversion of protein-bound lysine and/or hydroxylysine to reactive aldehydes prior to cross-link formation in elastin and collagen, and the possible role of amine oxidase has been pointed out [109–111]. Partridge [75] reviewed his work in which copper deficiency in rats or addition of lathyrogen to aortic tissue cultures inhibited the formation of desmosines and their intermediates, but not the incorporation of lysine, in growing elastin. Under these conditions ^{14}C-lysine was recovered unchanged, indicating that the first step in cross-link formation was blocked, namely, the oxidation of lysine to α-aminoadipic acid semialdehyde. Partridge noted the similarities of the enzyme system apparently operative in elastic tissue with recognized diamine oxidases; both enzyme systems require copper and are inhibited by semicarbazide.

Pinnell and Martin [112] detected in extracts of embryonic chick bone an enzyme which converted protein-bound lysine residues in chick embryo aortas to its aldehyde, which they called allysine. They point out that additional enzymes may be concerned with synthesis of desmosines, because this cross-link did not contain labelled lysine under their conditions of incubation. Lysine incorporated into aortic protein, but not free lysine, was a substrate for the enzyme, whose activity was measured by determining the release of tritium from ^{3}H-lysine, or by the amount of ^{14}C-α-aminoadipic acid semialdehyde formed from ^{14}C-allysine. This enzyme which catalyzes the lysyl to allysyl conversion is inactivated by levels of β-aminoproprionitrile (BAPN) which have little or no effect on amine oxidase but which inhibit the synthesis of lysine cross-links in collagen [113] and elastin [76]. Pinnell and Martin point out that BAPN does not appear to inactivate amine oxidase but is in fact a substrate for this family of enzymes and competitively inhibits the metabolism of endogenous amines. Furthermore, the enzyme acting on peptide-bound lysine was found in the supernatant fraction, in contrast to the amine oxidases which are associated with cell particulates.

The first step(s) in the synthesis of cross-links derived from lysine is probably enzymic and results in the formation of reactive aldehydes. Condensation of the modified and unaltered lysine side chains to produce interchain bonds may, however, be spontaneous. It is known that aggregates of soluble collagen become insoluble with standing, apparently due to the formation of interchain covalent linkages [114, 115]. Spontaneous cross-link production *in vitro* probably involves aldehyde groups to some extent, since gels of aldehyde-deficient collagen from lathyritic animals (see Section 7.3.1) remain readily reversible [116–118], as do those from collagen treated with aldehyde reagents [94]. Tyrosine residues may also be converted *in vitro* to cross-linking entities in collagen gels or may merely serve to align the polypeptide chains; Bensusan [119] showed that iodination of tyrosine in soluble collagen markedly raised the rate of both fibril formation and development of insolubility. (The increase in fluorescence and corresponding stability of collagen gels that develop during standing [61] more likely involves oxidation of aromatic amino acids rather than lysine side chains.) Cross-links develop within the collagen and elastin fibers over several days, and Piez [22] believes it unlikely that enzymes could operate in the confines of the collagen triple helix. He also suggests that some special associations between peptide chains in the proteins drives the condensation of the precursors. Schiff base formation between collagen chains has been shown to occur spontaneously *in vitro* and requires the presence of aldehyde groups on the protein (see Sections 7.2.1 and 7.3.1).

7.2.2   Other Potential Cross-links

Dityrosine

Dityrosine, a biphenolic compound formed by two molecules of tyrosine, was first found in nature by Andersen [120, 121] in acid hydrolysates of resilin, a rubberlike protein from the wing ligaments of locusts. Resilin is brilliantly fluorescent when viewed under ultraviolet light, a property which is probably due to the relatively abundant dityrosine in the protein. Andersen estimated the dityrosine content of resilin to be approximately 8 residues (16 tyrosine residues) per 1000 total amino acid residues. He also reported the presence of smaller amounts of trityrosine and traces of tetratyrosine (Fig. 7.5). Andersen established the chemical identity of the compound by titration, functional group reactions, and other methods of establishing the presence of multiple reactive groups. Synthetic dityrosine, prepared by the method of Gross and Sizer [122] who incubated tyrosine with peroxidase plus hydrogen peroxide, was indistinguishable from the natural material by chemical and physical criteria. Andersen also showed the derivation of dityrosine and trityrosine from either tyrosine or phenylalanine by administration of ^{14}C-amino acids to developing locusts. Tyrosine is incorporated into

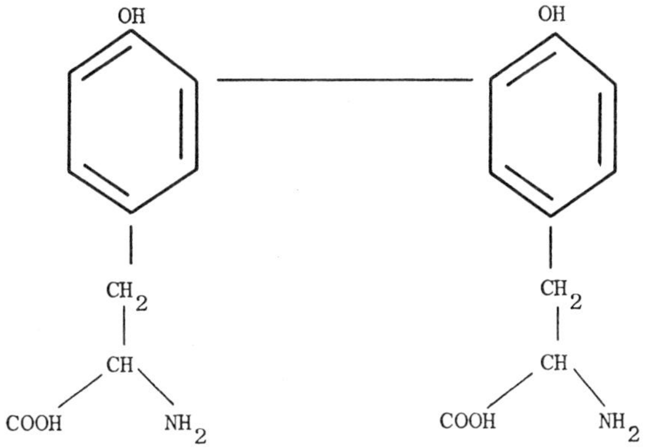

DITYROSINE

Figure 7.5.

resilin and the biphenyl linkage is apparently produced on the protein, because with time label is lost from tyrosine per se and appears in dityrosine.

During a study of the incorporation of ^{14}C-tyrosine into elastin of chick embryo aortic cultures, LaBella et al. [48] detected radioactivity in tyrosine and two other regions of the amino acid chromatogram of elastin hydrolysates. One radioactive fraction was in the alkali wash used to regenerate the ion-exchange column; the other was localized to a fraction eluted between lysine and histidine. Because the radioactivity of the latter fraction was associated with an unknown ninhydrin-positive component, it was believed that a single compound was responsible for both ninhydrin reactivity and ^{14}C label; up to 4.6 residues of the ninhydrin material were calculated to be present. However, it was subsequently found that by altering the temperature of the eluting buffer ^{14}C could be dissociated from the ninhydrin-reactive component. The radioactive component isolated from chick elastin labelled with ^{14}C-tyrosine showed chromatographic properties identical to those of dityrosine reported by Anderson [120, 121] and to authentic dityrosine synthesized with peroxidase. The amount of dityrosine present in chick embryo elastin was too small to give a ninhydrin-positive peak on the amino acid chromatogram, but it could be identified, isolated and partially characterized by virtue of its ^{14}C-label or by its specific intense fluorescence.

LaBella and co-workers [5, 49] subsequently identified dityrosine by several rigorous criteria in an alkali-soluble protein isolated from chick aorta and bovine ligamentum nuchae. Dityrosine in chick aorta was present at about 10 and 3 residues per 100,000 total amino acids in the alkali soluble protein and in elastin, respectively. Relative to other cross-linking candidates, the content of dityrosine in elastin is extremely low. This alkali-soluble protein is probably derived from the microfibrils identified electron microscopically in fetal bovine ligament by Ross and Bornstein [70] and which they extracted and analyzed chemically. Dityrosine was detected consistently in immature elastin from chick aorta but was usually absent from mature elastin. Two possible explanations: dityrosine is found only in the polar portion of the elastin precursor which is eventually removed (see Section 7.1.2), or it is converted to another compound, perhaps an aromatic polymer.

In an extensive study LaBella et al. [123] were unable to detect the presence of dityrosine in acid hydrolysates of a large number of purified proteins, with the exception of a few preparations of soluble collagen derived from rat skin. The reason for the infrequent and inconsistent presence of dityrosine in highly purified collagen is unknown, but it is significant that this apparent cross-link has been found, thus far, only in certain structural fibrous proteins. LaBella (unpublished findings) has not detected dityrosine in hydrolysates of eye lens albuminoid, keratin, or shark fin elastoidin.

Although a cross-link involving tyrosine residues has been demonstrated only rarely in soluble collagen, that collagen fraction most readily purified and therefore most amenable to meaningful chemical analysis, a number of observations suggest a potential role for such cross-links in this protein. These tyrosine cross-links, if they do exist, may play a role in stabilizing collagen through intermolecular bonding, and, as a consequence, be absent from the extractable fraction. Incubation of purified soluble collagen with tyrosinase [124] or peroxidase plus hydrogen peroxide [123] results in polymerization of the protein by covalent interchain bridges apparently due to specific conversion of phenolic residues to reactive cross-linking species. With suitable proportions of peroxidase, peroxide, and soluble collagen, a rigid, clear insoluble gel develops within a few minutes [123]. Amino acid analysis demonstrated the appearance of dityrosine in the enzyme-treated protein, with no detectable change in the number of tyrosine or other amino acid residues. Gel formation apparently resulted from formation of one dityrosine cross-link for approximately five collagen chains [123]. Marked gel stability, in this case, was apparently due largely to noncovalent associations between the polypeptide chains. Prior treatment with trypsin or pepsin inhibited collagen polymerization by either tyrosinase [124] or peroxidase [123]. These observations support the concept that tyrosine residues involved in cross-linking are located on the terminal nonhelical telopeptides, whose removal precludes subsequent cross-linking of the polypeptide chains.

Fujimori [66] irradiated solutions of acid soluble collagen with ultraviolet light and obtained physical evidence for the formation of new cross-links in the protein. Fluorescent photoproducts of tyrosine and phenylalanine were believed to constitute the radiation induced cross-links. It is likely that the photoproducts included dityrosine, which has been isolated from irradiated tyrosine peptides [125].

Disulfides

Mammalian collagen does not appear to contain cysteine, and trace amounts of this amino acid occasionally reported are believed to represent contaminating substances. On the other hand, collagen from the cuticle of the round worm, Ascaris has about 25 residues of cysteine per 1000 amino acids and is solubilized by reagents which split disulfides [126, 127]. Nimni [116] extracted soluble collagen from rat skin with several thiol compounds, and pointed out [116, 117] that, because of the absence of disulfides in collagen, other types of stabilizing bonds might be thiol sensitive. Schiff bases formed between peptide chains in collagen have been shown to be cleaved by these reagents (see Section 7.2.1). On the other hand, because of the intimate relationships among the fibers and ground substance of connective tissues, rupture of disulfide bonds in surrounding proteins may in some way labilize a certain fraction of the tissue collagen.

Elastin, isolated by a procedure which gives the most reproducible preparation and one with the lowest content of polar amino acid residues, namely extraction with hot 0.1 N NaOH, contains no cysteine. One may argue, as in the case of collagen, that disulfides in compounds extraneous to the protein may contribute to anchoring the elastin network in the tissues. Miller and Fullmer [128] attempted to isolate elastin by less drastic procedures and used prolonged extraction with salt, proteolytic enzymes, and denaturing agents. The product contained significant amounts of cysteine, which, however, may reflect extraction-resistant contaminants.

Phosphate Bridges

Glimcher et al. [129], identified organically bound phosphate in purified acid soluble and neutral salt soluble collagen from skin. The phosphate was not extracted with acids, was nondialyzable, and was estimated to be present in less than 1 mole per alpha chain. Peptides from enzymic digests of collagen contained more phosphate than could be accounted for by assuming it to be bound to serine hydroxyls, suggesting the presence of phosphorylated carbohydrate attached to collagen. Incubation of gelatin with acid phosphatase liberated inorganic phosphate, indicating an ester linkage [130]. Studies using electron paramagnetic resonance were interpreted as supporting the thesis that in bone a direct physical bond exists between the apatite crystallites and collagen fibers [131].

Covalently bound phosphate was found in completely demineralized dentin [132] and could not be removed by nonhydrolytic or other non-degradative procedures. Veis and Perry [133] isolated a protein of molecular weight 38,000, which represented only about 2% of the total dentin matrix but contained 34 phosphate groups per molecule, apparently attached to the hydroxyl groups of hydroxylysine. This phosphoprotein was in turn covalently bound to collagen molecules in a molar ratio of about 1 to 5, respectively. Veis [15] suggests that the phosphate groups participate directly in the formation of diester cross-links, and they may also be involved in the *in vivo* nucleation required for mineralization. Periodate treatment liberated a phosphate-rich peptide which appeared to be derived by main-peptide-chain degradation. Veis proposes the possibility that the phosphopeptide represents a telopeptide unique to hard tissue collagen. Since dentin and skin collagens dissolve at the same rate during periodate treatment, other types of susceptible cross-links must be common to both types of collagen.

Partridge [134] and LaBella [46] found organically-bound phosphate in purified elastin, about 0.02% by weight, and the latter noted its very rapid turnover in aortas of rats given inorganic P^{32}.

Di-enosaline

Blumenfeld and Gallop [135] identified another aldehydic compound in collagen, and, on the basis of a number of analytical procedures, proposed a structure for the isolated compound which they called di-enosaline. They propose a cross-linking role for this compound and suggest its possible formation through a series of reactions leading to conversion of lysine residues on each of two chains to enosaline with subsequent dimerization. A requirement for this reaction is the linkage of lysine in the peptide backbone through its side chain amino group only.

$$NH_2-CH_2-CH_2-CH_2-C{=}CH-CH{=}O$$
$$O{=}CH-CH{=}CH-CH_2-CH-CH_2-NH_2$$

Di-enosaline

This same laboratory has identified very small amounts of aldehydes of several other amino acids in collagen [135, 136]. Bornstein and Piez [23] believe that most of the aldehyde in the soluble collagens is accounted for by the lysine-derived aldehyde precursor of the aldol condensation product, and that other aldehydes are present only in trace amounts. Conceivably even traces of aldehydes might contribute to fiber stabilization, perhaps by forming Schiff Bases or more stable bonds at critical locations. Gustavson [55] has pointed out that even chemically undetectable amounts of certain tanning agents can markedly influence the physical properties of hides or purified collagen.

Quinones

LaBella [3, 42–44] drew an analogy between the fluorescence and pigmentation in elastin and the presumed quinone tanning processes indicated in hardening of insect cuticles. Quinone tanning of structural protein, which is complexed with chitin in the cuticle, is widespread in invertebrates. It has been postulated that, in cuticle tanning, dihydroxyphenolic compounds are enzymically oxidized to quinones and subsequently form covalent links with amino groups on adjacent peptide chains [137, 138]. Blocking of free amino groups led to subsequent failure of the protein to harden [139]. Sclerotin, one of these highly cross-linked proteins, yielded a fluorescent fraction containing an aminophenol and apparently formed from a protein-derived nitrogen atom linked to a benzene ring [140, 141]. Dennell [140] believes that the aminophenol is 1:4 diamino hydroquinone, resulting from acid hydrolysis of the cuticle protein cross-linked by a circulating tanning agent, and he proposes a structure for the *in situ* protein cross-link. More recent work by Karlson [142–144] indicated that hydroquinone-C^{14} was not incorporated into the cuticle of the blowfly larva, thus casting doubt on Dennell's proposal for paraquinone tanning. On the other hand, N-acetyldopamine was rapidly incorporated into the cuticle (Fig. 7.6). This and other findings, such as the presence of a specific phenolase and the correlation between enzyme and substrate levels and cuticle hardening, strongly indicate that, at least in the insects studied, N-acetyldopamine is oxidized to the active quinone tanning agent. These workers also showed the synthesis of the tanning agent from ^{14}C-tyrosine.

In cases where quinone tanning was suspected in the absence of detectable 0-dihydroxyphenols, self-tanning, that is, covalent linkages formed between quinone-yielding residues and amino or sulfhydryl groups on the protein itself, has been postulated [145]. Pryor [146] concluded that sclerotin consisted of a meshwork of protein, cross-linked by a mass of polymerized quinone that fills the interstices between the

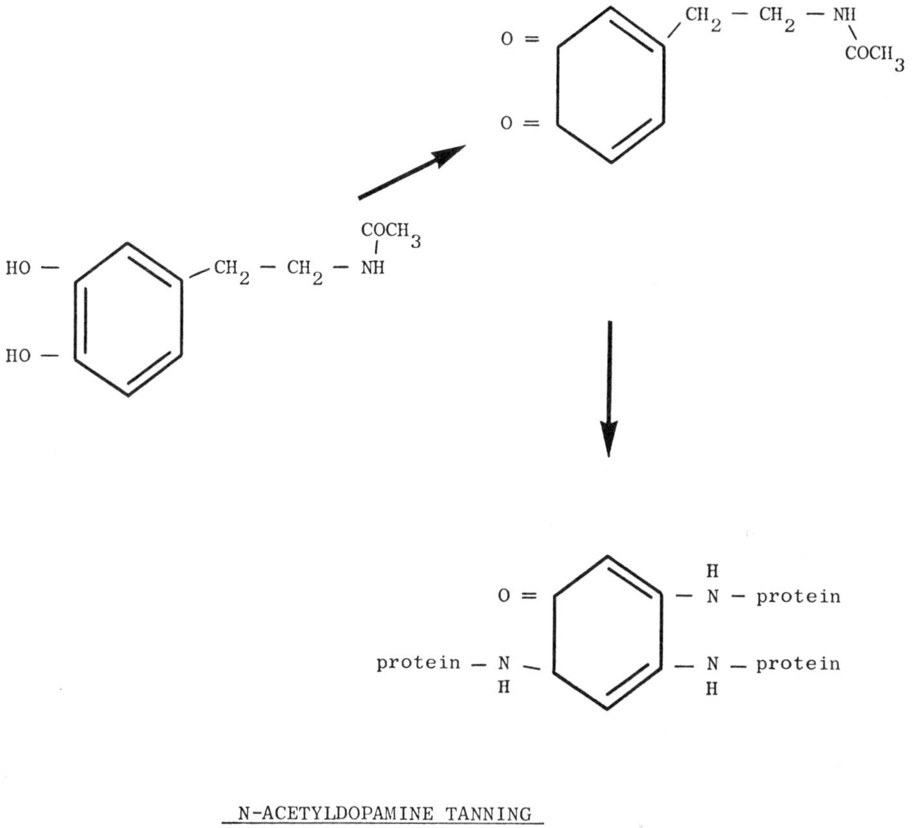

N-ACETYLDOPAMINE TANNING

Figure 7.6.

protein chains. Quinone tanning, occurring by autotanning or by deposition of circulating quinones or quinone precursors, darkens and toughens the protein, rendering it insoluble and inert. In the human, elastin and insoluble matrix collagen become increasingly pigmented and fluorescent with age [3, 42, 68]. Furthermore, the pigment and fluorescence in elastin is associated with the elastase-resistant, and presumably cross-linked, region of the protein [42, 147]. Acid-hydrolyzed elastin yields yellow, fluorescent compounds which darken and polymerize rapidly in air, adhere to Sephadex and polystyrene ion-exchangers, and are derived from tyrosine, properties compatible with a quinone structure.

Furthermore, in both collagen and elastin the fluorescent material shows spectra similar to those of quinones [3, 43, 44], increases with age in correspondence to a decreasing tyrosine content [42, 68], and ultraviolet irradiation converts tyrosine residues to a product with fluorescent, visible, and ultraviolet properties identical to that in the original proteins [43]. The changes in the physical and chemical properties of collagen and elastin as a function of age have been universally interpreted to reflect increased cross-linking in the proteins (see Section 7.3.2). All of these observations are compatible with a continuous process of tanning by quinones formed from phenolic residues in collagen and elastin. However, additional tanning by circulating agents cannot be ruled out. A precedent for the occurrence of cross-linking mechanisms in structural proteins, common to both invertebrates and vertebrates, has been demonstrated for dityrosine in insect resilin and in mammalian elastin, two rubberlike proteins (see Section 7.2.2).

Several polyhydric phenols have been found to enhance the state of aggregation of purified neutral salt soluble collagen [148]. Warming solutions of soluble collagen causes precipitation or gel formation, which is reversed by cooling; pyrogallol, catecholamines, hydroquinone, and homogentisic acid were active in preventing redispersion of the aggregates, whereas resorcinol and gentisic acid were not. The effectiveness of the compounds in promoting gel stability was related to their ability to form quinones, which presumably cross-linked the collagen chains. An oxidative step was required for the polyphenols to promote gel insolubility, since they were ineffective in a nitrogen atmosphere. Tyrosine plus tyrosinase were also effective, supporting the cross-linking role of quinones. Dabbous [124] induced aggregation of soluble collagens by incubation with tyrosinase and demonstrated the formation of covalent interchain cross-links in the telopeptide region. On the basis of the products formed by the enzyme, he concluded that quinones, formed from protein-bound tyrosine residues, were involved.

Although there is no evidence that quinone cross-links exist in extractable collagen which consists primarily of single chains and covalently linked double chains, the progressive increase with age in pigmentation, decrease in tyrosine content, and increased fluorescence of insoluble collagen, at least allow for the possibility of this form of *in vivo* tanning.

γ-Glutamyl Bonds

The possible presence of γ-glutamyl bonds in collagen was extensively reviewed by Harding [149]. He concluded that this type of bond is present in considerable amount in collagen. The bond is apparently not involved in interchain cross-linking but serves as an alternative mode for linking amino acids in the main polypeptide chains. In the vertebrate blood-clotting process, the formation of stable fibrin gels from soluble fibrinogen has been shown to be due to interchain cross-links involving ϵ-amino groups of lysine and γ-glutamyl groups [150, 151]. The ubiquitous glutathione is γ-glutamylcysteinylglycine. Gallop [152, 153] estimated that in ichthyocol gelatin at least 31 of the 71 glutamyl residues per 1,000 total amino acids were present in γ-glutamyl linkage, and 10 per 1,000 in acid soluble collagen of calf skin. Peptides containing glutamic acid in this type of linkage were isolated [154].

Mechanic and Levy [156] isolated a tripeptide, containing glutamic acid and lysine linked through the γ-carboxyl and ϵ-amino groups, from partial hydrolysates of bovine skin collagen. The α-carboxyl of glutamic acid was in peptide linkage with glycine. Thus, it appears likely that glutamic acid and lysine can form interchain bonds in collagen, although the frequency and significance of these bonds is uncertain. It has been suggested that these bonds serve to disrupt the helical structure and introduce regions of flexibility at specific intervals [155].

Esterlike Bonds

Gallop [152] showed that under defined conditions hydroxylamine reacts with "esterlike" bonds to form protein-bound hydroxamic acids. In the reaction 6 acyl hydroxamic acids were bound to each chain of soluble collagen and the polypeptide chain was cleaved into 6 subunits. Gallop concluded that three different subunits existed, each of about 17,000 molecular weight, and that 3A, 2B, and 1C were united by ester bonds to form the basic collagen chain. Because he detected no new amino groups liberated by hydroxylamine, there was apparently no significant cleavage of peptide bonds. Evidence was obtained from analysis of hydrazine peptides that the β-carboxyl of aspartic acid contributed to some ester bonds, although the alcoholic function was unknown [157]. However, there is no evidence that ester bonds are involved in *interchain* cross-links in collagen. Hormann [158] suggested that hexoses might constitute the hydroxylamine sensitive bonds, but Gallop's group [159] reported that hexose in soluble ichthyocol collagen was attached to the protein at only one point.

Butler [54] concluded that at least one type of hydroxylamine sensitive bond in the $\alpha 1$ chain of rat skin collagen was a peptide, asparaginylglycine, bond. Bornstein [160] treated a peptide derived from the α chain of rat collagen with hydroxylamine. He concluded that the fragments had been joined through a cyclic imide, formed by condensation of an aspartyl side chain and an adjacent amide nitrogen on the polypeptide chain. He proposes that hydrolysis of bonds of this type by

$$
\begin{array}{c}
\text{—NH—CH—C} \\
\end{array}
$$

Cyclic imide

hydroxylamine causes the fragmentation of the collagen chain as reported by Gallop. Cyclic imides of this type may be formed during isolation or hydrolysis of peptides [98]. However, whether or not they are naturally occurring or arise artifactually, they could well be the hydroxylamine sensitive regions of the collagen chains. This finding indicates that the peptide chains of the collagen molecule probably contain backbones comprised only of peptide bonds, and that no unusual "esterlike" bonds are present.

Carbohydrate

Purified collagen from all sources contains carbohydrate in covalent linkage, the amount varying from less than 1% in vertebrates to as much as 13 to 18% in certain invertebrates. Butler and Cunningham [161] solubilized matrix collagen from skin by digestion with collagenase and trypsin and isolated peptides in which glucose and galactose were in 0-glycosidic linkage with hydroxylysine. They suggest that the hexoses may control the rate of interchain cross-linking by preferentially rendering those hydroxylysine residues with which they unite susceptible to deamination. Hörmann [158] suggested that hexoses might be the hydroxylamine-sensitive ester bonds in collagen and proposed possible intramolecularly and intermolecularly bridging structures (Fig. 7.7 and 7.8).

Although the hexoses in the soluble ichthyocol collagen characterized by Gallop's group [159] are not involved in a two-point covalent attachment, they are potential cross-linking groups and may be operative in matrix collagen. Another mechanism has been proposed whereby cross-linking of proteins occurs by means of hexoses [162, 163]. Support for the feasibility of the reaction was provided by characterizing the products resulting from incubation of glucose with various amino acids at physiological pH and temperature. In addition, fibrils reconstituted from soluble collagen became insoluble in 6 M urea-0.1 M acetic acid after 4 to 7 days in the presence of glucose, compared to 12 to 19 days for the control fibrils. Bannister [164] found no statistically significant

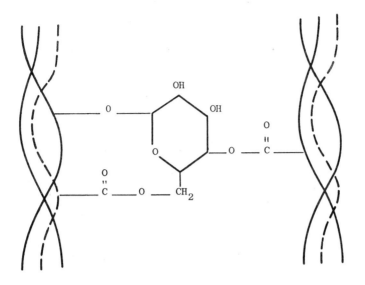

INTERMOLECULAR HEXOSE CROSSLINK

Figure 7.7.

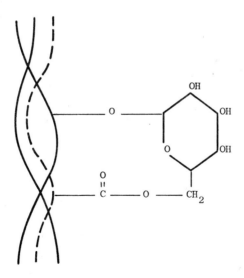

INTRAMOLECULAR HEXOSE CROSSLINK

Figure 7.8.

281

increase in the *in vitro* conversion of α chains to β and γ components in the presence of glucose.

The presence of carbohydrate influences the morphological appearance, for example, the banding of collagen fibers examined microscopically [10]. In collagens with high carbohydrate content, normal periodicity is indistinct or absent, or an abnormal banding pattern is seen. These observations suggest that there is more than one type of association between carbohydrate and the collagen molecule. Precipitation of collagen solutions generally results in formation of fibrils with the usual 640 Å spacing; in the presence of glycoprotein, a long spacing of 2300 Å is produced, indicating that the normal bonding zones of the collagen molecules are blocked by associated glycoprotein [26].

Circulating "Tanning Agents"

Both collagen and elastin become pigmented with age. This is seen most clearly in the human where tissues are available from very old individuals. The proteins retain the pigmentation following conventional purification procedures [3, 42, 68]. They also become increasingly fluorescent with age [3, 42, 68]. In the case of elastin it is clear that with time contaminating protein becomes more firmly associated, probably covalently, with the elastin fiber [3]. Accretion of various substances on collagen and elastin, obvious in old individuals, probably begins at the time the proteins are consolidated into the tissue mass, and perhaps earlier.

Both collagen and elastin have been reported to be associated with a number of substances which resist extraction, and, thus, appear to be in covalent linkage. Mucopolysaccharides and mucroproteins constitute the connective tissue ground substance in which collagen and elastic fibers are normally embedded. Lipids are another class of substance intimately associated with the fibrous proteins. Windrum [165] reported that reticulin consists of 85% collagen, about 4% carbohydrate, and the remainder as bound lipid, the lipid apparently contributing to the organization and stability of the fibrils. Melcher [166] reported that collagen previously extracted for fat is stained with Sudan Black B in mature, but not developing connective tissue. Other substances are apparently bound to collagen. As mentioned earlier, collagen contains several aldehyde groups per molecule. Although some of these can be attributed to modification of amino acids in the primary structure of collagen, others may be of extraneous origin. Veis [15] has reviewed reports on noncollagen proteins which may be covalently linked to collagen. Organic phosphorus in collagen has been referred to earlier. Collagen from all sources contains significant amounts of carbohydrate in covalent linkage [167]. This amounts to less than 1%, generally, in vertebrate collagens, but as much as 13–18% in certain invertebrates.

Elastin appears to contain lipid which is intimately associated with the protein, because it resists extraction with organic solvents. Much of this lipid may be trapped within the elastin fibrils, for Lansing [168] reported that alkali purified, fat extracted ligamentum elastin, subsequently solubilized by elastase, released globules of fat. Lipid was also recovered from acid hydrolysates of elastin, the protein having been previously extracted with fat solvents [46, 169]. One of these lipids was apparently bound in a plasmalogen-like linkage (α, β unsaturated ether bond) to the protein, since its activation and blockade in the staining reaction paralleled those of typical lipid plasmalogens [170]. Keller et al. [171] isolated peptides from an enzymic digest of elastin, one of which was rich in polar amino acids and contained 7% carbohydrate and 50% lipid. The possibility exists, however, that the protein, carbohydrate, and lipid were liberated from the interior of the fiber and were not covalently linked to elastin. Even after removal of lipid aldehyde, elastin still gives an apparent aldehyde-staining reaction with Schiff's reagent [170], and with a more specific aldehyde reagent [172]. As with collagen, at least some of the aldehydes may be derived from amino acids in the protein. It would appear that the most satisfactory means of determining whether or not a particular substance, for example, cysteine or lipid, is covalently linked to native elastin is the isolation of a peptide containing the substance in question together with a component typical of elastin. The desmosines appear to be ideal markers for elastin-derived peptides.

It appears likely that over the lifespan of the individual, interactions occur between the inert, ubiquitous connective tissue fibrous framework and a host of circulating metabolites. Indeed, the changes in the physical and chemical properties of collagen and elastin that take place with age (see Section 7.3.2) no doubt reflect the cumulative effects of these interactions. Chemical substances which have been found most effective in the leather industry for artificially cross-linking, that is, tanning, of animal hides include quinones, lipid oxidation products, polyvalent metals, unsaturated lipids, and aldehydes [173]. These same materials are present in abundance in tissues and are strong candidates for an *in vivo* tanning role. Milch [174] incubated collagen with a large number of aldehydic compounds known to be metabolic intermediates. There were a number of compounds which cross-linked collagen, but the most efficient were aliphatic aldehydes with a maximum of four carbon atoms, having a terminal formyl group, and with carbon atom 1 or 2 having an active hydrogen. Cross-linking of structural proteins by incorporation of tanning substances is widespread in invertebrates as a mechanism for hardening protective or supporting tissues (see Section 7.2.2). Evolutionary retention of some of these processes may account for the changes occurring with time in collagen and elastin. The major structural proteins of higher animals, permanently consolidated into the tissues early in life, are subject to persistent chemical attack throughout the life span of the individual. It is possible that certain of these tanning reactions, implicated in age-associated degenerative sequelae, may be designed into the maturation phase of collagen and elastin fiber formation.

7.3   FACTORS WHICH MAY INFLUENCE CROSS-LINKING OF ELASTIN AND COLLAGEN

Essentially all of the conclusions which have been reached with respect to changes in cross-linking density of elastin and collagen, as a function of age, disease, and other influences, are based on indirect evidence. The chemical nature of some of the cross-links in these proteins has only recently been elucidated. Thus, very few reports are available in which the amounts of specific cross-links, in situations other than during the period of their formation in the newly synthesized protein, are estimated. The greatest portion of these indirect data is derived from measurement of physical properties such as thermal shrinkage, tensile strength, swelling in aqueous solutions, thermal degradation, x-ray diffraction pattern, and elasticity of tissues rich in elastin or collagen. Additional indirect evidence, in the case of collagen, is obtained from estimates of the relative proportions of the "soluble" and "insoluble" fractions which reflect the degree of intermolecular cross-linking. In addition, changes in the behavior of artificially cross-linked proteins or tissues have frequently been shown to parallel that measured for the components presumably cross-linked *in situ*, as for example, during the aging process.

The mechanical properties of tendons, ligaments, strips of skin and arteries, and other connective tissue structures are determined by a large number of factors which may vary independently with age or other influences. Thus, changes in relative proportions of collagen, elastin, polysaccharides, and other substances, fiber arrangement, and cross-sectional diameter of component fibers, for example, may confound attempts to determine cross-linking density specifically in collagen or elastin in tissues as a function of age, disease or other condition.

7.3.1   Lathyrogens

Over the past decade a major stimulus to investigations into the chemistry of connective tissue proteins, and into the chemical nature of cross-links in particular, was provided by the finding that a group of related compounds administered to young animals produces a profound adverse change in the structural integrity of connective tissues. The drugs cause "lathyrism," characterized by the occurrence of skeletal deformities, dissecting aortic aneurysms, and other abnormalities. The first of these "lathyrogens" to be described was β-aminopropionitrile (BAPN), isolated from a variety of sweet pea, *Lathyrus odoratus*. Young grazing animals feeding on the plant subsequently developed the abnor-

$$NH_2—CH_2—CH_2—C\equiv N$$
BAPN

malities just described. The basic defect was gradually elucidated and shown to be a failure in the processes which govern formation of cross-links derived from lysine in both collagen and elastin [76, 112, 199–203]. Collagen in tissues of lathyritic animals remains largely in the "soluble" form, in contrast to the normal growing animal in which the soluble fraction is rapidly converted to matrix collagen. Lathyritic collagen and elastin from BAPN-treated animals contain abnormally low amounts of aldehyde groups [23, 175, 176], and gels of soluble collagen from these animals fail to achieve the state of insolubility reached by collagen from normal animals [114, 115]. It has been shown that aldehydes in collagen are necessary for spontaneous *in vitro* intramolecular and inter-molecular cross-linking that leads to covalent bonding and gel stability [94, 116–118]. There is abundant evidence that cross-linking reactions within the collagen triple-helix and between collagen molecules involve the same types of functional groups and are continuous, competing processes [11–13]. (There may be additional cross-links, however, that are specific to either intramolecular or intermolecular union.) It was subsequently demonstrated that BAPN inhibits the enzyme(s) that convert the side chain of lysine in the proteins to the aldehyde precursor of certain covalent cross-links. Thus there is failure of collagenous and elastic tissues to attain the structural integrity necessary for withstanding the mechanical stresses applied to bones, the aorta, and other organs.

Penicillamine also induces lathyrism but acts in a different manner than does BAPN. Nimni and co-workers [116–118] carried out a series

$$NH_2—CH——C\begin{matrix} SH \\ \diagup \\ —CH_3 \\ \diagdown \\ CH_3 \end{matrix}$$
$$\underset{COOH}{|}$$
Penicillamine

of studies demonstrating that collagen from animals treated with penicillamine (1) had an apparently normal content of aldehyde but, in contrast to collagen from normal animals, failed to form insoluble gels

upon standing at 37°, (2) contained an abnormally low proportion of
β-components which did not increase upon standing *in vitro*, and (3)
after dialysis, aggregated normally *in vitro*. Their work indicated that
administered penicillamine chemically combines *in vivo* with aldehyde
groups on the collagen molecule, thereby precluding spontaneous *in vitro*
cross-link formation. A similar action of the drug is indicated on elastin,
in which desmosine biosynthesis is blocked by administration of penicillamine and is accompanied by an abnormally high content of α-amino-
adipic acid semialdehyde [76, 102]. Thiosemicarbazide, another lathyrogen, appears to act like BAPN, in that it inhibits the enzymic formation
of aldehyde in collagen, and like penicillamine in combining with preexisting aldehydes on collagen *in vitro*, and perhaps *in vivo* as well
[94].

$$\begin{array}{c} \text{S} \\ \| \\ \text{NH}_2\text{---C---NH---NH}_2 \end{array}$$
Thiosemicarbazide

The discovery of the lathyrogens and elucidation of their mechanisms
of action suggest possible ways in which cross-linking of the fibrous
proteins may be physiologically modulated.

7.3.2   Aging

The fibrous connective tissue proteins are estimated to make up 30
to 40% of total body protein, and the bulk of the fibrous elements
become permanently affixed to the tissues early in life. Aging in animals
and man is manifested to a large extent in the connective tissue components of all tissues, and it is quite apparent that deleterious change,
for example in arteries, skin, and joints, is continually taking place
in the fibrous proteins. Sobel [177] has emphasized another possible,
more general role of connective tissues in the aging process, in postulating
that the increased fiber to gel ratio and other changes in the ground
substance lead to diminished nutrient exchange between blood and paren-
chyma. The cross-linking hypothesis of aging assigns a major causative
role in the process of human aging to the "tanning" of body proteins
and other macromolecules and nucleic acids [173]. It appears quite likely
that covalent union between peptide chains, and other chemical changes,
continually take place on the less metabolically active proteins. The
significance of connective tissue aging as a possible determinant of
human aging is yet to be elucidated.

There is almost universal agreement that the physical properties of
collagen-rich tissues, such as tendons and skin, change with aging in

a manner that is consistent with the gradual accumulation of covalent cross-links between polypeptide chains of the protein. Thus, with aging, solubility, extensibility, and swelling of the proteins decrease, and tensile strength and the temperature for shrinkage increase. In addition, artificial cross-linking of tissue proteins, usually performed with formaldehyde and other aldehydes, influences the physical properties of the tissue in a manner comparable to the aging process. This aspect of collagen biochemistry has been considered in a number of reviews [41, 173, 178–180], and only a few selected areas will be discussed here. A discordant note in this unanimity concerning the behavior of old collagen was struck by the suggestion of Ciferri and Rajagh [83] that the complexity of tendon organization and its variation with age could account for the changes that have been attributed to increased covalent cross-linking. Fewer studies have been carried out with elastin-rich tissues such as ligament and aorta, but conclusions similar to those for collagen have been drawn [27, 41, 178, 181].

It is not clear what time period in the human, in terms of connective tissue aging, corresponds to the two or three year life span of the rat, the species from which most of our information is derived. For example, Verzar [179] demonstrated a progressive decrease with age in the amount of labile, hydroxyproline-containing peptide released during thermal contraction of tail tendon isolated from the rat. Stabilization of certain intermolecular bonds in collagen appears to take place during the "aging" process in the rat [182]; however, similar studies which might indicate whether these changes are in fact age-related (as opposed to time-related processes), have not been carried out in man or other animals. Over a 9-month period in the rat, there was reported to be a progressive decrease in the number of labile bonds in tail-tendon collagen, corresponding to an increased tension during thermal contraction. Reduction with borohydride stabilized and penicillamine treatment labilized the heat-labile bonds, indicating that the major intermolecular links were Schiff bases [182, 183]. In man, cross-link stabilization of this type may be of significance only during the fiber maturation phase which occurs, for the most part, early in life.

LaBella and co-workers [3, 42, 43, 68] correlated age-related increased insolubility, decreased aromatic amino acid content, and increased fluorescence and pigmentation of elastin and collagen with an increase in cross-links. In elastin a given desmosine cross-link is probably formed over a period of a few weeks or less. Hence, even at birth the proportion of newly synthesized elastin is only a small part of the total elastin, and the desmosine content has almost reached a maximum; this is true for the chick [5, 80], the ox [81], and the human [4] (see Table 7.3).

The desmosine content of human aortic elastin is constant up to age 90 years [3]. The indicated increased cross-linking of aging elastin must be due to other, as yet unknown, types of bonds, and may involve auto-tanning or deposition of circulating tanning agents (see Section 7.2.2).

LaBella and Thornhill [43] showed that ultraviolet irradiation of alkali-purified elastin powder from human aorta produced alterations in the protein, similar in many respects to those occurring naturally in the aging human. There was a decrease in the number of unaltered aromatic amino acid residues, an increase in the characteristic fluorescence, and an increased yellowing. Furthermore, the insoluble elastin became progressively more susceptible to elastase upon continued irradiation. Several investigators had reported that elastin in histological sections from aged humans is more rapidly solubilized by elastase then is that from young individuals [184–186]. Mull and Ram [187] reported similar observations on human aortic elastin demineralized with formic acid extraction. In contrast, LaBella and Lindsay [42] reported increased resistance to the enzyme with age; this last investigation was validly criticized on the grounds that measurement of solubilization was determined by means of the changes in optical density of elastin suspensions which also contained insoluble mineral salts [187]. Thus, assuming the correctness of an increased rate of dissolution by the enzyme with age, the oxidative environment of living tissues and of ultraviolet irradiated aqueous elastin suspensions lead to strikingly similar changes in the physical properties of the protein. As mentioned earlier, increased cross-linking with age is indicated for elastin on the basis of changes in certain physical parameters estimated on gross tissue structures. Ayer [188] reported that the rate of solubilization of aortic elastin with formic acid was inversely related to age. However, increased susceptibility to elastase with age may reflect denaturation and/or rupture of the polypeptide chain at various points, both processes rendering elastin more vulnerable to the enzyme. Certainly, fragmentation of elastic fibers is a very common histological finding in aged human tissues.

Matrix collagen, of course, is the only collagen fraction capable of undergoing aging. Because of the complexity of this component, due in part to progressive association with other substances, the exact functional groups of the molecule which may be tied up with age will be difficult to determine. The probable derivation of the fluorescent substance from aromatic residues in collagen and elastin, and its association with the enzyme-resistant portion of elastin has already been discussed. Serial extracts of collagen from Achilles tendon from individuals aged 1 to 90 years, and from presumably progressively deeper portions of the collagen fiber, showed increased fluorescence, as did the original tendon powder. Tendon from young individuals was most soluble and this decreasing solubility was correlated with age [68].

If cross-linking of the abundant and ubiquitous connective tissue proteins is indeed a causative factor in animal aging, then interference with cross-linking processes should prolong life. Kohn [189] and LaBella [190, 191] treated rats chronically with lathyrogens, because these agents interfere with intramolecular and intermolecular cross-linking in collagen. Although, at the time these studies were initiated, the specific chemical groups affected by the drugs were unknown, it was postulated that increased cross-linking that appears to occur with age may be a continuation of maturation processes in the fibrous proteins [190]. Kohn [189] reported no effect of BAPN on rat survival in an experiment involving relatively few animals. LaBella [191] reported an increased mean life span in experiments involving several hundred rats, treated with varying doses of BAPN, semicarbazide, and penicillamine for varying periods of time; the effectiveness of the treatment was shown for animals started on the drug as young as 2 months and as old as 16 months. Harman [192, 193] reported an increase in mean, but not maximum, life span of mice treated with drugs that are known to "trap" free radicals. The free-radical hypothesis of aging would appear to be concerned with at least some of the concepts inherent in the cross-linking hypothesis. Reactive free radicals, which are continually being produced in the body tissues and fluids, are capable of effectively cross-linking macromolecules including collagen and elastin. Also, LaBella [194] showed that labyrogens form covalent bonds with aromatic amino acid residues in elastin during ultraviolet irradiation of the purified protein *in vitro,* presumably due to the formation of free radical intermediates.

McCay [195], in his classic experiments, promoted an approximate doubling of the life span of rats by severe caloric restriction. That inhibition of connective tissue protein cross-linking may have contributed to life prolongation is suggested by the report that the apparent age of tail tendon from rats subjected to dietary restriction was similar to that of much younger control animals [196]. A proponent of the cross-linking hypothesis of aging might postulate a diminished body concentration of potential tanning metabolites, as a result of the reduced food intake. Conversely, a high fat, atheroma-promoting diet appeared to accelerate the aging process in rats, at least on the basis of changes in the physical properties of the tail tendon [197]. In this instance, one could postulate increased cross-linking of tendon collagen through lipid metabolites.

7.3.3 Disease

Certain disease processes, either congenital or occurring later in life, may, of course, direct the pathways of collagen and elastin biosynthesis, maturation and consolidation, and resorption in a number of ways, including interference with cross-linking reactions. Many conditions have been shown to affect the fibrous protein synthetic processes. There are suggestions that consolidation of the proteins into permanent supporting frameworks is sometimes inhibited. Also, fiber degeneration is a common histological finding in several disease states.

A number of pathological conditions are associated with disturbances in the ratio of soluble to insoluble collagen in a given tissue. Obviously, these situations involve deviations from the normal sequence of the intermolecular cross-linking reactions which determine the conversion of soluble collagen to matrix collagen. With the exception of experimental lathyrism in animals, in no instance has it yet been directly demonstrated that there is either absence of a known cross-link in collagen and elastin or occurrence of unusual types or numbers of cross-links.

Because at least some of the cross-links in both elastin and collagen appear to be formed through the mediation of several enzymic steps, one might anticipate the occurrence of genetic defects in cross-link formation. Failure of enzymic deamination of protein-bound lysine, for example, would preclude the formation of lysine-derived cross-links. A defect in tissue peroxidase might prevent formation of dityrosine cross-links. Genetically determined lack or defectiveness of other enzymes, necessary for hydroxylation of proline or lysine, or for scission of preliminary, reversible bonds during tissue remodelling, might also arise. Thus, there might exist one or more "molecular diseases" in which specific defects occur in elastin and collagen. On the other hand, because of the importance of the connective tissue proteins in the development and maintenance of the integrity of the animal body, genetic defects of this type may be incompatible with survival.

Brief reference will be made here only to some of the pathological states for which disturbances in protein cross-linking or tertiary structure have been suggested, implicated, or suspected. Many of the observations in this area are contradictory, sketchy, and lack independent confirmation.

Marfan's syndrome is a heritable disorder of connective tissue and is characterized by aortic dilation and dissecting aneurysm, skeletal deformities, hernia, lens detachment, and other complications. Histological observation suggests the presence of abnormal, apparently weakened connective tissue. The similarities between Marfan's syndrome and experimental lathyrism have often been noted [198]. Administration of lathyrogens to young growing animals, in which vigorous synthesis of all body proteins is occurring, leads to a general weakening of the connective tissue framework. The biosynthesis of at least one class of major cross-links in collagen and elastin has been shown to be inhibited by these agents. In both proteins oxidative deamination of lysine is inhibited, resulting in the inhibition of desmosine formation in elastin and the aldol condensation product in collagen [76, 112, 199–203]. LaBella (unpublished observations) found that the amino acid composition, including lysine and the desmosines, of purified elastin from aorta and skin from several patients with diagnosed Marfan's syndrome was normal. Histological studies of tissues from afflicted individuals, have implicated defects in both collagen and elastin, but the problem may derive from subtle disturbances in fiber organization rather than a gross chemical abnormality [204]. It has been suggested, also, that the acquired defect may reside in the connective tissue ground substance, intimately concerned with establishing fiber stability [205]. There are histological reports that suggest abnormalities of the mucoprotein matrix in aorta, epiphysial plate, and other tissues (see review, [206]).

The Ehlers-Danlos syndrome (rubber-skin) is another genetically acquired disease of connective tissue and is characterized by hyperextensibility of the skin and joints, among other things. A number of workers have reported excessive amounts of elastica-staining fibers in afflicted individuals, but others have denied this [198]. Again, disorders of either collagen or elastin have been implicated. Defects in major cross-links of the proteins are probably not involved, since the amino acid composition of elastin is reportedly normal [207], as is the shrinkage temperature of Achilles tendon [208]. Jansen [209] reported that there was no histological evidence of excessive collagen or elastic fiber formation and proposed failure of collagen fibrils to form into bundles. Examination of teeth from afflicted individuals showed gross abnormalities in dentine, which contains collagen but no elastin. Wechsler and Fisher [210] rejected the suggestion of Jansen that abnormal collagen organization was the key. They found no tinctorial derangements in collagen or elastin, and their histological work implicated excessive collagen content as the basis of the disease.

Matrix collagen fibrils solubilized from the knee joint of rheumatoid arthritics by treatment with a mixture of proteases and saccharases were reported to be "kinked" as determined by electron microscopy [211]. Furthermore, the reported abnormal susceptibility of rheumatoid collagen to proteases [211] suggests an *in vivo* denaturation of the protein polymer in the region of the kinks.

Alcaptonuria is a heritable disease of man in which there is deposition of brown-black (ochronotic) pigment in connective tissues, particularly in cartilage. Afflicted individuals very often exhibit degenerative arthritis of the spine and peripheral joints. The "inborn error" is the absence of homogentisic acid oxidase, resulting in the accumulation of homogentisic acid. Homogentisic acid is derived from tyrosine and is normally metabolized in a series of reactions to fumaric acid and acetoacetic acid. Arthropathy appears to be the major specific morbid process resulting from ochronotic pigment deposition, although other organs may be afflicted in some individuals [212]. It has been demonstrated, also, that tissues contain enzymes which convert homogentisic acid to quinones [213]. These observations suggest that tanning of tissue proteins by accumulated quinones leads to degenerative changes which are confined largely, but not entirely, to cartilaginous connective tissues. Milch [214] demonstrated that auto-oxidized, polymerized homogentisic acid effectively cross-linked collagen *in vitro* as determined by decreased swelling and increased resistance to collagenase, and he proposed quinones as the cross-linking chemical species.

7.3.4   Other

There is little doubt that the rate and extent of cross-linking in collagen and elastin is determined by a host of nutritional, hormonal, and other endogenous and exogenous factors. With the exception of the few examples discussed in earlier sections, direct chemical determination of cross-links has not been achieved. In the case of collagen, the degree of intramolecular and intermolecular cross-linking is inferred from the relative proportions of soluble and matrix fractions. Generally, one cannot determine whether tissue structure and composition in a given condition reflects altered cross-linking of the fibrous proteins or a change in the rate of their synthesis and/or removal. Only a very few observations which bear on the factors which may influence cross-linking reactions will be cited here as examples.

Severe caloric restriction apparently retards [196] and an atheroma-inducing diet apparently enhances cross-linking of collagen in the tail tendon of the rat, as determined indirectly by thermal shrinkage and tensile strength [197]. The role of copper deficiency in the biosynthesis of cross-links formed from lysine residues in collagen and elastin has been cited. Vitamin B_6 deficiency has been reported to promote arteriosclerotic changes in monkeys [215] and in chicks to result in diminished levels of amine oxidase, mature aortic elastin, and ^{14}C-lysine incorporation into the desmosines [216]. Magnesium deficiency also causes localized fragmentation of arterial elastic lamellae in growing animals [217], although the molecular defect is unkown. Vitamin E is among the most important naturally occurring antioxidants. It is of significance that tissue levels of potential cross-linking free radicals and lipid peroxides are elevated in vitamin E-deficient animals and in other pathological conditions, such as inflammation induced by chemicals and ionizing radiation. (See review, [218].)

Hormonal influences are no doubt exerted at all stages of fibrous protein biosynthesis, maturation, and consolidation. These effects are most clearly reflected in the relative proportions and total amounts of soluble and matrix collagens. The high incidence of aortic rupture in young turkeys, treated for a few weeks with estrogen [219], is a dramatic example of probable hormonal interference in cross-linking reactions. Hypophysectomy reportedly retards the apparent aging of collagen in the rat [220, 221]. The breaking time for rat tail tendon in urea at 40° increases logarithmically with age; 25 days after hypophysectomy there is a transient increase in breaking time, but 200 to 800 days after the operation there occurs a below normal reduction. The biological age of the tendon in the 800-day old hypophysectomized rat corresponds to that of a 400-day old sham-operated control. Earlier studies [222] had indicated an inhibition of interchain cross-links in collagen of hypophysectomized animals. A decreased tensile strength of tendon fibers was reported for adult rats of both sexes castrated early in life [223].

The effects of sunlight on exposed skin in man leads to a number of changes, some of which appear to be duplicated by experimental ultraviolet irradiation of animal skins and other tissues. At least initially, ultraviolet irradiation appears to promote interchain cross-links in skin collagen, since the soluble fraction is diminished with irradiation [224–226]; in addition, shrinkage temperature is elevated, indicative of increased cross-linking [226]. However, prolonged irradiation *in vitro* results in hydrolysis of peptide bonds and amino acid destruction in collagen [227] and elastin [54]. Ionizing irradiation of rat tail tendon is reported to apparently increase cross-linking, as indicated by diminished solubility of the collagen [228] and to have no apparent effect as determined by thermal contraction [229]. Obviously, many factors, including total dose and duration of radiation, influence the process and are reflected in the large number of contrasting reports dealing with the physical properties of connective tissues in various physiological, pharmacological, and pathological states.

The rate of collagen fibrogenesis *in vitro* [230, 231] and the stability and ease of dispersion of the fibers [232] are markedly altered by many simple substances such as salts and amino acids, known to be present in tissues. L-Ascorbic acid prevents aggregation (gel formation) of soluble collagen under conditions of temperature, pH, and ionic strength similar to those *in vivo* [233]. There is some question whether the concentrations of these compounds, shown to be effective *in vitro*, are ever approached *in situ*. However, since fiber stability can be drastically altered by the insertion of an extremely small number of cross-links, specific interaction between functional groups on a fibrous protein with any of a large number of reactive metabolites cannot be excluded.

REFERENCES

1. K. Hannig and A. Nordwig, *Treatise on Collagen*, G. N. Ramachandran, Ed., Academic Press, New York, 1967.

2. K. Piez, *Treatise on Collagen*, G. N. Ramachandran, Ed., Academic Press, New York, 1967.

3. F. S. LaBella, S. Vivian, and D. P. Thornhill, *J. Gerontol.*, **21**, 550 (1966).

4. F. S. LaBella and S. Vivian, *Biochim. Biophys. Acta*, **133**, 189 (1967).

5. F. W. Keeley, Ph.D. Thesis, University of Manitoba, 1970.

6. J. P. Bentley and A. N. Hanson, *Biochim. Biophys. Acta*, **175**, 339 (1969).

7. K. H. Gustavson, *Nature*, **188**, 419 (1960).

8. K. A. Piez, *J. Amer. Chem. Soc.*, **82**, 247 (1960).

9. W. F. Harrington and N. V. Rao, *Conformation of Biopolymers*, G. N. Ramachandran,Ed., Academic Press, London, 1967.

10. K. M. Rudall, *Treatise on Collagen*, G. N. Ramachandran, Ed., Academic Press, New York, 1968.

11. A. Veis and J. Anesey, *J. Biol. Chem.*, **240**, 3899 (1965).

12. P. Bornstein, G. R. Martin, and K. A. Piez, *Science*, **144**, 1220 (1964).

13. P. Bornstein, and K. A. Piez, *J. Clin. Invest.*, **43**, 1813 (1964).

14. J. Gross, *Biochim. Biophys. Acta*, **74**, 314 (1963).

15. A. Veis, *Treatise on Collagen*, G. N. Ramachandran, Ed., Academic Press, New York, 1967.

16. A. Veis, J. Anesey, and S. Mussell, *Nature*, **215**, 931 (1967).

17. A. J. Hodge, J. H. Highberger, G. G. Deffner, and F. O. Schmitt, *Proc. Nat. Acad. Sci.*, **46**, 197 (1960).

18. A. L. Rubin, D. Pfahl, P. T. Speakman, P. F. Davison, and F. O. Schmitt, *Science*, **139**, 37 (1963).

19. A. L. Rubin, M. P. Drake, P. F. Davison, D. Pfahl, P. T. Speakman, and F. O. Schmitt, *Biochemistry*, **4**, 181 (1965).

20. J. Rosmus, Z. Deyl, and M. P. Drake, *Biochim. Biophys. Acta*, **140**, 507 (1967).

21. Z. Deyl, J. Rosmus, and S. Bump, *Biochim. Biophys. Acta*, **140**, 515 (1967).

22. K. A. Piez, *Ann. Rev. Biochem.*, **37**, 547 (1968).

23. P. Bornstein and K. A. Piez, *Biochemistry*, **5**, 3460 (1966).

24. P. Bornstein, A. H. Kang, and K. A. Piez, *Biochemistry*, **5**, 3803 (1966).
25. F. R. Partington and G. C. Wood, *Biochim. Biophys. Acta*, **69**, 485 (1963).
26. R. A. Grant, R. W. Cox, and R. W. Horne, *J. Roy. Microscop. Soc.*, **87**, 143 (1967).
27. T. P. Ayer, *Intern. Rev. Conn. Tissue Res.*, D. A. Hall, Ed., Academic Press, New York, 1964.
28. N. M. Wiederhorn and G. V. Reardon, *J. Polymer Sci.*, **9**, 315 (1952).
29. N. M. Wiederhorn, G. V. Reardon, and A. R. Broune, *J. Amer. Leather Chemists' Assoc.*, **48**, 7 (1953).
30. L. Gotte, G. Pezzin, and G. D. Stella, *Biochimie et Physiologie du Tissu Conjunctif*, Ph. Comte, Ed. Soc. Orméco et Imprimérie du Sûd-Est à Lyons, 1965, p. 145.
31. S. O. Anderson, *Biochim. Biophys. Acta*, **69**, 249 (1963).
32. P. J. Flory, *Principles of Polymer Chemistry*, Cornell University Press, Ithaca, N.Y., 1953, Chapter 11.
33. J. H. Bowes and C. W. Cater, 27th Meeting of Res. Panel, Gelatin and Glue Res. Assoc., 1964. Cited by A. Veis, *Treatise on Collagen*, G. N. Ramachandran, Ed., Academic Press, New York, 1967.
34. C. W. Cater, *J. Soc. Leather Trades' Chem.*, **47**, 259 (1963).
35. V. Mohr and J. R. Bendall, *Nature*, **223**, 404 (1969).
36. E. Heikkinen, L. Mikkonen, and K. Kulonen, *Exptl. Gerontol.*, **1**, 31 (1964).
37. K. H. Gustavson, *The Chemistry and Reactivity of Collagen*, Academic Press, New York, 1956.
38. R. A. Milch, *J. Amer. Leather Chemists' Assoc.*, **57**, 581 (1952).
39. F. Verzar and K. Huber, *Gerontologia*, **2**, 81 (1958).
40. D. S. Jackson, *Advan. Biol. Skin*, **6**, 219 (1964).
41. H. R. Elden, *Intern. Rev. Conn. Tissue Res.*, D. A. Hall, Ed., Academic Press, New York, 1968, p. 283.
42. F. S. LaBella and W. G. Lindsay, *J. Gerontol.*, **18**, 111 (1963).
43. F. S. LaBella and D. P. Thornhill, *Studies of Rheumatoid Disease*, Proc. 3rd Canad. Conf. Res. Rheum. Dis., Canad. Arthr. Rheum. Soc., Toronto, 1965, p. 246.
44. F. S. LaBella, *J. Gerontol.*, **17**, 8 (1962).
45. D. P. Thornhill and F. S. LaBella, *Studies of Rheumatoid Diseases*, Proc. 3rd Canad. Conf. Res. Rheum. Dis., Canad. Arthr. Rheum. Soc., Toronto, 1965, p. 236.
46. F. S. LaBella, *Nature*, **180**, 1360 (1957).
47. F. J. Loomeijer, *J. Atheroscler. Res.*, **1**, 62 (1961).
48. F. S. LaBella, F. Keeley, S. Vivian, and D. Thornhill, *Biochem. Biophys. Res. Commun.*, **26**, 748 (1967).
49. F. W. Keeley, F. S. LaBella, and G. Queen, *Biochem. Biophys. Res. Commun.*, **34**, 156 (1969).
50. F. S. LaBella, *Arch. Biochem. Biophys.*, **93**, 72 (1961).
51. R. L. Walford, D. L. Moyer, and R. B. Schneider, *Arch. Pathol.*, **72**, 40 (1961).

52. S. M. Partridge, D. F. Elsden, and J. Thomas, *Nature*, **197**, 1297 (1963).

53. S. M. Partridge, *Advan. Protein Chem.*, **17**, 227 (1962).

54. R. T. Butler, *J. Biol. Chem.*, **244**, 3415 (1969).

55. K. H. Gustavson, *The Chemistry of Tanning Processes*, Academic Press, New York, 1956.

56. W. S. Pierpoint, *Biochem. J.*, **112**, 609 (1969).

57. W. S. Pierpoint, *Biochem. J.*, **112**, 619 (1969).

58. F. W. Keeley and F. S. LaBella, *Federation Proc.*, (1968).

59. P. C. Brown, R. Consden, and L. E. Glynn, *Ann. Rheumat. Diseases*, **17**, 196 (1958).

60. F. S. LaBella, *Sec. Canad. Conf. Res. Rheumat. Dis.*, Canad. Arthr. Rheum. Soc., Toronto, 1961, p. 221.

61. R. Consden and J. A. Kirrane, *Nature*, **215**, 165 (1967).

62. J. M. Landucci, *Bull. Soc. Chem.*, **21**, 120 (1954).

63. J. Rosmus and Z. Deyl, *Experientia*, **23**, 610 (1967).

64. S. Ayad, F. S. Steven, and D. S. Jackson, *Biochim. Biophys. Acta*, **188**, 302 (1969).

65. J. F. Woessner, *Collagen*, B. S. Gould, Ed., Vol. 2B, Academic Press, New York, 1968, p. 253.

66. E. Fujimori, *Biochemistry*, **5**, 1034 (1966).

67. D. R. Cooper and R. J. Davidson, *Biochem. J.*, **97**, 139 (1965).

68. F. S. LaBella and G. Paul, *J. Gerontol.*, **20**, 54 (1965).

69. J. Blomfield and J. F. Farrar, *Cardiovasc. Res.*, **3**, 161 (1969).

70. R. Ross and P. Bornstein, *J. Cell Biol.*, **40**, 366 (1969).

71. M. D. Haust, *Amer. J. Pathol.*, **47**, 1113 (1965).

72. H. E. Karrer, *J. Ultrastruct. Res.*, **4**, 420 (1960).

73. E. G. Cleary, D. S. Jackson, and L. B. Sandberg, *Biochimie et Physiologie du Tissu Conjunctif*, Ph. Comte, Ed., Soc. Orméco et Imprimérie du Sûd-Est à Lyons, 1966, p. 167.

74. F. S. Steven and D. S. Jackson, *Biochim. Biophys. Acta*, **168**, 334 (1968).

75. S. M. Partridge, *Gerontologia*, **15**, 85 (1969).

76. E. J. Miller, G. R. Martin, C. E. Mecca, and K. A. Piez, *J. Biol. Chem.*, **240**, 3623 (1965).

77. D. W. Smith, N. Weissman, and W. H. Carnes, *Biochem. Biophys. Res. Commun.*, **31**, 309 (1968).

78. J. Thomas, D. F. Elsden, and S. M. Partridge, *Nature*, **200**, 651 (1963).

79. S. M. Partridge, D. F. Elsden, J. Thomas, A. Dorfman, A. Telser, and Ho Pei-Lee, *Nature*, **209**, 399 (1966).

80. E. J. Miller, G. R. Martin, and K. A. Piez, *Biochem. Biophys. Res. Commun.*, **17**, 248 (1964).

81. M. Ledvina and F. Bartos, *Exptl. Gerontol.*, **3**, 171 (1968).

82. R. A. Anwar and G. Oda, *Biochim. Biophys. Acta*, **133**, 151 (1967).

83. A. Ciferri and L. V. Rajagh, *J. Gerontol.*, **19**, 220 (1964).

84. L. L. Salcedo, B. Faris, and C. Franzblau, *Biochim. Biophys. Acta,* **188,** 324 (1969).

85. E. J. Miller, S. R. Pinnell, G. R. Martin, and E. Schiffmann, *Biochem. Biophys. Res. Commun.,* **26,** 132 (1967).

86. W. Shimada, A. Bowman, N. R. Davis, and R. A. Anwar, *Biochem. Biophys. Res. Commun.,* **37,** 191 (1969).

87. S. M. Partridge, *Nature,* **213,** 1123 (1967).

88. S. M. Partridge, *Biochim. Biophys. Acta,* **140,** 132 (1967).

89. C. Franzblau, F. M. Sinex, B. Faris, and R. Lampidis, *Biochem. Biophys. Res. Commun.,* **21,** 575 (1965).

90. B. C. Starcher, S. M. Partridge, and D. F. Elsden, *Biochemistry,* **6,** 2425 (1967).

91. C. Franzblau, B. Faris, and R. Papaioannou, *Biochemistry,* **8,** 2833 (1969).

92. R. Lent and C. Franzblau, *Biochem. Biophys. Res. Commun.,* **26,** 43 (1967).

93. R. W. Lent, B. Smith, L. L. Salcedo, B. Faris, and C. Franzblau, *Biochemistry,* **8,** 2837 (1969).

94. M. Tanzer, L. D. Monroe, and J. Gross, *Biochemistry,* **5,** 1919 (1966).

95. M. Rojkind, L. Rhi, and M. Aguirre, *J. Biol. Chem.,* **243,** 2266 (1968).

96. M. Rojkind, A. M. Gutienez, M. Zeichner, and R. W. Lent, *Biochem. Biophys. Res. Commun.,* **36,** 350 (1969).

97. A. H. Kang, B. Faris, and C. Franzblau, *Biochem. Biophys. Res. Commun.,* **36,** 345 (1969).

98. R. L. Hill, *Advan. Protein Chem.,* **20,** 37 (1965).

99. M. L. Tanzer, *J. Biol. Chem.,* **243,** 4045 (1968).

100. A. J. Bailey, *Biochim. Biophys. Acta,* **160,** 447 (1968).

101. A. J. Bailey and D. Lister, *Nature,* **220,** 280 (1968).

102. S. R. Pinnell, G. R. Martin, and E. J. Miller, *Science,* **161,** 475 (1968).

103. M. Rojkind and H. Juarez, *Biochem. Biophys. Res. Commun.,* **25,** 481 (1966).

104. A. J. Bailey and C. M. Peach, *Biochem. Biophys. Res. Commun.,* **33,** 812 (1968).

105. A. J. Bailey, L. J. Fowler, and C. M. Peach, *Biochem. Biophys. Res. Commun.,* **35,** 663 (1969).

106. A. J. Bailey and L. J. Fowler, *Biochem. Biophys. Res. Commun.,* **35,** 672 (1969).

107. R. C. Page, E. P. Benditt, and C. R. Kirkwood, *Biochem. Biophys. Res. Commun.,* **33,** 752 (1968).

108. E. J. Miller, G. R. Martin, K. A. Piez, and M. J. Powers, *J. Biol. Chem.,* **242,** 5481 (1967).

109. D. W. Bird, J. E. Savage, and B. L. O'Dell, *Proc. Soc. Exptl. Biol. Med.,* **123,** 250 (1966).

110. C. H. Hill, B. Starcher, and C. Kim, *Federation Proc.,* **26,** 129 (1967).

111. R. C. Page and E. P. Benditt, *Biochemistry,* **6,** 1142 (1967).

112. S. R. Pinnell and G. R. Martin, *Proc. Nat. Acad. Sci.,* **61,** 708 (1968).

113. C. I. Levene and J. Gross, *J. Exptl. Med.,* **110,** 771 (1959).

298 Cross-links in Elastin and Collagen

114. J. Gross, *Biochim. Biophys. Acta*, **71**, 250 (1963).

115. E. Hausmann, *Arch. Biochem. Biophys.*, **103**, 227 (1963).

116. M. E. Nimni, *Biochem. Biophys. Res. Commun.*, **25**, 434 (1966).

117. K. Deshmukh and M. Nimni, *Biochim. Biophys. Acta*, **154**, 258 (1968).

118. A. D. Deshmukh and M. E. Nimni, *Biochem. Biophys. Res. Commun.*, **35**, 845 (1969).

119. H. B. Bensusan and A. Scanu, *J. Amer. Chem. Soc.*, **82**, 4990 (1960).

120. S. O. Andersen, *Biochim. Biophys. Acta*, **93**, 213 (1964).

121. S. O. Andersen, *Acta Physiol. Scand.*, **66**, Suppl. 263 (1966).

122. A. J. Gross and I. W. Sizer, *J. Biol. Chem.*, **234**, 1611 (1959).

123. F. S. LaBella, P. Waykole, and G. Queen, *Biochem. Biophys. Res. Commun.*, **30**, 333 (1968).

124. M. K. Dabbous, *J. Biol. Chem.*, **241**, 5307 (1966).

125. S. S. Lehrer and G. D. Fasman, *Biochemistry*, **6**, 757 (1967).

126. O. W. McBride and W. F. Harrington, *J. Biol. Chem.*, **240**, pc 4545 (1965).

127. O. W. McBride and W. F. Harrington, *Biochemistry*, **6**, 1484 (1967).

128. E. J. Miller and H. M. Fullmer, *J. Exptl. Med.*, **6**, 1097 (1966).

129. M. J. Glimcher, C. J. Francois, L. Richards, and S. M. Krane, *Biochim. Biophys. Acta*, **93**, 585 (1964).

130. R. J. Schleuter, PhD. Thesis, cited by A. Veis, *Treatise on Collagen*, G. N. Ramachandran, Ed., Academic Press, New York, Vol. 1, 1967, p. 367.

131. A. A. Marino and R. O. Bicher, *Nature*, **213**, 697 (1967).

132. A. Veis and R. J. Schleuter, *Biochemistry*, **3**, 1650 (1964).

133. A. Veis and A. Perry, *Biochemistry*, **6**, 2409 (1967).

134. S. M. Partridge, H. F. Davis, and G. S. Adair, *Biochem. J.*, **61**, 11 (1955).

135. O. O. Blumenfeld and P. M. Gallop, *Proc. Nat. Acad. Sci.*, **56**, 1260 (1966).

136. A. Schneider, E. Henson, O. O. Blumenfeld, and P. M. Gallop, *Biochem. Biophys. Res. Commun.*, **27**, 546 (1967).

137. P. C. J. Brunet and P. W. Kent, *Proc. Roy. Soc. (B)*, **144**, 259 (1955).

138. P. C. J. Brunet, *Biochem. Soc. Symp. (London)*, T. W. Goodwin, Ed., **25**, 49 (1965).

139. M. G. M. Pryor, *Proc. Roy. Soc. (B)*, **128**, 378 (1940).

140. R. Dennell, *Biol. Rev.*, **33**, 178 (1958).

141. J. H. Kennaugh, *J. Insect Physiol.*, **2**, 97 (1958).

142. P. Karlson, *Z. Physiol. Chem.*, **318**, 194 (1960).

143. P. Karlson and C. E. Sekeris, *Nature*, **195**, 183 (1962).

144. P. Karlson and H. Lieban, *Z. Physiol. Chem.*, **326**, 135 (1961).

145. C. H. Brown, *Nature*, **165**, 275 (1950).

146. M. G. M. Pryor, *Comparative Biochemistry*, Vol. 4, M. Florkin and U. S. Mason, Eds., Academic Press, New York, 1962.

147. F. S. LaBella, *Arch. Biochem. Biophys.*, **93**, 72 (1961).

148. N. H. Grant and H. E. Alburn, *Biochemistry*, **4**, 127 (1965).

149. J. H. Harding, *Advan. Protein Chem.*, **20**, 109 (1965).

150. J. Pisano, J. S. Finlayson, and M. P. Peyton, *Science,* **160,** 892 (1968).
151. L. Lorand, J. Downey, T. Gotok, A. Jacobsen, and S. Tokura, *Biochem. Biophys. Res. Commun.,* **31,** 222 (1968).
152. P. M. Gallop, O. O. Blumenfeld, and S. Seifter, *Treatise on Collagen,* G. N. Ramachandran, Ed., Academic Press, New York, Vol. 1, 1967, p. 339.
153. C. Franzblau, P. M. Gallop, and S. Seifter, *Biopolymers,* **1,** 71 (1963).
154. M. Rojkind and P. M. Gallop, *Collagen Currents,* **4,** No. 542 (1963).
155. S. Seifter, C. Franzblau, E. Harper, and P. M. Gallop, *Structure and Function of Connective and Skeletal Tissue,* Butterworths, London, 1965, p. 21.
156. J. Mechanic and M. Levy, *J. Amer. Chem. Soc.,* **81,** 1889 (1959).
157. O. Blumenfeld and P. M. Gallop, *Biochemistry,* **1,** 947 (1962).
158. H. Hormann, *Leder,* **13,** 79 (1962).
159. O. O. Blumenfeld, M. A. Paz, P. M. Gallop, and S. Seifter, *J. Biol. Chem.,* **238,** 3835 (1963).
160. P. Bornstein, *Biochem. Biophys. Res. Commun.,* **36,** 957 (1969).
161. W. T. Butler and L. W. Cunningham, *J. Biol. Chem.,* **3882,** 241 (1966).
162. H. B. Bensusan, *Structure and Function of Connective and Skeletal Tissue,* S. F. Jackson, R. D. Harkness, S. M. Partridge, and G. R. Tristam, Eds., Butterworths, London, 1965, p. 42.
163. H. B. Bensusan, S. McKnight, and M. S. R. Naidu, *Federation Proc.,* **25,** 716 (1966).
164. D. W. Bannister, *Biochem. J.,* **114,** 509 (1969).
165. G. M. Windrum, P. W. Kent, and J. E. Eastoe, *Br. J. Exptl. Pathol.,* **36,** 49 (1955).
166. A. M. Melcher, *Gerontologia,* **15,** 217 (1969).
167. J. E. Eastoe, *Treatise on Collagen,* G. N. Ramachandran, Ed., Academic Press, New York, Vol. 1, 1967, p. 1.
168. A. I. Lansing, T. B. Rosenthal, M. Alex, and E. W. Dempsey, *Anat. Record,* **114,** 555 (1952).
169. F. J. Loomeijer, *J. Atheroscler. Res.,* **1,** 62 (1961).
170. F. S. LaBella, *J. Histochem. Cytochem.,* **6,** 260 (1958).
171. S. Keller, M. M. Levi, and I. Mandl, *Arch. Biochem. Biophys.,* **13,** 565 (1969).
172. K. Nakao and A. A. Angrist, *Amer. J. Clin. Pathol.,* **49,** 65 (1968).
173. J. Bjorksten, *J. Amer. Geriatrics Soc.,* **16,** 408 (1968).
174. R. A. Milch, *J. Ann. Leather Chemists' Assoc.,* **57,** 581 (1962).
175. P. Bornstein, A. H. Kang, and K. A. Piez, *Proc. Nat. Acad. Sci.,* **55,** 417 (1966).
176. R. C. Page and E. P. Benditt, *Proc. Soc. Exptl. Biol. Med.,* **124,** 459 (1966).
177. H. Sobel, *Adv. Gerontol. Res.,* B. L. Strehler, Ed., Academic Press, New York, Vol. 2 1967, p. 205.
178. R. A. Milch, *Monographs in the Surgical Sciences,* Williams and Wilkins Co., Baltimore, 2, 1965, p. 261.
179. F. Verzar, *Intern. Rev. Conn. Tissue Res.,* D. A. Hall, Ed., **2,** 244 (1964).

180. J. Gross, *Structural Aspects of Aging* G. H. Bourne, Ed., Pitman Medical Publication, 1961, p. 178.

181. G. Hass, *Arch. Pathol.*, **35**, 29 (1943).

182. A. J. Bailey and D. Lister, *Nature*, **220**, 280 (1968).

183. A. J. Bailey, *Biochim. Biophys. Acta*, **160**, 447 (1968).

184. J. Balo and I. Banga, *3rd Internatl. Congr. Biochem.*, 120 (1955).

185. H. Saxl, *4th Internatl. Congr. Gerontol.*, **2**, 67 (1957).

186. R. E. Tunbridge, *Ciba Found. Colloq. Aging*, Little, Brown & Co., Boston, Vol. 3, 1957, p. 92.

187. J. D. Mull and J. S. Ram., *J. Gerontol.*, **20**, 201 (1965).

188. J. P. Ayer, G. M. Hass, and A. Philpott, *Arch. Pathol.*, **65**, 519 (1958).

189. R. R. Kohn and A. M. Leash, *Exptl. Molec. Pathol.*, **7**, 354 (1967).

190. F. S. LaBella, *Gerontologist*, **6**, 46 (1966).

191. F. S. LaBella, *Gerontologist*, **8**, 13 (1968).

192. D. Harman, *J. Gerontol.*, **12**, 257 (1957).

193. D. Harman, *J. Gerontol.*, **23**, 476 (1968).

194. F. S. LaBella, *Proc. 7th Internatl. Congr. Gerontol.*, Vienna, **1**, 153 (1966).

195. C. M. McCay, *Amer. J. Publ. Health*, **37**, 521 (1947).

196. M. Chvapil and Z. Hruza, *Gerontologia*, **3**, 241 (1959).

197. Z. Hruza and M. Chvapil, *Physiol. Bohemosl.*, **11**, 423 (1962).

198. V. A. McKusick, *Heritable Disorders of Connective Tissue*, C. V. Mosby, Co., St. Louis, 1960.

199. B. L. O'Dell, F. Elsden, J. Thomas, and S. M. Partridge, *Nature*, **209**, 401, 1966.

200. E. J. Miller, and H. M. Fullmer, *J. Exptl. Med.*, **123**, 1097 (1966).

201. M. E. Nimni, *J. Biol. Chem.*, **243**, 1457 (1968).

202. C. I. Levene and J. Gross, *J. Exp. Med.*, **110**, 771 (1959).

203. G. R. Martin, J. Gross, K. A. Piez, and M. S. Lewis, *Biochim. Biophys. Acta*, **53**, 599 (1961).

204. J. S. Kennedy and G. D. C. Kennedy, *Proc. Soc. Exptl. Biol. Med.*, **98**, 843 (1958).

205. D. S. Jackson and J. P. Bentley, *J. Insect Physiol.*, **2**, 189 (1958).

206. R. Rybach, *Gerontologia*, **11**, 120 (1965).

207. D. P. Varadi and D. A. Hall, *Nature*, **208**, 1224 (1965).

208. C. Nordschow and E. B. Marsolias, *Arch. Pathol.*, **88**, 65 (1969).

209. L. H. Jansen, *Dermatologica*, **110**, 108 (1955).

210. H. L. Wechsler and E. R. Fischer, *Arch. Pathol.*, **77**, 613 (1964).

211. F. Steven, *J. Insect Physiol.*, **2**, 46 (1958).

212. W. N. O'Brien, B. N. La Du, and J. J. Bunin, *Amer. J. Med.*, **34**, 813 (1962).

213. V. G. Zannoni, N. Lomtevas, and S. Goldfinger, *Biochim. Biophys. Acta*, **177**, 94 (1969).

214. R. A. Milch, *Clin. Orthoped.*, **24**, 213 (1962).

215. J. F. Rhinehart, *Connective Tissue in Health and Disease*, G. Asboe-Hansen, Ed., Munksgaard, Copenhagen, 1954, p. 239.

216. C. H. Hill and C. S. Kim, *Biochem. Biophys. Res. Commun.*, **27**, 94 (1967).

217. J. J. Vitale, E. E. Hellerstein, M. Nakamura, B. Loun, *Circulation Res.*, **9**, 387 (1961).

218. A. A. Barber and F. Bornheim, *Advan. Gerontol. Res.*, **2**, 355 (1967).

219. C. F. Simpson and R. H. Harms, *Proc. Soc. Exptl. Biol. Med.*, **123**, 604 (1966).

220. A. V. Everitt, G. G. Olsen, and G. R. Burrows, *J. Gerontol.*, **23**, 333 (1968).

221. F. Verzar and H. Spichtin, *Gerontologia*, **12**, 48 (1966).

222. Z. Deyl, A. V. Everitt, and J. Rosmus, *Exptl. Gerontol.*, **2**, 249 (1967).

223. Z. Hruza, M. Chvapil, and V. Kobrle, *Physiol. Bohemosl.*, **10**, 290 (1961).

224. A. J. Bailey, D. Rhodes, and C. W. Cater, *Radiat. Res.*, **24**, 606 (1964).

225. E. Bottoms and S. Schuster, *Nature*, **199**, 192 (1963).

226. R. Consden and J. A. Kirrane, *Nature*, **215**, 165 (1967).

227. D. R. Cooper and R. I. Davidson, *Biochem. J.*, **98**, 655 (1966).

228. A. J. Bailey and W. J. Tromans, *Radiat. Res.*, **23**, 145 (1964).

229. E. B. Darden and A. C. Upton, *J. Gerontol.*, **19**, 62 (1964).

230. G. C. Wood, *Biochem. J.*, **76**, 598 (1960).

231. J. Gross and D. Kirk, *J. Biol. Chem.*, **233**, 355 (1958).

232. J. K. Candlish and G. R. Tristram, *Biochim. Biophys. Acta*, **88**, 553 (1964).

233. J. C. Caygill, *Biochim. Biophys. Acta*, **181**, 334 (1969).

8

Structure and Hydration of Mucopolysaccharides

FREDERICK A. BETTELHEIM

Department of Chemistry, Adelphi University, Garden City, New York

The name mucopolysaccharides was coined by Meyer [1] to describe "hexosamine containing polysaccharides of animal origin." While this terminology adequately describes the physical properties of solutions containing such substances, in the present parlance, the name glycosaminoglycans is used more often because it relates to the chemical structure of these compounds. Since in the medical literature the term mucopolysaccharide is used almost exclusively, it is retained here.

The mucopolysaccharides occur mostly as extracellular material. Their main physiological role is to bind together cells and organs. In this sense their function is structural, providing toughness and flexibility (together with fibers) in the connective tissues of animals, and largely acting as the cementing material of ground tissues between cells. Since all substances going from cell to cell must pass through such ground substances, the chemical composition and physical state of the muco-polysaccharides may well influence the metabolism of cells. Physiological and pathological processes such as control of electrolytes and water in extracellular fluids, lubrication, calcification, and wound healing have been associated with the mucopolysaccharide matrix.

Most of the mucopolysaccharides occur in nature as protein complexes. In the present treatment, first the attention is focused on the carbohydrate moieties only.

The polysaccharide parts of protein-mucopolysaccharide complexes have been isolated and studied to a great extent and their chemical structures (primary, secondary, and tertiary) are known. In contrast, there is very little known on the protein moieties of these complexes. Currently, however, a large amount of work is being done on the carbohydrate-protein linkage. This will constitute the second part of the discussion of the structure of mucopolysaccharides together with the meager knowledge we possess on the nature of the protein moieties.

The overall view of the protein-mucopolysaccharide complex may be the macromolecular view. In this sense we deal with biological polyelectrolytes. Moreover, since the preponderance of the charge of the protein-mucopolysaccharide complex is anionic (although some cationic groups may be present on the protein moieties), these macromolecules can be considered polyanions.

The polyanions are characterized by (1) their polysaccharidic and protein backbones and (2) the special anionic groups (mainly $-COO^-$ and $-SO_3^-$) and their spatial charge distribution along the backbone of the polymer. Most of the physical-chemical properties arise from these two features. The polysaccharide backbone can be considered as a condensation polymer of monosaccharides. The resulting glycosidic linkage (α or β) will partly determine the intrinsic stiffness of the backbone, since the monosaccharidic units largely exist in the ring form (pyranose, etc.) and, therefore, the only rotational possibility of the polysaccharide backbone is around the glycosidic bond.

In contrast to this, the protein backbone consisting of more flexible peptide linkages will have an intrinsic stiffness or flexibility depending on the amount of steric hindrance the bulky side chains of amino acids provide and/or the type of interaction (hydrophylic and hydrophobic) among these side chains. These interactions will determine the tertiary structure (coiling, helix formation, etc.). It is believed that the protein moiety in most cases occupies a central position, sort of a core of the molecule, and the polysaccharide moieties are on the outside as long side chains [2] (Fig. 8.1). The spatial distribution of the anionic groups and their degree of ionization will contribute to the conformation of

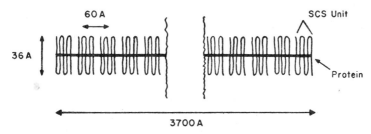

Figure 8.1. Schematic representation of protein-mucopolysaccharide complex. (Reproduced from Mathews and Lozaityte, *Arch. Biochem. Biophys.*, **74**, 158 (1958), through the courtesy of the *Arch. Biochem. Biophys.*, Academic Press, N.Y.)

the molecules due to the mutual electrostatic repulsion of the negative charges along the polysaccharidic backbone. In addition, both the conformation of a single molecule and the tertiary structure of the mucopolysaccharides in concentrated solutions, gels, and in the solid state will be influenced by the large amounts of inter- and intramolecular hydrogen bonding among the abundant polar sites such as —OH, —C—O—C—, —C=O, —NH$_2$, COO$^-$, —SO$_3$$^-$, and so on. Similarly, hydrophobic interactions of the protein moiety may also influence the structure.

8.1   STRUCTURE OF THE POLYSACCHARIDE CHAINS

Hyaluronic acid is one of the most important mucopolysaccharides of the connective tissues. It was first isolated by Meyer and Palmer [3] from vitreous humor of cattle eyes. It is widely distributed in different connective tissues, synovial and vitreous fluids of animals, and in some bacteria [4–6]. Meyer has demonstrated [7] that it consists of equimolar quantities of D-glucuronic acid and 2-acetamido-2-deoxy-D-glucose. Subsequent work, mainly by Meyer and his group [8] and Jeanloz and co-workers [9], have established the primary structure (Fig. 8.2). The repeating unit of the chain polymer is a disaccharide, hyalobiuronic acid, in which the glucosamine moiety is linked with a β-glycosidic linkage to the C-3 position of the glucuronic acid [2-acetamido-2-deoxy-3-O-(β-D-glucopyranosyl uronic acid)-D-glucose]. The polymer is made up of the 1 → 4-β-glycosidic linkages of the hyalobiuronic acid repeating group [4].

Bettelheim [10] has purified a hyaluronic acid fraction from umbilical cords with no protein content. This proved to be semicrystalline, hence,

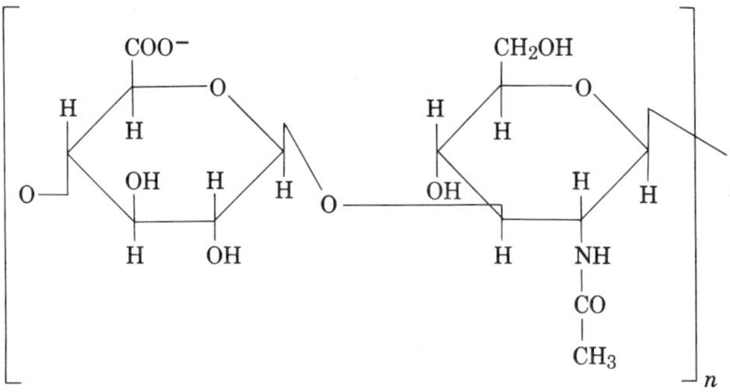

Figure 8.2.   The structure of the repeating unit of the hyaluronic acid chain.

amenable to structural analysis by x-ray diffraction. Fiber diagram of sodium hyaluronate [11] indicated that in the solid state the hyalo-biuronic acid repeating unit is a very stiff segment of the chain. The length of this disaccharidic repeating unit is 11.98 Å as compared to 10.3 Å in the case of the disaccharide in the relatively stiff cellulose molecule.

The mucopolysaccharide chondroitin is closely related to hyaluronic acid from the structural point of view. It is similar to the hyaluronic acid in primary structure except that the hexosamine moiety is galactosamine instead of glucosamine. It was isolated by Meyer et al. [12], from bovine cornea and on the basis of acidic enzymatic hydrolysis products proved to be a polymer of $(1 \rightarrow 4)$-O-β-D-glucopyranosyluronic acid-$(1 \rightarrow 3)$-2-acetamido-2-deoxy-β-D-galactopyranose.

More frequent acidic polysaccharides of the connective tissues are chondroitin-4-sulfate and chondroitin-6-sulfate, which are also called chondroitin sulfate A and C, respectively. Chondroitin is thought to be the biological precursor [4] of chondroitin sulfates A and C. Chondroitin-4-sulfate (A) was first isolated from cartilage [13]. Structural studies by Levine [14], Wolfrom [15], and Meyer [16] proved that the repeating unit is a disaccharide, chondrosin, in which the glucuronic acid is bound in a $1 \rightarrow 3$-β linkage to the galactosamine moiety and the galactosamine is sulfated at the C-4 position (Fig. 8.3).

A partially sulfated chondroitin-4-sulfate was isolated by Bettelheim and Philpott [17] from bovine trachea. It was proposed that this highly crystalline chondroitin sulfate fraction was stereospecifically sulfated on an every third chondrosine moiety [18].

Chondroitin-6-sulfate C was first isolated by Meyer and Palmer [19] from umbilical cord. The only difference between chondroitin-4-sulfate

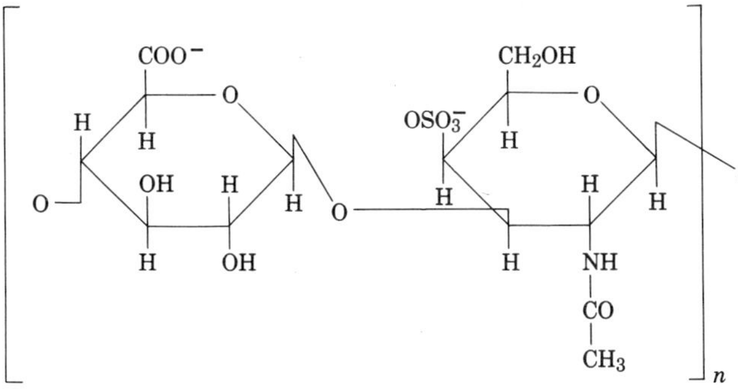

Figure 8.3. The structure of the repeating unit of the chondroitin-4-sulfate chain.

and chondroitin-6-sulfate is the position of the sulfate on the galactosamine moiety; in the first case this is in the C-4 position, in the second case in the C-6 position [20–22].

A chondroitin-6-sulfate preparation, which contained higher sulfate concentrations than the regular chondroitin sulfate C was isolated from shark cartilage [23, 24]. This shark cartilage chondroitin sulfate is also called chondroitin sulfate D [4].

Another acid polysaccharide of the connective tissue is called dermatan sulfate but in earlier literature it may appear under the name of chondroitin sulfate B or β-heparin. Since it is different both chemically and physiologically from the chondroitin sulfates, the name dermatan sulfate is less confusing. It was first isolated from pig skin by Meyer and Chaffee [27]. It differs from the chondroitin sulfates in that the uronic acid moiety is not a D-glucuronic acid but L-iduronic acid [28–30]. The repeating unit of the dermatan sulfate is, therefore, $(1 \rightarrow 4)$-O-α-L-idopyranosyluronic acid-$(1 \rightarrow 3)$-2-acetamido-2-deoxy-4-O-sulfo-β-D-galactopyranose (Fig. 8.4).

However, recent evidence shows that dermatan sulfate is not composed solely of iduronic and N-acetylgalactosamine residues. Hyaluronidase action on pig-skin dermatan sulfate indicated the presence of glucuronic acid in the chain [31]. A tetrasaccharide was isolated from pig-skin dermatan sulfate by Fransson and Rodén [32] which had a composition of glucuronic acid–N-acetylgalactosamine-4-sulfate–iduronic acid–N-acetylgalactosamine-4-sulfate. This proves that some of the dermatan sulfate chains, especially far away from the protein-carbohydrate linkage, may be block copolymers of two kinds of disaccharidic units.

A highly sulfated acidic polysaccharide, heparin, was isolated in 1916 by McLean from liver [33]. It had very high anticoagulant activity. It

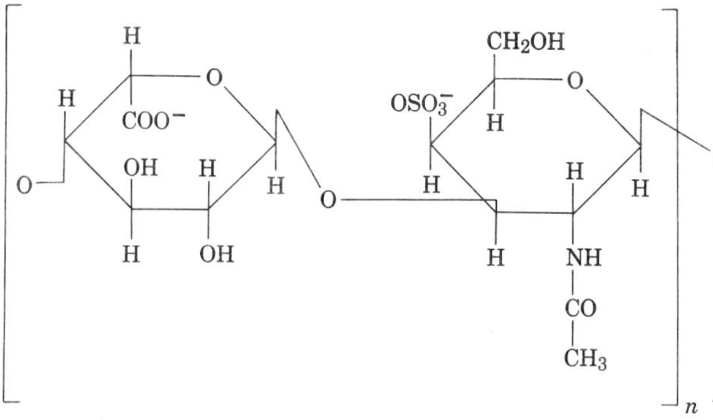

Figure 8.4.   The structure of the repeating unit of the dermatan sulfate chain.

also occurs in skin, muscles, lung, heart, kidney, spleen, and blood. In spite of the large amount of structural investigation performed on heparin, its primary structure is still not fully known (Fig. 8.5). The repeating unit is composed of equimolar quantities of D-glucosamine and D-glucuronic acid residues. Its sulfate content varies from 5 to 6.5 sulfate residues per tetrasaccharide [34, 35]. One of the sulfate groups is the glucosamine-N-sulfate moiety [36, 37]. The other sulfate groups are most probably located as O-esters. The glucosamine moiety is considered fully O-sulfated at the C-6 position [38]. On the basis of the behavior of heparin toward alkali hydrolysis it was suggested that the remaining O-sulfate groups may be located at the C-2 position of the uronic acid residue and at the C-3 position of the hexosamine moiety. However, the degree of sulfatation on these two positions varies from sample to sample and this may cause the variability of the total sulfate content reported in the literature [34]. The glycosidic linkage in heparin is mainly the $(1 \rightarrow 4)$-α-glycosidic linkage [39, 40]. However, there is still a possibility that some glycosidic linkage at $1 \rightarrow 6$ position provides branched structure, and some β configuration cannot be completely excluded. In heparin, besides the D-glucuronic acid, iduronic acid is also present. While the iduronic acid may be sulfated, the D-glucuronic acid is not [38].

Jorpes and Gardell [41] have isolated a dextrorotatory mucopolysaccharide from beef liver after the removal of heparin. This mucopolysaccharide, which is called heparitin sulfate, contained equimolar amounts of glucosamine, uronic acid, acetyl, and sulfate residues (Fig. 8.6). On the basis of its composition, it was suggested that the repeating unit may be a tetrasaccharide which contains one N-acetyl, one N-sulfate, and one O-sulfate group [42]. Heparitin sulfate, thus, may be a block

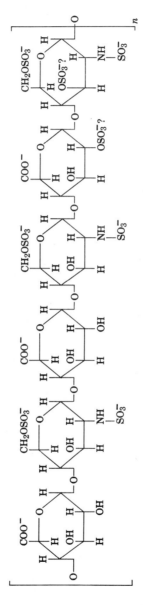

Figure 8.5. The structure of the repeating unit of the heparin chain.

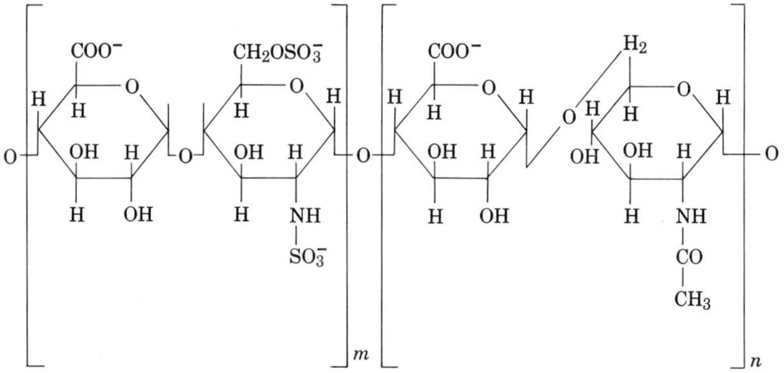

Figure 8.6.   The structure of the repeating unit of the heparitin sulfate chain.

co-polymer of disaccharides in which the glucosamine moiety carries O-sulfates and of disaccharides having N-acetylglucosamine moiety only [43]. It was reported that the heparitin sulfate may contain $(1 \rightarrow 6)$-uronylhexosamine linkage besides the usual $(1 \rightarrow 4)$ linkage [44]. Cifonelli [45] has suggested that the $1 \rightarrow 6$ linkages are branching points and the outer branches are composed of predominantly N-sulfate glucosamine groups and the inner core, principally N-acetylglucosamine groups. This suggestion has been confirmed by isolating two fractions of heparitin sulfates when eluting them from Dowex Cl⁻ column with NaCl. The fraction eluted with 1.0 M NaCl exhibited lower sulfate and N-sulfate but higher N-acetyl content than the fraction eluted with 1.3 M NaCl [46].

Keratan sulfate (Fig. 8.7) was first reported in bovine cornea [47], where it constitutes about half of the total mucopolysaccharide content. The repeating unit was shown to be N-acetyllactosamine which is sulfated in C-6 of the glucosamine moiety. It is polymerized through $1 \rightarrow 3$

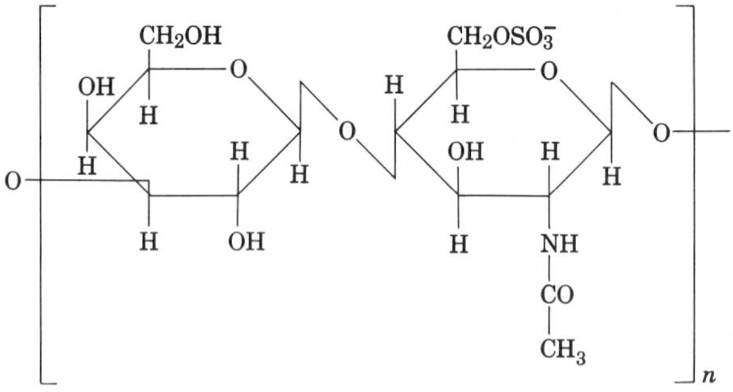

Figure 8.7.   The structure of the repeating unit of the keratan sulfate chain.

glycosidic linkages [48]. The corneal keratan sulfate, also called keratan sulfate I, differs from skeletal keratan sulfate II in its relative stability toward alkali. Keratan sulfate I and II differ slightly in their minor constituents, keratan I having smaller sialic acid and methylpentose content than keratan II [49]. Some keratan sulfate preparations from senile human cartilage have a sulfate to hexosamine ratio greater than one. In these cases the galactose moiety is also sulfated at the C-6 position [50]. On the other hand, Wortman [51] reported that a fraction of corneal keratan sulfate contains about half as much sulfate as the regular keratan sulfate. This variability in degree of sulfation was confirmed by Cifonelli et al. [52], who surveyed keratan sulfates isolated from various embryonic and adult tissues and found that the range of sulfate to hexosamine ratio varies from 0.46 to 1.51.

Further structural studies on keratan sulfate II indicated that about 50% of the galactose residues and 60% of the glucosamine residues are substituted on the C-6 position. The major portion of the substitution is a C-6 sulfate group. But an appreciable amount of the C-6 also serves as a branching point in the polymer, the substituent being another sugar moiety of the branching chain [53]. The authors' opinion is that the minor constituents such as sialic acid, fucose, and so on, are part of these branches.

Almost all of the above-mentioned polysaccharides have been found in the skin of different animals. However, the main mucopolysaccharides are hyaluronic acid, dermatan sulfate, heparin with smaller amounts of chondroitin-4-sulfate and heparitin sulfate. Keratan sulfates and chondroitin-6-sulfates are found in minute quantities only. The mucopolysaccharide composition of skin has been examined in pigs [54], bulls [55], embryo pigs [56], rats [57, 58], rabbits [59], and humans [60].

These polysaccharides have been isolated after digestion of the skin with proteolytic enzymes using two kinds of separation techniques. Before 1960 [54–56, 60] the acidic polysaccharides were separated by fractional ethanol precipitation. Since 1960 [57, 58] the favored technique is to use quaternary ammonium salt precipitation on a column and selective elution with different normality of electrolytes: NaCl or $MgCl_2$. Other separation techniques used are electrophoresis in zinc sulfate or zinc acetate solution [61] and fiberglas chromatography [62].

8.2 PROTEIN MOIETY OF MUCOPOLYSACCHARIDES AND THE CARBOHYDRATE-PROTEIN LINKAGE

Different hyaluronic acid preparations contain different amounts of associated protein depending on source and technique of isolation. The

range of these protein contents vary from 0 to 38% and the most important of these preparations have been reviewed by Preston et al. [63].
These authors also analyzed the amino acid content of a hyaluronic
acid preparation obtained as ultrafilter residue of synovial fluid having
a total protein content of 15.5%. Glutamic acid, aspartic acid, threonine,
serine, proline, glycine, alanine, leucine, valine, and lysine account for
more than 60% of the protein present. Swann [64] analyzed a low protein content (0.35%) hyaluronic acid preparation for rooster comb and
found that serine, glycine, alanine, aspartic, and glutamic acid accounted
for 65% of the total amino acid present. Wardi et al. [65] isolated
a hyaluronate-peptide which contained arabinose besides glucuronic acid
and glucosamine. The inference is that arabinose may take part in the
carbohydrate-protein linkage of hyaluronic acid.

Chondroitin-4-sulfate also appears as a covalently linked protein complex. Muir was the first to point out that the carbohydrate-protein linkage point is at the serine residue [66]. Schubert and his co-workers
[67–69] isolated two fractions from nasal septa which were separated
by centrifugation. The protein-polysaccharide complex that sedimented
first was designated as PPH, the H standing for heavy. The light fraction, on contrast, is referred to as PPL. The protein content of PPL
is 15% while that of PPH is 56% [58]. 75% of the total protein-polysaccharide complex was isolated as PPL and 13% as PPH, making
a total recovery of 88%. The nonrecoverable material is left as insoluble
residue of the aqueous extract and it contains collagen, hexosamine,
and a high percentage of neutral sugars [70].

Most of the subsequent work has been done on PPL. It was shown
that in addition to chondroitin-4-sulfate it also contains some keratan
sulfate [71]. Gregory et al. [72] have shown that the chondroitin-4-
sulfate protein linkage in PPL is a galactose-galactose-xylose-serine
sequence.

Later the correct linkages were established by isolating the trisac-
charides participating in the chondroitin-4-sulfate-protein linkage region
[73]. The sequence proved to be glucuronic acid $(1 \rightarrow 3)$-N-acetylgalac-
tosamine-4-sulfate-$(1 \rightarrow 4)$-glucuronic acid $(1 \rightarrow 3)$-galactose $(1 \rightarrow 3)$-
galactose $(1 \rightarrow 4)$-xylose-O-serine.

The most frequent amino acids of the PPL were glutamic acid, aspartic
acid, serine, proline glycine, leucine, and arginine. On the other hand,
PPH had glutamic acid, glycine, alanine, aspartic acid, arginine, proline,
hydroxyproline, and leucine as the most abundant amino acids. The
presence of hydroxyproline in PPH indicated to the authors that this
fraction may contain collagen [74].

Anderson et al. [75] suggested that PPL presents different accessibilities towards different proteolytic enzymes; namely that the papain-digested remnants have only one polysaccharide chain while the trypsin-digested fragment has two chains. This was later confirmed by Luscombe and Phelps [76].

On the basis of equimolar concentrations of certain amino acids, Serafini-Fracassini et al. [77], suggested that the protein core of the chondroitin-4-sulfate PPL complex is made up of a number of peptide subunits, the sequential arrangement of which in the macromolecule is not strictly determined. A further study of the fragments of PPL obtained by acid hydrolysis indicated that there may be three different subunits. One peptide subunit has aspartic on its N-terminal, another peptide subunit has valine. Both subunits carry two chondroitin-4-sulfate side chains of 15,000–18,000 mol wt. The third subunit has an N-terminal amino acid of leucine or isoleucine. If it is leucine, it carries two chondroitin-4-sulfate side chains as the other subunits. If it is isoleucine, the side chain is keratan sulfate [78].

Other chondroitin-4-sulfate protein preparations have been isolated and separated into fractions by electrophoresis [79] and disruptive and dissociative techniques [80].

The protein-polysaccharide complex of chondroitin-6-sulfate isolated from shark cartilage has been studied by Mathews [81]. The total protein content of the complex varied from 8 to 17%. The amino acid composition of different fractions varied, the most abundant being aspartic acid, glutamic acid, serine, histidine, arginine, and proline. The carbohydrate-protein linkage is similar to that found in chondroitin-4-sulfate; namely, glucuronic acid-galactose-galactose-xylose-serine-peptide [82].

The dermatan sulfate-protein complex has a carbohydrate-protein linkage similar to the two chondroitin sulfates mentioned previously [83]. This is especially interesting since 90% of the uronic acid in dermatan sulfate is iduronic acid and only 10% is glucuronic acid. It seems that most of these glucuronic-acid moieties are participating in the protein-carbohydrate linkage area. The most important amino acids in the glycopeptides near the protein-carbohydrate linkage are serine, glycine, alanine, glutamic, and aspartic acid.

The universality of the glucuronic acid-galactose-galactose-xylose-serine linkage has been demonstrated by finding it in heparin [84] and also in heparitin sulfate [85]. The heparin-protein complex contains 13% protein, the most important amino acids being aspartic, glutamic acid, leucine, and lysine [86]. In heparitin sulfate glycopeptide, serine was the most abundant amino acid. The inner core of principally N-acetylated groups being linked to the protein while the outer branches of N-sulfate glucosamine groups are farther away from the protein core [46].

Seno et al. [49] have found that the carbohydrate-peptide linkage in keratan sulfate II is bond via an O-glycosidic bond to threonine and serine while in keratan sulfate I there is either a glycosylamine linkage between carbohydrate and asparagine and glutamine or an amide linkage between the glucosamine and aspartic and glutamic acids.

An interesting effect of aging has been demonstrated on the peptide content of mucopolysaccharides. Manley et al. [87] studied chondroitin-4-sulfate and heparitin sulfate-protein complexes from human aorta. In both polymers the number of amino acids remaining attached to the polysaccharide chain after papain hydrolysis was twice as much in the case of old aorta than the one isolated from young aorta.

Anderson, Hoffman, and Meyer [75] also reported the remaining peptide composition for chondroitin-4-sulfate isolated from rib cartilage. The difference between aorta and cartilage chondroitin-4-sulfate peptide is that, in the case of cartilage, proline was one of the major amino acids instead of aspartic acid. Similar organ-specific replacement is also found in keratan sulfates. Keratan sulfate of cartilage has proline, while that of cornea has aspartic acid [49].

8.3 MACROMOLECULAR PROPERTIES

The most important macromolecular properties that describe the structure of a compound are the molecular weight, the size of the molecule, and the shape of the molecule. In discussing these properties one has to be aware of the fact that all mucopolysaccharide preparations (whether free of protein or in the protein-polysaccharide complex form) proved to be polydisperse. Polydispersity simply means that there is a distribution of molecular weight, size, and so on, in any batch, and therefore, the property which is measured is an average property. Furthermore, the averaging process depends on the type of measurements. For example, osmotic pressure measures a number-average molecular weight in which each particle contributes equally in the averaging process. Light scattering and ultracentrifugal technique, for example, measure a weight-average molecular weight in which the heavier particles contribute more than the light ones to the average. Similarly, with the Z-average molecular weights obtained (also in ultracentrifugal experiments), the heavier particles contribute even more to the average than in the weight-average molecular weight.

An average property such as molecular weight really does not adequately describe the system; some other dispersion indices (rarely given in the literature) would be required in addition.

Since, however, it was shown that the degree of polydispersity varies with source, isolation technique, and so on, complete fractionation and characterization of each fraction of a preparation is rarely done. For this reason, the macromolecular properties here will be discussed in general terms giving the ranges that were found for a certain property rather than quoting exact values for certain preparations.

Hyaluronic acid isolated from different sources with different protein contents shows a molecular-weight range of 7.7×10^4–28×10^6 daltons. Usually the lower the protein content, the smaller the average molecular weight [10, 63, 88, 89]. There is some controversy in the literature about the shape of hyaluronic acid. The small molecular weight compounds with less protein are presumed to be rod-shaped molecules with a length varying from 250 to 1,000 Å. The larger molecules with high-protein content assume more of a random coil shape with radii of gyration 540–4540 Å [63, 88, 90]. The larger the molecular size and the more assymetrical a molecule, the more it will contribute towards the viscosity of solution. There is ample evidence from birefringence [91, 92], electron microscopy [93], and x-ray diffraction [11] measurements that the hyaluronide chain is intrinsically stiff, which would lead to rod-shaped molecules. It was thought that the protein may serve as a core from which long, relatively rigid, hyaluronate side chains originate. However, it seems that there is more interaction between and possibly branching on the hyaluronate chains themselves. Preston et al. [63] found that the rigidity of high molecular weight protein-hyaluronate complex is such that it cannot be taken as a random coil rather than as a spongelike structure. Balazs [94] showed that molecular weights higher than 10^5 daltons form viscoelastic putty within pH 2.5–2.7 which bounce, although they are not truly cross-linked gels. Swann reported recently [95] that high-viscosity hyaluronate preparations do not lose their viscosity upon pronase digestion of the protein part. Therefore, in the aggregation of stiff chains into random coillike shapes, the covalently linked protein core may not play such an important role after all. On the other hand, electrostatic interactions between proteins (especially collagen) and hyaluronic acid may further complicate the structure of aggregates [96, 97].

The chondroitin-4-sulfate and its protein complexes present an even more complicated picture. The preparations from different tissues are not only polydisperse, but they usually contain more than one fraction which can be separated by physical means such as centrifugation, gel filtration, and electrophoresis [69].

The macromolecular structure is described by the Mathews-Partridge model [2, 98, 99] in which a central protein core contains carbohydrate side chains. For the PPL fractions of chondroitin-4-sulfate protein complex, the central core had a reported molecular weight of 3.2×10^6 daltons and 20% protein content. This would mean that on the average there 4–5 protein cores present in the molecule [76]. Each of the protein cores would carry 20–25 chondroitin-4-sulfate chains, each composed of about 29 disaccharidic repeating units, which means a total of 100 chains per "molecule," the molecule being the whole protein-polysaccharide complex. Such a structure was proposed by Luscombe and Phelps and is reproduced here in Fig. 8.8. Most probably the complex aggregate is held together by electrostatic and hydrogen bonds [2].

A somewhat different picture is presented by Serafini-Fracassini and co-workers [77, 78]. Their total molecular weight for the PPL fraction is about a fifth (6.3×10^5 daltons) of that given in the Luscombe-Phelps

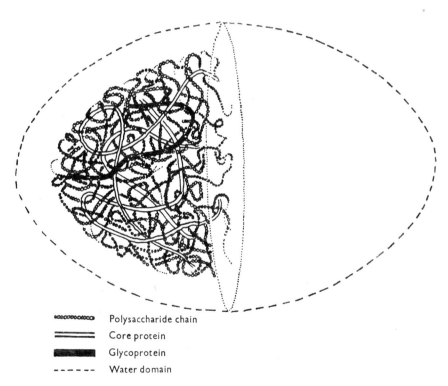

●○○○○○○○○	Polysaccharide chain
═══	Core protein
▬▬	Glycoprotein
- - - - -	Water domain

Figure 8.8. The proposed macromolecular structure of the PPL fraction of chondroitin-4-sulfate according to Luscombe and Phelps [76]. Courtesy of *J. Biochem.*

model. The protein core consists of three peptide subunits in lateral arrangement. The subunits bearing valine and aspartic acid as N-terminal amino acids each carry two, laterally extending chondroitin-4-sulfate side chains. The third subunit, if its N-terminal amino acid is leucine, carries two chondroitin-4-sulfate chains; if it is a subunit having isoleucine as its N-terminal amino acid, it carries two keratan-sulfate side chains. The total length of the protein core is about 1100–1500 Å, probably a triple-chain core. The mucopolysaccharide side chains, a total of 20–24, are lined up along the protein core in more or less random-coil arrangements [100].

The chondroitin-4-sulfate protein complex isolated from pig laryngeal cartilage was separated into two fractions by electrophoresis by Muir and co-workers [79, 101]. A fast-moving fraction contained only 2% protein and had a weight-average molecular weight of 2.3×10^5 daltons and was rather polydisperse. A slow-moving component resembled the PPL preparations and had 10% protein content. The same kind of separation was achieved by gel chromatography. The side chains of chondroitin-4-sulfate contained 28 disaccharidic repeating units [102]. The fast-moving and low molecular weight protein-chondroitin-4-sulfate complex contained no keratan sulfate, while the slow-moving and high molecular weight material always showed keratan sulfate.

Both fractions were antigenic due to their protein cores; the small molecular weight, fast-moving fraction carried a single antigen while the other fraction contained a number of species specific antigens in the protein core [103].

The chondroitin-6-sulfate-protein complexes are similar to the complexes of chondroitin-4-sulfates. The protein content varies from 10 to 12% [81]. The molecule is rod-shaped, having a length of 3500 Å, with a total molecular weight of 4×10^6 daltons. The chondroitin-6-sulfate side chains are flexible random-coil polymers ranging between 2.5×10^4 and 4.0×10^4 daltons molecular weight.

The dermatan-sulfate-protein complex differs from the previous sulfated mucopolysaccharide complexes. It was reported to have 60% protein [104] and average molecular weights in the range of 2–2.5×10^5 daltons. The dermatan-sulfate side chains are of the order of 1–2×10^4 daltons [105]; hence, about 8–10 dermatan-sulfate side chains per protein core. Thus, the dermatan-sulfate-protein is smaller in molecular weight and less dense than the other sulfated mucopolysaccharide complexes. It appears as a rigid rod, 1000 Å long and 22 Å wide.

Heparin isolated by different techniques contains different amounts of proteins. Some of these proteins are associated, others are covalently linked. Although the molecular weight of heparin chains has been established [106] (being of the order of 0.8–1.6 $\times$ 10^4 daltons), the macro-molecular structure of covalently linked protein-complex has been studied very little [107].

The polysaccharide moiety is a random coil with a radius of gyration of 36 Å [108]. Based on dye-binding properties, Stone suggested that it may behave like helical polypeptides [109].

8.4 HYDRATION OF MUCOPOLYSSACHARIDES

Mucopolysaccharides in tissues are in different states of hydration. Most of the time they form gels or viscous concentrated solutions. The water content of such tissues may vary from 30 to 98%. In tissue matrix, the mucopolysaccharides are mostly responsible for water imbibition and retention. Thus, the part they play in tissue hydration and the transport of metabolites through these tissues is a function of many variables, among which the structure is only one factor.

The following parameters are of significance when talking of hydration:

1. *Water-sorptive capacity* simply describes the amount of hydration a solid mucopolysaccharide sample will achieve at a certain relative vapor pressure (relative humidity). It is best described by a sorption isotherm which gives the amount of hydration in grams or moles of H_2O per gram or per repeating unit of the polymer as a function of water vapor pressure at a set temperature. Most of the water vapor-sorption isotherms of mucopolysaccharides have a general S shape (Fig. 8.9). Such an S-shaped sorption isotherm can be interpreted in the following way: At the beginning, the solid matrix is hydrated on the available polar sites which are the most energetic from the point of view of (dipole-dipole or ion-dipole) interactions. When all these available energetic sites are covered (saturated) with a molecular layer of water, we talk of a "monolayer" coverage. The isotherm can be analyzed in terms of the Brunauer, Emmett, and Teller (BET) equation when the monolayer coverage has been completed [110].

$$\frac{P/P_0}{a(1 - P/P_0)} = \frac{1}{A_m C} + \frac{(C - 1)P/P_0}{A_m C} \tag{1}$$

where P/P_0 is the relative vapor pressure, a is the amount of water sorbed at each specific relative vapor pressure, A_m is the amount of water sorbed at "monolayer" coverage, and C is a term that is related to the net heat of sorption. Thus, the monolayer can be evaluated by

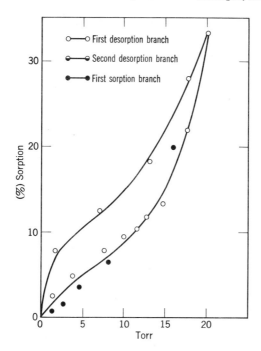

Figure 8.9. Sorption isotherm and hysteresis of semicrystalline sodium hyaluronate at 24°C.

plotting $[P/P_0]/a[1 - (P/P_0)]$ against P/P_0. Up to about 0.3–0.5 relative vapor pressure a straight line is obtained and one can evaluate the "monolayer" coverage from the slope (S) and the intercept (I) of such a plot.

$$A_m = \frac{1}{S + I} \tag{2}$$

$$C = 1 + \frac{S}{I} \tag{3}$$

In swelling polymers, such a "monolayer" does not have the usual molecular surface area interpretation as in the original Brunauer, Emmett and Teller equation because the surface is heterogeneous and even may have discontinuities. Rather it means the amount of water bound most energetically to the polymer matrix.

After the completion of the monolayer, the isotherm usually flattens out and a gradual increase is exhibited with increasing vapor pressure.

This is associated with multilayer sorption; that is, water molecules are sorbed on the previously sorbed water molecules at the primary polar sites. This is a swelling process in the polymer.

Finally, a sudden upward trend is noticeable in the sorption isotherm; that is, a large amount of water sorbed for every little change in the water vapor pressure. This process is associated with either capillary condensation of the water in millipores of the solid matrix or, in the case of a swelling polymer, with a solution process. If the polymer network is not entangled and there is no limit to the swelling and/or to the solution process, the amount of water vapor sorbed is infinite at relative vapor pressure of 1.0. However, chain entanglement, hydrogen and hydrophobic bonds, as well as ionic bridges, and ion-dipole interactions limit the swelling properties of the network.

The vapor-sorptive capacity just described is related to the swelling capacity of the network from solution. However, the latter is much harder to determine in the case of mucopolysaccharides because of the change in shape of gels during swelling and disintegration in many cases. Thus, water vapor-sorptive capacity, "monolayer" coverage, and so on, are used as indications of swelling capacity as well.

2. *The retentive capacity of mucopolysaccharides* is the second parameter of importance. The hydration and dehydration process does not follow the same path and the difference in path is referred to as hysteresis (Fig. 8.9). The water content at a certain relative vapor pressure is higher if we proceed on a desorption path than on the sorption path. This means that the hydration and dehydration process is not a reversible one and the mucopolysaccharides retain more water than they sorb at a specified vapor pressure. The hysteresis loop is the measure of the degree of irreversibility of the process. The following model can explain this behavior. The water vapor sorbed in the polymer matrix is tightly bound by neighboring chains. The swelling polymer exerts a physical constraint on the sorbed water molecule; hence it cannot be removed at the same vapor pressure as it was sorbed, but a higher vacuum must be applied to remove it. Thus, the hysteresis is a result of the changes in the structure of the swelling network.

3. *The energetics of the sorption process* is a third parameter of importance. It is assumed that the heat of sorption of the first molecules of water on the polar sites of the polymers is greater than the heat of condensation of the water. (Both heats of sorption and condensation are negative, since they correspond to exothermic processes.) This assumption is usually fulfilled, although in the case of water as opposed to other sorbents this need not be so. In liquid water, on the average, there are 2–3 hydrogen bonds per molecule. In order to get a heat of

sorption greater than the heat of condensation, interactions with polar sites should occur, the interactions having magnitudes greater than that equivalent to 2–3 hydrogen bonds.

It is plausible that in an open polymer matrix the polar sites are far from each other and the incoming water molecule establishes only 1–2 hydrogen bonds per molecule with the matrix. Under such a condition, the heat of sorption in the "monolayer" coverage may be less than the heat of condensation. However, as mentioned before, in most cases the heat of sorption before completion of monolayer is higher than the heat of condensation and it is increasing up to "monolayer" coverage. This could be explained if we assume that, just before "monolayer" completion, the incoming water molecule will enter into the tightest part of the matrix and thus establish 3–4 or more hydrogen bonds or the equivalent in ion-dipole bonds.

The usual calculations of the heats of sorption are based on the Clausius-Clapeyron equation [111].

$$\frac{d \ln P}{d(1/T)} = \frac{\overline{\Delta H}}{R} \tag{4}$$

where P is the vapor pressure at a certain water content and T is the absolute temperature, $\overline{\Delta H}$ being the isosteric heats of sorption, and R the gas constant. Thus, a plot of $\ln P$ versus $1/T$ gives a slope from which $\overline{\Delta H}$ can be calculated for each water content. However, this treatment assumes a reversible process and the water vapor sorption is an irreversible process. Thus, the $\overline{\Delta H}$ calculated is actually an overestimated value and it includes a $T \overline{\Delta S}_{irr}$ term; namely, the entropy production of the system. This $\overline{\Delta S}_{irr}$ is the measure of irreversibility, the structural change that occurs in the polymer matrix during swelling. In order to evaluate the true heats of sorption, calorimetric measurements should be made. A comparison of the calorimetric and isosteric heats of sorption then provide a value for the $\overline{\Delta S}_{irr}$.

Knowing the heat of sorption and the free energy of sorption, $\overline{\Delta G}$, from the relative vapor pressure, P/P_0,

$$\overline{\Delta G} = RT \ln P/P_0 \tag{5}$$

one can estimate the entropy of sorption from Equation 6 at each water content.

$$\overline{\Delta S} = \frac{\overline{\Delta H} - \overline{\Delta G}}{T} \tag{6}$$

This entropy of sorption is a complex term. It involves the entropy change due to the loss of two degrees of freedom in localizing water from vapor to its sorbed state; it includes the configurational entropy of the probability of finding an energetically favorable sorption site; it includes the entropy change due to the structural change in the polymer.

4. *The spectroscopic results of the perturbations a sorbed water molecule may exert on individual polar groups of the matrix* and vice versa is the final-critical parameter of the hydration. This usually pinpoints what extent the individual polar groups of the macromolecule influence the hydration process.

The water-sorptive capacity of a mucopolysaccharide depends on the primary, secondary, and tertiary structures of the molecule as well as on the physical state.

For example, in the case of hyaluronic acid [112] the sodium salt had greater sorptive capacity than the potassium salt which had in turn greater sorptive capacity than the acid form. It seems that the protein content does not influence the sorptive capacity to any appreciable extent, indicating that most of the water is sorbed by the polyuronide part of the molecule. The molecular weight has an effect on the sorptive capacity only if it falls below a minimum level of 2×10^5. The physical state of the polymer is of great importance. A low molecular weight (7.7×10^4 daltons) sodium hyaluronate sorbed less water than the high molecular weight (5.8×10^6 daltons) amorphous compound at the same relative vapor pressure. However, the amount of water sorbed in the monolayer is the same in both samples. This means that the crystalline polymer is able to swell, and therefore, all the available polar sites will be covered with water just as in the case of the amorphous polymer except that this happens at a higher vapor pressure with the crystalline sample than with the amorphous sample.

The retentive capacity of hyaluronates is also influenced by the ionic species of the compound. The retentive capacity of the sodium salt is also greater than that of the potassium salt. This may represent the more open structure of the matrix with the larger K^+ ion than with Na^+ ion. Since the acidic form showed a nonreproducible isotherm in which the sorptive capacity increased with the number of cycles of the experiment, one cannot say much about the retentive power of the acid form except that the matrix in this form is the most prone to structural changes due to a "zippering" effect of the chains.

The calorimetric heats of sorption [Fig. 8.10] of sodium hyaluronate indicated that below monolayer coverage (10% H_2O content) the heat of sorption was less than the heat of condensation, indicating an open

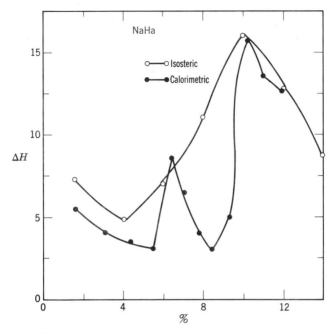

Figure 8.10. Isosteric and calorimetric heats of sorption of water vapor by sodium hyaluronate as a function of water content.

spongelike structure of the matrix [63]. A difference between the isosteric and calorimetric heats was evident only below the "monolayer" coverage. This again indicates an open structure in which most of the swelling is done up to "monolayer" coverage [113].

Among the calcium salts of sulfated mucopolysaccharides, the chondroitin-6-sulfate has the highest sorptive capacity, followed by heparin, dermatan sulfate, and chondroitin-4-sulfate in this order [114]. However, the monolayer coverage was highest with heparin, having the largest number of polar groups; less with chondroitin-6-sulfate; still less with dermatan sulfate; and the least with chondroitin-4-sulfate.

The hysteresis, and hence the water retentive capacity, showed the opposite order. Chondroitin-4-sulfate retains most of the water and sorbs the least, indicating a tight polymer matrix, while chondroitin-6-sulfate retains the least and sorbs the most, indicating a loose matrix.

The isosteric heats of sorption showed a similar trend among the monosulfated mucopolysaccharides. Chondroitin-4-sulfates had the highest heats of sorption, followed by dermatan sulfate and finally chondroitin-6-sulfate. This again indicated that the tightest matrix had the greatest interaction with water and the loosest, the least. Heparin, which has about 2.5 sulfate groups per repeating unit and a relatively open structure, had a heat of sorption somewhat less than that of chondroitin-4-sulfate.

To answer the question of which polar group is the most important in the hydration of mucopolysaccharides, the infrared spectra of the hydration process was studied. As was expected, the numerous —OH groups were primarily responsible for water vapor sorption in each of the mucopolysaccharides [115]. In chondroitin-4-sulfate, the next most important group was the —NH, followed by —SO₃⁻ and —COO⁻ in this order. In the case of dermatan sulfate the order was —OH > —COO⁻ > —NH > —SO₃⁻, while with chondroitin-6-sulfate it was OH > —COO⁻ ≥ —NH ≅ —SO₃⁻.

For heparin the order was —OH > —SO₃⁻ > —N—S > —COO⁻.

The mode of sorption of the water molecule in chondroitin-4-sulfate was studied by microwave absorption spectroscopy. It was found that there were two energetically different sites and the water sorbed on the —OH group had a potential barrier for orientation of the order 2600 cal mole⁻¹, while that of the molecules sorbed on —NH groups were more free to orient in the electrical field having a barrier of 2340 cal mole⁻¹ [116].

Measurement of the dielectric properties of chondroitin-4-sulfate at different degrees of hydration indicated that the polymer chains themselves have very little freedom of movement even in the highly hydrated state. The bound water behaved very much like ice providing a conductance band together with the dissolved counter-ions of the gel [117].

REFERENCES

1. K. Meyer, *Cold Spring Harbor Symp. Quant. Biol.,* **6,** 91 (1938).
2. M. B. Mathews and I. Lozaityte, *Arch. Biochem. Biophys.,* **74,** 158 (1958).
3. K. Meyer and J. W. Palmer, *J. Biol. Chem.,* **107,** 629 (1934).
4. J. S. Brimacombe and J. M. Webber, *Mucopolysaccharides,* Elsevier, Amsterdam, 1963.
5. K. Meyer, E. Davidson, A. Linker, and P. Hoffmann, *Biochim. Biophys. Acta,* **21,** 506 (1956).
6. E. A. Balazs, T. C. Laurent, U. B. G. Laurent, M. H. DeRoche, and D. M. Bunney, *Arch. Biochem. Biophys.,* **81,** 464 (1959).
7. K. Meyer, *Physiol. Rev.,* **27,** 335 (1947).
8. B. Weissmann and K. Meyer, *J. Amer. Chem. Soc.,* **74,** 4729 (1952); **76,** 1753 (1954).

9. R. W. Jeanloz and H. M. Flowers, *J. Amer. Chem. Soc.*, **84,** 3030 (1962); *Biochemistry,* **3,** 123 (1964).

10. F. A. Bettelheim, *Nature,* **182,** 1301 (1958).

11. F. A. Bettelheim, *J. Phys. Chem.,* **63,** 2069 (1959).

12. K. Meyer, A. Linker, E. A. Davidson, and P. Weissmann, *J. Biol. Chem.,* **205,** 611 (1953).

13. G. Fischer and D. Boedeker, *Ann. Chem.,* **117,** 111 (1861).

14. P. A. Levene, *Hexosamines and Mucoproteins,* Longmans, Green and Co., London, 1925.

15. M. L. Wolfrom and B. O. Juliano, *J. Amer. Chem. Soc.,* **82,** 1673 (1960); **82,** 2588 (1960).

16. E. A. Davidson and K. Meyer, *J. Amer. Chem. Soc.,* **76,** 5686 (1954).

17. F. A. Bettelheim and D. E. Philpott, *Nature,* **188,** 654 (1960).

18. F. A. Bettelheim, *Biochim. Biophys. Acta,* **83,** 350 (1964).

19. K. Meyer and J. W. Palmer, *J. Biol. Chem.,* **114,** 689 (1936).

20. S. F. D. Orr, *Biochim. Biophys. Acta,* **14,** 173 (1954).

21. M. B. Mathews, *Nature,* **181,** 421 (1958).

22. P. Hoffmann, A. Linker, and K. Meyer, *Biochim. Biophys. Acta,* **30,** 184 (1958).

23. O. Furth and T. Bruno, *Biochem. Z.,* **294,** 153 (1937).

24. T. Soda, F. Egami, and P. Harigome, *J. Chem. Soc., Japan,* **51,** 43 (1940).

25. S. Suzuki, *J. Biol. Chem.,* **235,** 3580 (1960).

26. M. B. Mathews and M. Inouye, *Biochim. Biophys. Acta,* **53,** 509 (1961).

27. K. Meyer and E. Chaffee, *J. Biol. Chem.,* **138,** 491 (1941).

28. T. J. Stoffyn and R. W. Jeanloz, *J. Biol. Chem.,* **235,** 2507 (1960).

29. R. W. Jeanloz, P. J. Stoffyn, and M. Tremege, *Federation Proc.,* **16,** 201 (1957).

30. P. Hoffmann, A. L. Linker, V. Lippman, and K. Meyer, *J. Biol. Chem.,* **235,** 3066 (1960).

31. L. Fransson and L. Rodén, *J. Biol. Chem.,* **242,** 4161 (1967).

32. L. Fransson and L. Rodén, *J. Biol. Chem.,* **242,** 4170 (1967).

33. J. McLean, *Amer. J. Physiol.,* **41,** 250 (1916).

34. G. J. Durant, H. Hendrickson, and R. Montgomery, *Arch. Biochem. Biophys.,* **99,** 418 (1962).

35. A. B. Foster, R. Harrison, T. D. Inch, M. Stacey, and J. M. Webber, *J. Chem. Soc.,* 2279 (1963).

36. J. E. Jorpes, H. Bostrom, and V. Mutt, *J. Biol. Chem.,* **183,** 607 (1950).

37. K. H. Meyer and Z. E. Schwartz, *Helv. Chim. Acta,* **33,** 1651 (1950).

38. M. L. Wolfrom, P. Y. Wang, and S. Honda, *Carbohyd. Res.,* **11,** 179 (1969).

39. I. Danishefsky, H. B. Eiber, and A. H. Williams, *J. Biol. Chem.,* **238,** 2895 (1963).

40. M. L. Wolfrom, J. R. Vercellotti, H. Tomomatsu, and D. Horton, *J. Org. Chem.,* **29,** 540 (1964).

41. J. E. Jorpes and S. Gardell, *J. Biol. Chem.,* **176,** 267 (1948).

42. A. Linker, P. Hoffmann, B. P. Sampson, and K. Meyer, *Biochim. Biophys. Acta*, **29**, 443 (1958).

43. A. Linker and B. P. Sampson, *Biochim. Biophys. Acta*, **43**, 366 (1960).

44. J. A. Cifonelli and A. Dorfman, *Biochim. Biophys. Res. Commun.*, **4**, 328 (1961).

45. J. A. Cifonelli, *Federation Proc.*, **23**, 2206 (1964); **24**, 364 (1965).

46. J. Knecht and A. Dorfman, *Biochim. Biophys. Res. Commun.*, **21**, 509 (1965).

47. K. Meyer, A. Linker, E. A. Davidson, and B. Weissman, *J. Biol. Chem.*, **205**, 611 (1953).

48. S. Hirano, P. Hoffmann, and K. Meyer, *J. Org. Chem.*, **26**, 5064 (1961).

49. N. Seno, K. Meyer, B. Anderson, and P. Hoffmann, *J. Biol. Chem.*, **240**, 1005 (1965).

50. V. P. Bhavanandan and K. Meyer, *Science,* **151**, 1404 (1966).

51. B. Wortman, *Biochim. Biophys. Acta*, **83**, 288 (1964).

52. J. A. Cifonelli, A. Saunders, and J. I. Gross, *Carbohyd. Res.*, **3**, 478 (1967).

53. V. P. Bhavanandan and K. Meyer, *J. Biol. Chem.*, **243**, 1052 (1968).

54. K. Meyer, E. Davidson, A. Linker, and P. Hoffmann, *Biochim. Biophys. Acta,* **21**, 506 (1956).

55. P. Hoffmann, A. Linker, and K. Meyer, *Arch. Biochem. Biophys.*, **69**, 435 (1957).

56. G. Loewi and K. Meyer, *Biochim. Biophys. Acta,* **27**, 453 (1958).

57. S. Schiller and A. Dorfman, *Nature*, **185**, 111 (1960).

58. S. Schiller, A. Slover, and A. Dorfman, *J. Biol. Chem.*, **236**, 983 (1961).

59. E. A. Davidson, W. Small, P. Perchemlides, and W. Baxley, *Biochim. Biophys. Acta,* **46**, 189 (1961).

60. G. Loewi, *Biochim. Biophys. Acta,* **52**, 435 (1961).

61. F. Haruki and J. E. Kirk, *Biochim. Biophys. Acta,* **136**, 391 (1967).

62. G. S. Berenson and E. R. Dalferes, *Biochim. Biophys. Acta*, **58**, 34 (1962).

63. B. N. Preston, M. Davies, and A. G. Ogston, *Biochem. J.*, **96**, 449 (1965).

64. D. A. Swann, *Biochim. Biophys. Acta*, **160**, 96 (1968).

65. A. H. Wardi, W. S. Allen, D. L. Turner, and Z. Stary, *Arch. Biochem. Biophys.*, **117**, 44 (1966).

66. H. Muir, *Biochem. J.*, **69**, 195 (1958).

67. I. Malawista and M. Schubert, *J. Biol. Chem.*, **230**, 535 (1958).

68. B. R. Gerber, E. C. Franklin, and M. Schubert, *J. Biol. Chem.*, **235**, 2870 (1960).

69. B. M. Scheinthal and M. Schubert, *J. Biol. Chem.*, **238**, 1935 (1963).

70. J. Rotstein, M. Gordon, and M. Schubert, *Biochem. J.*, **85**, 614 (1962).

71. J. D. Gregory and L. Rodén, *Biochem. Biophys. Res. Comm.*, **5**, 430 (1961).

72. J. D. Gregory, T. C. Laurent, and L. Rodén, *J. Biol. Chem.*, **239**, 3312 (1964).

73. L. Rodén and R. Smith, *J. Biol. Chem.*, **241**, 5949 (1966).

74. R. D. Campo and D. D. Dziewiatkowski, *J. Biol. Chem.*, **237**, 2729 (1962).

75. B. Anderson, P. Hoffmann and K. Meyer, *J. Biol. Chem.*, **240**, 156 (1965).
76. M. Luscombe and C. F. Phelps, *Biochem. J.*, **103**, 103 (1967).
77. A. Serafini-Fracassini, T. J. Peters, and L. Floreani, *Biochem. J.*, **105**, 569 (1967).
78. A. Serafini-Fracassini, *Biochim. Biophys. Acta*, **170**, 289 (1968).
79. H. Muir and S. Jacobs, *Biochem. J.*, **103**, 367 (1967).
80. S. W. Sajdera and V. C. Hascall, *J. Biol. Chem.*, **244**, 77 (1969).
81. B. M. Mathews, *Biochim. Biophys. Acta*, **58**, 92 (1962).
82. T. Helting and L. Rodén, unpublished work.
83. L. A. Fransson, *Biochim. Biophys. Acta*, **156**, 311 (1968).
84. U. Lindahl, *Arkiv f. Kemi*, **26**, 101 (1966); *Biochim. Biophys. Acta*, **130**, 368 (1966); *ibid.*, **156**, 203 (1968).
85. J. Knecht, J. A. Cifonelli, and A. Dorfman, *J. Biol. Chem.*, **242**, 4652 (1967).
86. A. Serafini-Fracassini, J. J. Durward, and L. Floreani, *Biochem. J.*, **112**, 167 (1969).
87. G. Manley, R. N. Mullinger, and P. H. Lloyd, *Biochem. J.*, **114**, 89 (1969).
88. T. C. Laurent, M. Ryan, and A. Peitruszkiewicz, *Biochim. Biophys. Acta*, **42**, 476 (1960).
89. B. S. Blumberg and A. G. Ogston, Ciba Foundation *Symp. on the Chem. and Biol. of Mucopolysaccharides*, 1958, p. 22.
90. T. C. Laurent, *J. Biol. Chem.*, **216**, 263 (1955).
91. B. Sylvén and E. J. Ambrose, *Biochim. Biophys. Acta*, **18**, 587 (1953).
92. V. DerSarkissian and F. A. Bettelheim, *J. Polymer Sci.*, A, **1**, 725 (1963).
93. F. A. Bettelheim and D. E. Philpott, *Biochim. Biophys. Acta*, **34**, 124 (1959).
94. E. A. Balazs, *Federation Proc.*, **25**, 1817 (1966).
95. D. A. Swann, *Biochem. Biophys. Res. Comm.*, **35**, 571 (1969).
96. F. A. Bettelheim, T. C. Laurent, and H. Pertoft, *Carbohyd. Res.*, **2**, 391 (1966).
97. W. Niedermeier and E. S. Gramling, *Carbohyd. Res.*, **8**, 317 (1968).
98. S. M. Partridge, H. F. Davis, and G. S. Adair, *Biochem. J.*, **79**, 15 (1961).
99. E. Buddecke, W. Kroz, and E. Lanka, *Hoppe-Seyl. Z.*, **331**, 196 (1963).
100. A. Serafini-Fracassini and J. W. Smith, *Proc. Roy. Soc.*, B, **165**, 440 (1966).
101. C. P. Tsiganos and H. Muir, *Biochem. J.*, **113**, 879 (1969).
102. C. P. Tsiganos and H. Muir, *Biochem. J.*, **113**, 885 (1969).
103. G. Loewi and H. Muir, *Immunology*, **9**, 119 (1965).
104. B. N. Preston, *Arch. Biochem. Biophys.*, **126**, 974 (1968).
105. C. F. Tanford, E. Marler, E. Jury, and E. A. Davidson, *J. Biol. Chem.*, **239**, 4043 (1964).
106. G. H. Barlow, L. J. Coen, and M. M. Mozen, *Biochim. Biophys. Acta*, **83**, 272 (1964).
107. A. Serafini-Fracassini, J. J. Durward, and L. Floreani, *Biochem. J.*, **112**, 167 (1969).
108. J. S. Stivala, M. Herbst, O. Kratky, and I. Pilz, *Arch. Biochem. Biophys.*, **127**, 795 (1968).

109. A. L. Stone, *Biopolymers,* **2**, 315 (1964).

110. S. Brunauer, P. H. Emmett, and E. Teller, *J. Amer. Chem. Soc.,* **60**, 309 (1938).

111. F. A. Bettelheim, *J. Colloid, Interface Sci.,* **23**, 301 (1967).

112. A. Block and F. A. Bettelheim, *Biochim. Biophys. Acta,* **201**, 69 (1970).

113. F. A. Bettelheim, A. Block, and L. Kaufman, *Biopolymers,* **9**, 1531 (1970).

114. F. A. Bettelheim and S. H. Ehrlich, *J. Phys. Chem.,* **67**, 1948 (1963).

115. S. H. Ehrlich and F. A. Bettelheim, *J. Phys. Chem.,* **67**, 1954 (1963).

116. I. Lubezky, F. A. Bettelheim, and F. Folman, *Trans. Faraday Soc.,* **63**, 1794 (1967).

117. L. Kaufman, Ph.D. Thesis, Adelphi University, 1969.

9

The Physical Chemistry
of Multicomponent Salt
Solutions

FRANK J. MILLERO

Contribution No. 1206 from The Institute of Marine and Atmospheric Sciences, University of Miami, Miami, Florida 33149

The knowledge of ionic interactions in multicomponent aqueous salt solutions like the oceans and body fluids is necessary for an understanding of the chemical properties of these systems. Most of the studies of the physical chemistry of electrolytes in aqueous solutions have been made on single electrolyte solutions. In recent years, the physical chemistry of multicomponent electrolyte solutions has been stressed due to the increasing interest in the chemical properties of the oceans and biological systems.

In this chapter, we will review the thermodynamics of multicomponent electrolyte solutions. Since the properties of multicomponent or mixed salt solutions are generally dependent on the interactions of salts with water in a binary salt system, in the first section of this chapter we will examine ion-water interactions in dilute single-electrolyte solutions. In the second section of this chapter we will review the thermodynamics of mixed salt solutions. Since the activity coefficients of mixed salt solutions have been discussed in great detail elsewhere [1–4], we will stress the effect of temperature (heat effects) and the effect of pressure (volume effects) on the activity coefficients. In the third section of this chapter we will briefly review the physical chemistry of seawater.

9.1 ION-WATER INTERACTIONS

Water is a very complex and ill-understood substance. It is anomalous in many of its physical and chemical properties. To mention a familiar example, water is a liquid at room temperatures, while its sister compounds (i.e., H_2S, H_2Se, and H_2Te) of higher molecular weight are gases. The cause of the structural complexties of water and its anomalies is the ability of water molecules to associate with one another by forming hydrogen bonds. The structure of liquid water has caused considerable controversy in recent years. Several reviews [5–10] and monographs [11–13] have appeared recently summarizing the current status of research on the structure of water. The reader is also referred to earlier water structure theories reviewed briefly in connection with various treatments of the structure of water [14–19].

The current models of water structure can be divided into two major categories. The first category is the "uniformist" or "average" models. In the "uniformist" models no local domains of structure exist in water different from that of any other domain. The individual water molecules behave at any time in the same manner as any other water molecule. Bernal and Fowler [14] and Pople [16] have adopted this theory. The recent study by Wall and Hornig [20] indirectly lends support to this theory. The second major category is the "mixture models." Frank and co-workers [15, 17, 18] have adopted this model. The mixture models have received more attention than the "uniformist" models. The mixture models can be divided into the following: (1) broken-down ice lattice

models ("icelike" structural units in equilibrium with monomers) [21];
(2) cluster models (clusters in equilibrium with monomers) [6, 17];
(3) models based on clathrate-like cages (again, in equilibrium with
monomers) [18, 22]; and (4) the significant structure theory [23, 24]
and Eucken's polymer [25] model (bulky species is not necessarily a
monomer).

In each case, at least two species of water exist, namely, a bulky
species representing some type of structural units and a dense species
such as monomeric water molecules.

Most workers [11] in the field find the mixture model to be most
useful in explaining the thermodynamic properties of water (i.e., the
expansibility and compressibility behavior) and we will use this general
model as a starting point. We will not go into detail concerning the
exact form of the minimum of two types of water present (i.e., whether
the structural form is "icelike," a cluster or a clathrate or the unstructured form is a monomer or some other high-density form). Since we
will be concerned mainly with relative effects of ion-water or ion-ion
interactions, the exact structure of water will not be a limiting factor.

The addition of an electrolyte to water multiplies the complexity of
the system. Before reviewing the thermodynamics of mixed electrolyte
solutions, it is appropriate to examine the interactions that occur between
ions and water molecules devoid of other interactions (i.e., ion-ion interactions). We will use the partial molal volume of ions, $\bar{V}^0$, at infinite
dilution to examine the interactions between ions and water molecules.
This thermodynamic property, $\bar{V}^0$, has been selected because volume
properties are easy to visualize.

The partial molal volume of a salt can be visualized by considering a
large reservoir of water, so large that the addition of one mole of salt
will not appreciably alter the concentration. The increase in volume of
the water upon the addition of one mole of salt to this large reservoir is
the partial molal volume of the salt. The usefulness of the concept of the
partial molal volume of a salt lies in the additivity of the partial molal
volume of salts at infinite dilution. By additivity we mean that the
partial molal volume of the salt, $\bar{V}^0(MX)$, is equal to the sum of the
partial molal volume of the ions, $\bar{V}^0(M^+) + \bar{V}^0(X^-)$, that make up that
salt. The division of the partial molal volume of a salt into its ionic
components cannot normally be made by experimental thermodynamic
methods [26]; thus, empirical methods have been used to make the
division. The various methods have been reviewed [27, 28] and in general
the empirical techniques [28] yield results that agree with the experimentally determined values recently made by Zana and Yeager [26].
When the $\bar{V}^0$ of one ion is estimated the $\bar{V}^0$s of the other ions are fixed.

Table 9.1 The Partial Molal Volume and Expansibility of Ions at Infinite Dilution in Water at 25°C

Ion	Crystal Radii, Å[a]	$\bar{V}^0$(cryst), ml mol^{-1}[b]	$\bar{V}^0$(ion), ml mol^{-1}[c]	$\bar{E}^0$(ion), ml mol-deg^{-1}[d]
H$^+$	0.00	0.0	-5.4	-0.012
Li$^+$	0.60	0.5	-6.3	-0.014
Na$^+$	0.95	2.1	-6.6	0.032
K$^+$	1.33	5.9	3.6	0.023
Rb$^+$	1.48	8.2	8.7	0.016
Cs$^+$	1.69	12.2	15.9	0.012
NH$_4^+$	1.48	8.2	12.4	-0.028
Me$_4$N$^+$	3.47	105.3	84.2	0.033
Et$_4$N$^+$	4.00	161.3	143.7	0.054
Pr$_4$N$^+$	4.52	232.7	209.0	0.095
Bu$_4$N$^+$	4.94	303.8	270.3	0.177
Mg^{2+}	0.65	0.7	-32.0	-0.105
Ni^{2+}	0.72	0.9	-34.8	—
Co^{2+}	0.74	1.0	-34.8	—
Zn^{2+}	0.74	1.0	-32.4	—
Fe^{2+}	0.76	1.1	-35.5	—
Mn^{2+}	0.80	1.3	-28.5	—
Cu^{2+}	0.96	2.2	-35.0	—
Cd^{2+}	0.97	2.3	-30.8	—
Ca^{2+}	0.99	2.4	-28.7	-0.042
Hg^{2+}	1.10	3.4	-30.1	—
Sr^{2+}	1.13	3.6	-29.0	-0.010
Pb^{2+}	1.20	4.3	-26.3	—
Ba^{2+}	1.35	6.2	-23.3	-0.012
Al^{3+}	0.50	0.3	-58.4	—
Fe^{3+}	0.64	0.7	-59.9	—
Cr^{3+}	0.69	0.8	-55.7	—
La^{3+}	1.15	3.8	-55.3	—
Th^{4+}	1.10	3.4	-75.1	—
F$^-$	1.36	6.3	4.2	0.035
Cl$^-$	1.81	14.9	23.2	0.046
Br$^-$	1.95	18.7	30.1	0.050
I$^-$	2.16	25.4	41.6	0.069
OH$^-$	1.38*	6.6	1.4	—
CH$_3$COO$^-$	2.21*	27.2	45.9	—
NO$_3^-$	2.03*	21.1	34.4	0.100
HCO$_3^-$	1.92*	17.8	28.8	—
H$_2$PO$_4^-$	2.03*	21.1	34.5	—
SO$_4^{2-}$	2.05*	21.7	24.8	0.107
CO$_3^{2-}$	1.73*	13.0	6.5	—
HPO$_4^{2-}$	1.96*	18.9	18.5	—

[a] Pauling crystal radii are given for all the simple monatomic ions. Since the polyatomic ions have an uncertain geometry, it is difficult to assign a reliable value for the radii. We have, thus, estimated the radius (given by *)
[b] $\bar{V}^0$(cryst) = 2.52 r^3
[c] Taken from Ref 28
[d] Taken from Ref 29

Table 9.1 contains the partial molal volume of the major ions of importance in seawater and body fluids [28].

Since the Frank and Wen model [17] for ion-water interactions has been so successful in describing the thermodynamic properties of aqueous solutions, we will use it to examine the $\bar{V}^0$(ions). The Frank and Wen model [17] divides ions into three classes: (1) "structure-breakers," which have a net effect of breaking the water structure, (2) "electrostrictive structure-makers," which order the water molecules by their high electrostatic field, (3) "hydrophobic structure makers," which induce more hydrogen bonding in the water near their nonpolar surface. Using this model for ion-water interactions, the partial molal volume of an ion at infinite dilution, $\bar{V}^0$(ion), can be attributed to [28, 29]

$$\bar{V}^0(\text{ion}) = \bar{V}^0(\text{cryst}) + \bar{V}^0(\text{elect}) + \bar{V}^0(\text{disord}) + \bar{V}^0(\text{caged}) \qquad (1)$$

where $\bar{V}^0$(cryst) is the crystal partial molal volume, $\bar{V}^0$(elect) is the electrostriction partial molal volume, $\bar{V}^0$(disord) is the disordered partial molal volume, and $\bar{V}^0$(caged) is the caged or structure partial molal volume (Fig. 9.1).

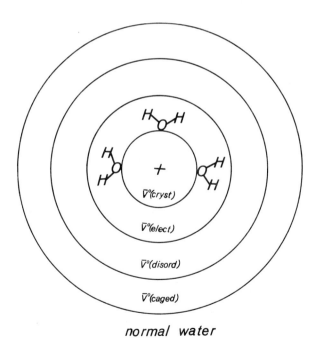

normal water

Figure 9.1. The Frank and Wen model for ion-water interactions. $\bar{V}^0$(ion) = $\bar{V}^0$(cryst) + $\bar{V}^0$(elect) + $\bar{V}^0$(disord) + $\bar{V}^0$(caged); *"Structure-Maker"* $\bar{V}^0$(ion) − $\bar{V}^0$(cryst) is negative; *"Structure-Breaker"* $\bar{V}^0$(ion) − $\bar{V}^0$(cryst) is positive.

In the electrostricted region, the ionic charge on the ion predominates and the water dipoles are completely oriented toward the central ion. Although the water molecules in this region are rapidly exchanging, they are immobilized to a considerable extent compared with bulk water; and the volume is decreased. For an ion with a large electrostricted region (i.e., ions of high charge and small radius) or when this region predominates the ion is called an "electrostrictive structure-maker." Water in the second and third solvation layer will be less immobilized or tightly packed. In the intermediate region between the electrostricted region and the bulk water, the effect of the ionic charge has diminished to such an extent that it can only partially orientate the water molecules; but the orientations are still large enough to interfere with the formation of the normal structure of water. Water in this region has a lower degree of hydrogen bonding and structure and, consequently, if this region is very large, the ion is said to be a net "structure-breaker." For ions with a large hydrophobic surface it is necessary to consider another effect. Water molecules at the surface of these large ions are influenced very little by either the ionic charge or the inert hydrocarbon. Thus, the water-water interactions appear to have a higher degree of hydrogen bonding or structure. This type of ion can be considered to be a "hydrophobic structure-maker."

Since the various components of Equation 1 may be small when compared to the absolute size of the ion (i.e., the crystal volume), it is difficult to determine the importance of the individual components of $\bar{V}^0(\text{ion})$ or separate overlapping effects. In recent work [29–32] we have tried to solve this problem by examining the effect of temperature on the $\bar{V}^0(\text{ions})$ of different charge and size type. Upon differentiation of Equation 1 with temperature, we obtain the partial molal expansibility of an ion, $\bar{E}^0(\text{ion})$,

$$\bar{E}^0(\text{ion}) = \bar{E}^0(\text{cryst}) + \bar{E}^0(\text{elect}) + \bar{E}^0(\text{disord}) + \bar{E}^0(\text{caged}) \quad (2)$$

Table 9.1 contains the partial molal expansibility of various ions [29] at 25°C.

We will now examine the various components of $\bar{V}^0(\text{ions})$ and $\bar{E}^0(\text{ions})$, given in Table 9.1 in further detail.

9.1.1   The Intrinsic Partial Molal Volume $\bar{V}^0(\text{int})$

The true "nonhydrated" volume of an ion in solution cannot be measured directly and is usually evaluated from the crystal volume, $\bar{V}^0(\text{cryst})$, by assuming the ions are perfect hard spheres

$$\bar{V}^0(\text{cryst}) = \frac{4}{3}\pi N \times 10^{-24} \times r^3 = 2.52r^3 \quad (3)$$

where r is the crystal radius in angstrom (Å) units. Table 9.1 contains $\bar{V}^0(\text{cryst})$ for various ions calculated from Equation 3 using Pauling crystal radii [33]. As can be seen from the examination of the $\bar{V}^0$ of the large monovalent ions, $\bar{V}^0(\text{cryst})$ is smaller than the measured $\bar{V}^0(\text{ion})$. For example, $\bar{V}^0(\text{cryst})$ of Cs^+ is calculated to be 12.2 ml mol^{-1} compared to a measured value of 15.9 ml mol^{-1}. The experimental estimates of the "nonhydrated" volume from compressibility measurements [34] and those calculated by various semiempirical correlations [35–38] of $\bar{V}^0(\text{ions})$ are also larger than the crystal volume. In general, the results indicate that the $\bar{V}^0(\text{int})$ of an ion in solution is 77 % larger in water than $\bar{V}^0(\text{cryst})$. This discrepancy can be caused by (1) the radius of the ion in solution being 21 % greater than the radius in the crystal or (2) the void space around the hydrated ion or some other positive disorder effect.

Since the internal pressure in water will be comparable to that in the ionic crystal because both are condensed phases and pairs of ions enter water with energies of hydration which are almost equal to their lattice energies in the solid salt [39], it is reasonable to suppose that the radius of an ion in solution is equal to the crystal radius [39–41]. Benson and Copeland [41] have estimated the change of the radius of an ion when going from the crystal to water and show that at best the radius increases by only 0.01 Å. Thus, there is no basis for believing that ions in solution are under less electrostatic pressure than are ions in the crystal and we can equate $\bar{V}^0(\text{int})$ with the crystal volume $\bar{V}^0(\text{cryst})$. The apparent increase in $\bar{V}^0(\text{int})$ for ions in solution is therefore caused by void space-packing effects around the nonhydrated ion (i.e., in the $\bar{V}^0(\text{elect})$ region) or around the hydrated ion (i.e., the $\bar{V}^0(\text{disord})$ region) [29, 42].

The effect of temperature on $\bar{V}^0(\text{int})$ or $\bar{V}^0(\text{cryst})$ is positive and very small for normal ions; however, it may be large for ions with hydrocarbon portions (e.g., the R_4N^+ ions).

9.1.2   The Disordered Partial Molal Volume, $\bar{V}^0(\text{disord})$

Various workers [36–38, 42–45] have attempted to separate the crystal volume, $\bar{V}^0(\text{cryst})$ and the disordered or void-space effects, $\bar{V}^0(\text{disord})$, by using equations of the form

$$\bar{V}^0(\text{int}) = \bar{V}^0(\text{cryst}) + \bar{V}^0(\text{disord})$$

$$= Ar^3 = 2.52r^3 + (A - 2.52)r^3 \tag{4}$$

$$= 2.52r^3 + A'r^2 \tag{5}$$

$$= 2.52(r + a)^3 = 2.52r^3 + [2.52(r + a)^3 - 2.52r^3] \tag{6}$$

Equation 4 [36–38, 42] assumes that $\bar{V}^0(\text{int})$ is equal to the crystal volume times some constant (i.e., $A = 2.52 \times$ constant and $A > 2.52$) or $\bar{V}^0(\text{disord}) = (A - 2.52)r^3$. Values for the constant $A = 4.35$ [38], 4.48 [37], 4.6 [36], 4.9 [35], and 5.3 [36] have been obtained by various workers. These values are nearly twice the theoretical value of 2.52. Using the average value (4.72), $\bar{V}^0(\text{int})$ is found to be 1.86 times greater than $\bar{V}^0(\text{cryst})$, and $\bar{V}^0(\text{disord}) = 2.2r^3$.

Conway et al. [43, 44] have calculated the void space or disordered volume using Equation 5. They calculate a value of $A' = 3.15$ by making the assumptions: (1) the crystal radius = the radius in solution; (2) when $r(\text{ion}) \gg r(\text{water})$ Equation 3 holds; (3) when $r(\text{ion}) = r(H_2O)$, $\bar{V}^0(\text{int}) = (2r)^3 N$ holds and the ion-water molecules are locally, cubically (or probably) hexagonally packed; (4) there is a smooth transition between these limiting conditions.

Glueckauf [45] postulated that the void-space volume can be represented by a hollow sphere of radius $(r + a)$ (Equation 6). He calculates a value of $a = 0.55$ Å by assuming the void space of an ion with the same radius as a water molecule (1.38 Å) has the same void volume as that for pure water.

$$a = \left[\frac{\bar{V}^0(H_2O)}{2.52} \right]^{1/3} - r(H_2O) \tag{7}$$

His results for large ions seem reasonable, but for small ions (e.g., Li+ and Na+) $\bar{V}^0(\text{int})$ is larger than $\bar{V}^0(\text{cryst})$ which is not reasonable when $r(\text{ion}) < r(H_2O)$. Although Glueckauf [45] feels that void-space effects are the cause of the large $\bar{V}^0(\text{int})$ of ions, the addition of a constant a to the crystal radius in effect is similar to assuming that all ions expand by a constant amount.

Recently [42] we have examined the $\bar{V}^0(\text{ions})$ in the solvents, water, N-methylpropionamide (NMP) and methanol by the semiempirical equations:

$$\bar{V}^0(\text{ion}) = Ar^3 - \frac{BZ^2}{r} \tag{8}$$

$$\bar{V}^0(\text{ion}) = 2.52(r + a)^3 - \frac{B'Z^2}{r} \tag{9}$$

$$\bar{V}^0(\text{ion}) = 2.52r^3 + A'r^2 - \frac{B''Z^2}{r} \tag{10}$$

It was found that the constants A, A', and a of Equations 4, 5, 6 and 8, 9, 10 were not proportional to the dielectric constants or compressibilities of the solvents (as might be expected if the radius of the ion increased in solution). It was found, however, that the constants were proportional to the structure of the solvent, that is, $A(H_2O) > A(NMP) > A(MeOH)$. Thus, the $\bar{V}^0$(disord) appears to be related to the disordered region surrounding the solvated ion. This disordered effect may be visualized as the void space caused by the solvated ion (i.e., including the electrostricted region) rather than improper packing in the electrostricted region.

The effect of temperature on $\bar{V}^0$(disord) or $\bar{E}^0$(disord) appears to be different for cations and anions of the same size due to the different orientation of the water molecules in the electrostricted region [28, 29]. The relative size of the disordered region depends on the temperature and magnitude of the electrostricted region. For ions with a large electrostricted region (large Z^2/r) the disordered region is very small; however, for ions with a small electrostricted region (small Z^2/r, like the large monovalent ions), this region is very important. The disordered region appears to become relatively less important at high temperatures causing the maximum in the $\bar{V}^0$ of the simple salts near 50°C. At low temperatures or near room temperatures, $\bar{V}^0$(disord) is large enough to cause the $\bar{V}^0$ of the large monovalent ions to appear to be larger in solution than $\bar{V}^0$(cryst). Thus, when $\bar{V}^0$(ion) $-$ $\bar{V}^0$(cryst) is positive this is due to $\bar{V}^0$(disord) and the ion can be classified as a "structure-breaker" ($\bar{V}^0$(disord) $>$ $\bar{V}^0$(elect)).

The $\bar{E}^0$(disord) accounts for the positive values of $\bar{E}^0$ for the monovalent ions at room temperature and the difference between the cation and anion $\bar{E}^0$ dependence on size [30]. The $\bar{E}^0$(disord) is positive and becomes less important at high temperatures (as the structure of water is broken).

9.1.3   The Electrostriction Partial Molal Volume, $\bar{V}^0$(elect)

The theoretical prediction of the electrostriction caused by various ions is difficult because of the uncertainty in the form of the interaction between an ion and the water molecule. Drude and Nernst [46] were the first to calculate the electrostriction of an ion. The electrical free energy, $\Delta \bar{G}^0$(elect) of a charged sphere in a continuous dielectric medium is given by the relation

$$\Delta \bar{G}^0(\text{elect}) = \frac{NZ^2e^2}{2Dr} \tag{11}$$

where N is Avagodros' number, Z is the charge on the ion, e is the electrostatic charge, D is the dielectric constant, and r is the radius of the ion (usually taken as the crystal radius). Upon differentiation of this equation with respect to pressure, one obtains the Drude-Nernst equation

$$\frac{\partial \Delta \bar{G}^0(\text{elect})}{\partial P} = -\bar{V}^0(\text{elect}) = \frac{NZ^2e^2}{2Dr}\left[\frac{\partial \ln D}{\partial P}\right] = \frac{BZ^2}{r} \tag{12}$$

This equation is valid only for large isolated ions (at infinite dilution) and serves only as an approximation. Using the most recent value for $d \ln D/dP$ and D [47], a value of 4.2 is obtained for the constant B in pure water. Benson and Copeland [41] have used a modified version of the Drude-Nernst equation and obtain a value of $B = 6.0$. Other authors [48–53] have attempted to calculate $\bar{V}^0(\text{elect})$ by more elaborate methods by considering dielectric saturation effects; however, normally the equations are complex functions and $\bar{V}^0(\text{elect})$ must be evaluated for each individual ion or charge type (in the limit when r is large, most of these complex functions approach the Drude-Nernst equation). These theoretical B values can be compared to a value of $B = 8.0$ found by Mukerjee [37] by correlating the partial molal volume of monovalent ions using Equation 8 (where $A = 4.48$). If Equations 9 and 10 are used [42], slightly different values are obtained; $B' = 10$ and $B'' = 11$ when $A' = 4.0$, $a = 0.45$.

For polyvalent ions the partial-molal volume is negative indicating that the electrostriction term is the predominate component of $\bar{V}^0(\text{ion})$. Using the Frank and Wen model for ion hydration these ions would be classified as "electrostriction structure-makers."

The effect of temperature on $\bar{V}^0(\text{elect})$ or $\bar{E}^0(\text{elect})$ appears to be predictable in sign and order of magnitude from the simple continuum model [29]. Since $\bar{V}^0(\text{elect})$ of the divalent cations (Mg^{2+}, Ca^{2+}, Sr^{2+}, and Ba^{2+}) is mainly due to electrostriction [29], one would expect that $\bar{E}^0(\text{elect})$ would be the important contribution of $\bar{E}^0(\text{ion})$ for the divalent ions and also $\bar{E}^0(\text{ion})$ to be proportional to Z^2/r. The expansibility for the divalent ions have been fit to the equation [29]

$$\bar{E}^0(\text{ion}) = -0.31\frac{Z^2}{r} + 0.092 \tag{13}$$

The value of the slope agrees very well with the theoretical value (0.027) obtained by Noyes [54] by differentiating the Drude-Nernst equation with respect to temperature

$$\bar{E}^0(\text{elect}) = \frac{\partial \bar{V}^0(\text{elect})}{\partial T} = \frac{-\partial}{\partial T}\left[\frac{1}{D}\frac{(\partial \ln D)}{\partial P}\right]\frac{Ne^2Z^2}{2r} \tag{14}$$

The positive intercept indicates that there is a positive contribution to the $\bar{E}^0$ of the divalent ions (and probably other polyvalent ions) similar to nonelectrolytes and the monovalent ions. This is probably due to a contribution to $\bar{E}^0(\text{ion})$ due to $\bar{E}^0(\text{disord})$—although $\bar{E}^0(\text{caged})$ may cause the same effect. Further $\bar{E}^0$ studies on other polyvalent ions are needed to examine the causes of the positive intercept.

9.1.4 The Caged or Structured Partial Molal Volume $\bar{V}^0$(caged)

The tetraalkylammonium ion (R_4N^+) is a typical example of an ion that causes structural effects that are different compared to the simple monovalent ions. One would expect the large R_4N^+ ions to have little or no electrostriction (i.e., $\bar{V}^0$(elect) ≈ 0); thus, one would expect $\bar{V}^0$(ion) $\approx$ $\bar{V}^0$(cryst) $+ \bar{V}^0$(disord). An examination of the $\bar{V}^0$ (R_4N^+) ions in Table 9.1 compared to the crystal volume indicates that $\bar{V}^0$(ion) $- \bar{V}^0$(cryst) is negative for these ions. The $\bar{V}^0$ of the R_4N^+ ions is similar in this respect to the polyvalent ions. The negative effect decreases in magnitude for the polyvalent ions as the radius increases; however, for the R_4N^+ ions the negative effect increases in magnitude as the radius increases. The $\bar{V}^0$(caged) term of $\bar{V}^0$(ion) is needed to explain this negative effect for the R_4N^+ ions. (This behavior is similar to that observed for the aliphatic alcohols) [30].

Measurements of heat capacity [17], dielectric relaxation times [55], viscosities [56–57], soret coefficients [58], NMR relaxation times [59], conductivities [60], and heats of dilution and solution [61, 62] also indicate that the R_4N^+ ion become "hydrophobic structure-makers" as the size of the alkyl group increases. The evidence is quite strong in indicating that the nBu_4N^+ and nPr_4N^+ ions are strong "hydrophobic structure-makers." The evidence is not so conclusive about the Me_4N^+ and Et_4N^+ ions. Wen and Saito [63] have pictured the Me_4N^+ ion as being a slight structure-breaker and the Et_4N^+ ion as a slight structure-maker. They visualize a competition between the charge effect and the hydrophobic effect, where the Me_4N^+ ion was just small enough so that the water structure around the ion was still under the influence of its charge, while the Et_4N^+ ion was just large enough that the effect of charge on the water structure was slightly overshadowed by the hydrophobic or clathrate effect.

Recent measurements of conductivities [64] and the viscosities [65] of Kay and co-workers indicate that the Me_4N^+ ion is a structure-breaker, but that the Et_4N^+ ion is in the transition region between a structure-maker and a structure-breaker.

An examination of the $\bar{V}^0$ of the R_4N^+ ions compared to their crystal volume (i.e., $\bar{V}^0$(ion) $- \bar{V}^0$(cryst), indicates that the Me_4N^+ ion may behave as an electrostriction structure-maker as well as a hydrophobic structure-maker. The similarity of the $\bar{V}^0$ behavior of the R_4N^+ ions and the aliphatic alcohols has been discussed elsewhere and it has been postulated that the abnormal properties of the R_4N^+ salts may be normal for all solutes able to cause hydrophobic bonding [30].

Since the large R_4N^+ ions are not hydrated in the normal sense (i.e., electrostrictive hydration), Conway et al. [43, 44] have used the $\bar{V}^0$ of these salts to determine the absolute $\bar{V}^0$ value of the halide ion. They found that the $\bar{V}^0$ of the R_4N^+ halides is a linear function of the molecular weight of the cation (R_4N^+) and by plotting $\bar{V}^0(R_4NX)$ versus the molecular weight of R_4N^+ and extrapolating to zero, they found values for the $\bar{V}^0$ of Cl^-, Br^-, and I^- that agree within experimental error with those calculated by other methods [27, 28]. Recently we attempted to determine the absolute expansibility of the Cl^- ion by a similar technique [30]. We found that a linear relation is not obtained. A smooth curve is obtained with the $\bar{E}^0$ of the Pr_4NCl and Bu_4NCl salts appearing to be high compared to the lower molecular weight R_4NCl. At higher temperatures (30°) a linear relation is obtained for the Me_4N^+, Et_4N^+, and Pr_4N^+ chlorides with the Bu_4N^+ salt appearing to be high. The high values of the Bu_4N^+ and Pr_4N^+ at low temperatures indicates that the caged or structural term of $\bar{E}^0$(ion) is causing a higher value for $\bar{E}^0$ than expected (by comparison with the lower molecular weight R_4NCl). The results at higher temperatures indicate that $\bar{E}^0$(caged) decreases with temperature. These results indicate that $\bar{E}^0$(caged) is positive; increases with increasing size of the hydrocarbon portion of the ion and decreases or becomes less important at high temperatures. Although the linearity does not exist for all of the R_4NCl salts, it is possible to estimate $\bar{E}^0(Cl^-) = 0.048$ ml mole^{-1} deg^{-1} at 25°. Using the method of Conway et al. for the $\bar{V}^0$ (R_4NBr) at two temperatures [66], we have determined $\bar{E}^0$ (Br^-) = 0.035 ml mole^{-1} deg^{-1}. Thus, $\bar{E}^0(H^+)$ was found to be between -0.010 to -0.014 ml mole^{-1} deg^{-1} (using $\bar{E}^0$(KBr), $\bar{E}^0$(KCl), $\bar{E}^0$(HCl)).

The $\bar{E}^0$ of the R_4N^+ salts increase with increasing temperature in a manner similar to the behavior of aliphatic alcohols [30]. The $\bar{E}^0$ of other electrolytes (salts), however, decrease with increasing temperature. Comparison [30] of the $\bar{E}^0$ of the R_4N^+ cations and aliphatic alcohols indicates that a common line is obtained when plotted versus $\bar{V}^0$ with the exception of Bu_4N^+. Since $\bar{E}^0$(elect) ≈ 0, the $\bar{E}^0$ of these solutes can be attributed to $\bar{E}^0$(int), $\bar{E}^0$(caged), and $\bar{E}^0$(disord). It appears that $\bar{E}^0$(ion) is proportional to $\bar{V}^0$ and as the volume increases $\bar{E}^0$(caged) becomes important.

The cause of the R_4N^+ ions behaving as hydrophobic structure-makers (i.e., whether it is due to void-space effects, $\bar{V}^0$(disord), or changes in the structure of water, $\bar{V}^0$(caged), cannot be exactly stated). Further studies are needed on nonelectrolyte hydrocarbons in water and other solvents.

In summary, the examination of the various components of $\bar{V}^0$(ions) conforms with the Frank and Wen model [17] for ion-water interactions.

It should be emphasized, however, that the division of ions into "structure-breakers" and "structure-makers," although being useful, is not a rigid division. For example, at temperatures above 50°C, the $\bar{V}^0$ of all ions approach negative values, indicating that even the so-called "structure-breaking ions" (i.e., Cs^+, Rb^+, and I^- become electrostatic "structure-makers" at high temperatures). Thus, $\bar{V}^0$(disord) is not important (i.e., relative to $\bar{V}^0$(elect)) at high temperatures when the structure of water is broken down. By saying that the structure of water is broken down it is not meant that water exists as only monomers, but that one structured form responsible for the anomalous thermodynamic behavior disappears at high temperatures (e.g., the temperature coefficient of the isothermal compressibility of water above 50°C is positive as for other solvent systems; however, at temperatures from 0 to 45°C the temperature coefficient is negative [67]).

9.2 THERMODYNAMICS OF MIXED ELECTROLYTE SOLUTIONS

Although most of the thermodynamic studies of electrolytes in aqueous solutions have been made on single electrolyte solutions, recent work has stressed mixed-salt solutions due to their importance in oceanography and physiology. Earlier work on mixed-salt solutions have been concerned with the determination of activity coefficients [1–4]. In Section 9.2 we will review some of the recent experimental results on the effect of temperature (ΔH) and pressure (ΔV) on the activity coefficients of mixed-salt solutions.

The Debye-Hückel theory of interionic attraction [1–4] works very well for very dilute electrolyte solutions in which long-range interactions are important. However, when ions move closer together the Debye-Hückel theory is no longer valid.

The theory gives for the mean activity coefficient ($f_{\pm}$) of an electrolyte in water [1]

$$- \log f_{\pm} = \frac{S_f \mu^{\frac{1}{2}}}{1 + A a \mu^{\frac{1}{2}}} \tag{15}$$

$$S_f = \frac{1}{\gamma} \sum_i \gamma_i Z_i^2 \, (DT)^{-\frac{3}{2}} \, 1.8243 \times 10^6 \tag{16}$$

$$A = \frac{50.29 \times 10^8}{(DT)^{\frac{1}{2}}} \tag{17}$$

where γ is the total number of ions formed when one molecule of electrolyte dissociates of which γ_i is the kind i of charge Z_i; μ is the volume ionic strength $\mu = \frac{1}{2}\Sigma C_i Z_i^2$, D is the dielectric constant, T is the absolute temperature, and a is the ion-size parameter. For a 1–1 electrolyte in water at 25°C, $S_f = 0.5091$ and $A = 0.3286 \times 10^8$. Equations for other thermodynamic properties can be derived from Equation 15 by the appropriate differentiation. Two such equations [1] representing the relative partial molal volume and the relative partial molal heat content are

$$\bar{V} - \bar{V}^0 = \frac{S_v \mu^{\frac{1}{2}}}{1 + Aa\mu^{\frac{1}{2}}} + \frac{W_v \mu}{(1 + Aa\mu^{\frac{1}{2}})^2} \tag{18}$$

$$\bar{H} - \bar{H}^0 = \frac{S_H \mu^{\frac{1}{2}}}{1 + Aa\mu^{\frac{1}{2}}} + \frac{W_H \mu}{(1 + Aa\mu^{\frac{1}{2}})^2} \tag{19}$$

where the theoretical limiting slopes

$$S_v = 2.303\gamma RTS_f^{\frac{3}{2}} \left[\frac{\partial \ln D}{\partial P} - \frac{\beta}{3} \right] \tag{20}$$

$$S_H = -2.303\gamma RT^2 S_f^{\frac{3}{2}} \left[\frac{\partial \ln D}{\partial T} + \frac{1}{T} + \frac{\alpha}{3} \right] \tag{21}$$

are derived by differentiation of $S_f \mu^{\frac{1}{2}}$. The symbols α and β represent the expansibility and compressibility, respectively. $S_v = 2.802$ and $S_H = 707.1$ at 25°C for a 1–1 electrolyte in water. The terms for the coefficients

$$W_v = -2.303\gamma RTS_f Aa \frac{1}{2} \left[\frac{\partial \ln D}{\partial P} - \beta - \frac{2\partial \ln a}{\partial P} \right] \tag{22}$$

$$W_H = 2.303\gamma RTS_f Aa \frac{1}{2} \left[\frac{\partial \ln D}{\partial T} + \frac{1}{T} - \alpha - \frac{2\partial \ln a}{\partial T} \right] \tag{23}$$

result from the $(1 + Aa\mu^{\frac{1}{2}})$ term and cannot normally be evaluated since the effect of temperature and pressure on the ion size parameter is unknown (i.e., $\partial \ln a/\partial T$ and $\partial \ln a/\partial P$).

These equations give reasonable results [1, 2] up to about $\mu = 0.1$; however, at high concentrations they are no longer valid. The magnitude and sign of the added linear term in μ that is normally added to extend these equations cannot be estimated theoretically. Furthermore, at higher concentrations the whole concept of the ionic-strength principle breaks down; that is, the principle stating that the properties of the ion depend on the ionic strength only and not on the specific ions that constitute the mixture.

There are many strong electrolytes for which the Debye-Hückel formula requires absurdly small or even negative values for the ion-size parameter a.

Two types of approaches have been used to describe the effects of short-range interactions using activity coefficient data. The first is based on the association model of Bjerrum [68]. The basic assumption in this approach is that short-range interactions in mixed salt mixtures can be represented by the formation of ion-pairs. The ion-pair is formed by ions of opposite sign and they may be separated by one or more solvent molecules. The ion association of an electrolyte (MA) may be represented by

$$M^+ + A^- = M^+A^-$$ (24)

A characteristic association equilibrium constant is given by

$$K_A = \frac{(M^+A^-)}{(M^+)(A^-)}$$ (25)

where the brackets enclose activities of the species. Bjerrum [68] defined, from electrostatic grounds, the distance between oppositely charged ions which can be classified as being associated. This distance, q, the ionic separation of which the mutual potential energy is equal to $2kT$ represents the position of minimum probability of finding ions of opposite charge within a spherical shell of radius surrounding the central ion

$$q = \frac{|Z_+Z_-|e^2}{2DkT}$$ (26)

In this treatment, two oppositely charged ions between a (the ion-size parameter) and q are considered to form an ion-pair. Bjerrum's equation [68] predicts greater ion-pair formation the higher the valancies and the smaller the dielectric constant, (which is in agreement with experimental results) [1]. The theory has been criticized, however, due to the somewhat arbitrary cutoff distance q and it has now been superceded by the theories of Denison and Ramsey [69] and by Fuoss and Kraus [70]. These workers argue that the association constant is given (to a first approximation) by

$$\ln K = \ln K^0 - \frac{|Z_+Z_-|e^2}{aDkT}$$ (27)

and regard only ions in actual contact as forming ion pairs.

An alternate approach to short-range interactions, the specific interaction model, can be exemplified by the equations of Brønsted [71] and

Guggenheim [72]. Robinson and Stokes [2] have shown that the empirical equation known as Harned's rule can be obtained from Guggenheim's equation [72]. Activity coefficients of binary ionic components in a mixed ternary solution have been determined by various workers by emf and isopiestic measurements [1–4]. The activity coefficients have been found to obey Harned's rule [1] in many cases

$$\log \gamma_2 = \log \gamma_2(o) - \alpha_{23} m_3 \tag{28}$$

$$\log \gamma_3 = \log \gamma_3(o) - \alpha_{32} m_2 \tag{29}$$

where γ_2 and γ_3 are the activity coefficients of electrolytes 2 and 3 in the presence of each other, $\gamma_2(o)$ and $\gamma_3(o)$ are the activity coefficients of the single component electrolyte solutions at molality $m = m_2 + m_3$, α_{23} and α_{32} are functions of the total molality m, but are independent of the individual molalities m_2 and m_3. In some instances [73, 74], it is necessary to modify these equations by considering higher order terms:

$$\log \gamma_2 = \log \gamma_2(o) - \alpha_{23} m_3 - \beta_{23} m_3{}^2 \tag{30}$$

$$\log \gamma_3 = \log \gamma_3(o) - \alpha_{32} m_2 - \beta_{32} m_2{}^2 \tag{31}$$

Various workers have concluded that ion association does not occur in mixed solutions when Harned's rule is obeyed. This conclusion is open to question; however, as shown by the work of Pytkowicz and Kester [75]. They found that Harned's rule can be derived not only from Guggenheim's equation, but also from the association model. Also, the interaction terms in the Guggenheim equation which are present in the α_{23} term, includes the effects of ionic association (Ref. 1, p. 516). The association model also provides a better formal representation of short-range interactions than can be done by a specific interaction model.

Compared to solutions of single electrolyte, solutions of several electrolytes have received little study. Many systems of importance (e.g., seawater and biological fluids) contain mixtures of electrolytes. The measurement of the heats and volumes of mixing of electrolyte solutions is an excellent way to study the interactions of ions in aqueous solutions. If the measurements are made at constant ionic strength, effects of the ionic atmosphere are (supposedly) cancelled. If the measurements are made between electrolytes with a common ion, the effects of oppositely charged ion-pairs cancel. Thus, the pair-wise and triplet interactions of like-charged ions can be conveniently studied.

Brønsted's theory of specific ion interactions [71] assumes that like-charged ions do not have specific interactions. This means that replacing one ion by another of similar charge should not produce specific effects so that the excess free energy, heat and volume of mixing two electrolytes with a common ion should be zero. Guggenheim [72] and Scatchard and Prentiss [76] have extended the Brønsted theory while keeping the assumption that like-charged ions have no specific interactions. Scatchard and Prentiss [76] derived equations for mixed electrolytes which include both oppositely charged pair and triplet interactions. Guggenheim's equations for mixed electrolytes [72] include only oppositely charged ion-pair interactions and have been shown to be quite accurate below 0.1 m [1–3].

Recently, Friedman [77], using Mayer's ionic solution theory [78], predicted that like-charged ions should have specific interactions and these interactions should be more important than triplet interaction for many systems. The most sensitive-free energy measurements have not shown deviations from Brønsted's principle if triplet interactions are included [79]. Since calorimetric and volumetric measurements are capable of measuring the smaller energies and volumes of interaction in the 0.1 to 1.0 m region, the measurements of ΔH and ΔV of mixing have been used to test the Brønsted principle.

The excess free energy of mixing two electrolyte solutions, ΔG_m^{ex} is given by the equation

$$\Delta G_m^{ex} = \Delta G_m - \Delta G_m^i \tag{32}$$

where ΔG_m is the total free energy of mixing and ΔG_m^i is the ideal free energy of mixing—when the mixture is formed from its component solutions at constant total molality, temperature, and pressure.

The excess heat of mixing ΔH_m^{ex} is defined in a similar manner

$$\Delta H_m^{ex} = \Delta H_m - \Delta H_m^i \tag{33}$$

For an ideal solution ΔH_m^i is equal to zero and ΔH_m^{ex} is equal to the heat of mixing, ΔH_m. These and other excess properties of state show the same functional relationships as the fundamental variables of thermodynamics. Thus, for the excess entropy, ΔS_m^{ex}, we have

$$\Delta S_m^{ex} = \frac{\Delta H_m - \Delta G_m^{ex}}{T} \tag{34}$$

and for the excess volume of mixing $\Delta V^{ex} = \Delta V_m$ (since $\Delta \bar{V}_m^i = 0$)

$$\Delta V_m = \frac{\partial \Delta G_m^{ex}}{\partial P} \tag{35}$$

It can be shown [3] that ΔG_m^{ex} takes the following form for mixing two univalent electrolytes obeying Harned's rule

$$\Delta G_m^{ex} = -2.303RTm_2m_3 \Bigg[(\alpha_{23} + \alpha_{32}) + 2(m_3\beta_{23} + m_2\beta_{32}) +$$

$$\frac{2}{3}(\beta_{23} - \beta_{32})(m_2 - m_3) \Bigg] \quad (36)$$

Both electrolytes are initially at molality m and yield a final solution of total molality m containing $m_2 + m_3$ moles of each solute per kilogram of solvent. Using the Gibbs-Helmoltz equation the ΔH_m can be calculated from the temperature dependence of ΔG_m^{ex}

$$\Delta H_m = \frac{\partial(\Delta G_m^{ex}/T)}{\partial(1/T)} \quad (37)$$

In practice this indirect method of obtaining ΔH_m does not yield accurate results and direct calorimetric measurements are made to obtain results of high precision. By combining Equations 36 and 37 we obtain the relationship for ΔH_m

$$\Delta H_m = 2.303RT^2m_2m_3 \frac{\partial}{\partial T} \Bigg[(\alpha_{23} + \alpha_{32}) + 2(m_3\beta_{23} + m_2\beta_{32}) +$$

$$\frac{2}{3}(\beta_{23} - \beta_{32})(m_2 - m_3) \Bigg] \quad (38)$$

and by combining Equations 35 and 36 we obtain the relationship for ΔV_m

$$\Delta V_m = -2.303RTm_2m_3 \frac{\partial}{\partial P} \Bigg[(\alpha_{23} + \alpha_{32}) + 2(m_3\beta_{23} + m_2\beta_{32}) +$$

$$\frac{2}{3}(\beta_{23} - \beta_{32})(m_2 - m_3) \Bigg] \quad (39)$$

In practice ΔV_m is determined directly since ΔG_m^{ex} at different pressures is not easily determined. Alternate forms of Equations 38 and 39 may be expressed in terms of the total molality m and the solute mole fraction $m_2 = X_2m$ and $m_3 = (1 - X_2)m$. Substitution yields the equations

$$\Delta H_m = 2.303RT^2X_2(1 - X_2)m^2 \frac{\partial}{\partial T} \Bigg[(\alpha_{23} + \alpha_{32}) + \frac{2m}{3}(2\beta_{23} + \beta_{32}) +$$

$$\frac{2mX}{3}(\beta_{32} - \beta_{23}) \Bigg] \quad (40)$$

and

$$\Delta V_m = 2.303RTX_2(1 - X_2)m^2 \frac{\partial}{\partial P} \left[(\alpha_{23} + \alpha_{32}) + \frac{2m}{3}(2\beta_{23} + \beta_{32}) + \right.$$

$$\left. \frac{2mX}{3}(\beta_{32} - \beta_{23}) \right] \quad (41)$$

The excess thermodynamics of mixing of electrolyte solutions may be examined in relation to the Brønsted-Guggenheim theory of mixed electrolytes based on Brønsted's principle of the specific interaction of ions [2, 3]. This principle assumes that specific short-range interactions in solutions of constant total molality are limited to ions of opposite charge only. Ions of like charge influence each other uniformly without regard to their species. The theory leads to a very simple result for mixing two binary electrolytes with a common ion at constant total molality. No net changes in specific interactions are predicted and consequently ΔG_m^{ex}, ΔH_m, and ΔV_m are zero for such systems. Equations 36 through 41 are consistent with the theory when $\alpha_{23} = -\alpha_{32}$ and all the higher terms are zero. Nonzero values of ΔG_m^{ex}, ΔH_m, and ΔV_m can thus be considered as a measure of the deviations from the Brønsted-Guggenheim assumptions and attributed to differences in interaction between like-charged ions or three ion interactions.

Friedman [77] has derived the excess free energy of mixing

$$\Delta G_m^{ex}(y, I) = I^2RTy(1 - y)[g_0 + g_1(1 - 2y) + g_2(1 - 2y)^2 + \cdots] \quad (42)$$

where I is the molal ionic strength ($I = \frac{1}{2}\Sigma m_i Z_i^2$), y is the solute molefraction ($y = m_2/(m_2 + m_3)$), that is, the fraction of the ionic strength due to one electrolyte in a mixture of two electrolytes and g is the interaction parameter. Friedman's theory [77] predicts that the leading term, g_0, is the major term for 1–1 common-ion mixtures and the major interactions contributing to g_0 are those of like-charged ion-pairs (M^+–M^+, A^-–A^-). Using the Gibbs-Helmholtz equation, ΔH_m can be given by

$$\Delta H_m(y, I) = I^2y(1 - y)[h_0 + h_1(1 - 2y) + h_2(1 - 2y)^2 + \cdots] \quad (43)$$

where $h_0 = -RT^2(\partial g_0/\partial T)$, $h_1 = -RT^2(\partial g_1/\partial T)$, and so on. For ΔV_m we have

$$\Delta V_m(y, I) = I^2y(1 - y)[v_0 + v_1(1 - 2y) + v_2(1 - 2y)^2 + \cdots] \quad (44)$$

where $v_0 = RT(\partial g_0/\partial P)$, $v_1 = RT(\partial g_1/\partial P)$, and so on, and where h_0 and v_0 are a measure the magnitude of the interaction and h_1 and v_1

are a measure of the asymmetry or skew of ΔH_m and ΔV_m plotted versus $y \cdot \Delta H_m$ at $y = 0.5$ equals $h_0/4$ and ΔV_m at $y = 0.5$ equals $v_0/4$, when ΔH_m and ΔV_m plotted versus y is a perfect parabola (i.e., the maximum in ΔH_m and ΔV_m occurs at $y = 0.5$).

9.2.1 Heats of Mixing, ΔH_m

Young and co-workers [80–82] have measured the heats of mixing at 25°C of several 1 m uni-univalent electrolyte pairs. They found that ΔH_m is a parabolic and approximately symmetrical about the solute mole fraction y. At $y = 0.5$, the values ranged from 32 cal mole^{-1} for HCl-NaCl to -49 cal mole^{-1} for LiCl-CsCl.

Stern and Anderson [83] have measured the ΔH_m of the salt pairs KCl-NaCl and LiCl-NaCl over a wide range of ionic strength (0.5 to 4.8 or 6.0 m). They found that ΔH_m at $y = 0.5$ of both systems approach zero as the ionic strength approaches zero. The ΔH_m (at $y = 0.5$) for LiCl-NaCl approaches zero from the positive side and KCl-NaCl approaches zero from the negative side. Both systems appear to have ΔH_m effects that persist to very dilute solutions. Thus, deviations from the Brønsted-Guggenheim theory of specific interaction may be important for dilute solutions.

The work of Wood and Smith [84] has been extended to low concentrations (0.1 to 0.5 m). Their results show that like-charged ions do have specific interactions, even at low concentrations. The evidence indicates that these interactions are generally larger than triplet interactions, although smaller than oppositely charged pair interactions. It should be noted, however, that the specific effects are small at 0.1 m (less than 7 cal mole^{-1}). This is probably why previous experiments have tended to verify Brønsted's principle.

In most cases studied [80–84] the skew term (h_2) was very small or zero. The values of the h_0 term showed no general trend with concentration; some decreased while others increased. In cases of mixing with a common ion, the ΔH_m results are contrary to the Brønsted principle.

Scatchard and Prentiss [76] predicted that both g_0 and h_0 have the form

$$g_0 = AI = BI^{3/2} + \cdots \qquad (45)$$

where A and B are functions of the triple ion interactions (i.e., M$^+$X$^-$M$^+$). They found that the first two terms of Equation 45 are enough to represent the ΔG_m of the Li$^+$, K$^+$, Cl$^-$, NO$_3^-$ reciprocal salt pairs up to 1 m. The first two terms of this equation cannot represent Wood and Smith's data [84] for any of the salts within two to five times the estimated experimental error. The errors are always in the direction to be expected if h_0 is finite at zero concentration. A plot of h_0/m versus $m^{1/2}$ cannot be represented by a straight line as required by Equation 45. They can, however, be represented by a single charged-pair interaction with a triplet contribution (necessary in some cases).

The fact that h_0 usually varies slowly with ionic strength indicates that like-charged ion-pair interactions are usually more important than triplet interactions. Young, Wu, and Krawetz [81] have shown that for many systems the heats of mixing is independent of the common ion. Friedman [85] has noted that this fact indicates that like-charge ion-pairs are responsible for the effect.

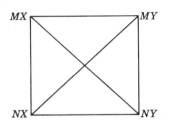

Figure 9.2.

Several observations of Young and co-workers [80–82] yield conclusions not generally derived from Friedman's theory [77].

1. In the presence of a common ion, ΔH_m of cations is much larger than the ΔH_m of anions (30 to 50 cal compared to 1 cal kg^{-1} of solvent).

2. Young, Wu, and Krawetz [81] have found that for common anion mixtures the cations can be divided into two groups (H$^+$, Li$^+$, Na$^+$ and K$^+$, Rb$^+$, Cs$^+$) and that mixing of two ions in the same group give positive values for h_0 and that mixing of two ions in different groups gives negative h_0 values. Division into these same groups holds for all the cations down to 0.1 m [84]. Since h_0 varies slowly this same division should also hold below 0.1 m for most salts.

3. For reciprocal salt pairs the sum of the heats of common-ion mixings equals the sum of the ΔH_m of the uncommon-ion mixings (the cross-square rule).

If one considers the number of mixings it is possible to make with four single electrolyte solutions (MX, MY, NX, NY) whose component ions are limited to two different cations and two anions, one finds six possible mixings as represented by the sides and diagonals of the square (Fig. 9.2). Krawetz [86] has shown that for the set LiCl, LiBr, KCl, KBr, the sum of the experimental heats of mixing represented by the sides of the square equals the sum of the heats of mixing represented by the diagonals. He calls this empirical relationship the cross-square rule ($\Sigma\square = \Sigma X$).

Bottcher [87] has shown that this rule will hold if the ΔH_m of the cations in the presence of each anion singly are nearly equal and the ΔH_m of the cations in the presence of an equal molal mixture of both anions has an intermediate value. Wu, Smith, and Young [82] have shown for several other sets of salts they studied at 1.0 m that the cross-square rule holds. Wood and Smith [84] have shown that the cross-square rule holds for the NaCl, NaBr, KCl, KBr mixed-salt pair. However, for the NaCl, NaNO$_3$, KCl, KNO$_3$ set, the sum of the common-ion mixing is more positive than the sum of the cross-mixing at every concentration (greater than experimental error). They noted that this test of the cross-square rule is the only one which contains an ion-paired salt, KNO$_3$ [88–89].

Wu [90] has shown how the individual heats of cross mixing (without a common ion) can be calculated from the cross-square rule and the relative apparent molal heat content, ϕ_L, of the four salts of a set.

$$\Delta H_m(NX - MY) = \frac{m}{4}\left[\phi_L(NY) + \phi_L(MX) - \phi_L(NX) - \phi_L(MY)\right]$$

$$+ \frac{1}{2}\Sigma\square \quad (46)$$

where ΔH_m and $\Sigma\square$ terms are in calories per kg of solvent.

Accurate ϕ_L data are needed to show the accuracy of this method of calculating cross mixing since the resultant ΔH_m for many salt pairs are the small differences between large ϕ_L values. Wood and Smith [84] have shown that for the salt pairs NaCl-KNO$_3$ and NaNO$_3$-KCl, excellent agreement is attained. For the salt pairs NaBr-KCl and NaCl-KBr the agreement is not as good.

Wood and Anderson [91] have investigated ΔH_m of the alkaline earth halides as a function of ionic strength (0.1 to 2.0 m). They found that h_0 decreases with decreasing concentration (unlike the simple alkali metal halides). They attribute this effect to triplet interactions due to the increased charge on the cations. They found, however, that it was not possible to use the Scatchard and Prentiss [76] Equation 45 to fit the experimental results, indicating that triplet interaction cannot be the total cause of the observed effect. The ΔH_m of the alkaline earth cations are, on the average, much smaller than ΔH_m of the alkali metal cations. (At 1 m, 7 cal for the alkaline earth halides and 20 cal for the alkali metal halides). This is in accord with the qualitative expectation that the higher the charge on the ions the less they will interact with ions of the same charge. The ΔH_m of the alkaline earth cations in the presence of a common anion are all endothermic. If ions are classified according to the groupings of Young, Wu, and Krawetz [81] according to size (large and small) the cations H^+, Li^+, and Na^+ are small "structure-making" ions (according to the Frank and Wen [17] model for hydration), and the cations K^+, Rb^+, and Cs^+ are all "structure-breaking" ions. Since the alkaline earth cations are "structure-making" ions, one would expect them to have positive ΔH_m in accord with the H^+, Li^+, and Na^+ ions. The heats of mixing of the Cl^- and Br^- ions in the presence of Mg^{++} and Ca^{++} (4.08 and 4.42 cal kg^{-1} of solvent) show fair agreement with the results of Wu, Smith, and Young [82] that the ΔH_m is relatively independent of the common ion. Mixtures which contain KNO_3 have considerable ion-pair character and deviate from this conclusion. The ΔH_m of Mg^{++} and Ca^{++} in the presence of Cl^- and Br^- ions also show deviations (3.50 and 2.76 respectively).

Wood and Anderson [91] have developed a set of general equations for the ΔH_m and the relative apparent molal heat content ϕ_L (mix) of a multicomponent aqueous solution containing electrolytes of the same charge type. These equations are based on the properties of single electrolyte solutions and common-ion mixtures. The equations were derived using Friedman's results [77] (including pair-wise and triple ion interactions, but excluding interactions of three like-charged ions). The cross-square rule is a special case of this general equation. Wood and Anderson [92] have tested these equations for the ΔH_m of $LiCl$-KCl-Me_4NCl-H_2O and $LiCl$-KCl-$NaCl$-H_2O systems at $25°$ and constant ionic strength. Their experimental results were in excellent agreement with those calculated from the general equations.

Wood and Anderson [93] have measured the ΔH_m of KF, KCl, KBr, and KAc at $25°C$ at 1 m constant total concentration. The purpose of this study was to examine the effect of anion size on the "structure-making" and "structure-breaking" relations of ΔH_m. They found ΔH_m from $+2.3$ to -3.5 cal $mole^{-1}$. These results include the largest heats of mixing observed for anion-common cation mixtures. If one neglects the ΔH_m of H^+ and Li^+ the ΔH_m for anions with a common anion ($+2$ to -12 cal $mole^{-1}$). As found with other ΔH_m studies, the mixing of two "structure-breakers" or two "structure-makers" gives negative ΔH_m while the mixing of the "structure-breaker" with a "structure-maker" gives a positive heat (F^- and Ac^- are "structure-makers"; Cl^- and Br^- are "structure-breakers") [94–97]. It is surprising that this simple classification will predict the sign of the ΔH_m when the mechanism of "structure-making" is probably quite different for F^- and Ac^-. In the case of F^- ion, the structure is created by the high electric field while for the Ac$^-$ ion the lack of specific interaction with the methyl group stabilizes a more highly hydrogen-bonded water structure around the hydrocarbon portion of the molecule. In addition, there is probably more structure near the oxygens where the electric field is concentrated (since the B coefficient of Ac$^-$ is larger than the B for HAc) [97]. The arguments used by Wood and Anderson [93] are similar to those used by Frank and Robinson [98] to explain heats of dilution of strong electrolytes.

Wood and Anderson's work [99] on the ΔH_m of the tetra-alkylammonium salts have also been explained by considering the detailed structure of water molecules around an ion of two like-charged ion interactions.

The ΔH_m of the R$_4$N$^+$ ions with a common anion are larger (-700 to $+100$) than for the alkali or alkaline earth metal ions (-200 to $+130$). Theoretical calculations using Friedman's hard sphere model indicate that the large interaction cannot be explained by the size parameters for the R$_4$N$^+$ ions [99]. Thus, it is due to the effect of the structure of water around the ions (even if only due to the way in which water structure influences the temperature dependence of the effective radius of the ions).

In conclusion, for all the common ion ΔH_m that have been measured, the sign of the heats of mixing follow a simple rule. The mixing of two "structure-makers" or two "structure-breakers" give positive ΔH_m, while a "structure-breaker" with a "structure-maker" gives negative ΔH_m. With the uncertainty of classifying the ions, it is not surprising to find that the simple correlation for the sign of ΔH_m runs into some exceptions. Assuming the structural classification for determining the sign of ΔH_m is valid, the Me$_4$N$^+$ ion acts as a "structure-breaker" toward the alkali cations. The Et$_4$N$^+$ ion also acts as a "structure-breaker." However, ΔH_m of Me$_4$N$^+$-Et$_4$N$^+$ is exothermic, indicating that they act as opposites when mixed with each other. The results for the Pr$_4$N$^+$ ion show that all the mixings of this ion give very large negative values for ΔH_m (-300 to -600 cal kg^{-1} solvent). This suggests that the Pr$_4$N$^+$ ions are responsible and that the large interactions of two Pr$_4$N$^+$ ions are masking other effects. In any common ion ΔH_m of MX with NX there are three like-charge interactions to consider: (1) the heat of diluting the M$^+$ ions and therefore, the reduction in the overlap of M$^+$ hydrating sheaths with each other, (2) the dilution of the N$^+$ ions and the reduction of N$^+$—N$^+$ overlap, and (3) the formation of some M$^+$—N$^+$ overlap. It is expected that at any given concentration the Pr$_4$N$^+$ ions will have more hydration-sphere overlap with neighbors because this is by far the largest ion studied. The Pr$_4$N$^+$ ion is a large hydrophobic structural maker and when the ion is mixed with another, the overlap of the hydration sheaths of the Pr_4N^+ ions is reduced. Wood and co-workers [100] have recently successfully extended their ΔH_m correlations to charge-asymmetrical mixtures (MgCl, with some alkali metal chlorides).

At present there have been only two studies [101, 102] of the ΔH_m of various salt pairs as a function of temperature. Stern and Passchier [101] have examined the ΔH_m of the HCl—NaCl salt pair from 0 to 40° (at the intervals, 0, 10, 25 and 40°C) from 1 to 3 total molality ionic strength. Their results indicate that ΔH_m at a constant ionic strength decreases with increasing temperature and ΔH_m increases as the ionic strength is increased at all the temperatures studied.

It thus appears that adherence to the Brønsted-Guggenheim theory improves with increasing temperature; that is, short-range repulsive interactions of hydrated like-charge ions diminishes. This may be due to effects of the structure of water around the ion or the structure of bulk water becoming less important at higher temperatures (that is, the solutions become more ideal).

9.2.2   Volume Change in Mixing ΔV_m

Young and Smith [80] showed that their mixture rule

$$\Phi = \frac{m_2\phi_2 + m_3\phi_3}{m_2 + m_3} \tag{47}$$

accurately represented the molal volume data of Wirth and co-workers [103, 104] for KCl—NaCl [103], KBr—NaCl [103], and $NaClO_4$—$HClO_4$ [104] mixtures. Φ, the mean apparent molal volume of a mixture of electrolytes is defined by

$$\Phi = \frac{V - n_1\bar{V}_1^0}{m_2 + m_3} \tag{48}$$

where V is the volume of solution containing 1000 g of water, $\bar{V}_1^0$ is the molal volume of pure water, n_1 is the moles of water (55.51) and $m_2 + m_3$ are the sum of the molalities of the two electrolytes. ϕ_2 and ϕ_3 are the apparent molal volumes of the electrolytes 2 and 3 in binary mixtures at an ionic strength I corresponding to $m_2 + m_3$. Wirth [105] and Young and Smith [80] found that a small correction term D had to be added to Equation 47 to give complete agreement for NaCl–HCl mixtures. The suggested form of D is

$$D = S_2S_3Ik \tag{49}$$

where $S_2 = m_2/(m_2 + m_3)$, $S_3 = m_3/(m_2 + m_3)$, I is the ionic strength, and k is a constant. Young's rule predicts that there should be no change in volume on mixing solutions of equal ionic strength.

The term D is calculated from the observed volume change, Δv, of mixing two electrolyte solutions, one containing n_2 moles of electrolyte 2 and n_1 moles of water and the other containing n_3 moles of electrolyte 3 and n_1' moles of water, as follows: The volume of the first solution $V_2 = n_1\bar{V}_1{}^0 + n_2\phi_2$ and the volume of the second solution $V_3 = n_1'\bar{V}^0 + n_3\phi_3$, where ϕ_2 and ϕ_3 are the apparent molal volume of the solutions. The total volume of the mixture, $V = V_3 + V_2 + \Delta v$, where Δv is the observed volume change of mixing. The mean apparent molal volume is defined by $\Phi = (V - n_1''\bar{V}_1{}^0)/(n_2 + n_3)$ where $n_1'' = n_1 + n_1'$. Substituting V into this equation yields $\Phi = (n_2\phi_2 + n_3\phi_3)/(n_2 + n_3) + \Delta v/(n_2 + n_3)$. The first term is Young's rule and the second term is equal to D. Using the notation of Friedman [77], $D = V_m$ and the k term is equal to v_0.

Wirth and co-workers [106] have recently examined the volume of mixing of electrolyte mixtures NaCl—HCl, NaCl—NaClO$_4$, NaCl—HClO$_4$, HCl—NaClO$_4$, HCl—HClO$_4$ and NaClO$_4$—HClO$_4$ at two concentrations, 1.000 and 4.1724 m. The results at 4.17 of D had to be represented by the relation $D = kS_2S_3 + k'S_2{}^2S_3$, since in all cases D was not symmetrical around a mole fraction of 0.5.

While this work is primarily concerned with deviations from Young's rule, it should be emphasized that the deviations are small (in the most unfavorable case the error is 0.6 ml mole^{-1} or 2%) and the rule gives a remarkably good first approximation. Only in heteroionic solutions or at high concentrations are the deviations larger than the errors of the equations representing Φ_v of pure salts.

Wirth and co-workers [106] showed that Young, Wu, and Krawetz's [81] cross-square rule holds for D at $X = 0.5$ as does the ΔH_m. For the set of electrolytes, NaCl, HCl, NaClO$_4$, and HClO$_4$, the net departure from additivity R is given by

$$R = \phi_v(\text{NaClO}_4) + \phi_v(\text{HCl}) + \phi_v(\text{NaCl}) - \phi_v(\text{HClO}_4) \qquad (50)$$

At a given ionic strength, the apparent molal volumes of the electrolytes can be given by their ionic components (i.e., $\phi v(\text{NaCl}) = \phi v(\text{Na}^+) + \phi v(\text{Cl}^-)$, etc.). The mean apparent molal volume of a mixture containing equal concentrations of all four ions as calculated by Young's rule for the pair, HCl-NaClO$_4$, is $\frac{1}{2}[\phi v(\text{H}^+) + \phi v(\text{Cl}^-) + \phi v(\text{Na}^+) + \phi v(\text{ClO}_4^-)]$ and $\frac{1}{2}[\phi v(\text{Na}^+) + \phi v(\text{Cl}^-) + \phi v(\text{H}^+) + \phi v(\text{ClO}_4^-)] - R$ for the pair NaCl—HClO$_4$. The difference between these two values is $0.5 R$ and is equal to the algebraic difference between the D values at $X = 0.5$ for HCl—NaClO$_4$ and NaCl—HClO$_4$. On this basis it is possible to design an equation which will represent the mean, Φ, for all possible combinations of the four electrolytes, using the constants obtained experimentally for all the four homoionic pairs. In a 50–50 mixture, one obtains

$$D_{0.5} = \pm 0.25\, R + 0.125\, \Sigma k + 0.0625\, \Sigma k' \qquad \text{I(5)}$$

where $\pm 0.25\, R$ is used for the cross or squared D. (This is similar to Anderson and Wood's [91] treatment for ΔH_m).

The values of Φ calculated from the original data on the HCl—NaCl and NaClO—HClO$_4$ mixtures agrees very well with those calculated from the equation

$$\Phi = S_2 \phi_2 + S_3 \phi_3 + S_2 S_3 k + S_2{}^2 S_3 k' \qquad (52)$$

They have been shown to agree to ± 0.012 to 0.015 ml mole^{-1} with a maximum deviation of 0.087 ml mole^{-1}.

Wirth and Mills [107] examined the volume changes at 25°C on mixing two solutions of equal ionic strength for the six combinations of the four electrolytes, LiCl, NaCl, Li$_2$SO$_4$ at ionic strengths of 1 and 4. Single mixing experiments were made at an ionic strength of 2.25 for the six combinations at ionic strengths of 0.25, 0.50, 1.5, and 3.0 for the Na$_2$SO$_4$—NaCl system in order to determine the concentration dependence of the volume changes. They expressed their results in terms of equivalents. For the mean equivalent volume one has

$$\Phi' = \frac{V - n_1 \bar{V}_1{}^0}{e_2 + e_3} \qquad (53)$$

where V is the volume of solution containing n_1 moles of water and e_2 and e_3 are the equivalents of the two salts (moles/number of equivalents) and $\bar{V}_1{}^0$ is the molar volume of pure water. Young's rule then becomes

$$\Phi' = \frac{e_2 \phi'_2 + e_3 \phi'_3}{e_2 + e_3} = E_2 \phi'_2 + E_3 \phi'_3 \qquad (54)$$

where ϕ'_2 and ϕ'_3 are the apparent equivalent volumes of the electrolyte (2 and 3) in the single component mixtures (i.e., containing only water) at the ionic strength (μ) corresponding to $(e_2 + e_3)$ equivalents per n_1 mole of water. For a 1-1 electrolyte $m = 55.51\, e/n_1$ and for a 2-1 electrolyte $m = 3 \times 55.51\, e/2n_1$. The equivalent fraction E_2 and E_3 are equal to $e_2/(e_2 + e_3)$, $e_3/(e_2 + e_3)$, respectively. The observed volume change (Δv)

gives the correction term for Young's rule

$$D' = \Phi' - (E_2\phi_2' + E_3\phi_3') = \frac{\Delta v}{(e_2 + e_3)} \tag{55}$$

At a given ionic strength

$$D' = kE_2E_3 + k'E_2{}^2E_3 \tag{56}$$

where k and k' are empirical constants. The cross-square rule was applied to the values of $D_{1.5}'$. They found that at each concentration the sum of $D_{0.5}'$ of the heteroionic electrolytes (ΣX) is slightly greater than the sum of the volume changes on mixing the homoionic electrolytes ($\Sigma \square$). The difference, however, is less than the experimental error so that the cross-square rule can be considered valid.

The values of R' were calculated for these systems by Wirth and Mills [107], where R' is given by

$$R' = \phi_v'(Na_2SO_4) + \phi_v'(LiCl) - \phi_v'(Li_2SO_4) - \phi_v'(NaCl) \tag{57}$$

and found to be in fair agreement with the differences between the $D_{0.5}'$ values for the heteroionic mixtures at $m = 1, 2.25$, and 4. The agreement between the predicted and experimental (R') values for the Li_2SO_4—$NaCl$ and Na_2SO_4—$LiCl$ salt pair was not as good as for their earlier study on the $HClO_4$—$NaCl$, and HCl—$NaClO_4$ systems. They suggested that this may be due to ion-ion interactions in the SO_4^{-2}—Cl^- system which are not present in the ClO_4^-—Cl^- system. They suggest that the observed behavior is due to $LiSO_4^-$ ion-pair formation.

The variation of $D_{0.5}'$ with ionic strength was also measured by Wirth and Mills [107]. They found that for $LiSO_4$—$NaCl$, Na_2SO_4—$NaCl$, Li_2SO_4—$LiCl$, and Na_2SO_4—$NaCl$, $D_{0.5}'$ increased with increasing ionic strength and for Li_2SO_4—Na_2SO_4 and $LiCl$—$NaCl$, $D_{0.5}'$ decreased with increasing ionic strength.

Recently Wirth and Lo Surdo [108] have determined the effect of temperature (5-45°C) on the ΔV_m of mixtures of Li_2SO_4—$LiCl$, Na_2SO_4—$NaCl$, and Li_2SO_4 at ionic strength 4. The cross-square rule did not hold as well as in their earlier work; the sum of $D_{0.5}'$ for the homoionic solutions is less than the cross-terms for the heteroionic solutions. In five of the six cases, the absolute value of $D_{0.5}'$ decreases with increasing temperature, as expected. The values of $D_{0.5}'$ for Na_2SO_4—$LiCl$ mixtures increases in value with increasing temperature. This can be explained if one assumes that $LiSO_4^-$ is formed by ion association. The resultant decrease in the ionic strength decreases the apparent equivalent volumes of the ions and compensates for the increase in volume owing to normal ion interaction. Decrease in the association constant with increasing temperature would decrease this effect and at higher temperatures $D'_{0.5}$ is approaching the values expected owing to ion interactions alone.

Wen and Nara [109] have measured the volume of mixing for systems which include the tetra-alkylammonium salts Me_4NBr, Et_4NBr, $n\text{-}Pr_4NBr$, and $(HO\text{---}Et)_4NBr$ with KBr and KCl with $n\text{-}Bu_4NCl$ at the ionic strengths 0.2 to 2.0 at 25°C. In addition [110] they measured the volume of mixing of these systems in D_2O at 25°C and in H_2O at 15°C (as well as ΔV_m of $Pr_4NBr\text{-}CsBr$, $Pr_4NBr\text{-}Me_4NBr$ at 25°C). Their results were analyzed in terms of Friedman's ionic-solution theory.

According to Friedman (Equation 44), we can derive the following equations for the mixing of two dilute solutions of AX and BX (for the systems under consideration, A denotes R_4N^+, B denotes K^+ or Cs^+ and X denotes Br^- or Cl^-).

$$\frac{\Delta V_m}{I^2 y(1-y)} = v_0 + \cdots = 2\bar{V}_{AB} - \bar{V}_{AA} - \bar{V}_{BB} + \cdots = Z \quad (58)$$

$$\frac{[V_m^{ex}(AX) - V_m^{ex}(BX)]}{I^2} = \bar{V}_{AA} + 2\bar{V}_{AX} - \bar{V}_{BB} - 2\bar{V}_{BX} \quad (59)$$

where

$$V_m^{ex}(AX) = I[\phi_v(AX) - \phi_v^0(AX)] \quad (60)$$

$$V_m^{ex}(BX) = I[\phi_v(BX) - \phi_v^0(BX)] \quad (61)$$

and y is the mole fraction of (AX) in the mixture. In these equations $\bar{V}_{ij}$ is the part of the volume changes on mixing due to the structural effects when ion i is in the neighborhood of ion j (the higher-order terms have been neglected for dilute solutions). Equation 59 (in contrast to Equation 58) relates the difference of excess volumes of two separate solutions at an identical ionic strength I. If $\bar{V}_{AA}$ is greater (comparing absolute values) than the other terms, then both Equations 58 and 59 will be large, while $\bar{V}_{AX}$ dominates then 59 will be larger than 58. A large absolute value of $\bar{V}_{AA}$ may be taken as an indication that the $R_4N^+\text{---}R_4N^+$ interaction is large. Wen and Nara found large values for the $\bar{V}_{AA}$ for Pr_4N^+ and Bu_4N^+ ions and concluded that the cation-cation interactions are responsible for the anomalous $\bar{V}$ of these ions in aqueous solutions. For the smaller cations Me_4N^+ and Et_4N^+ other terms become important (i.e., the $\bar{V}_{AX}$; $\bar{V}_{BB}$; and $\bar{V}_{BX}$). For the $(HO\text{---}Et)_4 NBr\text{---}KBr$ system, the values for ΔV_m were found to be zero at total ionic strengths 0.5, 1.0, and 2.0 in contrast to the $Pr_4NBr\text{---}KBr$ system. Their studies clearly indicate that the volume changes on mixing are strongly related to the effect of these ions on the solvent structure (see corrections in Ref. 111).

The contribution to the volume by the cation-cation interactions decreases with the cation size in the order

$$Bu_4N^+ > Pr_4N^+ > Et_4N^+ > Me_4N^+ > Na^+$$

The difference between Bu_4N^+ and Pr_4N^+ is relatively small compared to the large difference between Pr_4N^+ and Et_4N^+. A similar observation was made by Wood and Anderson [99] based on their heat of mixing studies.

The values obtained for the $Z = v_0 + \ldots$ term of Equation 58 is larger in D_2O than in H_2O for the Pr_4NBr—KBr system. Thus, the Pr_4N^+—Pr_4N^+ interactions are larger in D_2O than in water. The Z values in D_2O are found to be smaller than in H_2O for Et_4NBr—KBr and Me_4NBr—KBr systems. $Z(D_2O)/Z(H_2O)$ are 1.09, 0.90, and 0.59 for the systems Pr_4NBr—KBr, Et_4NBr—KBr, and Me_4Br systems. Since D_2O is thought to possess more structure than H_2O, a "structure-breaker" should break, more structure in D_2O than in H_2O (leading to a smaller partial volume in D_2O than in H_2O). The fact that the ratio for Pr_4NBr—KBr is larger than 1.0 is due to the structure promoting effect of Pr_4N^+ ions. For Me_4NBr—KBr the fact that the ratio is less than 1.0 may be taken as to imply that both Me_4N^+ and K^+ are structure-breakers. The Et_4NBr—KBr system has a value near 1.0, which may be taken as to imply a slightly structure-breaking effect of KBr and very little structure influence of the Et_4N^+ ion. These structural interpretations are in accord with the results of Kay and Evans [60].

The values of Z for the Pr_4NBr—KBr system are higher at 15° than at 25°C at constant ionic strengths 0.5, 1.0, 2.0. The increase in Z with the lowering of temperature indicates the existence of more structure at lower temperature (as expected). The Z value for the Pr_4NBr—$CsBr$ are about 8% greater than the values for the Pr_4NBr—KBr system (at $I = 1.0$). Wen and Nara interpret this as follows: Cs^+ ion is a greater "structure-breaker" than K^+; thus, the mixing of Cs^+ ions into Pr_4NBr will disrupt the "caging or hydrophobic effect" to a greater extent than K^+. The volume of mixing of Pr_4NBr and Me_4NBr is quite small $(Z = 0.9)$. Since the Me_4N^+ ion is classified as a "structure-breaker" by many criteria [99], one might expect a larger effect (i.e., similar to K^+ or Cs^+ ions) as shown by Wood and Anderson's ΔH_m results [99]. The difference in results of the ΔH_m and the ΔV_m on this system (as well as others) points out the fact that ΔH_m is largely a measure of changes in the number of hydrogen bonds, while ΔV_m is a measure in the geometric arrangement of water and ions. Thus, a more detailed model will be necessary to give a quantitative description of mixing effects.

Although we have stressed the use of volume of mixing data to study ion-ion interactions between like-charged species, volume of mixing of electrolyte solutions can also be a useful method of studying ion-complex formation or ion-pairing between unlike-charged species.

Many studies [1] have been made on the volume changes for the neutralization of protonic acids and bases; however, until recently, the volume changes for simple nonprotonic ion association reactions have received little attention. The volume changes for the neutralization of a strong acid with a strong base can be quite large (for example, $H^+ + OH^- = H_2O$, $\Delta \bar{V}^0 = 22.1$ ml mole^{-1} at 25°C, at infinite dilution) [112]. The volume changes associated with other proton-transfer reactions are also substantial (28).

Strauss and Leung [113] have measured the volume changes of mixing of anionic polyelectrolytes with alkali metal and alkaline earth metal cations. Their results show that the volume changes observed were very large and comparable with protonic reactions. They interpreted the results as evidence for site-binding of cations to the polyanions as opposed to ionic-atmosphere binding. Spiro, Revesz, and Lee [114] have examined the volume changes of various complex cations with various anions to study the formation of inner- and outer-sphere complexes. They found that the volume changes of both inner- and outer-sphere complexes were similar and also of the same order of magnitude as protonic reactions. Thus, the establishment of a general criterion for distinguishing between the two structural types, based on volume changes, is not possible. Nevertheless, their comparison for the volume changes for related systems under closely similar conditions have proved very useful and their methods of calculating association constants may offer a novel approach to studying ion-complex formation. Various other workers have examined the volume changes associated with the interaction of solutes with proteins [115, 116] and with the formation of micelles [117, 118]. The measurement of the volume changes for various processes can prove to be a very useful tool in studying ion-ion, ion-water, ion-nonelectrolyte, nonelectrolyte-nonelectrolyte, nonelectrolyte-water, and water-water interactions (28).

9.3 THE IONIC MEDIUM SEAWATER

Water is an essential constituent of all living things. It is the universal biological solvent, the phase in which most cellular reactions occur and the most necessary constituent to life in our environment. Since life undoubtedly began in the watery medium of the sea, one might expect a correspondence between sea-salt solutions and body fluids. The composition of the seas has remained relatively constant through animal evolution, although there may have been a small increase in Na^+ and total solids in the oceans (i.e., salinity) [119, 120]. The concentration of ions in body fluids are not present in exactly the same concentrations as in seawater [121]; however, the major ions of importance in seawater are also of importance in body fluids. It is hoped that this brief examination of the ionic medium seawater will be of interest to biochemists and physiologists as well as marine scientists.

The composition [122] of the major ions (99%) of average seawater (35 ‰ salinity or 19.0 ‰ chlorinity) is given in Table 9.2 at 25° and pH ≈ 8.2. Although our knowledge of the total element species in seawater is fairly complete, we know little about the composition and distribution of the chemical species in the sea. Various workers [123–127] have proposed chemical models for seawater based on specific interaction of ions and we will review these models in further detail.

At the high ionic strength of seawater (0.713 m) the Debye-Hückel theory of dilute solutions is not satisfactory and mean-salt methods must be used to calculate the activity of the various species. Table 9.3 gives the calculated and experimental activity coefficient of the major ions in seawater [128]. It can be seen that mass calculations for seawater that ignore activity coefficients are rather meaningless. Although some

Table 9.2   The Composition of the Major Species in Average Seawater (35 ‰ Salinity, pH = 8.2) at 25°C[a]

Ion	g kg⁻¹ Seawater[b]	Molality (mole kg⁻¹ of Water)
Na^+	10.794	0.48663
Mg^{++}	1.287	0.05487
Ca^{++}	0.412	0.01066
K^+	0.399	0.01058
Sr^{++}	0.008	0.00009
Cl^-	19.353	0.56577
SO_4^{--}	2.712	0.02926
Br^-	0.067	0.00087
H_3BO_3	0.026	0.00044
HCO_3^-	0.142	0.00241
F^-	0.001	0.00005
H_2O	964.810	53.554

[a] Ref. 122.
[b] From the total analytically determined concentrations including ion-pairs.

Table 9.3   The Calculated and Experimental Activity Coefficients of the Major Ions in Seawater[a]

Ion	Molality[b]	γ cal[c]	γ exp
Na^+	0.487	0.71, 0.70	0.68–0.73
Mg^{++}	0.054	0.36	0.17
Ca^{++}	0.010	0.28	0.22–0.24
K^+	0.010	0.64	0.64
Cl^-	0.566	0.64–0.70	0.68–0.73
SO^{--}	0.029	0.17	0.11
HCO_3^-	0.0024	0.68	0.36–0.55
CO_3^{--}	0.00027	0.20	0.019–0.020

[a] Results taken from Ref. 128.
[b] Total analytical concentration including ion-pairing.
[c] Values for the free, individual ions listed in first column.

discrepancies exist regarding the measurement, calculation, and interpretation of activity-coefficient data for seawater, it is nevertheless apparent that the calculated values for bibaronate, carbonate, and sulfate are considerably higher than the experimentally determined values; somewhat higher for magnesium and calcium and about the same for sodium, potassium, and chloride ions. The common approach used to describe these differences is the use of Bjerrum's model for the association of ions [68]. The basic assumption of this approach is that short-range interactions in seawater can be represented by the formation of ion-pairs and that there are standard solutions in which no association occurs. When the association model is used it is necessary to show that the concentration quotients (i.e., the stoichiometric association constants) for ion-pair formation are constant over a range of composition (at constant ionic strength) [129]. The procedure of using the association model has been described in detail by Pytkowicz and Kester [75]. The first step is the selection of a standard solution in which no ion-pairing occurs. Guggenheim [72] defined a standard solution as one that obeys the Debye-Hückel equation with an assigned value of the ion size parameter. The standard solution selected for most seawater work is aqueous NaCl, since there is little or no evidence for association between Na^+ and Cl^- [131, 132]. (Recent studies, however, indicate that ion-pairing may be important in NaCl solutions [F. J. Millero, *J. Phys., Chem.*, **74,** 356 (1970)].

The free ionic concentration or activity coefficient (which refers to the unpaired species) and the total quantities are separated when the association model is used. The following relations hold

$$a = \gamma_F m_F = \gamma_T m_T \tag{62}$$

where a is the activity of a single ion and m is its molal concentration, the subscripts F and T, respectively, refer to free and total quantities. Thus, the extent of ion-pair formation is characterized by the differences between the total and the free concentrations and by the concentration quotient [132], K^*,

$$K^* = \frac{(M^+A^-)}{(M^+)_F (A^-)_F} \tag{63}$$

for the ion association

$$M^+ + A^- = M^+A^- \text{ or } MA^0 \tag{64}$$

Some examples of the ion-pairs thought to be of importance in the sea are the following: $CaCO_3^0$, $MgCO_3^0$, $NaCO_3^-$, $CaHCO_3^-$, $MgHCO_3^-$, $NaHCO_3^0$, $CaSO_4^0$, $MgSO_4^0$, KSO_4^-, and $NaSO_4^-$. Using the association constants for these ion-pairs and the total concentrations of the various species given in Table 9.2, the speciation of the major ions in seawater can be determined. Table 9.4 gives the results obtained by various workers [123, 127] for the speciation in average seawater.

It can be seen from Table 9.4 that Mg^{2+} ions are the major ion-pair formers in seawater. The percent of Mg^{++} complexed is low because

Table 9.4   The Speciation of the Major Ions in 35‰ Seawater at 25°C

Ion	% Free	% SO_4^{--} Pair	% HCO_3^- Pair	% CO_3^{--} Pair
Ca^{2+}	88.5[a], 91[b]	10.8[a], 8[b]	0.6[a], 1[b]	0.07[a], 0.2[b]
Mg^{2+}	89.0[a], 87[b]	10.3[a], 11[b], 9.2[c]	0.6[a], 1[b]	0.13[a], 0.3[b]
Na^{2+}	97.7[a], 99[b]	2.2[a], 1.2[b]	0.03[a], 0.01[b]	—
K^+	98.8[a], 99[b]	1.2[a], 1[b]	—	—
		% Ca^{++} Pair	% Mg^{++} Pair	% Na^+ Pair	% K^+ Pair
SO^{2-}	39.0[a], 54[b]	14.0[a], 3[b]	19.4[a], 21.5[b]	37.2[a], 21[b]	0.4[a], 0.5[b]
HCO_3^-	70.0[a], 69[b]	3.3[b], 4[b]	17.8[a], 19[b]	8.6[a], 8[b]	—
CO_3^{2-}	9.1[a], 9[b]	6.4[b], 7[b]	67.3[a], 67[b]	17.3[a], 17[b]	—
Cl^-	100[a], 100[b]	—	—	—	—

[a] Results recently obtained by Pytkowicz and Kester [124] for 34.8‰ salinity seawater (these results are preferred due to the use of new values for the stoichiometric association constants for the $NaSO_4^-$ and $MgSO_4^0$ ion pairs.
[b] Results obtained by Garrels and Thompson [123] for 19‰ chlorinity seawater.
[c] Estimated by Fisher [127] from ultrasonic data.

the concentration is high compared to the complexing anions present. The interaction between Mg^{++} and SO_4^{--} are of particular importance in accounting for the large ultrasonic adsorption of seawater [126, 127, 133, 134].

The use of activity-coefficient data determined by various potentiometric techniques to study ion-complex formation yields values for the total association constant (or the total % of ion-pairs); however, little can be said about the cause of the interactions or the structure of the associated species (e.g., whether the species is an inner- or outer-sphere complex or the effect of pressure on the ion-pair). Various other techniques have been used to determine association constants or examine the structure of the ion-pair (e.g., conductance, solubility, spectrophotometric, UV, IR, and Raman, polargraphic, ion exchange, solvent extraction and freezing point, to name a few—Nancollas) [135]. Unfortunately, it is not possible to regard free energy changes (or association constants) as being diagnostic of the type of ion association, without considering the accompanying heat ΔH, entropy ΔS, and volume ΔV contributions.

In order to gain an insight into the factors which affect the formation of an ion-pair, the enthalpy ΔH, entropy ΔS, and volume $\Delta \bar{V}$, must be considered. The enthalpy ΔH is the property most directly related to changes in numbers and strengths of bonds as the system passes from reactants to products. The entropy change ΔS is a measure of the change of randomness and the driving force in the process (i.e., the tendency for the system to go to the most probably random state). The volume change $\Delta \bar{V}$ is a measure of the change in geometrial arrangement of water molecules and ions for the process. At present there are few $\Delta \bar{V}$, ΔH, and ΔS data for the ion-pair formation of the major ions in seawater.

Recently [136], we have examined the partial molal volume of salts in the ionic medium seawater [137] to obtain a better understanding of the ion-ion and ion-water interactions of importance. We will now briefly review these results.

As a first approximation one may assume that $\bar{V}^0(int)$ of ions in pure water and seawater and the major effects of transferring an ion from pure water to seawater is related to differences in $\bar{V}^0(elect)$. Thus, the volume change of an ion from infinite dilution in seawater, $\Delta \bar{V}^0(trans)$, is proportional to Z^2/r. It was found that for the simple monatomic ions that $\Delta \bar{V}^0(trans)$ could be represented by the equation (Table 9.5)

$$\Delta \bar{V}^0(trans) = \frac{0.37_2 Z^2}{r} + 0.83_3 \tag{65}$$

with a standard deviation of $\pm 0.1_6$ which is approximately within the

Table 9.5   The Partial Molal Volume of Ions in Water and Seawater (35.1‰) and the Partial Molal Volume of Transfer from Water to Seawater at 25°C

Ion	Z^2/r^a	$\bar{V}^0$(ion) in Water[b]	$\bar{V}^0$(ion) in Seawater[c]	$\Delta\bar{V}^0$(trans)
H^+	$0.72(A)^{-1}$	-4.5 ml mole^{-1}	-3.7 ml mole^{-1}	0.8 ml mole^{-1}
Na^+	1.05	-5.7	-4.4	1.3
K^+	0.75	4.5	5.9	1.4
Mg^{2+}	6.15	-30.1	-27.0	3.1
Ca^{2+}	4.04	-26.9	-24.6	2.3
Ba^{2+}	2.96	-21.5	-19.5	2.0
Cl^-	0.55	22.3	23.3	1.0
Br^-	0.51	29.2	30.3	1.1
I^-	0.46	40.8	41.4	0.6
OH^-	0.85	0.5	2.5	2.0
NO_3^-	0.49	33.5	34.8	1.3
HCO_3^-	0.52	27.4	31.4	4.0
CO_3^-	2.31	4.9	10.3	5.4
SO_4^-	1.95	22.9	29.3	6.4

[a] Calculated using radii given in Table 9.1, except $r(H^+)$ was assumed to be equal to $r(H_3O^+)$, 1.38 Å units.
[b] $\bar{V}^0$(ions) in water were taken from the review article by Millero [28].
[c] $\bar{V}^0$(ions) in seawater were taken from Refs. 136, 137, 103–105, and 141.

experimental error. The fact that the line does not have an intercept equal to zero indicates that $\bar{V}^0$(disord) effects are not exactly the same in pure water and seawater. The positive intercept may also be due to differences between pure water and the ionic medium seawater. For example, the partial molal volume of pure water $\bar{V}^0(H_2O)$ changes by 0.8 ml mole^{-1} when transferred from itself to seawater. The transfer of a monovalent ion from pure water to seawater should be 1.2 ml mole^{-1} according to the Debye–Hückel limiting slope. It appears that the intercept may be related to hydration differences of ions and nonionic solutes in pure water and seawater. The examination of the $\bar{V}^0$ of a greater variety of solutes in water and seawater will be needed to prove this postulation.

The positive slope of the straight line indicates that the magnitude of $\bar{V}^0$(elect) in seawater is smaller than pure water (or the constant B in the equation, $\bar{V}^0$(ion) $= Ar^3 - B Z^2/r$, in seawater is smaller by 0.4 ml Å ml^{-1}).

The A and B constants in seawater have also been determined by plotting $\bar{V}^0$(ion) $\times r/Z^2$ versus r^4/Z^2 (see Ref. 136). For the slope we obtain $A = 4.58 \pm 0.02$ Å-ml mole^{-1} and from the intercept we obtain $B = 7.5 \pm 0.1$ Å-ml mole^{-1}. As expected from the $\Delta \bar{V}^0$(trans) equation, A (water) $< A$ (seawater) and B (water) $> B$ (seawater).

The constant A in seawater (and water) is larger than the theoretical value of 2.52. In pure water the large A has been attributed to void-space effects caused by improper packing of water molecules around the unhydrated or hydrated ion (or some other positive disorder effect). The larger void-space effects in seawater may be due to the fact that seawater is more closely packed than pure water (i.e., seawater is less compressible than water [138]).

The constant B in pure water is larger than B in seawater. The smaller electrostriction of ions in seawater compared to pure water is what one would expect for a less compressible solvent and is in the right order for ion-pair formation (i.e., $\bar{V}^0$ is increased).

The $\Delta \bar{V}^0$(trans) of the anions OH$^-$, HCO$_3^-$, CO$_3^{2-}$, and SO$_4^{2-}$ show large deviations from Equation 65. Direct experimental measurements in seawater have been made for only the SO$_4^{2-}$ and HCO$_3^-$ ions and measurements in both 0.725 m NaCl and synthetic seawater have been made for only the SO$_4^{2-}$ ion. Thus, it is not possible at this time to state with certainty that this effect is independent of the ionic medium except for the SO$_4^{2-}$ ion. The $\bar{V}^0$ of these ions at infinite dilution in pure water of these ions have been shown to comply with the general model for ion-water interactions described earlier. Thus, it appears that the large $\Delta \bar{V}^0$(trans) for these ions is due to ion-pairing effects that occur in seawater (or 0.725 m NaCl), at least for the SO$_4^{2-}$ ion. Using the SO$_4^{2-}$ ion as an example, the ion-pairing effects can be described as follows: one can assume that when an ion pair is formed by two ions, the electrostricted waters of hydration of the individual ions is diminished and the volume of the system is increased. It is therefore possible to estimate the amount of ion-pair formation for the ions that deviate from the $\Delta \bar{V}^0$(trans) equation. The percent of SO$_4^{2-}$ complexed in seawater can be calculated as follows: the electrostricted volume of the SO$_4^{2-}$ ion in seawater can be estimated from the equation

$$\bar{V}^0(\text{elect}) = \frac{-7.5Z^2}{r} \qquad (66)$$

Using this equation and r(SO$_4^{2-}$) given in Table 9.1, we calculate $\bar{V}^0$(elect), in seawater $= -14.6$ ml mole^{-1} for the SO$_4^{2-}$ ion. Since the $\Delta \bar{V}^0$(trans) for SO$_4^{--}$ ion deviates by 4.9 ml mole^{-1}, the % contact ion-pair formation can be calculated from the equation

$$\% \text{ contact ion paired} = \frac{\bar{V}^0(\text{meas}) - \bar{V}^0(\text{cal})}{\bar{V}^0(\text{elect})} \times 100 \qquad (67)$$

We obtain from this equation a value of 34% of the SO_4^{2-} ion in seawater is in the form of a contact ion-pair.

Since the results of Hester and Plane [139] indicate that the sulfate-metal ion-pair complex is separated by at least one water molecule (i.e., they are not contact ion-paired), one should use $r = r(SO_4^{2-}) + r(H_2O)$ to calculate $\bar{V}^0(\text{elect})$ for the SO_4^{2-}. Using $r(H_2O) = 1.38A$, we obtain $\bar{V}^0(\text{elect}) = -8.75$ ml mole^{-1} and 56% of the SO_4^{2-} is complexed in seawater. This value agrees very well with the recent results of Pytkowicz and Kester [124] (given in Table 9.4). The agreement between the two results is fairly good considering the large number of assumptions made in our calculations. Since the Na^+, Ca^{2+}, and Mg^{2+} ions do not release large amounts of their electrostricted water (i.e., they do not show large deviations from the $\Delta\bar{V}^0(\text{trans})$ equation), it appears that the SO_4^{2-} ions are entirely responsible for the formation of the sulfate-metal ion-pairs in seawater. The examination of the $\bar{V}^0$ of ions in seawater thus offers a method of determining the ion responsible for ion-pair formation.

The examination of the $\Delta\bar{V}^0(\text{trans})$ of other ions by similar arguments can be a useful means of examining ion-pair formation in seawater and in other mixed salt solutions. The general methods and techniques applied to other ion-pairing systems will be discussed in further detail elsewhere. Further experimental $\bar{V}^0$ on mixed salt solutions by the methods described here and elsewhere is needed before the ion-complex formation of other ions in seawater can be examined. The method is strictly applicable for contact ion-pair formation (unless one has prior knowledge of the exact type of ion-pair formed) and cannot be used to differentiate between outer-sphere ion pairs and normally hydrated ions. It should be emphasized that the fact that other ions can be correlated by Equation 65 does not mean that they do not exist, at least, partly as ion-pairs (since ion-pair formation may also be proportional to Z^2/r). For example, if we assume that the difference between the $\bar{V}^0(Mg^{2+})$ in water and seawater is largely due to electrostricted water and one might postulate that the difference between $\bar{V}^0(Mg^{2+})$ in seawater and water is totally due to ion-pair formation. This argument suggests that 10% of the Mg^{2+} ions are paired in seawater (i.e., % ion paired = change in volume/volume expected when $\bar{V}^0(\text{elect})$ is constant) which agrees with the estimates made by Pytkowicz and Gates [140].

There are numerous ionic equilibria of importance in the ocean and the effects of pressure on these ionic equilibria are largely unknown. One of the primary uses of the $\bar{V}^0$ of ions or salts is in calculating the effect of pressure on ionic equilibrium [141]. The general relationship for the transfer of ions from water to seawater can be used to estimate the $\bar{V}^0$ of other ions in seawater from their value in pure water and the intrinsic properties of the ions. Using the $\Delta \bar{V}^0$(trans) equation based on direct experimental results, we arrive at the general equation for the $\bar{V}^0$(ion)^{sw}, the partial molal volume of an ion in seawater (ml mole^{-1})

$$\bar{V}^0(\text{ion})^{sw} = \bar{V}^0(\text{ion})^w + \frac{aZ^2}{r} + b \tag{68}$$

where a and b are constants equal to 0.37_2 Å-ml mole^{-1} and 0.83_3 ml mole^{-1} for 35.1 ‰ salinity seawater at 25°C. We have used this equation to calculate the $\bar{V}^0$(ions) in seawater [136]. The effect of temperature and salinity on $\bar{V}^0$(ions) in seawater has also been examined and shown to be predictable by the general model proposed for the ion-water interactions in seawater.

The dissolved nonelectrolytes (organic and inorganic) materials in natural waters and body fluids are of considerable importance and must be considered before these systems can be thoroughly understood. For example, organic nonelectrolytes in natural waters are important in the ecology of living organisms and also to many of the geochemical cycles. In recent years various workers have successfully characterized these organic materials in seawater; however, little is known about organic-mineral, organic-ion, and organic-water interactions in seawater. Thus, to thoroughly understand the physical chemistry of natural mixed-salt solutions, future work must stress the role that nonelectrolyte solutes play in the interactions of mixed-salt solutions.

ACKNOWLEDGEMENT

The author would like to thank Drs. T. F. Young, R. H. Wood, J. H. Stern, and Wen-Y. Wen for their comments and corrections; also, R. M. Pytkowitz and D. R. Kester for making their manuscript available of the office of Naval Research, Contract NONR 4008(02) and the National Science Foundation, GA-17386.

REFERENCES

1. H. S. Harned and B. B. Owen, *The Physical Chemistry of Electrolytic Solutions*, Reinhold Publishing Corp., New York, 1958.
2. R. A. Robinson and R. H. Stokes, *Electrolyte Solutions*, Butterworths, London, 1959.
3. G. N. Lewis and M. Randall, *Thermodynamics*, K. S. Pitzer and L. Brewer, Eds., 2nd Edition, McGraw-Hill, New York, 1961.

4. H. S. Harned and R. A. Robinson, *Multicomponent Electrolyte Solutions,* Pergamon Press, Oxford, England, 1968.

5. H. S. Frank, *Proc. Roy. Soc.,* **A247,** 481 (1958).

6. G. Nemethy and G. H. Scheraga, *J. Chem. Phys.,* **36,** 3382 (1962).

7. H. S. Frank, *Nat. Acad. Sci., Nat. Res. Council Pub.,* **42,** 141 (1963).

8. E. Wicke, *Angew. Chem., Internat. Ed.,* **5,** 106 (1966).

9. W. Drost-Hansen, *Equilibrium Concepts in Natural Water Systems,* **67,** 70, ACS Publications (1967).

10. E. S. Turner, *Structure and Properties of Liquid Water,* **124,** Technical Information Libraries, Bell Telephone Laboratories, 1968.

11. J. L. Kavanau, *Water and Solute-Water Interactions,* Holden-Day, San Francisco, 1964.

12. O. Ya Samoilov, *Structure of Aqueous Electrolyte Solutions and the Hydration of Ions,* D. J. G. Ives, trans., Consultants Bureau, New York, 1965.

13. D. Eisenberg and W. Kauzmann, *The Structure and Properties of Liquid Water,* Oxford University Press, Oxford, England, 1969.

14. J. D. Bernal and R. H. Fowler, *J. Chem. Phys.,* **1,** 515 (1933).

15. H. S. Frank and M. W. Evans, *ibid.,* **13,** 507 (1945).

16. J. A. Pople, *Proc. Roy. Soc.,* **A205,** 163 (1951).

17. H. S. Frank and W. -Y. Wen, *Disc. Faraday Soc.,* **24,** 133 (1957).

18. H. S. Frank and A. S. Quist, *J. Chem. Phys.,* **34,** 604 (1961).

19. W. Luck, *Fortschritte Chem. Forschung,* **4,** (1964).

20. T. F. Wall and D. F. Hornig, *J. Chem. Phys.,* **43,** 2079 (1965).

21. First proposed by Rowland and elaborated on by Röntgen in 1892. See Ref. 7.

22. L. Pauling, *Hydrogen Bonding,* Pergamon Press, London, 1959.

23. R. P. Marchi and H. Eyring, *J. Phys. Chem.,* **68,** 221 (1964).

24. M. S. Jhon, J. Grosh, T. Ree, and H. Eyring, *ibid.,* **44,** 1465 (1966).

25. A. Eucken, *Nach. Ges. Wiss. Gottingen,* **33,** (1947).

26. R. Zana and E. Yeager, *J. Phys. Chem.,* **70,** 954 (1966), **71,** 521 (1967), reported the first estimates of $\bar{V}^0$ (ion) based on direct experimental methods using an ultrasonic technique to determine $\bar{V}^0$ for neutral salts.

27. P. Mukerjee, *ibid.,* **70,** 2708 (1966).

28. F. J. Millero, Review article on Partial Molal Volumes, R. A. Horne, Ed. *Structure and Transport Processes in Water and Aqueous Solutions,* John Wiley & Sons, Inc., New York, 1970; *Chem. Rev.,* **70,** (1971) in press.

29. F. J. Millero, *J. Phys. Chem.,* **72,** 4589 (1968).

30. F. J. Millero and W. Drost-Hansen, *ibid.,* **72,** 1758 (1968).

31. F. J. Millero and W. Drost-Hansen, *J. Chem. and Eng. Data,* **13,** 330 (1968).

32. F. J. Millero, W. Drost-Hansen, and L. Korson, *J. Phys. Chem.,* **72,** 2251 (1968).

33. L. Pauling, *The Nature of the Chemical Bond,* Cornell University Press, Ithaca, N.Y., 2nd ed., 1945.

34. A. F. Scott, *J. Phys. Chem.,* **35,** 3379 (1931).

35. A. M. Couture and K. J. Laidler, *Can. J. Chem.,* **34,** 1209 (1956).

36. L. G. Hepler, *J. Phys. Chem.,* **61,** 1426 (1957).

37. P. Mukerjee, *ibid.,* **65,** 744 (1961).

38. R. H. Stokes and R. A. Robinson, *Trans. Faraday Soc.,* **53,** 301 (1957).

39. R. H. Stokes, *J. Amer. Chem. Soc.,* **86,** 979–982 (1964).

40. J. Burak and A. Treinin, *Trans. Faraday Soc.,* **59,** 1490 (1963).

41. S. W. Benson and C. J. Copeland, *J. Phys. Chem.,* **67,** 1194 (1963).

42. F. J. Millero, *ibid.,* **73,** 2417 (1969).

43. B. E. Conway, R. E. Verrall, and J. E. Desnoyers, *Z. Physik. Chem.,* **230,** 157 (1965).

44. B. E. Conway, R. E. Verrall, and J. E. Desnoyers, *Trans. Faraday Soc.,* **62,** 2738 (1966).

45. E. Glueckauf, *ibid.,* **6,** 914 (1965).

46. P. Drude and W. Nernst, *Z. Physik. Chem.,* **15,** 79 (1894).

47. B. B. Owen, R. C. Miller, R. C. Milner, and H. L. Cogan, *J. Phys. Chem.,* **65,** 2065 (1961).

48. T. J. Webb, *J. Amer. Chem. Soc.,* **48,** 2589 (1926).

49. H. M. Evjen and F. Zwicky, *Phys. Rev.,* **33,** 860 (1929).

50. J. Padova, *J. Chem. Phys.,* **39,** 1552 (1963).

51. E. Whalley, *ibid.,* **38,** (1963).

52. J. Padova, *ibid.,* **40,** 691 (1964).

53. J. E. Desnoyers, R. E. Verrall, and B. E. Conway, *ibid.,* **43,** 243 (1965).

54. R. M. Noyes, *J. Amer. Chem. Soc.,* **86,** 971 (1964).

55. G. H. Haggis, J. B. Hasted, and T. J. Buchanan, *J. Chem. Phys.,* **20,** 1452 (1952).

56. E. Huckel and W. Schaaf, *Z. Physik. Chem.,* **21,** 326 (1959).

57. E. R. Nightingale, *J. Phys. Chem.,* **66,** 894 (1964).

58. J. N. Agar, *Advan. Electrochem. Eng.,* **3,** 31 (1963).

59. W. G. Hertz and M. O. Zeidler, *Ber. Bunsenges Physik. Chem.,* **68,** 821 (1964).

60. R. L. Kay and D. F. Evans, *J. Phys. Chem.,* **69,** 4216 (1965).

61. S. Lindenbaum, *ibid.,* **70,** 814 (1966).

62. Y. C. Wu and H. L. Friedman, *ibid.,* **20,** 2030 (1966).

63. W. -Y. Wen and S. Saito, *ibid.,* **68,** 2639 (1964).

64. R. L. Kay and D. F. Evans, *ibid.,* **70,** 2325 (1966).

65. R. L. Kay, T. Vituccio, C. Zawoyski, and D. F. Evans, *ibid.,* **70,** 2336 (1966).

66. F. Franks and S. Smith, *Trans. Faraday Soc.,* **63,** 2586 (1967).

67. G. S. Kell and E. Whalley, *Phil. Trans. Roy. Soc. London,* **258,** 565 (1965); F. J. Millero and F. K. Lepple, *J. Chem. Phys.,* **54,** 946 (1971).

68. N. Bjerrum, *Kgl. Danske Videnskab. Selskab, Mat. Fys. Medd.,* (9) **7,** 1 (1926).

69. J. T. Denison and J. B. Ramsey, *J. Amer. Chem. Soc.,* **77,** 2615 (1955).

70. R. M. Fuoss and C. A. Kraus, *ibid.,* **79,** 3301 (1957).

71. J. N. Brønsted, *ibid.*, **44**, 877, (1922); **45**, 2898 (1923).
72. E. A. Guggenheim, *Phil. Mag.*, **19**, 488 (1935).
73. H. S. Harned, *J. Phys. Chem.*, **64**, 112 (1960); **63**, 1299 (1959).
74. R. A. Robinson, *ibid.*, **65**, 662 (1961).
75. R. M. Pytkowicz and D. Kester, *Amer. J. Sci.*, **267**, 217 (1969).
76. G. Scatchard and S. S. Prentiss, *J. Amer. Chem. Soc.*, **56**, 2315, 2320 (1934).
77. H. L. Friedman, *J. Chem. Phys.*, **32**, 1134 (1960); 1351 (1960); *Ionic Solution Theory*, Interscience Publishers, New York, 1962.
78. J. E. Mayer, *J. Chem. Phys.*, **18**, 1426 (1950).
79. G. Scatchard, *J. Amer. Chem. Soc.*, **83**, 2636 (1961).
80. T. F. Young and M. B. Smith, *J. Phys. Chem.*, **58**, 716 (1954).
81. T. F. Young, Y. C. Wu, and A. A. Krawetz, *Disc. Faraday Soc.*, **24**, 27, 77, 80 (1957).
82. Y. C. Wu, M. B. Smith, and T. F. Young, *J. Phys. Chem.*, **69**, 1868, 1873 (1965).
83. J. H. Stern and C. W. Anderson, *ibid.*, **68**, 2528 (1964).
84. R. H. Wood and R. W. Smith, *ibid.*, **69**, 2974 (1965).
85. H. L. Friedman, *Disc. Faraday Soc.*, **24**, 74 (1957).
86. A. A. Krawetz, *ibid.*, **24**, 77 (1957).
87. C. J. F. Bottcher, *ibid.*, **24**, 78 (1957).
88. C. W. Davies, *Trans. Faraday Soc.*, **23**, 354 (1927).
89. R. A. Robinson and C. W. Davies, *J. Chem. Soc.*, 574 (1937).
90. Y. C. Wu, Ph.D. Thesis, University of Chicago, 1957.
91. R. H. Wood and H. L. Anderson, *J. Phys. Chem.*, **70**, 992 (1966).
92. R. H. Wood and H. L. Anderson, *ibid.*, **70**, 1877 (1966).
93. R. H. Wood and H. L. Anderson, *ibid.*, **71**, 1869 (1967).
94. T. Ackermann and F. Scheimer, *Z. Electrochem.*, **62**, 1143 (1958).
95. J. N. Agar, *Advan. Electrochem. Eng.*, **3**, 31 (1963).
96. D. W. McCall and D. C. Douglas, *J. Phys. Chem.*, **69**, 2001 (1965).
97. C. D. Lawrence and J. H. Wolfenden, *J. Chem. Soc.*, 1144 (1934).
98. H. S. Frank and A. L. Robinson, *J. Chem. Phys.*, **8**, 933 (1940).
99. R. H. Wood and H. L. Anderson, *J. Phys. Chem.*, **71**, 1871 (1967).
100. R. H. Wood, J. D. Patton, and M. Ghamkhar, *ibid.*, **73**, 346 (1969).
101. J. H. Stern and A. A. Passchier, *ibid.*, **67**, 2420 (1963).
102. H. L. Anderson, Paper presented at Southeastern Regional Meeting of ACS, Tallahassee, Florida, December (1968); *J. Phys. Chem.*, **74**, 1455 (1970).
103. H. E. Wirth, *J. Amer. Chem. Soc.*, **59**, 2449 (1937).
104. H. E. Wirth and F. N. Collier, Jr., *ibid.*, **72**, 5292 (1950).
105. H. E. Wirth, *ibid.*, **62**, 1128 (1940).
106. H. E. Wirth, R. E. Lindstrom, and R. E. Johnson, *J. Phys. Chem.*, **67**, 2239 (1963).
107. H. E. Wirth and W. L. Mills, *J. Chem. and Eng. Data*, **13**, 102 (1968).
108. H. E. Wirth and A. LoSurdo, *ibid.*, **13**, 226 (1968).

109. W. -Y. Wen and K. Nara, *J. Phys. Chem.,* **71,** 3907 (1967).

110. W. -Y. Wen and K. Nara, *ibid.,* **72,** 1137 (1968).

111. W. -Y. Wen, K. Nara, and R. H. Wood, *ibid.,* **72,** 3048 (1968).

112. L. A. Dunn, R. H. Stokes, and L. G. Hepler, *ibid.,* **69,** 2808 (1965).

113. U. P. Strauss and Y. P. Leung, *J. Amer. Chem. Soc.,* **87,** 1476 (1965).

114. T. G. Spiro, A. Revesz, and J. Lee, *ibid.,* **90,** 4000 (1968); see also F. J. Millero, *J. Phys. Chem.,* **74,** 356 (1970).

115. W. Kauzmann, A. Bodanszky, and J. Rasper, *ibid.,* **84,** 1777 (1962).

116. J. Rasper and W. Kauzmann, *ibid.,* **84,** 1771 (1962).

117. J. M. Corkill, J. F. Goodman, and T. Walker, *Trans. Faraday Soc.,* **63,** 768 (1967).

118. L. Benjamin, *J. Phys. Chem.,* **70,** 3790 (1966).

119. E. J. Conway, *Proc. Roy. Irish Acad.,* **48,** 119 (1942).

120. W. W. Rubey, *Bull. Geol. Soc. Amer.,* **62,** 1111 (1951).

121. C. L. Prosser and F. A. Brown, Jr., *Comparative Animal Physiology,* 2nd Ed., W. B. Saunders Co., Philadelphia, Pa., 1965, pp. 57–80.

122. F. Culkin, *Chemical Oceanography,* J. P. Riley and G. Skirrow, Eds. Vol. I, Academic Press, London, 1965; D. Dryssen, **Chemical Oceanography,** Ed. R. Lange, Univeritetsforlaget, Norway (1969).

123. R. M. Garrels and M. E. Thompson, *Amer. J. Sci.,* **260,** 57 (1962).

124. R. M. Pytkowicz and D. R. Kester, *Limnol. Oceanog.,* **14,** 686 (1969).

125. D. R. Kester and R. M. Pytkowicz, *Limnol. Oceanog.,* **13,** 670 (1969).

126. F. H. Fisher, *J. Phys. Chem.,* **66,** 1607 (1962).

127. F. H. Fisher, *Science,* **157,** 823 (1967).

128. S. D. Morton and G. F. Lee, *J. Chem. Educ.,* **45,** 513 (1968).

129. L. G. Sillen, *J. Inorg. Nucl. Chem.,* **8,** 176 (1958).

130. C. W. Davies, *Ion Association,* Butterworth, London, 1962, p. 190.

131. L. G. Sillen and A. E. Martell, *Stability Constants of Metal Ion Complexes,* Burlington House, London, 1964, p. 754.

132. F. J. C. Rossotti and H. Rossotti, *Determination of Stability Constants,* McGraw-Hill, New York, 1961.

133. L. Lieberman, *Phys. Rev.,* **76,** 1520 (1944).

134. F. H. Fisher, *J. Phys. Chem.,* **69,** 695 (1965).

135. G. H. Nancollas, *Interactions in Electrolyte Solutions,* Elsevier, London, 1966.

136. F. J. Millero, *Limnol. Oceanog.,* **14,** 376 (1969).

137. I. W. Duedall and P. Weyl, *Limnol. Oceanog.,* **12,** 52 (1967).

138. W. Wilson and D. Bradley, *Deep-Sea Res.,* **15,** 355 (1968).

139. R. E. Hester and R. A. Plane, *Inorg. Chem.,* **3,** 769 (1964).

140. R. M. Pytkowicz and R. Gates, *Science,* **161,** 690 (1968).

141. B. B. Owen and S. R. Brinkley, Jr., *Chem. Rev.,* **29,** 461 (1941).

10

Sorption of Water by Collagen

J. R. KANAGY*

National Bureau of Standards, Washington, D.C.

The relation between water and skin is one of the most important phenomena of life on this earth. The fundamental purpose of the skin is protection of the organism and the great majority of the skin's activities contribute to this function. These include sensation, temperature regulation, secretion, excretion, and the ability to repel or neutralize various chemicals, bacteria, fungi, and other harmful agents.

The intimate association of water with the skin plays the most important role in temperature regulation and in secretion and excretion. The evaporation of sweat, which is largely water from the surface of the skin, is an important function in temperature regulation. Evaporation of one gram of water causes a heat loss of 0.54 kcal and enables us to endure temperatures of higher than 100°F, providing the humidity is low enough to allow evaporation of the sweat. The close association

* Deceased.

of water within the porous structure of skin is therefore a highly important process in animal metabolism.

Most of the results presented in this paper are for the protein collagen, which is by far the most predominant and most important protein of the skin. It is assumed that results obtained for collagen would also be obtained in a large part for skin itself.

At this point, a few words about the properties of water and its molecular structure are appropriate. It has been known for many years that life at any level must contain moisture. Although we are 50–60% water, relatively little of our total body water of 30–40 liters has fluid properties. This water is in the most part bound by little understood mechanisms in gels of connective tissue and the protoplasm of cells. Water is, in a sense, skeletal in that the physical properties of hard and dense tissues are altered very appreciably by both increases and decreases in this content of bound water. Tendon, ligament, bone, and the tough connective-tissue structures have physical properties dependent upon water of hydration.

The following remarks by J. H. Bland are pertinent to water in biological systems [1]. "Ice or solid water has a basic molecular arrangement in a hexagonal lattice, each molecule hydrogen-bonded to its neighbors. It is in a reasonable sense a complete polymer. Each hexagon has a hole in its center, a water cage, so that the density is relatively low and molecular packing is loose. Liquid water is also hydrogen-bonded but the polymer probably reaches no further than the molecules of one hexagon, and the hydrogen bonds are continually making and breaking in flickering clusters. With increasing temperature, hydrogen-bond breaking increases in rate and at the transition phase, the boiling point, all evidence of molecular structure disappears and the water is in monomeric form."

Other properties of water which make it important in biological life may be mentioned [1]. The fact that ice floats puts it in a class by itself. It is different in this behavior from practically everything else. Most materials increase in density on solidification. Life as we know it could not exist on this planet without solid water having this property. The heat capacity of water is also extremely high. This means the ability to absorb more heat than any other material with the same increase in its own temperature. Another property which has wide implications in biological systems is the property of "pulling itself together," intermolecular adherence. With the single exception of mercury, water has the highest surface tension of all liquids.

The most important bond energy of water with regard to absorption by collagen is without doubt that of hydrogen bonding. Frank and Wen

[2] consider that a hydrogen bond is formed only as the electrons are polarized. More important in their view, however, is the fact that the polarization of one pair leads to polarization of all the electrons on the molecule and therefore to all those on neighboring molecules so that there is a cooperative resonance effect over a large group which resonate together to form a large cluster.

Now we will consider the structure of collagen which makes it so receptive to a substance like water. It has been estimated that approximately 30% of the total protein of the mammalian body is collagen. A large part of this is in the skin. Collagen, physically, is a highly fibrous material. It is composed of twenty different simple amino acids. These amino acids are present in different percentages ranging from less than 1% for histidine and methionine to 26.2% for glycine. These amino acids are combined to form large units by virtue of the carboxyl of one unit combining with the amino group in another unit to form polypeptide chains containing a series of —CO—NH— linkages.

The reaction of the carboxyl and the amino groups to form the polypeptide chains leaves the other active polar groups of the amino acids free in the side chains which are rotated perpendicular to the polypeptide group in the oriented crystalline material. These side chains thus contain the most reactive groups of the polymerized protein. Active groups in the side chains are composed of guanidyl, amino, carboxyl, and hydroxyl. The amounts of these groups may be determined quantitatively from the known contents of the specific amino acids in the protein. Certain sites over a large part of the surface area of the collagen molecule may therefore be seen as a prolific hydrogen-bond forming substrate which is highly receptive to water.

10.1 REACTION OF WATER WITH COLLAGEN

Considerable work has been done on the reaction of water vapor with proteins in general. Broad studies on the adsorption of water vapor by collagen were made by Bull [3], Kanagy [4], and by P. Bhaskara Rao [5].

The work on the adsorption of water vapor by collagen and also other proteins shows that a typical S-shaped curve is obtained when the amount of water vapor adsorbed is plotted against the relative humidity. Typical isotherms showing the adsorption of water at 28°, 50°, and 70°C are given in Fig. 10.1. This characteristic adsorption curve may be divided into three segments. The first part at low-vapor tensions is typical of a Langmuir adsorption. The amount adsorbed in-

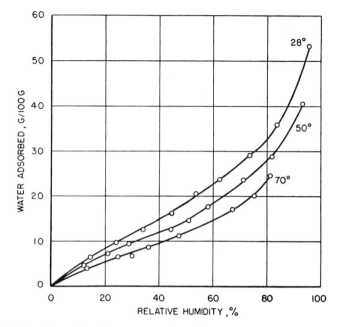

Figure 10.1. Adsorption of water vapor by collagen at different relative humidities at 28, 50, and 70°C.

creases rapidly with increase in vapor pressure. This is followed by a section which is more linear but has a gentle slope. It extends up to about 65% relative humidity. Beyond this is the third section where the curve rises sharply indicating greatly increased absorption. The up-take of water in this section has been explained in a number of ways, among them being capillary condensation and the multimolecular-layer theory as developed by Brunauer, Emmett, and Teller (BET) [6].

In the BET equation, calculations are made by plotting P/V $(P_0 - P)$ against P/P_0 where P is the vapor pressure and P_0 is the pressure at saturation; V is the volume. The straight line obtained from the plot will have a slope equal to $C - 1/V_mC$ and an intercept equal to $1/V_mC$. From these two quantities, values for V_m and C may be calculated. V_m is the volume of water vapor at 0°C and 760 mm required to form a unimolecular layer and C is a constant related to the heat of adsorption. By multiplying V_m by 2.705, a value for the surface area of the sample is obtained when water is used as the adsorbate [7].

By using this procedure, Kanagy [4] obtained values for surface area in excess of 300 m^2g^{-1} for collagen at 28 and 50°C. Bull's values [3] on collagen obtained by the same procedure were in good agreement. Values for C obtained by Bull and by Kanagy also were in agreement.

To explain the high adsorption of water by proteins, Bull made a comparison with the water absorption of montmorillonite as studied by Hendricks, Nelson, and Alexander [8]. They showed that this mineral forms a crystalline material with one lattice constant which depends upon the humidity. Adsorbed water penetrates between the molecular layers of the montmorillonite and pushes them apart. Similarly in moist proteins which do not have the hardness to support capillaries as they occur in silica gel, adsorption of water between lattices or chains occurs by pushing them apart.

Bull quotes further evidence on the lattice separation in the x-ray diffraction studies of Boyes-Watson and Perutz [9] on horse methemoglobin crystals and gives a plot of the increase in ΔH with increase in side-chain spacings from the work of Katz and Derksen [10].

Rougvie and Bear [11] made an x-ray diffraction investigation of swelling by collagen. The water-sorption isotherm was determined at 25°C for kangaroo-tail tendon and small- and wide-angle x-ray patterns were made at various water contents. Over the range 0–120 g H_2O/100 g collagen, the major equatorial spacing and the fiber macroperiod increase with increasing water content from 10.6 to 14.6 Å and from 603 to about 670 Å, respectively. The results are interpreted to indicate the following sequence of events: The initial water sorption by dry collagen involves primarily the fibrillar bands, at which the axis of the roughly parallel helical polypeptide chains straighten. Next the polar groups located in the interbands become hydrated and the chains begin to separate laterally in these regions.

These processes continue with multilayer sorption of water and further chain straightening and separation. At low and at high sorption values, the sorbed water contributes to the increase of apparent molar volume in the expected manner. At intermediate sorptions, large increases in sorbed water cause relatively little increase in molecular volume. This is because the water is largely sorbed at band-interband margins, where it causes chain incoherence without affecting the macroperiod or the equatorial spacing from which the molecular volume is calculated.

Sponsler, Bath, and Ellis [12] made x-ray diffraction studies on gelatin and determined the lattice separation as well as the number of molecules of water present. At 0.2% water, 4 or 5 molecules, the chain separation was 10.4 Å. At 15% water, 260 molecules, the chain separation was about 11.3 Å, and at 33% water, 750 molecules, the chain separation was 13.10 Å. In addition, agreement was shown between the number of coordinate water molecules potentially possible in a 35% water-65%

protein system and the number computed to be present. The location and distribution of the water molecules on the gelatin chain molecule are shown by x-ray analyses, and the manner in which the water molecules are bound to the protein chain is shown by infrared absorption studies to be, in all probability, through hydrogen bridges.

Pauling [13] in commenting on Bull's data and on the failure of the BET equation to satisfactorily explain moisture adsorption on proteins made a strong case for attributing water take-up to specific polar groups. There are two main types of hydrophilic groups in proteins: the polar side-chain groups from such amino acids as glutamic and aspartic acid, arginine, tyrosine, and lysine, and so on, and the carbonyl and imido groups of the peptide bonds. The latter are much more abundant than the former. Bull's data with nylon, however, indicates that the peptide bonds are not particularly attractive to water because most of their hydrogen-bonding capacity is apparently used in the configuration which holds the two groups together in the peptide chain.

On the assumption that a residue of an amino acid with a side chain would take up one water molecule, Pauling calculated the number of groups available for a number of different proteins and compared Bull's data. He also assumed one group would be available for water absorption from the proline and hydroxyproline content of the protein since these two amino acids leave one —CO— group unpaired with an —NH— in the chain.

Pauling's calculation checked well for silk and also compared favorably for most of the other proteins. For collagen, the number of water molecules adsorbed was greater than the number of polar groups available before the proline groups were included. After the groups for proline were included, the number of available attracting groups was greater than the number of water molecules present.

For Bull's data with the protein, salmin, Pauling also gave an explanation which may be significant in explaining water absorption in other proteins. Salmin contains many polar groups, and these groups may be so close together that the first step of adsorption of water is the attachment of one water molecule to two polar groups, which consist primarily of the side-chain groups of arginine.

He submitted the following mechanism of the water absorption procedure by salmin: One molecule is first bound tightly by two cooperating polar groups; a second molecule is then added, giving a total of one water molecule per polar group; next a complete layer of water is sandwiched into each space between the protein layers; and then other layers of water are similarly introduced. At 95% relative humidity, six or seven of these water layers have been introduced between each protein layer and each of its neighboring layers.

10.2   WATER ABSORPTION ON SYNTHETIC AND MODIFIED PROTEINS

Work by Mellon, Korn, and Hoover [14] on polyglycines which have no polar end groups except for one amino and one carboxyl group indicated that water was absorbed on the peptide groups. They assumed from this work on comparison of the absorption of the polyglycine peptides with the absorption of proteins that the absorption of the peptide-chain backbone is probably of the same magnitude, if not identical, for all long-chain polypeptides and proteins. Peptide groups appear to be responsible for about 45% of the vapor-phase water absorption by casein and 70% of the absorption by zein at 60% relative humidity.

From further work on water absorption with benzoylated caseins, Mellon, Korn, and Hoover [15] concluded that 24–33%, depending upon the relative humidity, of the water absorbed by casein is absorbed by the amino groups.

Frey and Moore [16] studied the absorption of water vapor on powdered crystalline samples of glycine, leucine, diketopiperazine, and diglycylglycine, at 15, 25, and 40°C. The water adsorption appeared to occur primarily on the ionic COO^- and NH_3^+ groups of the amino acids and on the peptide linkages in diketopiperazine. Diglycylglycine sorbed water to a much greater extent than the other crystals and appears to provide an intermediate case between surface adsorption and the extensive sorption observed with proteins.

Green and Ang [17] made water-vapor adsorption studies on acetyl derivatives of collagen and of silk fibroin. The number of acetyl groups which may be introduced are exactly equivalent to the number of lysine and hydroxylysine residues. After correcting for denaturing produced by the acetyl treatment, they found no effect of the treatment on water absorption. Contrary to the findings of Mellon et al. [14] in the benzoylation of casein, the acetylation of the ε-amino groups of the lysine residues has no specific effect on adsorption of water vapor by collagen.

10.3   ENERGY RELATIONS OF WATER AND COLLAGEN

The three most common ways of determining the energy relations between water and collagen are (1) direct determination in a calorimeter,

Table 10.1   Integral Heats of Wetting of Collagen,
Leather, and Textile Materials

Material	Heat of Wetting, cal g^{-1}
Collagen	37.1
Hide powder (formaldehyde-tanned)	33.9
Hide powder (deaminated)	30.9
Chrome leather	31.5
Chrome-retanned leather	25.2
Vegetable-tanned leather	21.7
Viscose rayon	21.4
Wool	20.8
Silk	13.7
Cotton	11.2
Acetate	8.6
Nylon	6.6
Glass fiber	0.5

(2) adsorption measurements made at two different temperatures, by means of the Clausius-Clapeyron equation, and (3) the BET equation.

Direct measurements of heats of wetting or heats of adsorption on either collagen or leather in a calorimeter have been made by Kanagy [18], Mitton, and Mawhinney [19], Wollenberg [20], and Cheshire [21].

Table 10.1 gives some of the data obtained by Kanagy. These are integral heats of wetting (total heat given off on submersing the dry material in water) for collagen, modified collagens, leathers, and other synthetic and natural fibers at 25°C. It may be observed that the heat of wetting of collagen is higher than that for any other material. Rayon, wool, and silk are intermediate and acetate, nylon, and glass fiber have the lowest heats of wetting. Figure 10.2 shows that the integral heats of wetting correlate with the amounts of water adsorbed at 65% relative humidity. Thus, the heat given off is directly proportional to the amount of water which combines with the material.

Figure 10.3 shows the integral heats of wetting as a function of the initial water content. It may be observed that the amounts of heat evolved decrease rapidly with the moisture content of the material indicating, of course, that the water molecules first combine with the more active groups.

From the slopes of the curves in Fig. 10.3, the differential heats of wetting were calculated. This was done by differentiating empirical equations derived by applying the method of least squares. These differential heats of wetting are presented in Table 10.2. These values also decrease rapidly with increasing water adsorption so that moisture adsorption by collagen beyond 10% takes place at low energy levels and is held only slightly above the energy required for evaporation.

Mitton and Mawhinney [19] made determinations of the heats of wetting with chrome and vegetable-tanned leathers. Their results were, of course, highly dependent upon the amount of hide or collagen in the leathers. For this reason under all conditions chrome leather had the highest heats of wetting. The integral heats for chrome leather were 40.64 cal g⁻¹ at zero moisture content and for vegetable-tanned leather 23.10 cal g⁻¹ at zero moisture. These values appear to agree closely with those obtained by Kanagy [18].

Wollenberg studied heats of wetting of hide substance at temperatures

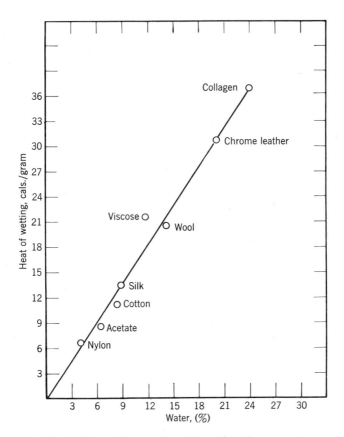

Figure 10.2. Correlation of heats of wetting with the percentage water vapor adsorbed at 65% relative humidity.

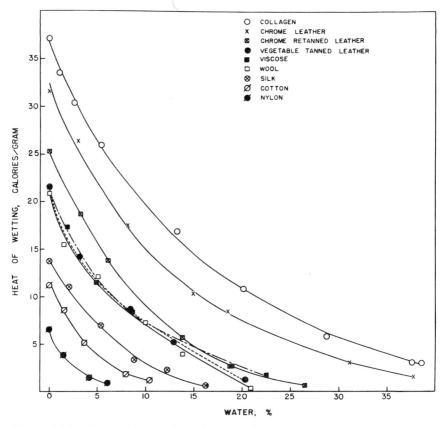

Figure 10.3. Integral heats of wetting of collagen and other materials as a function of the water content.

ranging from 0 to 60°C. His results are shown in Table 10.3, and they are most interesting since they show the decrease in the heat of wetting with increase in temperature. One explanation for these results is that less moisture combines at the elevated temperatures.

Cheshire [21] gave values of 40.0 cal g^{-1} for dry pelt and 21.9 cal g^{-1} for dry leather. These values are in agreement with those of Kanagy [18] Mitton and Mawhinney [19], and Wollenberg [20].

In Table 10.4, values are presented for the differential heats of adsorption which were obtained by means of the Clausius-Clapeyron equation from results obtained in the work of Kanagy [4] on the effect of temperature on adsorption. Results calculated by means of the BET equation are also given. These values are in fairly close agreement with some

Table 10.2 Differential Heats of Wetting of Collagen, Leather, and Textile Materials

H_2O, %	Collagen, cal mol^{-1} H_2O	Chrome Leather, cal mol^{-1} H_2O	Vegetable-tanned Leather, cal mol^{-1} H_2O	Chrome-retanned Leather, cal mol^{-1} H_2O	Viscose, cal mol^{-1} H_2O	Wool, cal mol^{-1} H_2O	Silk, cal mol^{-1} H_2O	Cotton, cal mol^{-1} H_2O	Nylon, cal mol^{-1} H_2O
0	4530	4920	6330	4170	5170	7050	2750	4260	3590
1	4140	4400	4640	3860	4260	4610	2590	3540	2950
2	3790	3960	3610	3580	3580	2830	2420	2930	2310
4	3210	3240	2460	3070	2630	1950	2100	1980	1030
8	2380	2270	1530	2240	1590	1330	1460	740	
16	1440	1260	990	1090	820	1030			
32	670								

Table 10.3   Heats of Wetting of Hide Substance 0–60°C, [20] (cal g^{-1})

	0.9°–0.4°C	18.2 ± 1.2°C	40.5 ± 0.3°C	59.8 ± 0.7°C
Limed normal	47.8	38.6	24.4	16.7
Green normal	41.9	34.4	25.9	18.6
Gelatin	44.0	35.2	20.4	14.5

of the high dilution results obtained directly from calorimetric measurements. The results from the BET equation are quite low since they are apparently the values of heats of adsorption after a monomolecular layer has been formed.

Bull [3] gives a value of 3,640 cal for the adsorption of water vapor on collagen. This figure was obtained by means of the Clausius-Clapeyron equation and is in good agreement with the results obtained by Kanagy [4], McLaren and Rowen [22] give values for collagen in calories per mole at 25°C. They give a value of 1,840 as calculated from the BET equation and a differential heat of 6,600 cal at zero moisture content. These values are also in agreement with those obtained by other workers.

In the past, considerable emphasis has been placed on the determination of surface areas of collagen and other proteins from results obtained

Table 10.4   Heats of Adsorption of Water Calculated from Adsorption Measurements

H$_2$O, %	Collagen, cal mol^{-1}	Hide Powder, cal mol^{-1}	Chrome Leather, cal mol^{-1}	Vegetable-tanned Leather, cal mol^{-1}	Chrome-retanned Leather, cal mol^{-1}
5	3540	2840	4940	6240	5940
6	3140	3040	4240	4640	3240
8	3040	3140	3140	3040	2440
10	3140	3140	2940	2540	2140
15	1940	1540	1640	1940	1340
20	1540	1240	640	1340	840
25	1040	1040	440	840	840
40	740	440	340	—	—
	1140[a]	1340[a]	1540[a]	1640[a]	1640[a]

[a] From BET equation.

on water-vapor adsorption. From similar experiments with nitrogen, it became obvious that the adsorption of these two different gases took place by entirely different mechanisms. Surface areas obtained with these two gases were in the ratio of 100 for water to 1 for nitrogen.

The work and conclusions of Benson and Seehof [23] who studied surface areas of proteins with both polar and nonpolar gases appear pertinent to this point. They summarized the differences in behavior between polar and nonpolar gases in protein sorption as follows: (1) The amount of polar gas sorbed is independent of the surface area of the protein. (2) At comparable partial pressures, the amount of polar gas sorbed is from 10^2–10^4 times greater than the amount of nonpolar gas. (3) Equilibrium is reached within 2–5 min with the nonpolar gases, within 30 min to 24 hr or more for the polar gases. (4) Isosteric heats of sorption are much greater than the heat of liquifaction for the polar gases, whereas they are close to the heat of liquifaction for the nonpolar gases. (6) There is considerable hysteresis on desorption with all polar gases and also some irreversible binding with some of the gases. The nonpolar gases show no hysteresis or irreversible binding. (7) The polar-gas isotherms do not fit any of the physical adsorption isotherms in a sensible manner. When pressed into such a fit, they give absurdly high values for surface area.

Joyner, Barrett, and Skold [24] have shown that the surface areas calculated from nitrogen adsorption agree quite well with those obtained by calculation from data with the mercury porosimeter. From data obtained by Kanagy [25] on collagen with a mercury porosimeter, he calculated that the adsorption of mercury corresponds to a surface area of about two square meters. This is the order of magnitude obtained by Zettlemoyer, Schweitzer, and Walker [26] for the internal surface area using nitrogen as the adsorbent. It is therefore assumed that a nonpolar gas such as nitrogen gives more nearly the correct surface area of collagen, whereas water vapor is apparently adsorbed in clusters on active groups in such a way that there is no relation to surface area.

10.4 SOLUTION THEORIES OF SORPTION OF WATER BY PROTEINS

In many protein systems including gelatin and collagen at high vapor pressures, there results a solution of the adsorbent in the vapor. Consideration of such systems has led to attempts to analyze sorption isotherms in terms of current solution theories. Rowen and Simha [27] have taken into consideration the partial-molal free energy change due to elastic deformation of the polymer in the course of sorption. They obtained for the partial-molal free energy

$$\Delta F_1(\text{el}) = K\bar{V}_1 \left(\frac{1}{v_2^{\frac{1}{3}}} - 1\right)\left(\frac{5}{3v_2^{\frac{1}{3}}} - 1\right) \tag{1}$$

where K is a constant having dimensions of an elastic modulus, $\bar{V}_1$ is the partial-molal volume of the liquid, and v_2 is the volume fraction of the polymer. The partial-molal free energy of the adsorbate in contact with the absorbent is given by:

$$\overline{\Delta F_1}(\text{sol}) = RT\left[\ln \bar{V}_1 + \left(1 - \frac{\bar{V}_1}{\bar{V}_2}\right)v_2 + \mu v_2^2\right] \tag{2}$$

where R is the gas constant, T the temperature, v the volume fraction of the absorbate, and v_2 the volume fraction of the absorbent. $\bar{V}_2$ is the partial-molal volume of the absorbate and μ is a semiempirical dimensionless parameter consisting of a heat and entropy term. Since

$$RT \ln X = \overline{\Delta F_1} = \overline{\Delta F_1}(\text{sol}) + \overline{\Delta F_1}(\text{el}) \tag{3}$$

the combination of Equations 1 and 2 leads to the isotherm:

$$\ln x = \ln \bar{V}_1 + \left(1 - \frac{\bar{V}_1}{\bar{V}_2}\right)v_2 + \mu v_2^2 + \frac{K\bar{V}_1}{RT}\left(\frac{1}{v_2^{\frac{1}{3}}} - 1\right)\left(\frac{5}{3v_2^{\frac{1}{3}}} - 1\right) \tag{4}$$

since the term

$$\frac{K\bar{V}_1}{RT}\left(\frac{1}{v_2^{\frac{1}{3}}} - 1\right)\left(\frac{5}{3v_2^{\frac{1}{3}}} - 1\right)$$

makes a relatively small contribution, Equation 2 may be used instead of 4 for testing the applicability of the solution theory to protein-water systems.

10.5   GRAPHICAL PRESENTATION OF WATER ADSORPTION DATA

The plot given in Fig. 10.4 shows the relation between the log of the moisture adsorbed and the inverse of the absolute temperature. It is possible to estimate from this relation the amounts of moisture adsorbed at equilibrium at temperatures and relative humidities not studied

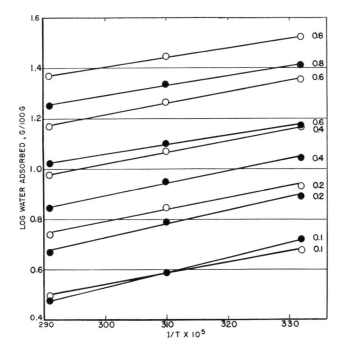

Figure 10.4.   Log of water absorbed by collagen ◯ and vegetable-tanned leather ● plotted as a function of the inverse of the absolute temperature.

experimentally. A similar relation was shown to exist for textile materials by Wiegerink [28].

Another valuable method for the representation of moisture relation data has been applied by Whitwell and Toner [29] to textile materials. They adapted this method from a basic relation first used by Othmer [30] for representing the vapor pressure of pure liquids. The Clausius-Clapeyron equation representing the equilibrium between pure water and its vapor may be written as follows:

$$\frac{dP_0}{P_0} = \frac{\Delta H_0 \, dT}{R T^2} \tag{5}$$

where P_0 is the vapor pressure of water, and ΔH_0 is the heat of condensation. For water vapor over the adsorptive material in question, the equation may be written as follows:

$$\frac{dP}{P} = \frac{\Delta H \, dT}{R T^2} \tag{6}$$

where P is the vapor pressure of water over the material, and ΔH is the heat of adsorption. These two equations may be combined to give the following relation:

$$\log P = \frac{\Delta H}{\Delta H_0} \log P_0 + C \qquad (7)$$

A plot of $\log P$ against $\log P_0$ should yield a straight line if ΔH is proportional to ΔH_0 in the temperature range of interest. Lines representing constant regains (constant moisture contents) over a range of temperatures and relative humidities are obtained in this way. The temperature dependence is expressed in terms of $\log P_0$.

In Fig. 10.5, the water-adsorption relations of collagen are plotted according to this method, and in Fig. 10.6 a similar plot is shown for vegetable-tanned leather. The graphs indicate that the water-adsorption data for both of these materials are accurately represented by Equation 7. Lines representing constant moisture contents are obtained. The water reference line is obtained by plotting the vapor pressure of water as a function of P against P_0. As the amount of water adsorbed increases,

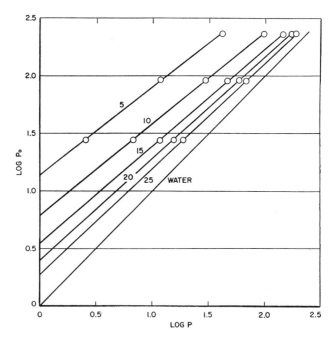

Figure 10.5. Equilibrium moisture contents of collagen plotted as a function of $\log P_0$ and $\log P$ as suggested by Whitwell and Toner [29].

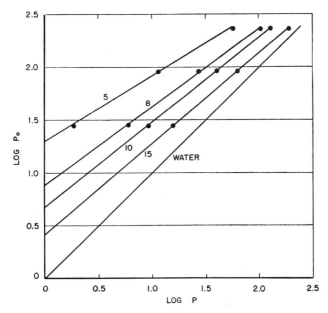

Figure 10.6. Equilibrium moisture contents of vegetable-tanned leather plotted as a function of log P_o and Log P as suggested by Whitwell and Toner [29].

the lines approach more closely the water reference line. It may be noted that the slopes of the lines change with increasing amounts of adsorption. This indicates changes in the heats of adsorption. These lines may be extrapolated as shown, and adsorption values obtained for other conditions for which no data were obtained.

The lines, when extended in the direction of increasing log P, approach intersection at a common point. The position of this point is assumed by Whitwell [29] to be related to the swelling characteristics of the material. It may readily be seen that the lines given for leather will meet in a common point at a lower value of log P than those for collagen. This can be demonstrated by observing the ratios of the distances between two corresponding lines at P values of log 0.5 and log 1.5. According to this hypothesis, collagen, as expected, shows the greater amount of swelling.

10.6   PERMEATION OF COLLAGEN BY WATER

Not only is water vapor adsorbed by collagen to maintain a steady state of equilibrium, but because of the porosity of the collagen substrate, it diffuses between active groups and permeates the membrane from the moist to the dryer side. Because of the use of leather in shoes where it is desired to have moisture permeation, there has been much interest in studies on the permeability of tanned hides which are, of course, composed of collagen.

According to Dacey [31], molecules which are adsorbed on the walls of the pores pass through more efficiently than those which are not adsorbed. He has concluded that the adsorbed phase contributes to the overall flow. It is obvious that in a porous solid if all the pores are filled, permeation will take place rapidly because passage occurs by hydrostatic flow.

Work by Kanagy and Vickers [32] has indicated a conduction of the moisture through leather by a surface mechanism which is indicated by an activated diffusion as shown by the existence of an energy of activation. Surface permeation of water vapor was also evidenced by a comparison of the flow rates of liquid water and water vapor through glass discs having different porosities. It was also shown that water vapor in a system of dynamic air streams will pass from the side of lower air pressure to the side of higher air pressure. This could not occur if the water vapor did not pass over the surface.

Mitton [33] made extensive studies on water-vapor permeability of leather and concluded that at least 97% of the water vapor passed through the pores by gaseous diffusion. He did, however, not compare leather with any other material whose walls do not adsorb moisture.

REFERENCES

1. J. H. Bland, *Federation Proc.* May–June 1966.
2. H. S. Frank and W. Y. Wen, *Disc. Faraday Soc.,* **24,** 133 (1957).
3. H. B. Bull, *J. Amer. Chem. Soc.,* **66,** 1499 (1944).
4. J. R. Kanagy, *J. Res. Nat. Bur. Stand.,* **44,** 31 (1950) RP2056.
5. P. Bhaskara Rao, Ph.D. Thesis, University of Madras. 1969.
6. S. Brunauer, P. H. Emmet, and E. Teller, *J. Amer. Chem. Soc.,* **60,** 309 (1938).
7. J. R. Kanagy, *J. Amer. Leather Chemists' Assoc.,* **42,** 98 (1947).
8. S. B. Hendricks, R. A. Nelson, and L. T. Alexander, *J. Amer. Chem. Soc.,* **62,** 1457 (1940).
9. J. Boyes-Watson and M. F. Perutz, *Nature,* **151,** 714 (1943).
10. J. R. Katz and J. C. Derksen, *Rec. Trev. Chim.,* **51,** 513 (1932).
11. M. A. Rougvie and R. S. Bear, *J. Amer. Leather Chemists' Assoc.,* **48,** 735 (1953).

12. O. L. Sponsler, J. D. Bath, and J. W. Ellis, *J. Phys. Chem.*, **44**, 996 (1940).

13. L. Pauling, *J. Amer. Chem. Soc.*, **67**, 555 (1945).

14. E. F. Mellon, A. H. Korn, and S. R. Hoover, *J. Amer. Chem. Soc.*, **70**, 3040 (1948).

15. E. F. Mellon, A. H. Korn, and S. R. Hoover, *J. Amer. Chem. Soc.*, **69**, 827 (1947).

16. H. J. Frey and W. J. Moore, *J. Amer. Chem. Soc.*, **70**, 3644 (1948).

17. R. W. Green and K. P. Ang, *J. Amer. Chem. Soc.*, **75**, 2733 (1953).

18. J. R. Kanagy, *J. Amer. Leather Chemists' Assoc.*, **49**, 646 (1954).

19. R. G. Mitton and R. J. Mawhinney, *J. Soc. Leather Trades' Chemists*, **39**, 206 (1955).

20. H. G. Wollenberg, *J. Soc. Leather Trades' Chemists*, **36**, 172 (1952).

21. A. Cheshire, *J. Soc. Leather Trades' Chemists*, **27**, 177 (1943).

22. A. D. McLaren and J. W. Rowen, *J. Polymer Sci.*, **7**, 289 (1952).

23. S. W. Benson and J. M. Seehof, *J. Amer. Chem. Soc.*, **73**, 5053 (1951).

24. L. G. Joyner, E. P. Barrett, and R. Skold, *J. Amer. Chem. Soc.*, **73**, 3155 (1951).

25. J. R. Kanagy, *J. Amer. Leather Chemists' Assoc.*, **58**, 524 (1963).

26. A. C. Zettlemoyer, E. D. Schweitzer, and W. C. Walker, *J. Amer. Leather Chemists' Assoc.*, **41**, 253 (1946).

27. J. W. Rowen and R. J. Simha, *J. Phys. Colloid Chem.*, **53**, 921 (1949).

28. J. G. Wiegerink, *J. Res. Nat. Bur. Stand.*, **42**, 557 (1949) RP1992.

29. J. C. Whitwell and R. K. Toner, *Textile Res. J.*, **16**, 255 (1946); ibid. **17**, 99 (1947).

30. D. F. Othmer, *Ind. Eng. Chem.*, **32**, 841 (1940).

31. J. R. Dacey, *Ind. Eng. Chem.*, **57**, 6 June (1965).

32. J. R. Kanagy and R. A. Vickers, *J. Res. Nat. Bur. Stand.*, **44**, 347 (1950) RP2082.

33. R. G. Mitton, *J. Soc. Leather Trades' Chemists*, **39**, 385 (1955).

11

Mechanical Properties of Skin in Relation to Its Biological Function and Its Chemical Components

R. D. HARKNESS

Department of Physiology, University College, London, England

393

This chapter deals primarily with mammalian skin, and considers principally two problems that cannot really be considered apart; first, what are the biologically important mechanical functions of skin, and, second, what part do the different components of skin play in mechanical properties?

11.1   RELATION BETWEEN BIOLOGICAL FUNCTIONS OF THE SKIN AND MECHANICAL PROPERTIES

The skin is a large organ forming up to 15–20% of the weight of the body [rat 103, 41; man 166]. Most of the solid tissue in mammals is collagen. It may contain up to half the total collagen in the body [mice, 85]. It is reasonable to assume, then, that skin has a mechanical function that is important to the animal. This function, however, is ill-defined compared to that of most organs. Perhaps this is partially because the skin is the boundary to the environment; knowledge of its function, therefore, involves observation of normal life of the animal and its relation to its environment—something that cannot be observed in the laboratory. Partly perhaps it is because the mechanical function of the skin seems so obvious. Because the relation between biological function and mechanical properties of skin has been rather neglected, we begin by considering it.

11.1.1   The Mechanical Functions of the Skin in Relation to its Other Functions

Sensation

In so far as the sensation involves displacement of the skin as in touch, vibration or pain, then presumably the mechanical properties of the skin must be involved in the transmission of the mechanical stimulus in the sense organ itself, or in the bed of tissue in which this lies, that may serve to restrict the effective stimuli to environmental ones [102]. The sense organ whose mechanical properties have received the most attention is the Pacinian corpuscle [99]. But the composition of its connective-tissue components has not been examined, though elaborate calculations have been made on the basis of considerable assumption about them [138].

Perhaps the most interesting sensation is pain. As the collagenous tissue of the dermis is its main, and probably most important, component, it would not be unreasonable to expect that this sensation might be related to its protection. Thermal pain is consistently induced by a temperature below that of thermal denaturation of collagen [74]. The mechanism of its production is obscure but the possibility of connective tissue being involved in this and other types of pain does not seem to have been considered.

Bodily Movement

During movement the skin changes shape, being stretched or wrinkled, and may move over the tissues underneath it; for example, it moves laterally over the knuckles (heads of metatarsals) when the fist is clenched. In so far as viscous, as opposed to elastic, elements in the tissue are concerned, these changes will involve an expenditure of energy, and reduce the speed of movement; so it is presumably advantageous to animals to keep them down. Speed of movement seems to play a more important part in survival from predators than mechanical protection by the skin. The disturbing effects of abnormalities in the flexibility of skin are apparent in, for example, scleroderma or in scar contracture in man, but the normal flexibility of the skin has been taken for granted. The only investigation appears to be that of Johns and Wright [105] who found that skin made little contribution to the stiffness of joints of cats compared to the connective tissues of the joints themselves. The accommodation of skin to movement of joints appears to be brought about largely by wrinkling, to a less extent by extension as one can see by looking at one's own joints. For example, flexing my own thumb increased the distance between two folds on the back of the last joint by about 50% but stretched the skin between by only about 10–15%. It is of interest that the direction of intraspecific attack against the sides of the body involves a part of the skin that is not much flexed in rapid mammalian movement, as galloping involves flexion in a different (dorso-ventral) plane. This part can be thickened it seems with little interference with movement (as similarly a saddle does not interfere).

The mechanical properties of the skin in relation to movement of aquatic animals through water is a special case, probably involving modification of the skin to improve performance [89]. Modification of the skin in relation to aerial flight is another special case, that will not be discussed.

Functional Contact with the Environment

The protective properties of the skin in relation to motion are considered separately elsewhere. Here we will consider other properties. Those of greatest potential interest seem to be the frictional and gripping properties of the surface and, in relation to them, perhaps the question of wastage of locomotive energy in surface contact. Whether this last question is of any biological importance is not clear. The security of a grip that does not slip between surfaces depends on surface irregularities and can be improved if these interlock, as they do if one surface is hard and the other deformable. If a surface is deformable, as soft-skin surfaces are, the deformation involves a loss of energy depending on the extent to which viscous flow is involved as opposed to elastic deformation. As the quality of the grip may be improved by the presence of viscous elements (as in car tires [200]) there is a potential conflict between requirements for greater speed and better gripping. In a car this raises no real problems because requirement for increased power is easily solved. One can, however, see the possibility that it might not be so easily solved biologically. This problem has not been investigated from this aspect.

Regarding the nature of specialized skin areas of environmental contact, there is a good deal of anatomical information but rather little functional, particularly in relation to the material or object to be gripped [*Hylidae* 13; some bats, see 63]. Apart from very specialized organs like the pads of some amphibia that enable them to grip smooth surfaces of large leaves or rock, there appear to be two common types of gripping or contact organs, soft tissue pads [216, 34, 55] and claws [64], the latter term being used in a general sense to include modified nails. Often the two are found together, for example in cats, and on the fingers and toes of some monkeys e.g., *Galagidae* (bush babies). Claws generally owe their effectiveness to their ability to penetrate a surface, and are used in this way by predatory mammals to grip skin. However, I have been unable to find any account of the mechanical design of claws in relation to the surfaces they act upon. The most familiar gripping pads to most people will be the tips of their fingers, though their properties in relation to grip do not appear to have been investigated, for example, frictional properties and the function of the epithelial ridges. This subject is of interest in relation to the design of artificial limbs and some ideas about how the normal grip works may be obtained from artificial ones. One design [193] consists of an inextensible, but flexible, bag containing a powder, enclosed in a thin elastic bag to maintain shape when the grip is loose, the whole being placed against a rigid flat backplate. When this is pressed against a surface, the powder behaves as a fluid, and allows the bag to adapt its shape to whatever it is pressed against. Under greater pressure the powder behaves as a solid and a firm even grip over the whole surface is established. It seems likely that the finger pads function in somewhat the same way. They appear to consist of chambers containing liquid fat enclosed in inextensible collagenous walls, the whole pad being backed by bone and the nail. The hypothetical function of the fingerprint epithelial ridges and sweat glands in gripping seems not to have been investigated. A mechanical function in relation to touch has been suggested, and it is here perhaps worth noting that ability to detect incipient slip between an object and the skin is important in adjusting grip so that the object is retained.

The function of the pads of the tips of the fingers and toes of monkeys seems also to be little understood. They do not appear to be used primarily in gripping round an object like a branch of a tree but on surfaces, the animals walking on them on tiptoe (e.g., the mouse lemur, *Microcebus murinus* [194]).

A rather specialized type of contact surface is found in animals like the polar bear and penguin that walk on ice [34]. Hairs are involved, but it is not clear how far these are concerned in frictional contact as opposed to insulation from the very cold ice (down to −30°C). Weasels in cold areas have more hairy under surfaces to their feet than in warmer areas [68]. The desert (*Jaculus*) shows the same adaptation, presumably as insulation from hot surfaces (up to 60°C or more).

11.1.2   The Mechanical Protective Function of Skin in Relation to the Body

The skin is generally assumed to have a mechanical protective function but there is no clear discussion in functional terms of the nature and origin of the forces it protects against or the method of protection.

There are two main sorts of protection to be considered. The first we might call self-protection, that is, the maintenance of the integrity of the structure for its own sake, and the protection of its own components from mechanical stresses that might disturb their function in other roles, for example, the function of glands or of cells of connective tissue concerned in the maintenance and production of extracellular substances. The second aspect is the one commonly understood, namely, the function of the skin as the boundary to the environment, as a container protecting the inner structures of the body. These two aspects of protective function are sufficiently different to be discussed separately.

The Protective Function of Skin in Relation to Its Own Functions Other than Mechanical

We may begin with the question whether skin structure is in any way designed to protect the cells in it. There seems no point in asking this question about the epidermis that consists only of cells, but the situation in the dermis is different. Here the cells are placed in cavities in an extracellular medium of much more robust qualities than their own. One might expect their position, and the arrangement of the extracellular material, would be such as to minimize the forces acting on them when the whole tissue was distorted, for example, they might be expected to be in positions where there were no large shearing stresses. There is, however, no evidence on this point. It is probably not important because it appears that fibroblasts can survive and recover rapidly from very severe mechanical trauma [4].

As regards the blood supply to the tissue, which is of great importance, and can be interrupted by stretching the skin (see below), there does not appear to be any specific feature in skin structure that might contribute to the protection of blood vessels. The same can be said of glandular structures. Sweat-gland ducts in the human skin do seem to be susceptible to trauma. Rapid deceleration through contact with the hard ground, as occurs in games like netball and squash, presumably by causing shear stresses may lead to haemorrhage into the ducts and their becoming blocked.

The Protective Function of the Skin in Relation to Tissues Under It

In general, it would seem that the skin has two sorts of protective functions; *enabling*, that is it enables its owner to move through his environment without undue surface injury from accidental or necessary contact with it; and *defensive*, that is against active mechanical attack from parasites, predators, and its own species. Skin may be subject to several forms of attack, penetrating from a sharp-pointed object moving along a line, cutting from a sharp object moving in a plane, and energetic from a blunt nonpenetrating object whose energy has to be absorbed. It is convenient briefly to discuss the nature of these different forms of attack first, and then the sources of such attack, their relative importance biologically and the defense the skin can provide against them.

Types of Attack. It is of interest that the classification of types of mechanical attack noted above is basically the same as has been used in the discussion of military combat of the direct personal type, as exemplified by the rapier (penetrating), the sabre (cutting) and the mace (energetic or percussive attack). Before discussing them it is useful to consider one general point relating to attack on the surface of an animal, namely, that the size of the animal is clearly going to determine to a great extent the factors involved. Thus, in a small animal the maximum force that can be applied to the skin from one side is limited to the amount that can move the whole animal (related to the velocity of application). Larger forces can be applied downwards as against the ground or from two opposite sides at once. In this connection it is interesting that horns do not seem to occur in small mammals.

Penetrating Attack. Penetrating attack by a sharp-pointed object moving along a line is the most effective in the sense that it is made over the smallest possible area and allows penetration with minimum applied force. On the other hand, its success is strongly dependent on the angle of incidence, the optimum for penetration being probably at right angles to the surface. Its damaging power after penetration is limited by the lesser chance of a line than a plane (as in a cut) going through a vital region of the interior. For the same reasons it is easier to avoid. Effective defense is primarily by the interposition of hard material, so arranged as to minimize the chance of the point attacking the surface orthogonally. If the surface is not hard then it should not fold too easily, as this can allow the surface to move into a position at right angles to the line of attack even though the original surface was not so related to it. So far as a layer of fibrous material is concerned, as in most skin, assuming the penetrating object to be circular in cross-section and increasing in diameter behind the point, as it usually is, penetration presumably involves pushing the fibers apart in the first instance; and subsequently on rupturing them, if the penetrating object is too large to go between them, in the case of mammalian skin presumably more than a few micra in diameter. One might then expect resistance to be related to the tensile strength of the fibers and to other factors less easily defined, for example, that they should be sufficiently easily deformed and movable as to prevent the hind part of the penetrating object assisting the point by transmission of force through the material to the region of the point (as happens when one is splitting a rigid material by extending a crack). It is of interest to note here that mammalian skin seems to provide rather poor defense against penetrating attack. It appears to be the standard method employed by primitive human predators against large animals, and perhaps the first person to realize this weakness and develop this method of attack deserves more credit as an inventor than he usually gets. This method of attack is used by mammals against one another, e.g., horns [56], walrus tusks [175]; and teeth of cats [134], and of course commonly by blood-sucking insects, (see below). Many plants have developed sharp spines and their functional relation of animals will be considered later.

Cutting. The characteristic of a cutting attack is that it moves through a plane, increasing its chance of hitting; on the other hand, it is easier to intercept, a linear object passing through the plane being enough. In fact, this sort of attack, in its pure form by a cutting edge, does not seem to have been developed by animals, though planar attack is used in catching prey, as with a line of teeth in *Pristis* (sawfish, 147a). Combined with a penetrating attack it can increase the effectiveness of the latter, as for example in the needle with two or three cutting edges (oval or triangular instead of circular cross-section) used in surgery to suture skin, or the modern hunter's arrow with cutting fins. Biologically it seems that it is probably less important than penetrating attack, certainly as between animals, though some plants appear to have developed cutting edges as opposed to spines (e.g., certain ferns and grasses).

Energetic or Percussive Attack. This type of attack, unlike the last, seems important, firstly in relation to accidental contact with the immovable part of the environment, and, secondly, in relation to animals attacking one another. As regards accidental contact the amount of energy to be absorbed without harm must be related to the weight and velocity of the moving part, to the square of the latter quantity. In movement of the whole body the maximum velocity of running is approximately constant in animals of different size, as might be expected from the properties of muscle and connective tissue, which limits the maximum force that can be exerted [93]. If the maximum velocity is constant, then one would expect the required protection to vary directly with weight, that is, the skin would be a constant proportion of body weight. However, the matter is complicated by other factors, in particular that in homoiothermic animals the requirements for temperature regulation vary with size in a different way and involve hair which may have a secondary protective function, as noted later.

Another circumstance in which protection from percussive damage may be important is in falling. It has been pointed out by Haldane [69] that the terminal velocity of free-fall in air and damage on landing decreases with body size so that a small animal may survive a fall that would kill a larger one. The spines on a hedgehog are said to be used to enable it to fall without damage from a height [25].

As regards animals' relations to one another, percussive attack certainly does occur, and can be very damaging—the very obvious example being the horse's use of its hind feet in this way; a rabbit can repel and even kill a weasel in a similar way [68]; giraffes also attack with their feet and with their heads [66]. Horned animals may also attack in this way with the flat surface of the horn [57]. In this last case, protection seems to be provided also by the horns, frequently with associated strengthening of the bone to which they are attached, and hair—the heavy growth on the head of the buffalo being reputed to act in this way [57]. The role of the skin in this form of attack is not clear, but it seems likely to be relatively unimportant since the major injury is produced often at a distance from the point of impact (e.g., head injuries in car accidents, percussive abdominal wounds leading to rupture of viscera like the liver or spleen). The energy-absorbing capacity of the human scalp has been measured and is not particularly great [206].

11.1.3   The Protective Function of Skin in Relation to the Environment

Having discussed briefly how the skin may be attacked we may now go on to consider the nature and biological importance of its mechanical protective function in real life. It is convenient to consider this in relation to the stationary environment, plants, and to other animals.

The Stationary Environment

The animal makes functional contact with the environment through the skin in locomotion and feeding and, in a rather restricted way, when it lies down to rest or sleep. I know of only one animal with parts of the skin specialized for a resting position—the camel. Its thick pads on the sternum and limbs support it when it lies down.

Regarding the skin and potentially damaging contact with the environment during locomotion, the most specialized contact is perhaps made through hooves, that is, hard, keratinized structures. But it is not clear what is functionally important here. Regarding less-specialized types of hand and foot, again there seems to be very little information. Keratinized digital appendages (claws, nails) are clearly used for hard contact as in digging. As regards the protective function of the skin in the gripping hand or sole of the foot, localized thickenings (callosities) of the epidermis may be formed over areas subjected to shearing stress, though the stimulus does not seem to have been investigated. Their effect would seem to be to spread shear-stress more evenly over a wider area. Such thickenings form (as a matter of observation and enquiry from personal experience) seemingly less readily on the fingertip pads than on the rest of the palmar surface, though they may form under severe stress, as in players of stringed instruments. In relation to protection it is of interest that the epidermis, in man at least, appears to have in it a plane of weakness where it ruptures under excessive shear-stress [155, 196]. This plane is above the layer from which the epidermis regenerates. It presumably acts, in effect, to produce a plane of slip so reducing the possibility of damage to the underlying dermis.

Plant Thorns

It is a reasonable hypothesis that the thorns found on many plants have a protective function in putting off browsing or grazing animals from eating them or, in a thicket, in making a structure into which such animals cannot enter [114, 204]; spines can be very damaging [172]. It seems clear, however, that this supposed protective mechanism is of limited effectiveness; for example, both the giraffe and black rhinoceros [65, 66] eat the thorny acacia (Acacia drepanolobia), though it is not clear in either case how this is made possible, by modification of the mechanical properties of the skin round the mouth and its lining, or by skill in manipulating the thorns between the teeth. I have seen a horse pick out a cut plant of the field thistle (Carduus arvensis) to eat from a heap of cut grass. In this connection it is interesting to note that land plants with spines, that probably were rigid as they are preserved in a three-dimensional state, not flattened, in sandy deposits, existed in early Devonian times before there is any evidence of the existence of browsing land vertebrates (Psilophytes [3]). These spines were near together (mm) and could possibly, though perhaps not very probably, have been concerned in resisting attack by invertebrate browsers (See Netolitsky [156] for discussion of the slight protective effect of plant hairs). I am told by my colleague, W. G. Chaloner, that the fossil record of thorny plants is very poor, so that it is impossible to correlate their occurrence with animal evolution (as, for example, it is possible to correlate the evolution of mammals and birds, presumably warm-blooded and needing a continuous supply of food, with the evolution of angiosperms and food storage in seed embryos [45]).

Regarding the question of spines inhibiting movement of animals, it seems again that they can be less effective than one would expect, and not necessarily because of any mechanical property of the animal's skin. A colleague, R. D. Martin, told me of the case of the Sifaka, a small primate that leaps about in an exceedingly prickly shrub (Dideria) apparently without injury and without special protection on its palms or soles. In another case, the desert pack rat (Neotomasp), adaptation to life amid spiny plants appears to be brought about not by a protective mechanism for preventing penetration of the skin, but by tolerance of this [189]. On the other hand, by repute, the resistant skin of an animal like the black rhinoceros, enables it to break through thickets of thorny plants. A protective function against plants has been attributed to the protuberances on the face of the wart hog. This and other pigs grub in the ground with their snouts [52] and it is reasonable to suppose that the skin must be specialized for this purpose, though there does not seem to be any information as to how.

It would be easier to consider this problem if more systematic information were available on the occurrence and nature of plant spines [36, 114]. One can see, for example, that the arrangement of spines in many cacti, in groups radiating from centres with those in adjacent groups overlapping, has the effect of making it impossible to approach the surface from any direction without meeting spines end on. A similar arrangement is found in the hairs of some lepidopterous larvae (*Saturnidae*). Though the inhibiting effect of such spines on the approach of animals seems obvious, their effectiveness seems to be much less easily demonstrable than that of taste or smell and other characteristics, [e.g., 1, 100]. Thus it is easy to observe avoidance of many soft plants by grazing animals, e.g., buttercups (*Ranunculus* species), ragwort (*Senecio jacobaea*) or elder (*Sambucus niger*) by horses; garden mint, spurge (*Euphorbia peplus*), fireweed (*Epilobium angustifolium*) and other species by guinea pigs (personal observations).

In conclusion it appears that the interactions between the skins of animals and plant organs apparently capable of producing mechanical damage (spines and the like) are as yet ill-defined. Possibly this is not an interaction that concerns the dermis and its mechanical properties. It is clear that quite minor penetrating damage to skin can produce pain and also in some cases major long-term effects by subsequent attack by microorganisms or other parasites, for example, flies whose larval stages attack living tissue, (warble flies, *Hypoderma* ssp, and screw worms [88]).

Parasites and Blood-sucking Animals

As a protection against invading organisms, the skin may be effective simply as an impenetrable barrier. Most microorganisms are held out by the epidermis, though some may live in it, as may small parasites (*Dermodex, Sarcoptes* in man [146]). They live there, it seems, probably rather because it suits their way of life than because they are unable to penetrate further. Other organisms can penetrate through the skin into the blood vessels and inner tissues. But even in these cases protection may be afforded by the skin delaying the organism until it can be destroyed by immune mechanisms, or until it dies naturally, for example, by the exhaustion of its food stores. Thus schistosomal larvae (cercariae) appear to penetrate into the epidermis readily, it seems, principally by direct mechanical means. They can move in it parallel to the surface.

But they appear to be delayed by the basement membrane which they attack enzymatically [130, 131]. The fact that this is a barrier may perhaps explain why few organisms make use of the ducts of glands or the spaces round hairs to penetrate the skin. Other organisms live for part of their life cycle in the connective tissue of the dermis (see, for example Refs. 88, 173) and can dissolve holes in it, for example, the larvae of warble flies (*Hypoderma* ssp). The interrelations between the tissues of the skin and parasites penetrating or living there are of great interest, but very little has yet been done to examine them in terms of modern knowledge of skin structure.

As a protection against blood-sucking organisms most skins seem relatively ineffective. Thus the skin area of the crocodile (*Crocodilus niloticus*) does not protect it against tsetse flies (*Glossina* ssp), though these attack it through the thinner flexible regions of skin and the inside of the mouth, which is frequently held open (94). Other blood-sucking organisms similarly tend to concentrate their attack on particular areas of skin, for example, ticks round the anus of the rhinoceros [65] where the skin is thin and sand flies (*Psychodidae*) on areas with only a sparse coating of hairs, the tails and ears of rodents [126a]. It seems probable that dense hair is an effective protection against many types of blood-sucking organisms. For example, the human crab louse (*Pythirus pubis*) will not live on the scalp, it seems, because of the high density of hair [26a]. The biological significance of this sort of partial protection that reduces the area of skin available to attack is not clear.

The most interesting feature of the relation between the skin and blood-sucking organisms is perhaps the mechanism by which they penetrate to obtain blood. There is a large literature on the structures of mouth parts [193a] from which deduction as to their probable mechanism of action can be made, but rather little direct observation of their function. The most notable contributions to this difficult subject have been made by Gordon and associates on mosquitos, tsetse, and tabanid flies [60a, 61, 61a, 62a]. These show clearly the astonishing effectiveness and apparent sophistication of the biting mouth parts, but still leave unclear the precise mechanism of penetration. The impression I have gained from this literature is that this generally involves first a parting of the tissues by chitinous blades acting in the same plane in opposition to one another and at right angles to the direction of penetration; then a drawing in of the mouth parts from the tip by the same or other blades or hooks. We may take the penetration of the mouth parts of the tsetse fly (*Glossina* ssp) as an example. These animals are viviparous, the larvae developing in the body of the mother to the stage at which it is ready to pupate, when it is expelled. The material for the growth of the larvae is provided by blood obtained by the mother, who has to feed 2 or 3 times a week for the purpose. A full meal of blood can be obtained in a matter of minutes or so, including the time required to penetrate. As might be expected, the mouth parts provide a beautiful example of a mechanical device built on a very small scale. Though made of several separable parts, the mouth parts consist essentially of a cylindrical tube 3–4 mm long and about 70 μ in diameter, swollen at the base, which contains the operating muscles, to 0.5 mm or so. This tube contains a canal of not much less diameter through which blood is sucked, and a smaller one which carries out saliva. In addition it contains two tendons about 5 μ in diameter that connect the muscle at the base to the penetrating machinery at the tip. This consists of a set of blades and another of hooks (called "rasps"), mounted, in effect, on a moving belt. Normally they lie enclosed in the tip facing inwards. Contraction of the muscle moves them forward to the tip, then outward, and finally back along the outside a little way toward the base. The movement appears to be something like that of the nails if one places his hands in front of him, back to back, and flexes the fingers. The movement it seems would first separate the tissues and then draw the tip forward into them.

This is a very brief outline of an interesting subject in which the role of the skin is little understood. Further information may be found in the following references: general information, 127a; mosquitoes, 28a, 30, 60a, 61a, and 62; tsetse flies, 26b, 60a; horse flies, 61; lice, 26a; and vampire bats, 21.

Predators

It seems clear that when the prey is sufficiently small in relation to the size of the predator, then nothing can protect it once the predator has made contact. The mammalian predator commonly kills its prey, if smaller, by biting it in the back of the head or neck, lacerating the spinal cord, or brain, (e.g., weasels [68], cats [134, 135], fox [119, 203], and mongoose [217]), though tigers frequently bite the front of the throat, strangling their prey, usually if the prey is larger than themselves, as it can be [187]. Predatory mammals learn by experience and modify their methods [134]. In general, the skin provides very little effective protection either to the penetrating canine teeth, or to the cutting carnassials [187], when the prey is of similar size or even larger than the predator; it can be several times heavier [weasels, 68; tigers, 187]. Initial attack on large animals seems usually to be made from the rear, and the prey bitten in the belly, rump, and hind legs, or knocked over. An account of an attack by lions on a buffalo that was filmed is given by Leyhausen [134]. Other accounts of methods of attack are given by Kühme [121], the hyaena dog, *Lycaeon pictus lupinus* and Schaller [187] tiger, *Panthera tigris*. The interesting problem here then seems not to be the protective function of the skin but the design of teeth and claws to grip it which they can do very effectively (e.g., polar bears catching seal with claws).

Thus, in many mammals the skin appears to provide no effective protection against predators. The exceptions are animals with specialized skins like the armadillo or pangolin (the plates of the scaly anteater, *Smutsia terminckii,* are recorded as deflecting the bullet of a 0.303 rifle at 100 yds [192]) or spines (porcupines and hedgehogs). But even spines may not put off predators despite the damage produced by them [90, 187], recording porcupine remains in tiger faeces. It is clearly more difficult to get evidence about the effectiveness as opposed to the ineffectiveness of a protective coat, because predators are intelligent and will no doubt tend to concentrate their attacks where they know they will be successful.

In conclusion, it appears that survival against predators depends mainly on avoidance (by alertness and superior speed) and mutual defence (in herds), the mechanical protective function of the skin in individuals being of relatively minor importance.

Intraspecific Fighting

There is evidence that the skin does have a protective function in fighting between individuals of the same species. The methods used by ungulates with horns, or specialized teeth (pigs) have been reviewed [57]. Commonly they fight side-by-side, each attacking the side of the other's body. This seems to be the primitive method of fighting with simple horns using the tips to produce puncture wounds and gashes [for a description of wounds see 56]. Such combat is largely between males and clearly must not be so damaging that they cannot reproduce. Wounded males have been observed not to mate [57]. The skin at the side of the body is thicker than elsewhere in some animals where it is attacked, for example, hogs [159, quoted in 57] and hippopotamus [78]. A uniquely interesting set of observations on this subject has been made by Geist [58], who gives the actual sites of puncture wounds together with their correlation with skin thickness in mountain goats (*Oreamnos americanus*); see Figure 11.1.

It seems likely the damaging effect of this fighting has been reduced more by the evolution of more elaborate horns, and change in behavior than by strengthening the skin [57]. Such horns appear to be more effective defensively than offensively, and are associated with frontal

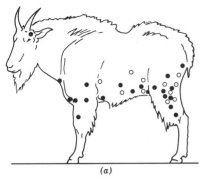
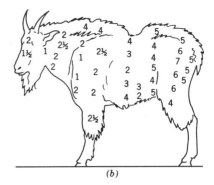

(a)   (b)

Figure 11.1.   (a) Shows the distribution of horn punctures on a three-year-old male goat, found in a moribund state; ○ punctures on *L*, ● on *R* side of body. (b) Shows the distribution of skin thickness in this species (in mm, 4-year-old male in rut) [58].

fighting, though this may occur with simple horns [187] and lead to wounding in the neck. With still more leaborate horns the conflict seems to turn progressively more to psychological, by display. It appears that the skin can have a mechanical protective function of some importance in intraspecific fighting.

The object of this discussion has been to try to set out at least some of the functional or biological problems related to mechanical properties of skin. If the discussion itself has been incomplete and to a great extent hypothetical and inconclusive, this is at least to some extent because the information needed for a more effective discussion is lacking. In general, these problems seem to have been approached in the past almost exclusively from one side, either the biological or the physical. It seemed better to have some discussion, however inconclusive, that might help to bring these two aspects together, rather than none at all.

11.2   STRUCTURE OF THE SKIN IN RELATION TO MECHANICAL FUNCTION

Outline of Skin Structure

Before going on to consider the chemical components of skin in relation to mechanical function, it is desirable to consider the general structure briefly.

The skin consists of two main layers, an outer *epidermis* lying on an inner *dermis*. The surface of the latter where it is in contact with the epidermis is a specialized region, the *basement membrane*, (basal lamina) forming a distinct layer in the electron microscope [e.g. 23], and containing a specialized form of collagen [108a, 176a, 193b].

The Epidermis. The epidermis, formed by continuous growth and division from its basal layer, consists principally of keratin, generally in the form of dead cells flattened in the plane of the surface, and arranged in the human skin in a rather regular fashion [140]. The strength of bonding between the cells is not high, at least in most regions, as they can be stripped off a layer at a time by application of Sellotape (Scotch tape) to the surface. The strength of the whole epidermis appears in general to be low in comparison with the dermis under it. It can be broken easily in most regions of the human body though in some (palms and soles of feet, for example) it is thicker and stronger than in others [34]. As noted elsewhere, the human epidermis appears to contain a plane of weakness where it ruptures differentially under shear-stress. Its main function seems to be that of preventing diffusion of water out from the body. The material from which the epidermis is made, keratin, is resistant chemically and also to enzymic attack by all but a very few pathogens.

The epidermis is flexible but appears to be relatively inextensible, as judged by the astonishing constancy of distances between recognizable points on fingerprints [35]. Its most interesting but largely unknown mechanical properties would seem to be frictional, at points of functional contact with the environment, as mentioned earlier.

The Dermis. The outermost layer of the dermis, the dermoepidermal junction, is a specialized region where (in the adult) a continuous distinct layer of material (basement membrane) can be seen in the electron microscope [23, 116]. The human epidermis, in some regions at least, seems to be attached rather loosely and can be loosened by simply stretching the whole skin [211, 60] or by reducing the pressure over the epidermis [20, 137, 115].

The dermis proper is made primarily of collagen (70–80% of dry weight up to 30% of wet [71]), and one can regard it as essentially similar to tendon except in the arrangement of the fibers of collagen in a three-dimensional weave instead of linearly. It is not, however, entirely homogeneous in structure. The most superficial layer contains a greater density of blood vessels than elsewhere, presumably related to the nutrition of the epidermis and in some skins to the thermoregulatory function. This layer, in man, appears to be looser than the deeper parts of the dermis. It is more easily distorted [observations on leather 212], and seems to carry little of the load when the whole skin is under tension [113].

The main bulk of the dermis (corium) consists, in mammals, of bundles of collagen fibrils running in many directions, that is, not only in the plane of the surface, but also between planes at different depth. This produces a structure that is resistant to shear. In this respect it is unlike the transparent cornea of the eye, that has fibrils running exclusively in the plane of the surface, though in different directions in successive layers [147]. This last condition, it seems likely, is a more primitive one. It is found in the skin of amphibian larvae [213, 214, 215] and a number of vertebrates other than mammals [153, 157]. Though a mammalian dermal arrangement shows no easily definable systematic organization, it seems very probable that such an organization exists, though difficult to detect.

The strength of strips of dermis under tension varies with the direction in which the strips are cut, which indicates that the distribution of fiber direction is similarly assymetrical. Thus, in cattle on the body, tensile strength is reported greater (up to 70%, belly) in a direction parallel to the long axis of the body than at right angles to it [32, 108, 107, 151, 150].

Collagen fibers in the dermis and tendons of some animals, for example cattle, are arranged in bundles, like tiny tendons, surrounded by sheaths of inextensible material, of apparently high strength [73, 74] that behaves differently from collagen under chemical treatment, for example, in acid solution [106, 37, 38, 126, 29, 49, 10]. The mechanical function of these sheaths is unknown. They appear to be strong [74] and may possibly be expected to prevent the fibers buckling under compression stress along their length as must occur on the inner side of a curve when the skin is flexed.

As well as collagen, many skins contain elastin (e.g., cattle [98, 149, 167, 168]; rat [2, 139]) generally distributed throughout the depth or sometimes in a particular layer, for example in the elephant's belly skin at the undersurface (personal observation). In human skin [42], elastin appears to be in higher concentration in the most superficial and deepest layers. The presence of elastin probably accounts for the fact, already mentioned, that many skins contract in area when removed from the body, indicating that the elastin is under tension in the normal state of the skin.

The total thickness of the skin varies considerably in different parts of the body as illustrated for the rat in Fig. 11.2, where it is measured in terms of structural material, collagen. In general, there is very little quantitative information on this point, nor about variation in skin thickness between species.

In general, investigations have been confined to the behavior of the skin under tension, and various formulae have been developed to describe this behavior under particular conditions of test ([73] and Chapters 1 and 12 in this volume). The behavior, in detail, is complex because both elastic and viscous elements are present. Also it is clear that there will be differences in different regions and between animals. The common elastic-type of skin that appears to be under tension in life, and contracts on removal from the body, has been mentioned. This is not the behavior

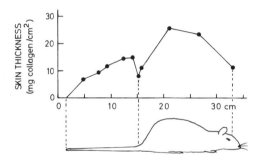

Figure 11.2. Thickness of a rat's skin (in terms of collagen). The figure gives the thickness of the skin as collagen per unit surface area of the back and tail. Collagen was estimated from the hydroxyproline content of the skin determined on an acid hydrolysate, by Stegemann's method. Samples from the back were cut out with a rotating punch, and rings were taken from the tail as described in the text [81].

of all types of skin and there is another type that alters little in shape on removal. The skin of the back and sides of the hippopotamus exemplifies this type, and the skin of the rat's tail appears to behave similarly.

Discussion of the strength of the collagenous framework of skin will be deferred until Section 11.1.4 in which the function of the different components and cross links in collagen are considered. Before going on to this it is well to discuss the mechanical state of the normal skin, that is, the range of its properties in which it normally works.

The Mechanical State of Normal Skin

It is a familiar fact that the human skin is potentially larger in area than the body it covers and can be lifted into folds. The relation of skin size to that of the body varies in different animals. Thus, the human skin is relatively a tight fit which limits the possibility of compensation for loss in wounding by drawing over remaining skin by contraction of the wound; on the other hand, a rabbit's skin seems to be relatively larger so that large areas can be recovered by drawing in skin from elsewhere. This question of the "size" of the collagenous framework of the skin has received little quantitative study and the biological significance of differences is not clear. Possibly an increase is involved in human Ehlers Danlos Syndrome [62]. Size can be a property of functional importance, as in the cervix of the uterus in pregnancy where a major change appears to be an increase in anticipation of the passage of the foetus at birth (rat, [76]). A similar change takes place in a nonpregnant horn in pregnancy of the other horn, in the rat [79]. The potential variation in skin area in a given animal is partly determined by the extent of folding, partly by the existence of elastic elements in the skin, that are discussed elsewhere. These elastic elements appear normally to be under tension in many types of skin as evidenced by contraction in the area of the skin after removal (10–20% in linear dimensions, human, hippopotamus belly [74]). The tension in normal human skin has been estimated from measurements of the pull required to bring together the edges of a fresh wound, and a figure of 2 g mm^{-1}-length of wound obtained [111 quoted erroneously as 20 g mm^{-1} in 73]. The tension needed to stop blood flow (blanching tension), which is important surgically, in human skin has been found to be of the order of 75 g mm^{-1} but varies with blood pressure [111].

11.2.1   Function of Different Anatomical Components in Mechanical Properties

The mechanical function of the *epidermis* will not be discussed. In the majority of mammal skins it seems to be relatively unimportant. There are exceptions as in the plantar surface of the foot of the camel that has a rubbery epidermis about a centimeter thick. In reptilian skins it may well be more important and in some it is obviously so; for example, *Chelonians* that have a horny shell associated with a bony carapace [15], but there seems to be no quantitative information about the mechanical properties of such skins.

Nothing really can be said either about the mechanical properties of the basement membrane. It is worth noting that chemical treatments that loosen the epidermis and therefore probably affect this region do not necessarily weaken the dermis—for example, treatment with solutions at pH 12–12.5 (our own observations on the special case of the skin of the rat's tail). The epidermis can be loosened in various ways, by raising the temperature to about 50°C, by enzymes and other reagents [78, 24, 195, 115, 116] though just what structure is involved in each case is not clear.

11.3   FUNCTION OF THE DIFFERENT CHEMICAL COMPONENTS OF THE DERMIS IN MECHANICAL PROPERTIES

Only in mammals is enough known about the composition of the skin for it to be possible to consider this problem. The discussion will be confined to the dermis in this group, but excluding dermal bone, such as found in some *Cetaceae,* and in specialized animals like the armadillo and pangolin. Dermal bone is common in reptiles, generally in association with scales (e.g., the slow worm, *Anguis fragilis Crocodilia* [15]; and collagenous hard tissue is found in fish scales [18, 19]. There seems to be little definite information about the function of these structures, generally considered as "protective."

11.3.1   Components Other than Fibrous Proteins

Cellular Components

There is little information either on the proportion of the volume of skin occupied by cells or their number or arrangement in the connective-tissue framework [74]. But they appear to account for only a small part, probably of the order of 10–20% of the bulk of the tissue. For many purposes it is reasonable to ignore their contribution to mechanical properties, but they may well be important in particular situations where the quantity of extracellular material is relatively small as in young developing tissues or in the early stages of wound healing, where there is evidence that they are directly concerned in wound contraction [104].

Extracellular Fluid

The largest single component of the extracellular dermal connective tissue is water. Estimates of the volume of the extracellular fluid space may be obtained from the distribution volume of substances that are differentially excluded from cells (Na^+, Cl^-, $SO_4^=$, thiocyanate, man, rat, rabbit, chicken [144, 51, 43, 44, 143, 148]. Figures so obtained are generally in the range of 50–70 ml per 100 g of fresh weight, which is of the same order as found in tendon. The state and detailed distribution of this fluid is not clear. Blood vascular space accounts for only a tiny proportion, about 1% of the skin weight [101]. Some water is very closely bound to the collagen as evidenced by examination of the relation between water content and water vapor pressure of air to which the collagenous tissue is brought into equilibrium [14, 184]. Removal of water may increase the tensile strength (at least $2 \times$ in rat-tail dermis, personal observation) presumably by allowing interactions that normally would not take place because of the presence of water masking sites of possible interaction. Though it has been recorded also as having no effect.

In cartilage the movement of fluid is restricted by the presence of fixed negatively changed groups and by limitation in the size of the spaces through which it can flow [145]. These restrictions are important in determining the mechanical properties of the material in maintaining its elasticity to rapidly applied stresses, as in running, while allowing adaptation in shape under prolonged stress of gravity, and also possibly in allowing cartilage to absorb energy when distorted by strong forces rapidly applied as in landing from a jump [218]. Such restriction of movement of fluid does not seem to be important in at least the bulk properties of skin, indeed it is reasonable to suppose its flexibility depends on the relative absence of restriction. The absence of gross restriction of fluid movements is clearly seen in oedema which is readily dispersed by local pressure. The main difference between normal and oedematous skin seems to be in the resting tension [42]. Whether restriction of fluid movement might play a part in localized environment, as in or round individual fibers or fibrils, is not known but the presence of structural materials (e.g., dermatan sulphate) with fixed-charge groups like those in cartilage makes this a possibility.

The extracellular fluid is involved in the functions of hyaluronic acid which will be discussed separately.

Glycosaminoglycans and Other Nonfibrous Extracellular Components

Plasma Protein. The extracellular compartment of the skin contains protein in solution, derived principally, it would seem, from plasma [86, 27, 101, 33, 141, 142, 50, 191]. The quantity is quite large, the distribution volume for albumen, assuming the same concentration as in plasma, being about 10 ml per 100 g fresh skin [101]. The state and location of the albumen is not clear but it appears from autoradiographic studies to penetrate right into the bundles of collagen [142]. Its function here, if any, is not known, but the fact that it penetrates into these structures suggests that they contain regions of free fluid and low resistance to shear.

Materials of Ill-defined Nature but Function Probably Structural. It has been known for a long time that skin contains a considerable amount of material of composition not clearly defined but probably playing a structural role, for example the periodic acid-Schiff staining material, presumably glycoprotein, associated with the superficial layer under the epidermis (light microscopic basement membrane [59]. Extracellular microfibrillar structures in this region can be detected electron-microscopically [171, 197, 163]. Glycoproteins [109] and noncollagenous protein closely associated with collagen have been described [22]. A number of antigenic components specific to skin connective tissue have been described [207] and an acidic protein has been isolated [208]. Though it is a reasonable possibility that some of these materials may have a structural role, at the moment nothing definite can be said about it. It is worth pointing out that mechanically resistant structures can be formed of noncollagenous material, for example, the vitelline membrane of the fowl's yolk [16] and the shell membranes [9].

Hyaluronic Acid. Hyaluronic acid is a large molecule that can fill an aqueous space in such a way as to exclude other large molecules, for example, plasma protein [127, 164]. By virtue of this same space-occupying property it can separate surfaces and thus act as a lubricant as in joints. It is found in skin, generally in small amounts (less than 1% wet weight) [188, 209, 174]. It can function mechanically as a material for holding up structures of a temporary nature like the cock's comb or the sex skin of monkeys [199]. Any mechanical function it may have in normal skin is less clear. As one would expect from its nature, it does not seem to be concerned in the maintenance of tensile strength, as judged by the evidence that hyaluronidase has little, if any, effect on this property (rats' skin) [77]. The question remains whether it may not have some lubricant function, between collagen fibers for example, but there is no evidence about this.

Dermatan Sulfate and other Glycosaminoglycans. Dermatan sulfate (in combination with its protein) is found characteristically in the dermis, like hyaluronic acid in relatively small amounts [209, 174]. It is closely associated with collagen for the most part, particularly with large collagenous fibers, and so is suspected of having a mechanical function, but there is really no evidence as to what this is. Other sulfated glyco-aminoglycans are present in skin (e.g. heparin, heparitin and sulfate [174] but the function of these is also little understood.

11.3.2   The Fibrous Proteins of Skin

Collagen is clearly much more important quantitatively than elastin as a component of skin, and more is known about it. So little really is known about elastin that one can only discuss it briefly. That many skins are under tension at rest has been mentioned, and the probability that the elastin present can account for this. There are, however, no quantitative measurements to substantiate this. Generally there appears histologically to be much less elastin than collagen in skin.

Role of Collagen and Its Relation to Other Materials

It seems clear that the principal role of collagen is to provide the material that determines the ultimate tensile strength of the skin and so, incidentally, a limit to its size as already discussed. The evidence for this function is of a general nature based on its presence in much larger quantity than any other material, and on the properties of the collagenous framework that, after removal of other material, forms the basis of leather. Direct evidence obtained by heating the skin for a short time at various temperatures up to and above the contraction temperature of collagen is shown in Fig. 11.3. It is clear that above this temperature the strength of this skin falls to a small fraction of its original. Differential heating of one side of the skin while the other was kept cool reduced strength when the heat was applied to the dermal side, but had little effect when it was applied to the epidermal [79]. These experiments give evidence at the same time of the relative unimportance of the epidermis in this mechanical property.

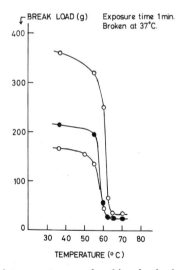

Figure 11.3. Effect of temperature on breaking load of rat-tail skins. The rings of skin (2.5 mm width) were exposed to the temperature stated on the abscissa for 1 min, then cooled and tested at 37°C. The three curves show experiments on three different rats [79].

Though collagen is clearly the primary structural material of skin, it appears to be laid down as a discontinuous structure of separate fibers and fibrils in a matrix. The analogy with artificial composite materials, like fiber glass, is obvious. The relation between fiber and matrix in determining mechanical properties has had a good deal of attention [109] and it is best to begin the discussion by considering briefly how this knowledge can be applied to collagenous structures. It seems reasonable to begin by considering these as consisting of discontinuous fibers (i.e., of finite length) in a plastic matrix, and to take the case where the

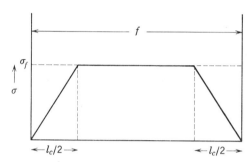

Figure 11.4. Expected variation of stress along a fiber within a plastic matrix. Abscissa, position along fiber of total length f; l_c = critical length; ordinate, shear stress at fiber surface, σ_f = flow stress of matrix [110].

fibers are all oriented in a single direction. If such a structure is subjected to tension along the axis of the fibers, the fibers are put under stress by the shear-stresses that develop at their surfaces. The tension in an individual fiber in theory should build up from the ends linearly towards the middle, up to a maximum determined by the yield-stress of the matrix (Fig. 11.4). When this is exceeded the fiber moves through the matrix. As stress builds up from the ends, there is a critical length of fiber below which its tensile properties are not fully utilized. For the same reason in a composite of fibers of uniform cross-section along their length there is a waste of material in this end region, in the sense that tension is always below the maximum reached beyond the critical distance. One cannot help observing that the ends of collagen fibers seem to be tapered [11], a feature that would avoid such a waste of material though it is perhaps fanciful to suppose this could have any biological significance.

When one tries to consider collagen fibers in terms of such a model, one finds one cannot progress far beyond the above theoretical ideas since there really is no information as to the length of the fibers, the nature of their surfaces or of the material between them. Tregear [210] has considered a model based on an array of rods (corresponding to fibers or fibrils) evenly spaced in a viscous medium; taking a measurement of the rate of viscous extensibility [78] and assuming slip was occurring between fibrils 500 Å in diameter and 100 Å apart in a medium of higher viscosity (10^4 c. poise, corresponding to 0.1–0.5% hyaluronic acid) he found a requirement of fibril length of 2 mm. Lower viscosity or larger fiber diameters would require longer fibrils. This is an interesting calculation. The weakest point is perhaps the assumption about interfibrillar distance. If the fibrils are not parallel but, as seems quite possible, arranged in helices then longitudinal tension will produce a force directly inwardly along the radius tending to press the fibrils together (as in wool or textile yarns); the important consideration then will be the frictional properties of the fiber surfaces.

Our first interest in the problem of the interrelationship between fibrils and interfibrillary material in mechanical properties arose from observations on the changes in the mammalian birth canal, in particular the cervix of the uterus, before parturition. One change was an increased plasticity in the connective tissue, that was assumed to be the result of a change in the matrix between the collagen fibrils [76]. The object of the experiments that will be discussed in the next sections was originally to try to find out about this matrix using a material that was easier to obtain and handle experimentally, namely, the skin. In fact, it appears difficult to interpret any of the experiments in terms of a matrix of known components of connective tissue, though a number can be interpreted in terms of cross-linkages in collagen. In the subsequent discussion then the initial hypothesis will be that the effects described are to be explained in terms of change in the collagen.

The collagen molecule is itself a stable structure of three polypeptide chains wound round each other and held together by many hydrogen bonds, and generally also by specific covalent intramolecular linkages [178]. However, it is difficult to believe these latter contribute materially to the mechanical stability of the structure though they might prevent proteolytic enzymes attacking the chains from the ends. When the molecules are associated together regularly as in native collagen [96], the stability of the structure mechanically will depend, one would expect, first on the intermolecular forces that lead to the formation of the regular structure and hold it together, and, second, on the later development of additional linkages including covalent ones. The contribution of these latter linkages to mechanical strength will be discussed later. The mechanical stability of the initial uncross-linked association has not been investigated.

Cross-linkages in Collagen

There is much evidence of a general nature about cross-linkages in collagen [70]. Direct information about their chemical nature is more limited. The linkages that are most thoroughly understood, largely owing to the work of Piez and his colleagues [177, 178] are intramolecular, between lysine molecules with their amino terminals converted to alde-hyde groups (allysine) near the *N*-terminal ends of the individual chains of the triple helix. In addition, recently, Bailey [5] has described inter-molecular linkages found in rat-tail tendon, of two sorts; first, in rat-

Intermolecular link   Intramolecular link

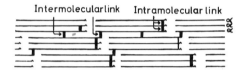

Figure 11.5. Diagrammatic representation of the structure of collagen. The three chains (α) of each helix are represented unwound with the amino head end marked so $\curlywedge$; cross-links are represented so $\mathbf{I}$; intramolecular links and two sorts of possible intermolecular links are shown, side-to-side near the middle of the molecule, head-to-tail near the end; the molecules are placed in a quarter-stagger arrangement, but, as it is a planar diagram, the true situation cannot be shown, nor can links in another plane, for example head-to-head; an irregular distribution of links is shown to illustrate variation in intramolecular linkage and the essentially unknown frequency and detailed position of intermolecular links [123].

tendon collagen, a Schiff-base (azomethine) link between a lysine derived aldehyde as above, and the ϵ-amino group of a hydroxylysine residue [8], and, second, in bone and dentine, a link resembling the intramolecu-lar ones, but formed between a hydroxylysine and a lysine derived alde-hyde [7]. In addition to this specific chemical information, there is electromicroscopical information [125], obtained from insoluble collagen brought into solution enzymically and then precipitated as segment long-spacing collagen that appeared in various forms, indicating the presence of linkages of three sorts, side-to-side, head-to-tail, and head-to-head (Fig. 11.5, showing the conventionalized quarter-stagger arrange-ment in one plane, and omitting head-to-head links that would have to be formed in another plane).

There is much presumptive evidence that cross-linkages in collagen are important in determining mechanical strength. In *lathyrism* [201], a condition produced by giving animals the seeds of peas of the genus lathyrus to eat or the active principle β-amino propionitrile or a number of other compounds [128], increased solubility of collagen is associated with tissue weakness [129, 54]. There is a failure in the formation of the lysine aldehydes, probably due to inhibition of the enzyme concerned by the lathyrogenic agent [179]. As it is not clear how these links could be concerned in mechanical properties, it seems likely that the mechanical defect is due to an accompanying failure in the formation of intermolecular links. As noted below, penicillamine applied *in vitro* to the skin [87] weakens it but leaves a substantial number of these links unbroken [159]. They are resistant to change of pH that markedly reduces strength as described below.

Administration of *penicillamine* to rats similarly leads to tissue weakness, particularly affecting skin [161]. In this case also intramolecular cross linking is inhibited [158]. The evidence is that the lysine derived aldehydes are formed but blocked by combination with the reagent [39]. The mechanical weakness is attributable probably to simultaneous blocking of aldehyde groups normally forming intermolecular links, possibly of the Schiff-base type, to be discussed later.

Nature of Links Concerned in Tensile Strength of Skin

Evidence about the nature of the changes that result in weakening of the tissue in lathyrism and after administration of penicillin is essentially circumstantial, and based on an association between mechanical and chemical changes. Particularly in the case of lathyrism it is clear a number of changes occur in the tissue, and the selection of those affecting cross-links in collagen to explain the mechanical defect, though reasonable, is to some extent arbitrary. In this section we consider first some further circumstantial evidence obtained by the direct action of various reagents on the tensile strength of skin, that seems to fit well the hypothesis that Schiff-base links play a critical part in this property. After this a number of other observations of effects of reagents that in some cases are strikingly large will be described, though at the moment their mechanism is obscure. Nearly all this evidence was obtained from experiments on rings of the tail skin of 30–50-day-old rats. These rings, or circular strips of skin, about 2.5 mm wide, were placed as a belt round two parallel cylindrical rods, and extended by pulling these rods apart [76, 79, 72]. The tension in the skin was increased at a constant rate to the point of rupture, the rate of loading being such as to give a break time in the region of 3–5 min for fresh untreated skin. The breaking load falls approximately linearly down the tail at a slightly greater rate than the taper in diameter, and to allow for this, rings were treated in pairs at equal distances above and below a point. Rings were in general treated with reagents dissolved in phosphate buffered (0.02 M) physiological saline at either 4 or 37°C. Most of the experiments were done with whole skin but the main effects have been checked on dermis freed from epidermis [72].

In vitro Effects Possibly Explicable in Terms of Intermolecular Azomethine Cross-Links in Collagen

Thiol Reagents. A number of reagents containing thiol groups can reduce the strength of skin markedly (to near zero) at neutral pH [81]. So far as the evidence goes, these fall into two groups according to whether or not there is an amino group on an adjacent carbon atom. For those without such a group (thioglycollic acid and mercaptoethanol) the weakening effect is less marked and differently pH dependent; at higher pH, 8 or over, they have little effect or may actually increase strength. Amino-thiols (cysteamine, cysteine, penicillamine) have a greater effect and it continues in regions of higher pH. The contrast between the two effects is seen most clearly by comparing the same reagent with and without the amino group blocked by acetylation (Fig. 11.6). A similar effect is obtained by comparing penicillamine and

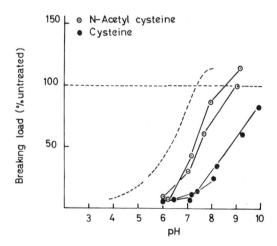

Figure 11.6. Effect of cysteine (●) and N-acetylcysteine (○) on strength in tension of skin of the rats tail: rings of skin were left overnight in 0.1 M solution of the reagent in phosphate (20 mM) buffered physiological saline (0.13 M NaCl), adjusted to various pH levels with HCl or NaOH; lines join means of pairs of rings from an individual tail; dotted line is the simple effect of pH (see Fig. 11.7) [87].

N-acetyl-penicillamine [87]. The effect is produced by concentrations down to between 1 and 10 mM. The effects of some of these reagents are at least partially reversible if they are removed, but that of penicillamine cannot be reversed in this way.

Among the thiol reagents described above as affecting the strength of the skin, cysteine occurs naturally. Other naturally-occurring reagents that have similar effects are glutathione and homocysteine. Gluthathione can reduce strength when applied in 2.5 mM concentration which is in the range of natural occurrence—for example in the liver.

It has been pointed out by Bailey [5] that this effect of amino thiols could be explained by their attacking Schiff-base links, as they might be expected to do. Another obvious hypothesis to explain the weakening effect of thiols in general is that it could be the result of their attacking disulphide links in a protein-containing cementing material between the fibers, but experiments to test this idea produced no confirmatory evidence [82].

Another possibility was that the effects were enzymic since thiol reagents activate many proteases. The reversibility of some of the effects makes this unlikely; previous treatment of skin in acetone does not prevent them; also a short treatment with the thiol followed by application of iodoacetamide which might be expected to inactivate an enzyme after previous activation to the —SH form, did not prevent the subsequent effect of further exposure to thiol reagents [81]. In general, the than an enzymic hypothesis, which could not be extended to cover the observations that will be described below.

Pyridoxal-5'-Phosphate. This reagent, which reacts rather specifically with amino groups [12], can reduce the strength of skin [83]. Treatment in the presence of lysine reduces the effect, which confirms that it is associated with this amino-reacting property. The effect is reversible on removing the reagent. Treatment of the tissue in the weakened state with hydroxylamine or hydrazine prevents this reversal. This effect is nicely explicable on the hypothesis that the reaction of the pyridoxal phosphate frees an aldehyde group, the blocking of which by the aldehyde-reacting agents prevents recovery.

In connection with this effect it is of interest that Page, Benditt, and Kirkwood [69] record that pyridoxal phosphate can react readily with some of the lysyl and hydroxylysyl side chains of collagen but only a small number (1 lysyl and 2 hydroxylysyl per chain).

Sodium Borohydride. Treatment of purified collagen, reprecipitated in native form, with sodium borohydride renders it insoluble [201], an effect which it was suggested could be explained by stabilization of Schiff-base (—C=N—) links by reduction. This reagent in tritiated form was used by Bailey & Peach [87] to isolate the link of this type referred to earlier. Treatment of whole rat-tail skin with sodium borohydride increases its strength, as much as doubling it. The reagent incidentally loosens the epidermis and causes it to fall off; the effect on strength is on the dermis. It also makes it resistant to the action of amino-thiols [82]. Conversely, previous treatment with penicillamine inhibits its effect in increasing strength as would be expected if both reagents reacted at the same point in the tissue.

Thus, the effect of sodium borohydride also fits the hypothesis that Schiff-base links are important in determining the strength of the dermis.

Effect of pH. One of the most striking effects on the strength of the skin of the rat's tail is that of pH shown in Fig. 11.7 [74]. The most interesting feature of the effect of pH is perhaps the strong reduction in strength in the range from physiological downwards to about pH 5. This effect is reversible on return to pH 7.5 (Fig. 11.8). Recovery of

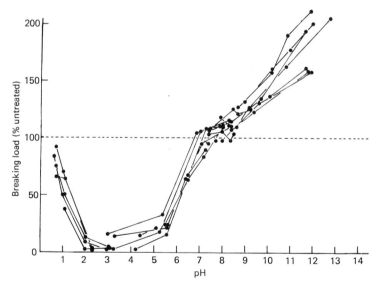

Figure 11.7   Effect of pH on strength of rat's tail skin. Rings of skin were left overnight at 4°C in phosphate-buffered physiological saline (see Fig. 11.6) adjusted to the required pH with HCl or NaOH. Lines join means of pairs of ring from the same tail [84].

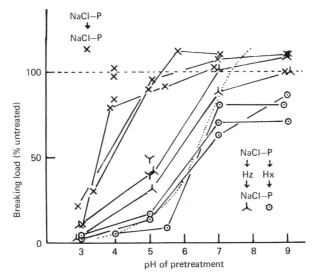

Figure 11.8. Effect of hydroxylamine and hydrazine after pretreatment in NaCl phosphate at different pH levels. Rings were treated with phosphate-buffered physiological saline (see Fig. 11.6) overnight at the pH on the abscissa; then with the same solution at pH 7.5, with (⊙⅄), or without (×) an intervening 2 hours' treatment with 0.1 M hydroxylamine (⊙) or hydrazine (⅄) at pH of 9. The lines join means of pairs of rings from the same tail; the dotted line gives the simple effect of pH [23a].

strength is inhibited by treatment in the weakened state with hydrazine or hydroxylamine (Fig. 11.8) as in the case of pyridoxal-5'-phosphate [83]. If the tissue is pretreated with sodium borohydride before being subjected to altered pH, the effect of the latter in this range is abolished (Fig. 11.9). These effects are compatible with the hypothesis that weakening produced by lowering pH, is associated with the breaking of Schiff-base links, either as a result of a configurational change or because they are labile to reduction in pH.

Summary. Experiments of the type we have been considering cannot give precise evidence on the nature of the linkages affected, but the hypothesis that Schiff-base links play a critical part in determining mechanical strength appears to form a reasonable basis for an explanation of the results. It seems probable that solubilization of collagen involves rupture of the same links. Amino thiols as well as weakening skin also solubilize collagen [87, 158, 160]. If, as seems probable, they act in virtue of a specific effect on a particular type of link, their solubilizing effect could be used perhaps as a test of its presence. At any rate their use in investigation of "solubility" of collagen would seem likely to provide more valuable evidence than the various buffers commonly used.

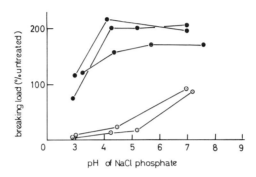

Figure 11.9. Effect of varying pH on breaking load for rat's tail skin after treatment with sodium borohydride. Pairs of rings were treated either with 0.1 *M* NaBH₄ or 0.1 *M* tris at pH 10, 4°C, and then put in phosphate buffered physiological saline (see Fig. 11.6) overnight (4°C) at the pH on the abscissa. Lines join means of pairs of rings from a single tail [82].

Other in vitro Effects

Effect of Amino-Group Reacting Substances Other Than Puridoxal Phosphate; Nitrite; Maleic Anhydride. Treatment with nitrite at pH 5, which might be expected to weaken the tissue, in fact has the opposite effect of increasing its strength to about twice the normal and making it insusceptible to pH. Maleic anhydride applied in an aqueous medium had almost no effect, presumably because it decomposes more rapidly than it diffuses into the solid tissue. Applied in alcohol or acetone, it altered the reaction of the tissue to pH in subsequent tests in aqueous solution. Strength at pH 7 was near zero but rose to a maximum about 50% of normal at about pH 5. These findings above are unpublished observations of our own.

Both these reagents clearly have widespread effects and one cannot without more information draw any useful conclusions from the above results.

Effect of Cyanide. If the tissue is treated with solutions of different pH in the presence of cyanide the strength at physiological pH is increased [80] and the effect of pH reduction is inhibited (Fig. 11.10,

[72]) rather in the same way as it is by pretreatment with sodium borohydride. This cyanide effect can be detected in concentrations down to between 10^{-5} and 10^{-4} M. It is reversible on removing the reagent. Though this rather dramatic effect of cyanide has been known for some time its explanation is still obscure. The fact that it can take place at low temperature (4°C) and low pH (down to pH 5) indicates that it is not the result of an action on the metabolic activity of the cells.

Effect of Halogenating Agents. Pretreatment with iodine has a similar effect to that of sodium borohydride on the subsequent reaction of the tissue to alteration of pH [87]. Bromine and hypochlorite also have a similar effect (unpublished observations). The explanation of these effects is obscure.

Effect of Aldehyde-Reacting Agents on Subsequent Reaction to pH. The effect of hydroxylamine and hydrazine in preventing recovery from reduced pH has been discussed. These reagents and phenylhydrazine have another effect when applied to fresh tissue. Brief treatment (at pH 9) inhibits the effect of reduction of pH in subsequent exposure to solutions at different pH levels [84]. This apparent stabilizing effect is difficult to understand in terms of the Schiff-base link hypothesis. One would expect these reagents if anything to rupture such links. There is evidence that they can do this [17]. The effect of the reagents is rapid with higher concentrations of reagent (0.1 M); with overnight treatment at 4°C the threshold level for demonstration of activity was between 10^{-5} and 10^{-4} M for hydrazine, though somewhat higher for

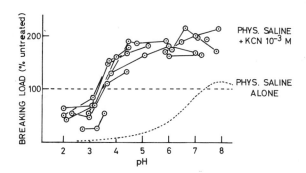

Figure 11.10. Effect of cyanide on breaking load for rat-tail skin at different hydrogen ion concentrations. Rings treated overnight at 4°C with 10^{-3} M KCN in phosphate (20 mM) buffered physiological saline, adjusted to different pH values with HCl. Lines join means of pairs of rings from a single tail [72].

hydroxylamine, possibly because this reagent decomposes quite rapidly in aqueous solution. Phenylhydrazine was also active but in higher concentration (10^{-2}–10^{-1} M), an effect which, however, cannot be accounted for by its contamination with hydrazine.

The effects of these reagents and of sodium borohydride interfere mutually; if the reagents are used in succession the effect is primarily that of the first used [84].

Other aldehyde reacting agents have different effects again to the above (semicarbazide, sulphite-bisulphite, dimedone) [84].

Effect of Dextran Sulfate. It was found by Milch [152] that exposure of skin to solutions of dextran sulfate reduced its strength. We have confirmed this observation and found additionally that the effect is reversible on removal of the reagent (unpublished). Unlike the effects previously described, it takes a long time (days). Though the mechanism of this effect is not known, this observation of Milch is interesting in view of the resemblances in structure between the reagent and the sulfated glycosaminoglycans of unknown function present in the tissue. It is also interesting that an effect of dextran sulfate *in vivo* has been described [47].

Effect of Enzymes on Mechanical Properties of Skin. The absence of effect of hyaluronidase on the strength of skin was discussed previously. Proteolytic enzymes trypsin and chymotrypsin on the other hand have been reported to have a large effect on skin of newborn rats [77], on the tensile strength and on the ability of the tissue to extend slowly under constant load. The effect of these enzymes appears to be considerably less in older animals (unpublished observations). The nature of these effects is not clear. They were originally interpreted as indicating a mechanical role for a noncollagenous protein. The role of noncollagenous peptides in collagen structure is still not clear [95, 186, 183, 40]. There is a great deal of evidence that enzymes can alter the properties of collagen [95, 122, 123, 124, 186, 67, 165].

Conclusions: Functional Aspects of Variation in Mechanical Properties of Skin

It is of interest, finally, to consider how the various factors found empirically to affect the strength of skin might enter its function in real life.

Effect of Age. The question of increased cross-linking of collagen with age and its effects has been much discussed in the literature. The strength of the skin per unit of collagen in cross-section appears, so far as there is any evidence [53] to increase with age by a factor of about 3 in the rat. This could be attributed to increased cross-linking for which there is other evidence. The effect of some of the reagents discussed above in rats diminishes with age (cysteamine, CN, unpublished observations), as has been found by Bailey [5] in tendon. The effect might be explained by Schiff-base cross-links becoming altered and stabilized as happens when they are reduced. But they are not apparently stabilized in this way *in vivo* since the cross-link obtained by borohydride reduction has not been found to occur naturally in older animals [8a]. It would be interesting to know whether the reported reduction with age in solubility of collagen in solutions sodium chloride (salt-soluble collagen) or mildly acid buffers is correlated with change in tensile strength, but the two properties do not appear to have been examined together in the same animals.

Regarding the question of increase in cross-linking with age, it is worth pointing out that even though some cross-linking between molecules may be critical for mechanical strength, a further increase may not necessarily improve the mechanical properties and might have the opposite effect. Thus, cross-linking collagen in leather may weaken it [31, 91]. The reason is probably that an excess of cross-linking increases the rigidity of a structure, and so may increase local stresses by reducing the ability of the structure to adapt to distribute them. It is possible to regard the carbohydrate groups that are found attached to many of the lysine residues in some collagens as anticross-linking agents, preventing these lysines from being utilized as cross-links [26].

Function of Labile Bonds Affecting Mechanical Properties. One of the most striking features of experiments *in vitro* on effects of reagents on tensile strength is the apparent lability of the links involved, whatever they may be, as judged by the mildness of some of the treatments that produce large effects. This introduces the possibility of their being involved in normal function. Thus, intracellular pH may be as low as pH 5, and extracellular pH in areas of inflammation nearly as low [136]. This would be low enough to reduce strength to about one fifth in the rat's tail skin. It is of interest that pain may be produced by injection of acid solutions intradermally, the intensity increasing with hydrogen ion concentration in a similar way to the effect in reducing strength, though solutions of high pH also induce pain. In connection with pH and normal function is of interest that simple incubation of the skin of the rat's tail in weakly buffered physiological saline containing glucose can drastically reduce its strength [78], without altering the pH of the solution

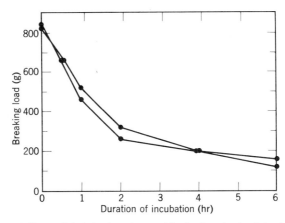

Figure 11.11. Effect of incubation in weakly buffered physiological saline containing glucose on breaking load of rings of rat-tail skin. Rings incubated at 37°C for the time given on the abscissa in buffered physiological saline (Lockes solution) at pH 7.5 in the presence of glucose (5.5 mM); lines join results for rings from an individual tail. The pH of the solution does not change [72].

(Fig. 11.11). This observation has not been fully examined but the effect was attributed to local reduction in pH because it was not found if the buffering power of the surrounding solution was increased. One can also see the possibility of cells using naturally occurring amino-thiols to release the collagenous structure to alter its shape. In this connection the observations of Klein [117, 118] on the metabolic "reutilization" of collagen are of particular interest. The process by which the new collagen is welded on to the old at the edge of a wound has never to my knowledge received any attention, and it is reasonable to suppose it might involve a local rearrangement of the old collagen. Though alteration of shape in hard collagenous tissues in development and growth is brought about by a combination of deposition and reabsorption, it is difficult to believe that change of shape by movements of parts of the framework relatively to one another play no part in soft tissues like the skin. Indeed, the hypothesis that such movement takes place would better fit the low turnover and long persistence of metabolic labelling [71], though admittedly a hypothesis of reutilization of a different sort would also fit.

Finally, perhaps it is worth mentioning that the production of change in mechanical properties by direct application of mild reagents raises the possibility of producing pharmacological effects on the connective-tissue framework by direct application of reagents to the skin surface.

ACKNOWLEDGEMENTS

I am very grateful to the following colleagues for advice and discussion: P. R. Bell, A. de A. Bellairs, W. G. Chaloner, P. A. Jewell, R. D. Martin, A. R. Ness, and K. Taylor.

REFERENCES

1. G. W. Arnold, "Factors within plant associations affecting the behavior and performance of grazing animals," in *Grazing in Terrestrial and Marine Environments,* Crisp, D. J., Ed., Blackwell, Oxford, pp. 133–154 (1964).

2. W. Andrew, *Amer. J. Anat.,* **89**, 283 (1951).

3. H. N. Andrews, *Paleobotany,* John Wiley and Sons, New York, (1961) p. 40.

4. S. C. Arya and F. Fulton, *J. Pathol. Bacteriol.,* **89,** 747 (1965).

5. A. J. Bailey, *Biochem. Biophys. Acta,* **160,** 447 (1968).

6. A. J. Bailey, Peach, C. M., and Fowler, L. J. In *Chemistry and Molecular Biology of the Intercellular Matrix,* E. A. Balazs, Ed., **1,** p. 385, Academic Press, London, (1970).

7. A. J. Bailey, L. J. Fowler, and C. M. Peach, *Biochem. Biophys. Res. Comm.,* **35,** 663 (1969).

8. A. J. Bailey and C. M. Peach, *Biochem. J.,* **111,** 12 (1969).

9. J. R. Baker and D. A. Balch, *Biochem. J.,* **82,** 352 (1962).

10. G. A. Balian and J. H. Bowes, *Nature,* **213,** 518 (1967).

11. W. G. Banfield, *Proc. Soc. Exptl. Biol. N.Y.,* **81,** 658 (1952).

12. B. E. C. Banks, In *The Chemistry of the Amino Group,* S. Patai, Ed., p. 499, Interscience, London, (1968).

13. T. Barbour, *Reptiles and Amphibians, their Habits and Adaptation,* Harrap, London, (1923).

14. R. S. Bear, *Adv. Protein Chem.,* **7,** 69 (1952).

15. A. d'A Bellairs, *The Life of Reptiles,* Weidenfeld and Nicholson, London, (1970).

16. R. Bellairs, M. L. R. Harkness, and R. D. Harkness, *J. Ultrastructure Res.,* **8,** 339 (1963).

17. H. B. Bensusan, S. D. McKnight, and M. S. R. Naidu, *Biochem. Biophys. Res. Comm.,* **23,** 128 (1966).

18. L. Bertin, In *Traité, de Zoologie,* P. P. Grassé, Ed., **13,** 482 Masson, Paris (1958).

19. L. Bertin, In *Traité de Zoologie,* P. P. Grassé, Ed., **13,** 505 Masson, Paris (1958).

20. I. H. Blank and O. G. Miller, *J. Invest. Dermatol.,* **15,** 9 (1950).

21. F. Bourlière, In *Traité de Zoologie,* P. P. Grassé, Ed., **17,** 1806 (1955).

22. J. H. Bowes, R. G. Elliot, and J. A. Moss, *Connective Tissue,* CIOMS Symp., R. E. Tunbridge, Ed., Blackwell, Oxford p. 264 (1957).

22a. R. Braams, *Internat. J. Radiation Biol.,* **2,** 229 (1960).

23. A. S. Breathnach, In *Progress in the Biological Sciences in Relation to Dermatology,* A. Rook and R. H. Champion, Eds., Cambridge University Press, Cambridge, p. 415 (1964).

23a. L. Brown, M. L. R. Harkness, and R. D. Harkness, *Acta Physiol. Hungary.*

24. J. P. E. Burbach, In *Progress in the Biological Sciences in Relation to Dermatology,* A. Rook and R. H. Champion, Eds., Cambridge University Press, Cambridge, p. 443 (1964).

25. M. Burton, *The Hedgehog.* Deutsch, London, p. 17 (1969).

26. W. T. Butler and L. W. Cunningham, *J. Biol. Chem.,* **241,** 3882 (1966).

26a. P. A. Buxton, *The Louse.* Edwards, London (1939).

26b. P. A. Buxton, *The natural history of tsetse flies.* London School of Hygiene and Tropical Medicine. Memoir No. 10 (1955).

27. W. O. Carter, A. B. Simon, and W. D. Armstrong, *Amer. J. Physiol.,* **183,** 317 (1955).

28. N. Cauna, *Anat. Rec.,* **119,** 449 (1954).

28a. S. R. Christophers. *Aëdes aegypti* (L) *The yellow fever mosquito* p. 484, Cambridge University Press (1960).

29. A. Ciferri and L. V. Rajagh, *J. Gerontol.,* **19,** 144 (1964).

30. A. N. Clements, *The Physiology of Mosquitoes,* Macmillan, London, p. 144, (1963).

31. E. D. Compton, *J. Amer. Leather Chemists' Assoc.,* **44,** 141 (1949).

32. G. O. Conabere and R. H. Hall, *J. Soc. Leather Trades Chem.,* **34,** 57 (1950).

33. D. R. Cooper and P. Johnson, *Biochim. Biophys. Acta,* **26,** 317 (1957).

34. M. J. Costello and R. C. Gibbs, *The Palms and Soles in Medicine,* Thomas, Springfield, (1967).

35. H. Cummins and C. Midlo, *Finger-prints, Palms and Soles,* Dover, New York, (1961).

36. C. Delbrouck, *Hansteins. Bot. Abhandl.,* **2,** (1875).

37. M. Dempsey and M. E. Garrod, *Ann. Appl. Biol.,* **34,** 435 (1947).

38. M. Dempsey, B. M. Haines, and J. H. Hitchborn, *J. R. Microsc. Soc.,* **75,** 176 (1955).

39. K. Desmukh and M. E. Nimni, *J. Biol. Chem.,* **244,** 1787 (1969).

40. Z. Deyl, J. Rosmus, and S. Bump, *Biochim. Biophys. Acta,* **140,** 515 (1967).

41. H. H. Donaldson, *The Rat,* Memorial Wistar Institute, **6,** 9184 (1924).

42. I. C. Dick, *J. Anat.,* **81,** 201 (1947).

43. L. Eichelberger, C. W. Eisele, and D. Wetzler, *J. Biol. Chem.,* **151,** 177 (1943).

44. C. W. Eisele and L. Eichelberger, *Proc. Soc. Exptl. Biol.,* **58,** 97 (1945).

46. H. R. Elden, this book in H. R. Elden, (Ed.), A Treatise on the Skin, Volume 1, Interscience, N.Y., p. 1, (1971).

47. H. A. Ellis, *J. Path. Bacteriol.,* **89,** 437 (1965).

48. Z. Felsher, *J. Invest. Dermatol,* **8**, 35 (1947).
49. Z. Felsher, *Anat. Rec.,* **154**, 513 (1966).
50. R. Fleischmajer, *J. Invest. Dermatol.,* **48**, 359 (1965).
51. L. J. Flemister, *Amer. J. Physiol.,* **135**, 430 (1942).
52. H. Frädrich, *Z. Tierpsychol.,* **22**, 328 (1965).
53. P. Fry, M. L. R. Harkness, and R. D. Harkness, *Amer. J. Physiol.,* **206**, 1425 (1964).
54. P. Fry, M. L. R. Harkness, R. D. Harkness, and M. Nightingale, *J. Physiol.,* **164**, 77 (1962).
55. M. Gabe, *Traité de Zoologie,* P. P. Grassé, Ed., **16**, 50 Masson, Paris, (1967).
56. V Geist, *J. Mammal.,* **45**, 551 (1964).
57. V. Geist, *Behavior,* **27**, 175 (1966).
58. V. Geist, *J. Wildlife Management,* **31**, 192 (1967).
59. I. Gersh and H. R. Catchpole, *Amer. J. Anat.,* **85**, 457 (1949).
60. D. Gilbert, P. D. Mier, and T. E. Jones, *J. Invest. Dermatol.,* **40**, 165 (1963).
60a. R. M. Gordon and W. Crewe, *Ann. trop. Med. Parasitol.,* **42**, 334 (1948).
61. R. M. Gordon and W. Crewe, *Ann. trop. Med. Parasitol.,* **47**, 74 (1953).
61a. R. M. Gordon and W. H. R. Lumsden, *Ann. trop. Med. Parasitol.,* **33**, 259 (1939).
62. R. Grahame and P. Beighton, *Ann. Rheum. Dis.,* **28**, 246 (1969).
62a. R. B. Griffiths and R. M. Gordon, *Ann. trop. Med. Parasitol.,* **46**, 311 (1952).
63. P. P. Grassé, In *Traité de Zoologie,* P. P. Grassé, Ed., **17**, 1729 Masson, Paris, (1955).
64. W. E. Le Gros, Clark, *Proc. Zool. Soc. London,* p. 1. (1936).
65. C. A. W. Guggisberg, *S.O.S. Rhino.,* Deutsch, London, (1968).
66. C. A. W. Guggisberg, *Giraffes,* p. 45, Barker, London, (1969).
67. R. Hafter and H. Hörmann, *Z. Phys. Chem.,* **330**, 169 (1963).
68. E. R. Hall, *American Weasels,* University of Kansas, Museum of Natural History, **4**, 1 (1951).
69. J. B. S. Haldane, *Possible Worlds and Other Essays,* Chatto and Windus, London, 1927.
70. J. J. Harding, *Advan. Protein Chem.,* **20**, 109 (1965).
71. R. D. Harkness, *Biol. Rev.,* **36**, 399 (1961).
72. R. D. Harkness, In *Wound Healing,* Sir C. Illingworth, Ed., Lister Centenary Symp. p. 243, Churchill, London, (1966).
73. R. D. Harkness, "Mechanical properties of collagenous tissues," in *Treatise on Collagen.* B. S. Gould, Ed., Vol. 2A, p. 247, Academic Press, New York, (1968).
74. R. D. Harkness, In *Chemistry and Molecular Biology of the Intercellular Matrix,* E. A. Balazs, Ed., **3**, 1309 Academic Press, London, (1970).
75. M. L. R. Harkness and R. D. Harkness, *J. Physiol.,* **132**, 492 (1956).
76. M. L. R. Harkness and R. D. Harkness, *J. Physiol.,* **148**, 524 (1959).
77. M. L. R. Harkness and R. D. Harkness, *Nature,* **183**, 1821 (1959).

78. M. L. R. Harkness and R. D. Harkness, In *Symposium on Biorheology,* A. L. Copley, Ed., p. 477, Wiley, New York, (1964).

79. M. L. R. Harkness and R. D. Harkness, In *The Structure and Function of Connective and Skeletal Tissues,* p. 376, Butterworths, London, (1965).

80. M. L. R. Harkness and R. D. Harkness, *Nature,* **205,** 912 (1965).

81. M. L. R. Harkness and R. D. Harkness, *Nature,* **211,** 496 (1966).

82. M. L. R. Harkness and R. D. Harkness, *Biochim. Biophys. Acta,* **154,** 553 (1968).

83. M. L. R. Harkness and R. D. Harkness, *Experientia,* **25,** 1048 (1969).

85. M. L. R. Harkness, R. D. Harkness, and D. W. James, *J. Physiol.,* **144,** 307 (1958).

86. R. D. Harkness, A. M. Marko, H. M. Muir, and A. Neuberger, *Biochem. J.,* **57,** 558 (1954).

87. R. D. Harkness and M. E. Nimni, *Acta Physiol. Hungary,* **33,** 325 (1968).

88. W. B. Herms and M. T. James, *Medical Entomology,* Macmillan, New York, (1961), p. 380.

89. H. Hertel, In *The Biology of Marine Animals,* H. T. Anderson, Ed., Academic Press, New York, (1969).

90. K. Herter, In *Hanbuch der Zoologie* (Kükenthal) VIII 10(10), Gruyter, Berlin, (1957).

91. J. H. Highberger, *J. Amer. Leather Assoc.,* **42,** 493 (1947).

92. J. H. Highberger, *The Chemistry and Technology of Leather.* Vol. 1. Reinhold, New York, (1956).

93. A. V. Hill, *Proc. Roy. Inst.,* **34,** 450 (1949).

94. C. A. Hoare, *Trans. Roy. Soc. Trop. Med. Hyg.,* **23,** 39 (1929).

95. A. J. Hodge, J. H. Highberger, G. G. J. Deffner, and F. O. Schmitt, *Proc. Natl. Acad. Sci. U.S.A.* **46,** 197 (1960).

96. A. J. Hodge, In *Treatise on Collagen,* G. N. Ramachandran, Ed., Vol. 1, p. 185, Academic Press, London, (1967).

97. A. J. Hodge, J. H. Highberger, G. G. J. Deffner, and F. O. Schmitt, *Proc. Nat. Acad. Sci.,* **46,** 197 (1960).

98. S. R. Hoover, S. J. Viola, A. H. Korn, and E. F. Mellon, *Science,* **121,** 672 (1955).

99. J. S. Hubbard, *J. Physiol.,* **141,** 198 (1958).

100. R. E. Hughes, C. Milner, and J. Dale, In *Grazing in terrestrial and marine environments,* D. J. Crisp, Ed., p. 189, Blackwell, Oxford, (1964).

101. J. H. Humphrey, A. Neuberger, and D. J. Perkins, *Biochem. J.,* **66,** 390 (1957).

102. A. Iggo and A. A. Muir, *J. Physiol.,* **200,** 763 (1969).

103. C. M. Jackson and L. G. Lowrey, *Anat. Rec.,* **6,** 449 (1912).

104. D. W. James, *Adv. Biol. Skin,* **5,** 216 (1964).

105. J. J. Johns and V. Wright, *J. Appl. Physiol.,* **17,** 824 (1962).

106. D. Jordan-Lloyd and R. H. Marriott, *Proc. Roy. Soc.,* **118,** 495 (1935).

107. J. R. Kanagy, *J. Amer. Leather Chemists' Assoc.,* **50,** 112 (1955).

108. J. R. Kanagy, E. B. Randall, T. J. Carter, R. A. Kinmouth, and C. V. Mann, *J. Amer. Leather Chemists' Assoc.*, **47,** 726 (1952).

108a. N. A. Kefalides, In *Chemistry and Molecular Biology of the Intercellular Matrix,* E. A. Balazs, Ed., **1,** p. 535, (1970).

109. A. Kelly and G. J. Davies, *Met. Rev.*, **10,** 1 (1965).

110. A. Kelly and W. R. Tyson, *Proceedings 2nd Internat. Materials Symposium,* Wiley, New York, 1964.

111. R. M. Kenedi, *Res. Devel.,* October, 18 (1963).

112. R. M. Kenedi, *Structural Eng.*, **42,** 101 (1964).

113. R. M. Kenedi, J. Gibson, and C. H. Daly, In *Structure and Function of Connective and Skeletal Tissues,* p. 388, Butterworth, London, (1964).

114. A. Kerner, von Marilaun and F. W. Oliver, *The Natural History of Plants,* Blackie, London, (1894), p. 430.

115. U. Kiistala, *J. Invest. Dermatol.*, **50,** 308 (1968).

116. U. Kiistala and K. K. Mustakallio, *J. Invest. Dermatol.*, **48,** 466 (1967).

117. L. Klein, *Proc. Eighth, Internat. Cong. Gerontol., II,* **14** (1969).

118. L. Klein, *Proc. Symp. on Biochem. Physiol. of Connective Tissue XII Cong. Rheumatol. Internat.,* p. 106, 1969.

119. H. Kruuk, *Behavior,* Supp. XI, (1964).

121. W. Kühme, *Z. Tierpsychol.*, **22,** 495 (1965).

122. K. Kühn, J. Kühn, and K. Hannig, *Z. Physiol. Chem.*, **326,** 50, (1961).

123. K. Kühn, P. Fietzek, and J. Kühn, *Naturwiss.*, **50,** 444, (1963).

124. K. Kühn, G. Schuppler, and J. Kühn, *Z. Physiol. Chem.* **338,** 10 (1964).

125. K. Kühn, J. Kühn, and P. Fietzek, *Biochem, Z.*, **344,** 418 (1966).

126. D. S. Kwon, P. Mason, and B. J. Rigby, *Nature,* **201,** 159 (1964).

126a. R. Lamson and J. J. Shaw, *Trans. Roy. Soc. Trop. Med. Hyg.*, **62,** 385, (1968).

127. T. C. Laurent, In *Chemistry and Molecular Biology of the Intercellular Matrix,* E. A. Balazs, Ed., **2,** p. 703, Academic Press, London, (1970).

127a. M. Leclerq, *Entomological Parasitology,* Pergamon: London, (1969).

128. C. I. Levene, *J. Expt. Med.*, **114,** 295 (1961).

129. C. I. Levene and J. Gross, *J. Expt. Med.*, **110,** 771 (1959).

130. R. M. Lewert, *Rice Institute Pamphlet,* **45,** 97 (1958).

131. R. M. Lewert and C. L. Lee, *J. Parisitol.*, **37,** 20 (1951).

132. R. M. Lewert and C. L. Lee, *J. Infect. Dis.*, **95,** 13 (1954).

133. R. M. Lewert and C. L. Lee, *J. Infect. Dis.* **99,** 1 (1956).

134. P. Leyhausen, In *Handbuch der Zoologie.* (Kükenthal) VIII, **10,** (21), (1956).

135. P. Leyhausen, *Z. Tierpsychol.*, **22,** 412 (1965).

136. O. Lindahl, *Acta Physiol. Scand. Suppl.*, **179,** 1 (1961).

137. B. L. Lowe and J. C. van der Leun, *J. Invest. Dermatol.*, **50,** 120 (1968).

138. W. R. Lowenstein and R. Skalak, *J. Physiol.*, **182,** 346 (1966).

139. T. H. McGavack and K T. Kao, *Expt. Med. Surg.*, **18,** 104 (1960).

140. J. C. Mackenzie, *Nature,* **222,** 881 (1969).

141. R. E. Mancini, *Int. Rev. Cytol.,* **14,** 193 (1963).

142. R. E. Mancini, O. Vilar, J. M. Dellacha, O. W. Davidson, C. J. Gomez, and B. Alvarez, *J. Histochem. Cytochem.,* **10,** 194 (1962).

143. J. F. Manery, *Physiol. Rev.,* **34,** 334 (1954).

144. J. F. Manery and A. B. Hastings, *J. Biol. Chem.,* **127,** 657 (1939).

145. A. Maroudas, *Biophys. J.,* **8,** 575 (1968).

146. M. J. Marples, *The Ecology of Human Skin,* Charles V. Thomas, Springfield (1965).

147. D. M. Maurice, In *The Eye,* H. Davson, Ed., Academic Press, New York, Vol. 1, p. 281. (1962).

147a. H. W. McCormick, T. Allen and W. E. Young. *Shadows in the Sea,* p. 281, Sidgwick Jackson: London, (1963).

148. R. Mellick and J. B. Cavanagh, *Expt. Neurol.,* **18,** 224 (1967).

149. E. F. Mellon and A. H. Korn, *J. Amer. Leather Chemists' Assoc.,* **51,** 469 (1956).

150. S. A. Mendoza and R. A. Milch, *Surg. Forum,* **15,** 433 (1964).

151. J. Menkart, J. H. Dillon, K. Beurling, J. G. Fee, and E. F. Mellon. *J. Amer. Leather Chemists' Assoc.,* **57,** 318, (1962).

152. R. A. Milch, *Biorheology,* **3,** 107 (1966).

153. V. Mizuhira, *Collagen Symp.,* **3,** 60 (1960).

154. E. Mohr, In *Die Neue Brehm Bücherii,* A. Ziemsen, Ed., Wittenberg-Lutherstadt, 1960.

155. P. E. D. Naylor, *St. John's Hosp., Trans., Dermatol. Soc.,* **31,** 29 (1952).

156. F. Netolitzky, In *Handbuch der Pflanzenanatomie,* K. Linsbauer, Ed., 1. Abt. 2. 2. Teil, Band IV. 1–253, (1932).

157. M. Niizuma, *Collagen Symp.,* **3,** 51 (1960).

158. M. E. Nimni, *Biochim. Biophys. Acta,* **111,** 576 (1965).

159. M. E. Nimni, *Biochem. Biophys. Res. Commun.,* **25,** 434 (1966).

160. M. E. Nimni, *J. Biol. Chem.,* **243,** 1457 (1968).

161. M. E. Nimni and L. A. Bavetta, *Proc. Soc. Expt. Biol. Med.,* **117,** 618 (1964).

162. M. E. Nimni and L. A. Bavetta, *Science,* **150,** 905 (1965).

163. F. Nürnberger and G. Müller, *Arch. Klin. Expt. Dermatol.* **232,** 345 (1968).

164. A. G. Ogston, In *Chemistry and Molecular Biology of the Intercellular Matrix.* E. A. Balazs, Ed., **3,** p. 1231, Academic Press, London, 1970.

165. B. R. Olsen, *Z. Zellforsch. mikrosk. Anat.* **61,** 913 (1964).

166. C. Oppenheimer and L. Pincussen, *Tabul. Biol.,* **2,** 469 (1925).

167. C. L. Ornes and W. T. Roddy, *J. Amer. Leather Chemists' Assoc.,* **55,** 124 (1960).

168. C. L. Ornes, W. T. Roddy, and E. F. Mellon, *J. Amer. Leather Chemists' Assoc.,* **55,** 600 (1960).

169. R. C. Page, E. P. Benditt, and C. R. Kirkwood, *Biochem. Biophys. Res. Commun.,* **33,** 752 (1968).

171. G. E. Palade and M. G. Farquhar, *J. Cell Biol.,* **27,** 215 (1965).
172. E. Palmer and N. Pitman, *Trees of South Africa,* Balkema: Cape Town, (1961), p. 153.
173. W. S. Patton and A. M. Evans, *Insects, Ticks, Mites and Venomous Animals,* H. B. Grubb, Croydon, (1929).
174. R. H. Pearce, In *The Amino Sugars,* E. A. Balazs and R. W. Jeanloz, Eds. Vol IIA., 149 (1965).
175. R. Perry, *The World of the Polar Bear,* p. 73, Cassell, London, (1966).
176. R. Perry, *The World of the Walrus,* Cassell, London, (1967).
176a. G. B. Pierce, In *Chemistry and Molecular Biology of the Intercellular Matrix.* E. A. Balazs, Ed., **1,** p. 471, Academic Press: London (1970).
177. K. A. Piez, Thule Internat. Symp., "Aging of Connective & Skeletal Tissue," A. Engel and T. Larsson, Eds., p. 15 (1968).
178. K. A. Piez, *Ann. Rev. Biochem.,* **37,** 547 (1968).
179. S. R. Pinnell and G. R. Martin, *Proc. Nat. Acad. Sci.,* **61,** 708 (1968).
180. R. I. Pocock, *Proc. Zool. Soc. Lond.,* 159 (1923).
181. K. R. Porter, *Biophys. J.,* **4,** 167 (1964).
182. G. N. Ramachandran, In *Treatise on Collagen,* G. N. Ramachandran, Ed., Vol. 1, p. 103, Academic Press, New York, (1967).
182a. G. G. Robinson, *Parasitology,* **31,** 212 (1939).
183. J. Rosmus, Z. Deyl, and M. P. Drake, *Biochim. Biophys. Acta,* **140,** 507 (1967).
184. M. A. Rougvie and R. S. Bear, *J. Amer. Leather Chemists' Assoc.,* **48,** 735 (1953).
185. A. L. Rubin, D. Pfahl, P. T. Speakman, P. F. Davison, and F. O. Schmitt, *Science,* **139,** 37 (1963).
186. A. L. Rubin, M. P. Drake, P. F. Davison, D. Pfahl, P. T. Speakman, and F. O. Schmitt, *Biochemistry,* **4,** 181 (1965).
187. G. B. Schaller, *The Deer and the Tiger,* p. 289, University of Chicago Press, Chicago, (1967).
188. S. Schiller and A. Dorfman, *Biochim. Biophys. Acta,* **15,** 305 (1955).
189. K. Schmidt-Nielsen, *Desert Animals,* Oxford University Press, London, (1964), p. 145.
190. S. D. Schultz-Haudt and N. Eeg-Larsen, *Biochim. Biophys. Acta,* **46,** 311, (1961).
191. A. C. Sellers, *J. Lab. Clin. Med.,* **68,** 177 (1967).
192. G. C. Shortridge, *The Mammals of South West Africa,* Vol 11, p. 664, Heinemann, London, (1934).
193. D. C. Simpson, Brit. Pat. 30169, (1969).
193a. R. E. Snodgrass, *Smithsonian Misc. Coll.,* **104,** No. 7, (1944).
193b. R. G. Spiro. In *Chemistry and Molecular Biology of the Intercellular Matrix* E. A. Balazs Ed., **1,** p. 511, Academic Press, London (1970).
194. F. Starmühlner, *Natur u. Volk,* **90,** 194 (1960).
194a. M. A. Stirewalt, In *The Biology of Parasites,* Ed. E. J. L. Soulsby, p. 41. Academic Press: New York (1966).

195. R. B. Stoughton, In *Progress in the Biological Sciences in Relation to Dermatology.* A. Rook and R. H. Champion, Eds. p. 431. Cambridge University Press, Cambridge, (1964).

196. M. B. Sulzberger, T. A. Cortese, L. Fishman, and H. S. Wiley, *J. Invest. Dermatol.,* **47,** 456 (1966).

197. J. L. Swanson and E. B. Helwig, *J. Invest. Dermatol.,* **50,** 195 (1968).

198. C. F. M. Swynnerton, *Proc. Zool. Soc. Lond.,* 180 (1923).

199. J. A. Szirmai, *The Amino Sugars* E. A. Balazs and R. W. Jeanloz, Eds., Vol. IIB. p. 129, Academic Press, New York, (1966).

200. D. Tabor, *Engineering,* **186,** 838 (1958).

201. M. L. Tanzer, *Biochem. Biophys. Acta,* **133,** 584 (1967).

202. M. L. Tanzer, *Int. Rev. Connective Tissue Res.,* **3,** 91 (1965).

203. G. Tembrock, In *Handbuch der Zoologie* (Kükenthal), VIII 10(15), (1957).

204. A. S. Thomas, *J. Ecology,* **31,** 149 (1943).

205. W. D'Arcy Thompson, *On Growth and Form,* Cambridge University Press, Cambridge, (1942).

206. S. J. Thurlow, *British J. Expt. Pathol.,* **44,** 538 (1963).

207. R. Timpl, and I. Pecker, *Z. ImmunForsch.,* **133,** 20 (1967).

208. R. Timpl, I. Wolff, H. Furthmayer, and M. Weiser, XII *Congressus Rheumatologicus Internationalis,* 1969, Prague, (1969).

209. B. P. Toole and D. A. Lowther, *Biochim. Biophys. Acta,* **121,** 135 (1966).

210. R. T. Tregear, *Physical Functions of Skin,* Academic Press, New York, 1966, p. 91.

211. E. J. van Scott, *J. Invest. Dermatol.,* **18,** 377 (1952).

212. A. G. Ward and F. W. Brooks, *J. Soc. Leather Trades Chem.,* **49,** 312 (1965).

213. P. Weiss, *J. Cell. Comp. Physiol.,* **49,** 105 (1957).

214. P. Weiss and W. Ferris, *Expt. Cell Res.,* **6,** 546 (1954).

215. P. Weiss and W. Ferris, *Proc. Nat. Acad. Sci.,* **40,** 528 (1954).

216. F. Wood-Jones, *Principles of Anatomy as Seen in the Hand,* Ballière, Tindall & Co., London, (1941).

217. F. Zannier, *Z. Tierpsychol.,* **22,** 672 (1965).

218. J. M. Zarek and J. Edwards, In *Biomechanics and Related Engineering Topics.* R. M. Kenedi, Ed., p. 187, Pergamon Press, Oxford, (1965).

12

Elasticity and Deformation of Skin

V. WRIGHT, M.D., F.R.C.P.

University Department of Medicine, General Infirmary at Leeds and Royal Bath Hospital, Harrogate.

Skin is a nonlinear, nonhomogenic, viscoelastic material. Its study is important from many angles. It is a readily accessible form of collagen and changes in this tissue may reflect changes elsewhere in the body; plastic surgery requires a knowledge of its biomechanics to determine the practical limits to which certain reconstructive techniques may be extended (such as the maximum practical angles for skin flaps, cut to relieve scarring); and it is involved in pathological conditions such as hereditable disorders of connective tissue, which exhibit a marked distensibility of skin. Considerable advances in the knowledge of the structure of rubber, plastics, and other polymers have been made through studies of their elastic and plastic properties. This has been convincingly demonstrated in the study of the creep behavior of a series of butyl rubbers differing in molecular architecture [1]. Connective tissue in normal and pathological situations studied similarly may yield information about alteration in elastic elements (collagen and elastin), in their crosslinking or wicker-work, and in the viscous medium (ground substance).

12.1 METHODS OF MEASUREMENT

Dick [2] tested skin by mounting a specimen as a circular diaphragm, one side of which was subject to hydrostatic pressure, which could be increased uniformly by raising the effective head. The deflection of the center of the diaphragm was amplified by a lever and read off a scale. This method has been modified for use *in vivo* recently [3]. There are certain disadvantages with this type of approach. The first is that tension in the specimen is calculated from the displacement of the center of the diaphragm, based on a theory for the deflection of diaphragms which holds for deflections considerably less than those obtained in the experiments. Moreover, the properties of skin vary in different directions which makes interpretation of the results difficult. The method precludes the determination of the humidity at which the specimen is being tested and this affects results considerably.

Another *in vivo* method has employed the Schade elastometer [4, 5, 6]. It consists of three small hemispheres arranged in a triangle. These are pressed lightly against the skin of a patient. The fourth hemisphere situated in the center of the triangle is then pressed against the skin under the action of a known force and the corresponding deflection observed. It is difficult to decide what is actually being measured by this apparatus since numerous factors influence the results, such as skin thickness, skin tension and the condition of the subcutaneous fat. A device for measuring the "resiliency" of skin has been described [7]. The system depends on measuring the force necessary to compress the skin of a patient into a fold. A similar system in the form of a spring-loaded caliper [8] has also been used. All these methods are subject to the criticism that it is difficult to tell what is actually being measured,

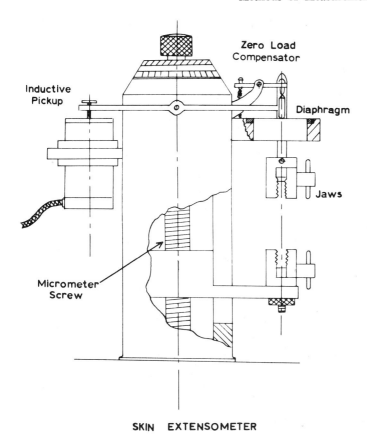

SKIN EXTENSOMETER

Figure 12.1. Skin extensometer.

although they may give useful comparative results. Another system employs two parallel lines drawn at a set distance apart on the surface of the skin of a patient. The two lines are forced together under the action of a light pressure, and their separation measured at the point where a fold is just about to form [9].

To give an indication of response to treatment of scleroderma, an apparatus has been used working on a principle similar to the Schade elastometer with displacement or depression of skin under the action of given weights [10].

We have used an extensometer (Fig. 12.1) having a constant rate of extension with which dumbell specimens of skin, obtained at biopsy or autopsy, could be tested [11]. This method has also been used by Daly [12], in parallel with tests done *in vivo*.

12.2   MECHANICAL PROPERTIES

12.2.1   Tensile Strength

The most complete study of the variation of tensile strength has been carried out by Rollhauser [13], who stated that in infants up to 3 months of age the value was only 0.25–0.3 kg mm^{-2}. In children 3 months to 3 years old it was 0.53–1.4 kg mm^{-2}. In adults from 15 to 50 years of age the value was 1.61 kg mm^{-2} and in persons from 50–80 years old 2.05 kg mm^{-2}. An average tensile strength of 1.8 kg mm^{-2} has been quoted by Wohlisch [14]. The tensile strength of epidermis plus dermis was greater than that of dermis alone. This suggests that in spite of its thinness the epidermis has appreciable tensile strength, although compared with the total tensile strength it is negligible.

Other qualitative results showed that tensile strength was very dependent on the rate of loading, rapid loading giving a value many times that of static loading [15]. Moreover, the tensile strength differed in the sexes and was altered by pregnancy and diseases such as Cushing's syndrome. The strength also varied with the direction in which the specimen was taken. Differences in tensile strength of skin between individuals were closely paralleled by differences in tensile strength of tendons, suggesting that the properties of collagen throughout the body varied similarly [15].

12.2.2   Distensibility

The distensibility of skin decreases with increasing age. Rollhauser [13] quoted values of extension of 50–59% for strips of skin taken from infants at birth. For children it varied between 37 and 52% and for adults 24–48%, a finding borne out by Dick [2].

12.2.3   Young's Modulus

It is difficult to quote a Young's modulus (stress/strain) for skin since, in common with many other biological tissues, the stress/strain curve is not linear, although some have claimed that after 5% strain is achieved Hooke's law applies [16]. The general form of the curve for various biological tissues is well established, commencing tangential to the extension axis, gradually bending toward the load axis. With a curve of this type it is imperative that the load at which the modulus is calculated be quoted. This, however, has not been done by many workers and makes their results difficult to compare.

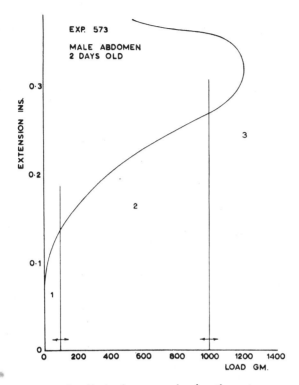

Load/extension curve showing three stages.

Figure 12.2.   Load-extension curve on skin from male abdomen.

A characteristic load-extension curve of skin is shown in Fig. 12.2. The extension process can be divided into three phases by boundaries at approximately 100 g and 1000 g. It has been shown histologically that the first phase corresponds to the straightening out and orientation of the collagen fibers of the specimen [17] and this process may be defined by the equation:

$$E = xy \log L \tag{1}$$

where E = extension and L = load and xy = constants.

The second phase is characterised by the equation:

$$E = c + kL^b \tag{2}$$

where c, k, b, = constants.

Tests on highly oriented collagen fibers from rat-tail tendon [18] produced a stress/strain curve characterized by a power law of exactly the same form as Equation 2. It seems likely therefore that the second phase of skin extension is attributable to the extension of orientated collagen fibers.

The third phase of extension concerns yielding, when the specimen gradually begins to extend more readily as individual fibers break down.

The significance of the constants in Equation 2 have been determined mathematically [19] and it has been shown that b reflected a specific property of the collagen fibers. This was shown theoretically and experimentally to be independent of the size of the specimen or the direction from which it was cut. The constant k was shown to represent the conditions of the fiber meshwork and was governed by the length and area of the fibers. The validity of this system was verified by using specimens cut at right angles to each other and by varying the width of the specimens.

Using a similar technique Daly [12] found that initial strains up to 20% of the unloaded length produced no significant increase in load, but that strains beyond about 40% required exceptionally high loads to produce further deformation. As an indication of the nonlinearity of skin it was interesting to note that the value of Poisson's ratio was generally in the region of unity. An elementary mathematical planar network model, incorporating viscoelastic features, was produced from this work.

The alignment of collagen fibers in the skin under stress has also been shown histologically by the workers at Strathclyde [20]. They found that when pieces of postmortem abdominal human skin were stretched, the collagen fibers of the dermis became orientated in the plane of stress, took an affinity for the red dye of the trichrome satin (fuchsinophilia, thus resembling smooth muscle), and eventually showed fracture lines and then complete disruption. Usually the fibers became oriented before the change in staining properties occurred. The greater the stress the greater the number of collagen fibers which became fuchsinophil. At low-load levels relaxation allowed the fibers to reassemble themselves in their normal random fashion but they retained their red staining. At slightly greater loads, although the orientation and affinity for the red dye remained on relaxation, yet the fibers assumed a wavy pattern. Greater stress produced changes of orientation and color that were not reversed by relaxing the tissue. It may be that in normal collagen fibrils only the mucopolysaccharide is stained and that this produces a blue reaction by any of the trichrome methods. On the other hand in stressed fibrils the mucopolysaccharide is disrupted, allowing access of the dye to the protocollagen which is fuchsinophil. It has been observed that the tinctorial changes in stressed collagen closely resemble those described as "fibrinoid degeneration of collagen" in some of the collagen diseases, but that it is entirely different from the fibrinoid exudate seen in the walls of blood vessels of renal glomenuli in cases of malignant hypertension, polyarteritis nodosa, and diabetic vasculosis [21].

The orientation of collagen fibers in the line of stress was obvious independent of which direction force was applied. The subepidermal deep zones of the dermis followed the same pattern of the midzone, but lagged somewhat behind. It was surprising to find that elastic and reticulin fibers seemed to be largely unaffected by stretching—they were merely displaced by and compressed between the orientated bundles of collagen.

This work has recently been extended by the use of scanning electron microscopy [22]. Detailed studies of the dermis indicated that the collagen fiber bundles run almost parallel to the epidermal surface. As expected random bundles that originally run close to a proposed line of loading fully align themselves in the direction of load. When the load is significantly out of line with the initial bundle orientation, the bundles only tend to the direction of the load axis. This appears to be the case even at high loads. Sometimes the bundles of two adjacent "layers" closed toward the load axis in a "scissor" action. It was shown that the lower dermis at its junction with the underlying fat consists of closely packed fibrous networks. There was a noticable initial orientation in a direction almost perpendicular to the line of the applied load and, in this case, loading had caused a splitting of this fibrous layer. As a result the larger collagen bundles in the middermis orientated themselves along the line of loading.

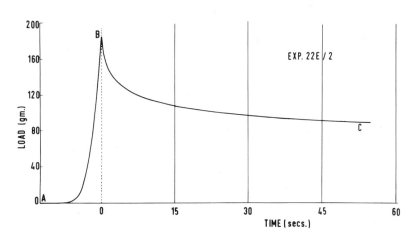

Figure 12.3. Stress relaxation of skin held at constant length (B to C) after stretching to peak force (A to B).

12.2.4   Other properties

That skin is a viscoelastic material is shown by its marked stress relaxation when subjected to a constant load for a period (Fig. 12.3). This has been confirmed by the work of Daly [12].

Skin in the body is permanently subject to a slight tension [2, 15, 23, 24]. This tension becomes less with advancing age and is found to differ in directions at right angles. This is readily demonstrated by marking a square on skin and then cutting around it [24].

12.3   PHYSIOLOGICAL VARIATION

12.3.1   Sex

The tensile strength of female skin is less than that of male skin [15]. Stress/strain measurements showed female skin to be more extensible [18], and the modulus of elasticity is significantly higher [3]. Wenzel investigated the shrinkage of excised skin due to the relaxation of the tension *in situ* and found it was greater in men than women, the respective values being 14% and 10.7%.

12.3.2   Age

When the skin of the relaxed hand of a medical student is pulled up between the finger and thumb and released it smacks back into place, whereas that of the senile instructor subsides slowly, because the elasticity is reduced [25]. This is verified by observing in a piece of skin removed from the body the shrinkage, which is decidedly more vigorous in young persons than in old ones. Conversely, there is a decrease with age of the compressibility of skin plus subcutaneous tissue [26].

Figure 12.4 demonstrates changes attributable to alterations in skin collagen with age. There is an increasing stiffness after 40 years of age. These findings agree well with those in rabbits [27] and in man [28]. The most likely explanation is that with advancing age the number of cross-links in the collagen fibers are increased. This is strongly supported by the fact that the tensile strength of skin increases with age [13]. Investigating the problem of the burst abdomen by subjecting sections of sutured aponeurosis to very rapid extensions and observing the loads required to rupture the specimens, we have demonstrated that specimens require a progressively greater load with increasing age up to 40 years. After this age the situation is reversed and the load required

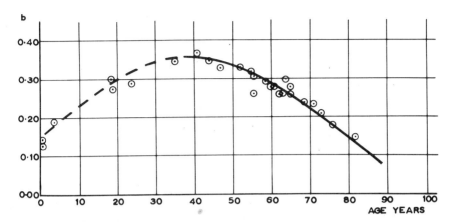

Figure 12.4. Variation of elastic stiffness b with age of skin isolated from male abdomen.

to rupture the specimen diminishes with age. There is a progressive rise in the modulus of elasticity of skin with age in both sexes, but in elderly subjects showing the condition known as "transparent skin", there is a significantly lower modulus of elasticity than in controls [3].

12.3.3   Site

Directional effects in skin were first noted by Dupuytren [29], who was called to treat a patient suffering from stab wounds. It was claimed that the wounds had been made with a circular-bladed stilletto. However, Dupuytren observed that the wounds, instead of being circular, were linear, suggesting that they had been made with a bladed instrument. This prompted him to carry out experiments on cadavers, in which he demonstrated that circular wounds did indeed assume an eliptical form. Langer [25] extended these observations and produced a system of lines for the whole body, known as Langer's lines.

Cox [30] showed histologically that Langer's lines follow the direction of preferential orientation of the fibers and this was confirmed by Ridge and Wright [24]. Langer's lines represent directions of principle tension and Ridge and Wright [24] postulated a theoretical lattice structure with a mean fiber angle to the direction of Langer's lines somewhat less than 45°. Differences were found in the stress-strain curve of specimens taken along and across Langer's lines (Fig. 12.5). This is explained

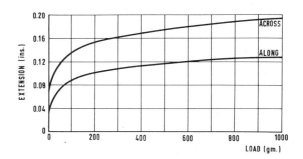

Figure 12.5. Stress/strain curves for abdominal skin from a woman age 88 taken along and across Langer's lines.

by the fact that extension of the specimen taken in the direction of Langer's lines will extend only a small amount before all fibers become orientated and parallel to each other, but the ones taken across Langer's lines will extend considerably before the fibers become orientated. Thus, across Langer's lines we are extending a smaller number of fibers, which have a greater orientated length than those in the direction along the lines. It is the architecture of the wicker-work which is changed, and this was demonstrated in the constant we proposed to characterize this aspect. The later work of Gibson et al. [31] using a method for measuring the stress/strain character of skin with a constant deformation rate *in vivo* [32] confirmed this.

The mechanical characteristics of skin varies with the part of the body in which it occurs. Changes due to aging were less pronounced in abdominal skin both with respect to changes in stiffness of the collagen and the architecture of the wicker-work [33]. Measurements of skin-fold compressibility at the arm, calf, scapula, and waist showed that while there was a decrease with age this decrement was not uniform over the body surface [26].

12.4   PATHOLOGICAL CONDITIONS

12.4.1   Ehlers Danlos Syndrome

Investigation of the *in vivo* elasticity of the skin of fourteen patients with Ehlers Danlos syndrome demonstrated that skin hyperextensibility occurred during the phase of taking up slack [34]. After this had been completed, further extension was achieved only by considerable increases in stress and values for the elastic modulus for intact skin in these patients did not differ from those obtained for control subjects. They showed that the skin thickness was significantly thinner than in control subjects. There was an inverse correlation between the thickness and the tendency to skin splitting, as evidenced by the degree of scarring.

12.4.2 Lathyrism

The tissues of lathyritic rats and chickens show the collagen unchanged, but the tensile strength considerably reduced in rat aorta, skin, and intestine [35]. The extensibility was normal for rat skin and intestine, but greater for chicken skin. We used protein-depleted rabbits to observe the effect of protein depletion and found that it reduced the thickness of skin and of aponeurosis but it made no difference to the values of the constants obtained, indicating that the amount, the meshwork, and the cross-linkage of collagen fibers were unchanged both in the skin and aponeurosis.

12.4.3 Transparent skin

McConkey et al. [36] introduced the term "transparent skin" to describe the appearance of the skin best seen over the hand, when the details of the smaller veins could be made out with ease. They found apparent correlation between this and senile osteoporosis, postulating that a generalized disorder of collagen may have been responsible for both disorders. In a pathological study of the skin [37] the collagen fibers were found to be loosely arranged, whereas in normal skin they were coarser and more closely packed. Furthermore their staining reactions were different. With the picropolychrome method, transparent skin collagen stained blue while opaque skin collagen stained deep-red. Transparent skin was shown to be more hydrated than opaque skin but biosynthesis as judged by the incorporation of ^{14}C proline was as active, if not more active, than normal skin. It was suggested that the defect was an arrested maturation of dermal collagen. The elastic modulus in a group of nine patients with transparent skin was significantly lower than in matched controls [16].

The skin thickness in untreated patients with rheumatoid arthritis was reduced compared with controls, and the skin thickness in patients with rheumatoid arthritis treated with prednisolone was reduced compared with untreated patients with rheumatoid arthritis [3]. Skin elasticity measurements, however, did not differ significantly in any groups.

This suggested that the qualitative change in skin collagen, observed in idiopathic, senile, transparent skin, did not occur in rheumatoid arthritis with or without the administration of steroid therapy. Interestingly ACTH therapy in rheumatoid arthritis did not cause skin atrophy and this would explain the almost complete absence of steroid bruising in ACTH-treated patients [38, 10].

REFERENCES

1. T. Alfrey and E. F. Gurnee, *Molecular Structure and Mechanical Behavior of Macro Molecules.* J. W. Remington, Ed., American Physiological Society, 1957, p. 12–32.
2. J. G. Dick, *J. Anat.,* **81,** 201 (1947).
3. R. Grahame, *Ann. Phys. Med.,* **10,** 130 (1969).
4. E. Kirk and S. A. Kvorning, *J. Gerontol.,* **4,** 273 (1949).
5. E. Kirk, *J. Gerontol.,* **5,** 387 (1950).
6. H. Schade, *Ztschr. F. Exper. Path. U. Therapie,* **11,** 369 (1912).
7. J. Joachimes, *Ztchr. F. Kiderheilk,* **56,** 81 (1943).
8. W. A. Sodeman and G. E. Burch, *J. Clin. Invest.,* **17,** 785 (1938).
9. G. Doerks, *Arch. F. Kinderheilk,* **136,** 1 (1949).
10. C. Tui, N. H. Kuo, and S. Simungço, *J. Invest. Dermatol.,* **15,** 181 (1950).
11. M. D. Ridge and V. Wright, *Med. Biol. Eng.,* **4,** 533 (1966).
12. C. H. Daly, *The Biomechanical Characteristics of Human Skin.,* Ph.D. Thesis, University of Strathclyde, Glascow (1966).
13. H. Rollhauser, *Gegenbaurs Morphol. Jahrb.,* **90,** 249 (1950).
14. E. Wohlisch, *Kolloid-Z.,* **104,** 14 (1943).
15. H. G. Wenzel, *Zentralbil, F. Aug. Path. U. Anat.,* **85,** 117 (1949).
16. R. Grahame and P. J. L. Holt, *Gerontologia,* **15,** 121 (1969).
17. V. Wright and M. D. Ridge, *Engineering,* **199,** 363 (1965).
18. M. D. Ridge and V. Wright, *Brit. J. Dermatol.,* **77,** 639 (1965).
19. M. D. Ridge and V. Wright, *J. Appl. Physiol.,* **21,** 1602 (1966).
20. J. E. Craik and I. I. R. McNeil, *Biomechanics and Related Bioengineering Topics,* R. M. Kennedi, Ed., Pergamon, London, 1964, pp. 159–164.
21. J. E. Craik and I. I. R. McNeil, *Nature,* **209,** 931 (1966).
22. B. Finlay, *Bio-med. Eng.,* **4,** 322 (1969).
23. R. Evans, E. V. Cowdry, and P. E. Neilson, *Anat. Research,* **86,** 545 (1943).
24. M. D. Ridge and V. Wright, *J. Invest. Dermatol.,* **46,** 341 (1966).
25. M. A. Ma, and E. V. Cowdry, *J. Gerontol.,* **5,** 203 (1950).
26. J. Brojek and W. Kinzey, *J. Gerontol.,* **15,** 45 (1960).
27. R. D. Harkness, *Biol. Rev.,* **36,** 399 (1961).
28. R. M. Kennedi, T. Gibson, and C. H. Daly, *Skin Research,* No. 2., Department of Bioengineering, University of Strathclyde (1963).

29. G. Dupuytren, quoted by H. T. Cox, *Brit. J. Surg.,* **29,** 234 (1942).

30. H. T. Cox, *Brit. J. Surg.,* **29,** 234 (1942).

31. T. Gibson, H. Stark, and J. H. Evans, *J. Biomechan.,* **2,** 201 (1969).

32. J. H. Evans and W. W. Siesennop, *Proc. 7th Intern. Conf. Med. Electron. Biol. Eng.,* Stockholm, 371 (1967).

33. M. D. Ridge and V. Wright, *Gerontologia,* **12,** 174 (1966).

34. R. Grahame and P. Beighton, *Ann. Rheum. Dis.,* **28,** 246 (1969).

35. P. Fry, M. L. R. Harkness, R. D. Harkness, and M. Nightingale, *J. Physiol.,* **164, 77** (1962).

36. B. McConkey, G. M. Fraser, A. S. Bligh, and H. Whitely, *Lancet,* **1,** 693 (1963).

37. B. McConkey, W. K. Walton, S. A. Corney, J. C. Lawrence, and C. R. Ricketts, *Ann. Rheum. Dis.,* **26,** 219 (1967).

38. O. Savage, W. S. C. Copeman, L. Chapman, M. V. Well, and B. L. J. Treadwell, *Lancet,* **2,** 22 (1962).

13

Tensile Strength of Healing Wounds

JOUKO VILJANTO

Department of Paediatric Surgery, University of Turku, Finland

The mechanical characteristics of the skin undergo gradual changes during the development of an individual. An injury, such as a skin wound, suddenly interrupts this natural development. Special reparative processes are needed for the continuity of the fibrous network to be restored. Wound healing and natural aging then take place coincidentally. Both of these processes follow their natural course and there is interaction between the intact and the regenerating tissue. The purpose of the new connective tissue which forms between the wound edges is to increase the strength of the wound from zero-point to a sufficient level whereas the surrounding tissue had some strength even at birth.

The thickness and the texture of the cutaneous connective tissue vary from one point to another. This variation may conceivably have developed according to the mechanical and functional demands of the area concerned. It is easy to think that the mechanical properties of the healing tissues accord with this variation. However, there is a great lack of knowledge on this point. We don't know precisely the "isomechanical" areas of the skin in our usual laboratory animals, to say nothing of isomechanically healing wounds. Except in bilaterally symmetrical parts there are virtually no areas of skin which have an exact counterpart elsewhere in the body.

Just as in the thickness of the skin, there is variation in skin tension. This is at a maximum in young animals, decreasing slowly with age until in very old subjects it has practically disappeared. Tension changes constantly with posture and is dependent on the internal environment. From the areas of connective tissue regeneration, where these tension lines are unidirectional, a similar arrangement of newly formed fibers can be seen.

Although the basic idea of tensile-strength measurement is simple, there are many obstacles to its detailed practical performance. The speed of wound healing can be evaluated from a number of parameters by morphological, cytochemical, chemical, and mechanical methods. All of these, with the exception of the last, are indirect methods, that is to say, they estimate one or several biologic parameters as a function of time. For some purposes, for example, forensic medicine, the first few minutes and hours after wounding may be of greatest value in drawing the conclusion [1–4]. In surgery the problem is different: Does the healing incisional wound, after a certain healing period, possess the strength it should normally have? Sometimes the contraction of open wounds is of great practical value, as in chronic leg ulcers and in healing gastric and duodenal ulcers. In some superficial wounds and in burns, epithelization is the essential process needed. But always when the incision penetrates the entire skin, fascia, tendon, muscle, intestine, vessel, and so on, the strength of the healing wound is, besides epithelization, the single requirement of practical importance.

None of the numerous methods of examining wound healing has super- seded the measurement of tensile strength and bursting strength. Unfor- tunately these and many other methods are useful in animal experiments only, and therefore investigators have long been trying to discover means capable of supplying, by histochemical or chemical methods, the same information in man as tensile-strength measurements now provide in the case of animals.

A number of excellent reviews and monographs have been published on various aspects of wound healing [1, 5–12]. They contain hundreds of investigations concerning many general and specific aspects of this subject. The tensile strength of healing wounds has been the main theme of many single articles but not of any of the reviews or papers that have come to my attention.

13.1   MECHANICAL FEATURES OF TISSUE REPAIR

Since the first report on tensile-strength studies by Paget in 1853 [13], concerned with the healing achilles tendon of rabbit, active interest has been aroused in the mechanical behavior of healing tissue. This is reflected in attempts to separate various phases of wound healing on the basis of increasing tensile strength. Howes, Sooy, and Harvey [14] distinguished the lag or latent phase during the first 1–4, sometimes 1–6 postoperative days, when the tensile strength decreased. They deter- mined that the period of fibroplasia lasted till the tenth or fourteenth day. During this phase the tensile strength increased rapidly with the number of fibroblasts. The period of maturation was not determined exactly. During that phase the scar received its final form. Dunphy and Udupa [15] stated that at the beginning of healing, there is a metabolically inert, initial shock phase lasting 12–24 hours. This is fol- lowed by the productive or substrate phase lasting 1–5 days postopera- tively. The collagen phase lasts from the fifth to the sixth day until the healing process is completed. Dunphy and Jackson [16] considered the increase in tensile strength to continue up to the twentieth day after wounding. Even these experiments show how uncertain the limits of the various healing periods are and, above all, how absolutely certain the mechanically inert "lag" or "latent" phase is during the first days of healing. In the light of the literature and in my own experience, some of the factors preventing the exact expression of the length of the healing period may be listed as follows:

1. The tensile strength of the wounds is so weak during the first 3 to 4 days that in the process of preparing the skin strip for measurement, tissue injury may easily ruin even the most accurate work.

2. Differences in experimental animals, in localization and direction of the wounds, in suture material and technique, and in healing conditions.

3. Differences in tensiometers and in measurement technique.

The fact that skin is a viscoelastic substance and thus has time-dependent properties [17] has not always been kept in mind. Unwounded rat skin has a mean breaking extension of over 50% of its original length. In the skin wounds of rats weighing about 350 g, the extension of the wound was only 20% after 10 days and about 35% at 40 days postoperatively [17]. The mean energy absorption was over 100 in. pounds per cubic inch (in. lb in^{-3}) for unwounded rat skin. In healing wounds the mean energy absorption was only 3.2% of the original value of unwounded skin at 10 days, and 52% at 150 days. From these results, we can assume that the healing wound tissue of the skin regains about one-third of the extensibility of unwounded skin at 10 days and about two-thirds at 100 days. Tensile strength of the wounds, as compared to the values of intact skin, was 4.5% at 10 days, 64% at 100 days, and about 70% at 150 days. This means that both the extension and tensile strength are restored to only two-thirds of their original values, the former earlier than the latter.

Most wounds involving skin, fascia, or tendon, never regain the initial strength of the tissue divided [16, 18, 19]. In contrast to wounds in fascia and skin, the tensile strength of an intestinal wound rapidly returns to normal and may even exceed the normal. The bursting strength of experimental intestinal wounds at 10 days exceeds that of normal, intact bowel wall. If the colon is wounded the entire colonic wall, both above and below the incision, undergoes a rapid and significant loss of collagen to as little as 40% of normal by the third day. From the fifth day on, the synthesis of new collagen results in a progressive rise in total collagen. At the same time the tensile-strength values of this intact part of the colon first decrease and later increase in relation to the content of collagen. Not only does the bursting strength of the incision exceed that of normal, uninjured bowel, but the bursting strength of the adjacent bowel rises above that of the normal, uninjured bowel [20].

In most healing tissues the need of sutures for approximation of the wound edges is only temporary. The strength of the vascular anastomosis and replacement is, however, almost entirely dependent upon the continued strength of the prosthesis and upon the sutures. Failure of the strength in the prosthesis or the sutures may lead to disruption and hemorrhage. The loss of tensile strength that occurs in the sutures or prosthesis used for vascular grafts has led to the discarding of a number of prosthetic materials [21].

Wound contraction is one essential feature in wound healing and one expression of the mechanical capacity of granulation tissue. There is strong evidence in favor of the hypothesis that wound contraction is mediated by the fibroblasts. Movement of the wound margins might be produced by shortening of the fibroblasts or their rearrangement [22]. The thickness of the granulation tissue and the tension developed in these wounds were well correlated. No significant association was found between tension and wound area. When contraction of open wounds has ceased, the surrounding skin was under abnormal tension, judged by the expansion occurring after excision of the wounded area [23].

A general trend towards more accurate, more detailed mechanical parameters incounting measurements is clearly to be seen. Despite a number of chemical and enzyme histochemical changes found in the very early phases of wound healing, the technique of tensile-strength measurements has mostly failed to demonstrate these changes. "It is quite possible that, were we able to measure tensile strength more accurately, a progressive increase from the very earliest phases of healing could be demonstrated" [24].

13.2   TENSILE STRENGTH AS A TEST METHOD OF HEALING WOUNDS

Conceptual differences in the term "tensile strength" have led to many difficulties in interpretation of the results. Parameters important in the determination of the mechanical properties of healing wounds can be listed according to Glaser et al. [25] as follows:

Maximum stress is defined as the maximum force at rupture divided by the initial cross-sectional area. It gives an indication of the ultimate strength of the specimen.

Work input into a specimen represents the work done on the specimen by the application of a force tending to elongate it. The work input may be computed for various predetermined stress levels or as the amount necessary to cause failure.

Maximum stiffness gives an indication of the elasticity of the skin and of the way in which the application of a change in strain affects the stress level in the specimen or vice versa. It can be calculated by measuring the slope of the almost linear portion of the specimen stress-strain curve. The larger the stiffness, the less elastic is the tissue.

Maximum strain is the total elongation of the specimen prior to the rupture, divided by the initial specimen gauge length. This quantity gives a measure of the total stretch a specimen can endure without rupturing.

Milch [26], in his nomenclature, gives the following definitions:

Nominal tensile stress (σ_t) is the force (tensile weight load $= W$) applied per unit original cross-sectional area A_0 to a test specimen at any given time t, expressed in terms of pounds per square inch (psi) or kilograms per square centimeter (ksc). Psi $= 14{,}223 \times$ (ksc)

$$\text{stress} = \sigma_t = \frac{W}{A_0}$$

Strain or unit extension is usually expressed as the dimensionless ratio of the observed extension, or the change in length of the specimen ΔL divided by the original longitudinal length:

$$\text{strain} = \epsilon_t = \frac{\Delta L}{L_0} = \frac{L_t - L_0}{L_0}$$

Total or ultimate unit extension $(\epsilon_u = \text{ultimate strain})$ is

$$\epsilon_u = \frac{L_u - L_0}{L_0}$$

where $L_u =$ ultimate longitudinal length of the specimen. The percentage elongation is then $\epsilon_u \times 100$.

The true ultimate tensile strength

$$\sigma_{ut} = \frac{W_u}{A}$$

where A is the minimal cross-sectional area determined immediately prior to rupture. The true ultimate strain

$$\epsilon_{ut} = \int_{L_0}^{L} \frac{dL}{L} = \ln \frac{L}{L_0}$$

Despite the accurate definitions of these terms, the detailed practical performance of tensile strength testing is unreliable in many respects.

It is never possible to prepare any type of test specimen entirely free of flaws. That is why the experimental data are always lower than the "actual strength" values. It is absolutely necessary to have specimens of uniform dimensions. In engineering practice, die-cut ring-shaped or preferably dumbbell-shaped specimens are employed. This shape of test specimens, only exceptionally used in wound-healing studies, provides the most reliable type for tensile-strength measurements [26]. In addition, it is important to realize that the properties of test specimens change after having been secured to the straining grips of the test instrument. The temperature, humidity, and the rate of straining exert their own effect on the end result. The biopolymer network present in connective tissue has both elastic and viscous components, which are not equally distributed in all directions. The non-Hookean behavior, in which strain is not directly proportional to stress, may be simulated by mechanical models like multiple Voigt-Kelvin elements in series, each having different retardation times, or multiple Maxwell elements, each with different relaxation times, in parallel.

The tissue tension around the wound and inside it is changeable and liable to sudden increases. Tensile strength measurement, in contrast, must be performed by increasing gradually the tension in wound tissue. Otherwise the rupture of the wound would occur too early with minor strain and major stress. In order to simulate conditions *in vivo*, a constant load of the specimen should be combined with sudden increases of the load of variable stress and duration.

13.2.1   Breaking Strength—Tensile Strength—Bursting Strength

Breaking Strength

Instead of the term tensile strength, which should be expressed as stress per cross-sectional area, breaking strength means the stress by which the wound edges are detached, independently of the cross-sectional area. However, tensile strength is often used incorrectly when the cross-sectional area has not been measured. Except in the usual technique of tensile-strength measurement by loading the specimen with continuously increasing weight, often in vertical direction, the term breaking strength has also been used in another sense. Harvey [27] used the term breaking strength for gastric wounds when inflating the stomach with air and recording by a mercury manometer the end point where the first leak of air was observed. To this we now apply the term bursting strength or bursting pressure. It is also possible to measure skin wounds in a similar manner. Huu and Albert [28] described a method in which the skin with a wound to be disrupted was placed between the plates with the wound exactly centered in the opening. A plastic ring prevented slippage as well as leakage. The wound was disrupted hydrostatically using flowing water. The pressure built up and disruption were recorded. Although breaking strength, wrongly termed tensile strength, is often used in mechanical studies of healing wounds, the selection of the experimental animals and the technique of making the wounds have been under such strict control that comparison of the results obtained has been justified. On the other hand, there is no sense in making a comparison of the results of various authors and experiments if no data are available on the cross-sectional area of the specimens measured.

Tensile Strength

The suitability of a tensile-strength measurement as a parameter of wound-healing studies is widely accepted [27–33].

These measurements are mostly used in studies of the strength of healing skin wounds, of sutured tendons, fascia, and muscle wounds [29, 32, 34–42].

Despite justified criticism, tensile strength is a fundamental tool of great interest to the surgeon. "Most of the confusion in tensile strength studies stems from the failure to recognize the specificity of repair. The rate of gain in tensile strength differs substantially in different tissues, in different species and at times in the same tissue in the same species" [24].

The greatest tensile-strength values, as calculated per cross-sectional area collagen, have been obtained in intact mammalian tendons and vary from 15 to 30 kg mm^{-2}. In human skin, tensile strength has varied with age from 0.25 kg mm^{-2} in infants to 1.6 kg mm^{-2} in adults [43]. This refers to about 10 kg mm^{-2} cross-sectional area collagen in the adult. The lower values obtained in skin than in tendon have been explained by the parallelism of the tendon fibers. In skeletal muscle, tensile strength is only 3–5 kg mm^{-2} collagen and in uterus, gut, and aorta 1–5 kg mm^{-2} [43]. The great differences in tensile strength values might be due, at least partly, to differences in collagen cross-linking. As from skin wounds, tensile strength can be measured from intestinal wounds too. The measurement recorded from colonic wounds reach the value for intact bowel at approximately 30 days [44]. Nelson and Anders [45], in studies of the small bowel, found that the discrepancy between bursting strength and tensile strength was related in part to the rate of distension. The circular wall tension produced on inflation of a segment of bowel was considerably lower at the anastomosis than in the normal bowel by virtue of the rigidity and limited distension of the anastomotic ring. Even taking this into account, the rate of gain in tensile strength of bowel wounds was more rapid than in the wounds of skin and fascia.

However, it is not generally known that the tensile strength of intestine behaves according to the formula of Laplace for a cylinder ($T = Pr$, where T = tension, P = pressure and r = radius). The bursting pressure of an intestinal segment may be measured in the usual manner by means of flowing water or inflation of air. When the maximum radius of the distended intestinal segment or abdomen is placed into the Laplace formula, the rupturing tension of the intestinal or abdominal wall is obtained. The radius of the intestine is directly related to the tension resulting from any given pressure [46].

Two phases were observed in the gain of tensile strength in healing tendon wounds [20]. The initial phase, lasting between 10 and 20 days, corresponded to the period of fibroplasia. Tensile strength during this phase was related to the amount of collagen present and partly to the adhesiveness contributed by as yet unidentified factors in the exudate and ground substance. A second and more significant gain in tensile strength began between 15 and 20 days and continued for many weeks or months. Studies with suture material [30] given an idea of the complexity of tensions existing in the connective-tissue texture and in the network of new granulation tissue. Although the main tension lies parallel to a number of collagen bundles (interrupted suture), a great many bundles are in oblique direction (continuous suture). These do not give the same support against the disrupting force of the wound edges. Their strength need not, however, be weaker in absolute terms than that of the other bundles. That is to say, if we want to know the real tensile strength of an incisional wound, we must test it in several directions both perpendicularly and obliquely to the wound edges. The distracting power should be both gradually increasing and suddenly increasing. Even this is not the whole truth about the effective forces. The skin often covers more or less curved surfaces. For instance the intraabdominal pressure produces forces which distract the wound tangentially and at the same time push it outwards. The latter component is theoretically similar in all parts of the cavity but the gastrointestinal tract and parenchyme organs may in certain areas damp the peak values for sudden pressure increases.

Bursting Strength

Bursting strength or bursting pressure means the intraluminal force, often expressed in mm Hg, which is needed to disrupt the abdominal or intestinal wall. When the first bubble of compressed air under the water level from the wound is noticed, the end point of the measurement is recorded [47–50]. The recovery of strength in colonic anastomosis was similar to that found by Howes et al. [14] in the healing stomach. During the first 3 or 4 days, the edges of the wounds were held together by sutures only. Then a rapid gain in strength occurred, so that by the tenth day, rupture no longer took place at the anastomosis but in the intact intestine. This finding was in accordance with Herrmann's observation [44] that the bursting pressure of a colonic anastomosis was higher after 10 days than in the normal colonic wall whereas the breaking strength as measured by a tensiometer did not reach the figure for the normal colon for two months. In end-to-end intestinal anastomosis of mongrel dogs, the healing curve was found to be similar to the healing curves reported for other tissues [49]. The supportive strength given by sutures to an anastomosis was of greatest importance during the lag phase of healing, which lasted for 3 to 4 days. The final resistance in the wounds of stomach, duodenum, ileum, and caecum of young adult rats was closely related to bursting pressure values of the corresponding intact gastrointestinal wall [50]. No definite correlation was observed between resistance of wound and thickness of intestinal wall. Gastrointestinal segments with a wide lumen, such as stomach and caecum, showed a low resistance to increased intraluminal pressure (according to the Laplace law).

13.2.2   Comparison of the Technical Details

In an unextended state the collagen fibers of the human skin form a disordered network. The single collagen fiber is highly resistant and responds under control of Hooke's law. Experiments with intact skin showed that, in a constant state of strain, the stress diminished according to the logarithm of the duration of the experiment. The relationship between the stress and the strain yielded characteristic curves which proved that the skin was not controlled by Hooke's law. Factors to be taken into consideration in tensile strength measurements are:

1. The procedure of tensile-strength measurement must be highly standardized.

2. The wounds should, in each case, be made, sutured, and prepared for tensile strength measurements using an identical technique, preferably by one and the same person.

3. All experimental animals in a study where the results are compared with each other should be of the same sex, age, and weight.

4. The investigator should have no knowledge of whether the animal being tested belongs to the experimental or the control group. Despite all these precautions there will still remain a wide biologic range in tensile-strength values unrelated to the method used [28].

Breadth of Strip

A frequently used breadth for the skin strip is 1 cm, with a piece of healing wound in the middle. In studies of human cadaver it was observed [52] that, if the breadth of the strip was less than 5 mm, the real strain rose rapidly in relation to the calculated strain. In skin strips 10 mm or more in breadth, this proportion remained unchanged. This is why the breadth of the strip should be at least 10 mm. In the case of strips 5–10 mm broad the results are uncertain. If the strips are 5 mm or less in breadth, then too large a number of collagen fibers, in relation to the whole number of fibers, will lie at the borders of the strips without any contact to the surrounding tissue [30].

Thickness of Strip

The thickness of the strip varies according to the age and size of the animal. It is not ideal to measure the thickness of the skin too close to the wound edges because of tissue edema. It is preferable to take the skin thickness of a different series of control animals and then to compare the weight of experimental animals to the standard curve thus obtained [33]. There may also be differences in the thickness of wound tissue due to the surgical technique. The depth of the wounds may vary; in some, the wound is deeper than the average. Some variation may be found in coaptation of the wound margins. Undermining may be unequal in various parts of the wound. Geever et al. [53] concluded that the shape of the wound is often so irregular that it cannot be determined by cross inspection. They found no method for skin-thickness measurement entirely satisfactory.

Curling Phenomenon

Curling of the skin specimen occurs because of the different properties of the dermal and epidermal layers [25]. The more curling a specimen exhibits, the greater are the stress concentrations at the dermis-epidermis interface. The viscoelastic nature of skin probably modifies these concentrations. The most important feature in this phenomenon is that curling introduces a nonuniform stress distribution within a specimen. Attempts to reduce this effect have led to the observation that, if the cross-sectional area of the strip to be measured is in the form of a square, the detrimental curling effect will be minimized. The primary disadvantage of narrow specimens is that they tend to dry out more rapidly than the larger ones when exposed to the atmosphere.

"Creep" Phenomenon

A careful analysis of strain rates has shown that those in the interval of 0.007 cm cm^{-1} sec^{-1} to 0.42 cm cm^{-1} sec^{-1} do not influence the elastic properties of skin tissue [25]. Strain rates smaller than 0.007 cm cm⁻¹ sec⁻¹, however, are not advisable since the "creep" phenomenon may be introduced during tensile testing. Thus, if the rate of extension is too slow, it will reduce the stresses placed upon it.

13.2.3   Reliability of Tensile-Strength Values

Considerable differences occur in the technical descriptions of various tensiometric methods [46, 51, 54–58]. Unfortunately a number of investigators have not reported on their measurement arrangements clearly enough. Although the name of the tensiometer or the main principles of the measurement, for example, flowing water, mercury, inflated air, gas, or liquid, may give an idea of the technique, it still remains unclear for the reader in many respects. It is to be hoped that forthcoming papers will contain further technical details on their own experiments. This is one reason why critical appraisal of the tensile strength values after the same observation periods is not possible. For the same reason there is no sense in trying to draw curves describing mean tensile-strength values for different healing tissues and for different animals.

Each investigator who has prepared test specimens for tensile-strength measurements knows that, during the first postoperative days, the strength of the skin wounds is so small that disruption of the wound may take place even before the measurement. Presumably this damage occurs to a certain extent in the preparation of wounds in general but proportionally the effect is most striking during the first days.

Healing skin wounds never regain the tensile strength of intact skin. However, the damage caused by the clamps at the fixing point is so great that disruption of the skin may take place outside the wound. A greater problem arises when tensile testing is performed in muscle or granulation tissue. This author has not found any rational method to test the strength of sponge ingrown granulation tissue after two weeks' implantation time.

13.3   TENSILE STRENGTH OF SKIN WOUNDS

13.3.1   Differences in Tensile Strength Between Experimental Animals

Considerable variability in tensile-strength values due to biologic variations in the animals is apparent [59, 60]. Young rats 70 days of age had nominal tensile strength values much lower than comparable values obtained in old rats 15 months of age. There was a highly significant difference in skin-breaking strength values between old male and old female animals. However, no such sex differences were found between young animals.

The mouse, in contrast to the rat, fails to demonstrate a rapid gain of tensile strength in secondary wounds [60].

Pikkarainen [61] has noted certain differences in the chemical composition of skin collagen. Studies of the amino acid composition revealed that the amount of hydroxyproline and proline increased whereas that of methionine decreased in the course of evolution. An evolutionary trend was detected also in the content of methionine, serine, and threonine, which all decreased. In general, the amino acid compositions of the collagens of the different species were related to the evolutionary ages of the species. Features common to all collagens were the constant total content of nonpolar amino acids (two-thirds, one-half of which glycine) and of acidic amino acids as well as the constant number of hydroxyl groups. The molar weights of the α-, β- and γ-components did not differ from each other in man [62] nor in rats [63]. Considerable differences were also found in the thermal shrinkage temperatures of vertebrate collagens determined for skins in water or physiological saline: in dogfish 35–41°C, in rat 59°C, in rabbit 60–62°C, in pig 62°C, and in man 60–67°C [64, 65–67]. On the basis of these differences in the composition of collagen and various nominal tensile-strength values for intact skin from man, dogs, rabbits, and rats [68], the differences in wound healing speeds in different species are natural. It is worth mentioning in this context that the tensile-strength values in the same animal differ depending on the direction in which the specimens are cut. This difference is entirely eliminated on boiling in water, which was associated with a significant decrease in nominal tensile strength [68]. No investigation has come to my notice in which the effect of heat denaturation was applied to tensile-strength studies of healing wounds.

13.3.2   Effect of Size, Shape, Number, and Localization of Incisional Wounds

Size

Usually the wounds have been made in the midline or symmetrically on both sides of the dorsal or abdominal skin of the animal. The length has varied from 2 to 6 cm depending upon the size of the experimental animal. By increasing the total length of the sutured skin wounds from 6 to 48 cm in rats, weighing 130–140 g, it was found that the strength values (g cm⁻¹) began to decrease when the total length of the wounds

exceeded 36 cm [69]. It may be concluded that the length of the incisional wound practically never exceeds the regeneration capacity of the
experimental animal provided that this is normally fed and otherwise
in good condition.

Shape

In all tensile-strength studies it is imperative that the shape of the
wound to be tested is rectilinear, otherwise, it is impossible to fix the
clamps parallel to the wound edges. If this is not done, the wound will
tear with a minor stress. The wound strips should be rectangular with
a minimum breadth of 1.0 cm, as stated earlier. It is not possible to
eliminate fully the curling effect because the preparation of narrower
strips increases the percentage of tissue damage per strip to be tested.

Number of Wounds

An increase in the number of wounds as a matter of fact has the
same effect as an increase in length of wounds. In our investigation
[69] the total number of wounds varied from 1 to 6 per experimental
animal. If the wounds are so located that vascularization is interfered
with, decreased tensile-strength values will result. It is also important
to note that too narrow necks or too long flaps between the wounds
may be deleterious.

Localization of Wounds

An essential requirement in wound-healing studies is to compare only
similarly located cutaneous wounds since the vascularity of different
regions of skin may differ markedly [70]. Besides differences in vascularity, the arrangement of collagen fibers must be taken into consideration. Connective tissue is capable of organizing in the manner best suited
to function in response to the existing stresses upon the tissue. In most
areas of skin the collagen fibers are arranged randomly. Instead, in
a tendon, for example, the bundles of collagen, viewed microscopically,
are aligned parallel to the lines of stress. In an experiment [71], increased extrinsic stress caused a significantly greater tensile strength
after a period of 14 days. According to Milch [26] the tensile strength
is directly related to the number of effective network chains per unit
volume, not to the total number of chains.

In the stretched skin the collagen fibers of the dermis lose their random
three-dimensional arrangement and become orientated along the line
of stress. Elastic and reticulin fibers seem to be largely unaffected by
stretching [72]. It is interesting to observe that normal, randomly located, and stressed collagen fibers stain differently. While the normal
collagen fibers stain blue, the stressed collagen fibers stain red, thus

resembling smooth muscle. The explanation for this fuchsinophilia is still obscure but it might be due to the disruption of the mucopolysaccharide matrix around the collagen fiber or to the active groups of the disrupted cross-links in the collagen molecule (see Chapter 7). In any case it must be based on some chemical alteration in the collagen fiber, which again may be related to the changed tensile strength. Even from this point of view the exactly symmetrical localization of the wounds for reliable results to be obtained, must be emphasized.

13.3.3   Role of Sutures

An ideal surgical suture should fulfill the following requirements: be easy to handle and use in any operation, cause minimal tissue reaction, not create situations favorable to bacterial growth, possess high nominal tensile strength in small calibre, and hold knots without fraying or cutting. It should be nonelectrolyte, noncapillary, nonallergenic, and noncarcinogenic. It should be easy to sterilize by boiling or autoclaving without alteration. If absorbable, absorption should cause minimal tissue reaction [27, 58].

Ferris and Henry [73] compared microporous tape, continuous subcuticular stainless steel wire, nylon, and silk thread suture, and stainless steel clips in 287 patients with abdominal surgical wounds. The number of dressing changes, infection rate, dehiscence rate, hematoma formation, and appearance of the skin two weeks following removal of the closure was observed. Tape closing was preferred, since it was associated with no foreign body reaction, with rapid healing, and with reduction of complications. In the case of an interrupted suture the effective tensile strength was over twice the British Pharmaceutical Codex (BPC) knot strength. In the case of continuous sutures the effective tensile strength may be up to ten times the BPC knot strength [30]. Persistently increased tensile strength and slightly higher hydroxyproline content was noted in the healing wounds of the rabbits sutured with aluminum for 5 days to 8 weeks, when compared with silk and stainless steel sutures [74]. Preston [29] in his study used the following eight suturing techniques: interrupted tight big-bite, interrupted loose big-bite, interrupted tight small-bite, interrupted loose small-bite, continuous tight big-bite, continuous loose big-bite, continuous tight small-bite, and continuous loose small-bite. After two weeks the strongest skin wounds were obtained by interrupted loose small-bite stitches. The wounds found to be the weakest had been closed with the continuous tight big-bite stitch. During the same time annealed stainless steel wire possessed the greatest average strength and showed the least local reaction to the suture material, less than plain catgut, chromic catgut, or silk. Douglas [30] pointed out the complexity of real tensile-strength values of sutures when measured by a tensiometer after specification of the BPC with the "straight-pull" and the "knot" method when compared with the tensile-strength values of the corresponding suture material after interrupted and continuous suture.

In young adult albino male guinea pigs it was observed [32] that normally healing abdominal wounds, closed and measured with nonabsorbable sutures *in situ* regained the strength of normal unwounded skin by the ninth day after wounding and exceeded it significantly by the forty-fifth day. Independently of the time of testing, all wounds with sutures in place were stronger than wounds without sutures. By the ninth day about 30% of the total strength of the wounds were still due to the sutures. From the third day on, the tensile-strength curves of skin measured with and without sutures ran parallel.

In vascular surgery, the strength of the sutures is most essential even weeks after the operation. It has been demonstrated that silk also does not maintain its tensile strength sufficiently well over a long period to ensure that false aneurysms do not develop at the suture line. The authors [21] have seen many cases in which there was breakage of the silk sutures several years after implantation of the graft. Accordingly the authors abandoned the use of silk sutures and used plastic sutures of similar composition to the prosthetic replacement in an attempt to eliminate this late complication.

13.4   BIOCHEMICAL ASPECTS OF HEALING WOUNDS

13.4.1   Production of Granulation Tissue in Sponge Implants

For many years investigators have tried to find means enabling them to determine from the same specimen both the mechanical and chemical properties of the granulation tissue formed. The preparation of poor granulation tissue from the wound for chemical study has been difficult because of the danger of healthy tissue being taken with the specimen. In order to avoid this fault, use has been made of granulating wound surfaces [75–77], foreign body granulomas [78–80], mesh wire cylinders and balls [81–83], carrageenin granulomas [84, 85], gauze and cotton wool pellets [86, 87], and various synthetic sponges [88–92].

I have used viscose cellulose sponge for ten years both in animal experimental and clinical trials [93–100]. The pores in this sponge are interconnected through gaps of variable size, forming an open-cell system. Microscopic measurements of sections have given a mean pore

radius of 0.25 mm, and a summed-up mean area of the pore walls of approximately 60 cm² cm⁻³ dry and 45 cm² cm⁻³ wet. One gram of this Visella* sponge yielded at 550°C 41 mg of ash. The following observations made at the Department of Medical Chemistry, University of Turku, Finland, are obtained using this implantation material solely.†
In my own experiment 340 white Wistar rats were used both for tensile strength studies and for production of granulation tissue [33]. A piece of Visella sponge measuring 10 × 10 × 20 mm was moistened and excess

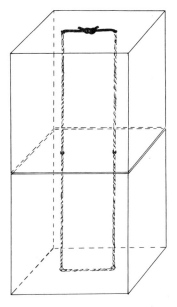

Figure 13.1. Outline of a piece of viscose cellulose sponge of which the two halves are sewn together with silk. After removal of the implant the thread is cut at the lower surface and drawn out through the opposite end [31].

water squeezed out. The piece was cut with scissors into two equal sections across its length. Using the technique shown in Fig. 13.1, the cut surfaces were sewn together in their original position. A median dorsal incision about 3-cm long was made through the skin and superficial fascia caudally from the scapulae. The implants, one on either side, were placed in position, and the wound was closed with continuous su-

* Registered trade name.
† The manufacturer Säteri Oy, Valkeakoski, Finland, has kindly prepared and given special proportions of this Visella sponge for our use.

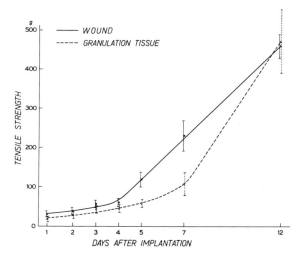

Figure 13.2.   Mean tensile strengths of skin wounds and granulation tissue and their standard deviations on the 1st–12th postoperative days. Note the maximal differences at 5 to 7 days [31].

ture. The 1st, 2nd, 3rd, 4th, 5th, 7th, 12th, 21st and 60th postimplantation days were selected as observation days. The removed sponges were enclosed in a connective tissue capsule varying in thickness with the implantation period. This capsule was carefully freed from the implants of the first days. Later the capsule was so strictly fixed to the surface of the sponge that removal was no longer possible. Tensile-strength measurements were performed both from the wounds and from the implants [33]. On the twenty-first postimplantation day the sponge ingrown granulation tissue was so strong that the halves stitched together could not be torn at the juncture and the pieces broke near the clamps. It was no longer possible with any of the methods employed to tear the granulation tissue between the halves. Tensile-strength measurements of granulation tissue could therefore be performed only on the first to twelfth days (Fig. 13.2).

13.4.2   Results of Chemical Analysis of Sponge Ingrown Granulation Tissue

Water-soluble Components

Soluble tissue proteins. The tissues were dialysed for three days against water, lyophilised, and redissolved in a small quantity of veronal-acetate buffer of pH 8.6. The electrophoretic runs were performed in the same buffer, ionic strength 0.1 for two hours at 120 V. Thus determined, the albumin: globulin ratio of water-soluble proteins in the sponge was 1.0 on the second and third days, 0.8 on the fourth–twelfth days, 0.6 on the twenty-first day and only 0.3 on the sixtieth day. The protein which had remained immobile at the point of application, that is, on the starting line, was interpreted as collagen. It averaged 5% on the first to third days, rising further up to the twenty-first day, when it was 20%. On the sixtieth day the proportion at the application site was only 9%.

Hemoglobin. The hemoglobin content of granulation tissue varied greatly with age. The initial value on the first day must be regarded as primarily due to blood oozing from small vascular lesions. On the second day it appeared to diminish but from the third day onwards it increased and the mean of the peak values 9.4 mg per piece was reached on the seventh day. The rich vascularity did not remain unchanged for long because by the twelfth day a fall of hemoglobin content to the final 6 mg per piece was already demonstrated.

Hexosamine. Only little variation was observed in the quantities of water-soluble hexosamine. On the first day most of this probably derived from tissue fluid. The peak value of 740 μg/piece was found on the fifth day. During the next two weeks the values again decreased to the original first-day level. The increase in hexosamine content concurrently with the volume of circulating blood is in agreement with the view that a part of the hexosamine in granulation tissue derives from plasma.

Uronic acid. There was an increase from the first-day value of 175 μg/piece to 216 μg/piece on the seventh day and then a decrease up to the sixtieth day, when there was only 150 μg/piece of uronic acid.

Free hydroxyproline. The amount of free hydroxyproline increased up to the fourth day to a peak value of 43 μg/piece and then remained at about this level. It is worth noting that the sharp growth of the total collagen quantity after the fifth day failed to cause any change in the amount of free hydroxyproline.

Imino acids. The content of proline and hydroxyproline in the water-soluble fraction increased during the first 7 days. The free imino acids represent only 3–4% of total imino acids. Neither free proline nor free hydroxyproline is dependent on the total amount of collagen.

Nonprotein nitrogen. An average of 0.3 mg/piece on the first day increased to 1.2 mg/piece on the sixtieth day. This must be mainly due to the protein metabolism of the granulation tissue itself.

Mucopolysaccharides

Lehtonen [101], using viscose cellulose sponges as implantation material and white Wistar rats as experimental animals, made the following findings concerning mucopolysaccharides during an observation period of 102 days: In saline-soluble mucopolysaccharides an early rise in the amounts of neutral sugars and of hexosamines was observed. Sialic acid was detected on the first and third day. Of acid mucopolysaccharides, both hyaluronic acid and chondroitin sulphates were present on the third day after implantation. The content of chondroitin sulphates subsequently increased rapidly until the twenty-fifth day. The content of hyaluronic acid likewise increased with age but remained relatively low. In addition, glycoproteins were detected at least during the first few days. The glucosamine content increased more rapidly than that of galactosamine in young granulomas.

In the saline-insoluble mucopolysaccharides, small amounts of amino sugars and neutral sugars were found on the first day after implantation. Chondroitin sulphate, first detected on the third day, increased in amount until the fortieth day and then remained approximately constant. No increase was observed with age in insoluble hyaluronic acid. The amount of neutral sugars was small on the first few days and then increased steadily. The content of insoluble mucopolysaccharides was about 10–20% of the soluble mucopolysaccharides on the third day and then increased steadily up to the fortieth day, when the amounts of both fractions were approximately equal. Further analysis showed that, of the chondroitin sulphates, chondroitin sulphate A predominated. The amount of chondroitin sulphate C was very small and chondroitin sulphate B was not found.

Nucleic Acids

In my own experiment [33] DNA reached a maximum on the twenty-first day whereas total RNA indicating protein synthesis in the cells continued to increase to the end of the test period of two months. The amount of free deoxyribonucleotides was doubled during the first three days and was then constant at 50–60 μg/piece. The amount of free ribonucleotides on the twelfth day was three times the first-day value. Peak values for transfer-RNA were also recorded on the twelfth day.

Ahonen [102], using the same implantation arrangement, showed that the rate of DNA biosynthesis, studied by incorporation of ^{14}C-glycine *in vitro*, was maximal during the first week of granuloma development (Fig. 13.3). The rate of RNA synthesis did not closely parallel the rate of synthesis of proteins. The extractability of RNA remained con-

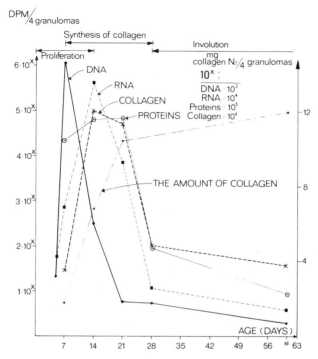

Figure 13.3. Development of experimental granulation tissue in the rat as indicated by the capacity to incorporate ^{14}C-glycine into nucleic acids and proteins *in vitro*. A modified scheme based on J. Ahonen, *Acta Physiol. Scand. suppl.*, **315**, (1968).

stant with increasing age of the granulation tissue while that of DNA decreased. On the basis of further investigation it was concluded that synthesis of ribosomal RNA dominates during the cell proliferation phase whereas emphasis is on the production of messenger-RNA during the phase of rapid synthesis of collagen.

Collagen Fractions

On the basis of the solubility of granulation tissue homogenate in neutral salt and acid solutions, the following schemes, seen in Figs. 13.4a and b, were obtained [33]. On the first three days the water-soluble fraction contained 70% of the total nitrogen in the granulation tissue and 45% on the sixtieth day. The absolute values rose from 6.0 mg/piece on the first day to a peak of 10.0 mg/piece on the twenty-first day. These high values come from the plasma proteins which were absorbed by the sponge. To a small extent this was due to the water-soluble

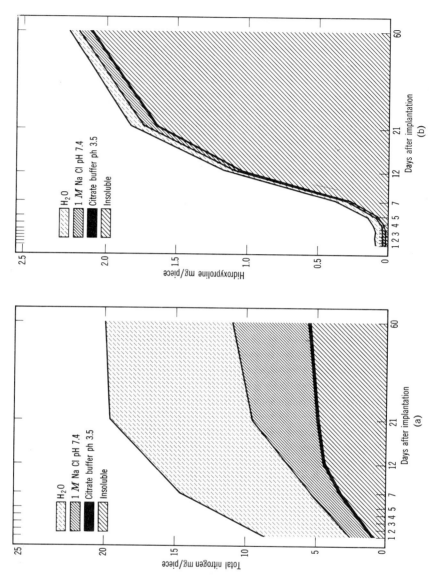

Figure 13.4. (a) Total nitrogen and (b) hydroxyproline contained in unpurified collagen fractions of the sponge-ingrown granulation tissue in the rat [31].

nitrogenous substances which were synthesized in the implant itself or were originally degradation products. The hydroxyproline of the water-soluble fraction was roughly doubled during the observation period. Approximately a half of this quantity was free hydroxyproline. Hydroxyproline in the neutral salt-soluble fraction rose slightly during the first five days. From the seventh day on, the increase was distinctly faster and at the sixtieth day it was seven times the first-day value. The acid-soluble fraction contained only minimal amounts of hydroxyproline per piece and remained such through the whole observation period. In insoluble-collagen fraction hydroxyproline was unchanged on the first three days, rose slightly on the fourth day and then very sharply up to the last observation day.

13.5   CHEMICAL BASIS OF MECHANICAL STRENGTH IN WOUND HEALING

13.5.1   Collagen

On the basis of their animal experiments Dunphy and Udupa [15] concluded that the tensile strength of the healing wound depends on the amount of collagen that has formed between the wound margins. To gain more accurate information about the role of various collagen fractions and about possible other components of connective tissue, correlation and regression analysis was performed between various analytical results of the sponge-ingrown granulation tissue and tensile-strength values of the wounds and poor granulation tissue (Fig. 13.5). The highest positive correlations with the tensile strength of the skin wound and granulation tissue were between the hydroxyproline of neutral salt-soluble, insoluble and total collagen ($r = +0.97$ or $+0.98$). The regression analysis showed that on the first to fourth days the tensile strength of healing skin wound depended directly on neutral salt-soluble and insoluble collagen in the ratio 2:3. From the twelfth day on this ratio varied from 1:8 to 1:10. Comparison between the calculated tensile-strength values and the measured values showed that the calculated values corresponded more closely to the tensile strength of the granulation tissue alone measured from the implants. Thus there must have been other factors operating at the time which increased the tensile strength of the healing-skin wounds. Water-soluble and acid-soluble components containing hydroxyproline had no positive effect on the tensile strength. An increase in acid-soluble collagen, on a purely mathematical basis, should result in a loss of tensile strength. Biochemically this might mean the breaking of the intermolecular cross-links of collagen when

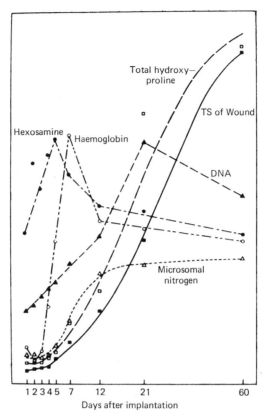

Figure 13.5. Graphic summary on the changes of tensile strength of healing rat wounds, and total hydroxyproline, hexosamine, hemoglobin, DNA, and microsomal nitrogen of sponge-ingrown granulation tissue during 1 to 60 postoperative days. The scale of the curves is the same in regard to time, not in regard to quantity [31].

converted into acid-soluble form. An increase in such a component would thus involve a relative decrease in insoluble collagen and hence, indirectly, loss of tensile strength.

Determinations of the molar ratios of α- and β-components in soluble collagens have shown that there are mainly α-components in collagen soluble in neutral-salt solution, whereas the ratios of α- and β-components in collagens soluble in acid-buffer solutions are equal. This is in agreement with the view that neutral salt-soluble collagen represents a recently synthesized collagen and that the number of cross-links in collagen increases with age as found, for example, by starch-gel electrophoresis [103]. An increase in the intermolecular attractive forces, perhaps an increase in the number of cross-links, might be the cause of the decreased solubility. The histological differences, laminated fiber structure versus three-dimensional, cannot alone explain the differences in solubility. No information is available on the relationship between the tensile strength and the number of cross-links *in vivo*. Even so, it is still under discussion whether similar cross-links exist between other proteins [104]. Significant for the stability of the collagen molecule are not only the numbers of hydrogen bonds and pyrrolidine rings, that is the content of proline and hydroxyproline, but also the distribution of these amino acids throughout the molecule [105, 106]. The way in which hydroxyl groups stabilize the collagen structure is unknown. The investigations of Bensusan and Nielsen [107] and Rao and Harrington [106] support the structure with two interchain hydrogen bonds to every amino-acid triplet. One hydrogen bond per triplet is, however, enough to produce triple helical conformation, as demonstrated by Traub and Yonath [108] on the synthetic polypeptides. Kühn et al. [109] distinguished three types of intermolecular cross-links, namely end-to-end, head-to-tail, and side-to-side bonds. No information is available as regards the bonds which (and the order in which they) stabilize the newly synthesized collagen in newly formed granulation tissue and give their support to the strength of healing wounds.

In this context it is worth mentioning the observations of Juva and Prockop [110], Kivirikko and Prockop [111], and Juva [112] on the hydroxylation of proline and lysine in the polypeptide (Fig. 13.6). In this process, together with a polypeptide of definite size and appropriate amino acid sequence, a hydroxylating enzyme, atmospheric oxygen, ferrous iron, and possibly ascorbate is required. Hutton et al. [113] have suggested that α-ketoglutarate might function as an allosteric activator of hydroxylating enzyme, and its concentration in the cell could regulate the activity of this enzyme and thus the synthesis of collagen.

Interesting are the relatively low-oxygen tensions in the wound tissue [114] and the beneficial effect of atmospheric oxygen on the synthesis of collagen [115–117]. Prolonged inhalation of 35–70 volumes % oxygen at 1 atm. increased the tensile strength of healing cutaneous wounds and of granulation tissue in the rats [117]. However, this treatment did not shorten the latent period of 1–5 days in the beginning of wound healing (Fig. 13.7).

13.5.2   Mucopolysaccharides

As already stated, collagen alone does not explain the rapid increase in tensile strength of the healing wounds. Some supporting factors must be present. For mucopolysaccharide to be effective as a binding agent it must have the following characteristics:

1. Inherent tensile strength
2. Ability to combine with collagen
3. Ability to augment collagen tensile strength when combined with it [60].

It is wrong to demand that some components should be stronger than collagen in order to give any additional support to the wound tensile

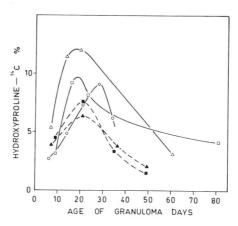

Figure 13.6. Hydroxylating activity in granuloma supernates of varying age. The hydroxylating mixtures contained, as a substrate, aliquots from a 100,000 x g supernate from chick-embryo tibia homogenate, labeled with L-proline-^{14}C in the presence of α, α'-dipyridyl, 0.05 M tris-buffer, pH 7.6, 0.02 M KCl, 1×10^{-5} M EDTA, 5×10^{-5} M FeSO$_4$, and 10 ml of granuloma supernate in a final volume of 15 ml. The samples were incubated at 37°C for 1 hr. Courtesy of K. Juva, [112] *Acta Physiol. Scand. suppl.*, 308 (1968).

strength [118]. On the other hand, it is proposed that alterations in the cohesive forces between collagen macrostructures (filaments, fibrils, fibers, and bundles) are directly related to the ratio of collagen to mucopolysaccharide [60]. Fessler [119] demonstrated that if there is a favorable collagen to mucopolysaccharide ratio (9.1:1 in the rat) in the wound, the mucopolysaccharide contributes to tensile strength gain by amalgamation of the larger collagen units (filaments, fibrils, fibers, and bundles). If the collagen to mucopolysaccharide ratio is unfavorable (3.8:1 in a mouse), the excess mucopolysaccharide interferes with aggregation and development of cohesiveness between the larger collagen units.

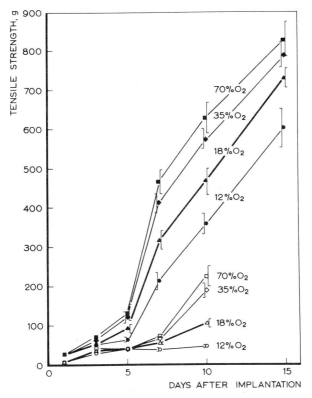

Figure 13.7. The tensile strengths of skin wounds and experimental granulomas at different atmospheric oxygen concentrations during the first 15 postoperative days. The tensile strengths of the skin wounds (dark symbols) are given in g cm^{-1} of healing wound width and the tensile strengths of the granulomas (open symbols) in g cm^{-2} of cross-sectional area. All values are means for 8–29 rats or 32–116 granulomas. The length of each vertical bar represents twice the standard error of the mean. Courtesy of J. Niinikoski [117], *Acta Physiol. Scand. suppl.*, **334** (1969).

As the excess mucopolysaccharide is resolved, a more favorable ratio is established, permitting tensile strength gain. Thus the ratio of collagen to mucopolysaccharide seems to be a decisive factor in tissue tensile strength.

Many other investigators have studied the interaction between mucopolysaccharides and collagen fibers. Hyaluronic acid, chondroitin sulphates A, B, and C, neutral polysaccharides, and polar polysaccharide-protein polymers have been beneficial in *in vitro* experiments to the precipitation and orientation of collagen fibers [119–130]. The interrelationship within healing wounds is not yet clear at all and much work remains to be done before this can be proved to play any role in stabilization of fibrils.

13.5.3 Noncollagenous Proteins

Geever et al. [131] treated the cut strips of guinea pig-skin wounds with mercuric chloride solution and determined their tensile strengths after 48-hr treatment. It is known that some reactive groups of proteins, such as primary amino and amido, guanidyl, indole and imidazole groups, mercapto radicals, and phenols, may take part in formaldehyde reactions. The authors assumed that mercury presumably reacts with different groups causing an additional bonding effect resulting from the successive treatment with both chemicals. The authors continued: "Similar opportunity for bonding probably exists in the margins between the wound proteins, cells, the preexisting dermal collagen, and noncollagenous proteins in the marginal ground substance." They considered that the reparative epidermis, fibroblasts, endothelial, adventitial, and inflammatory cells, and noncollagenous proteins within the wounds significantly contribute to the breaking strength of older wounds also.

13.5.4 Others

Heikkinen [104] stated the following order of the metal cations in the formation of insoluble collagen. The effectiveness decreased as follows; $Co^{2+} > Cu^{2+} > Cu^+ > Au^{3+} = Ni^{2+} > Fe^{3+} > Hg^{2+} > Cr^{3+} > Ca^{2+} > Fe^{2+} > Al^{3+} > Pb^{4+} > Sn^{4+} > Sr^{2+} = Ba^{2+} > Mn^{2+} = Mg^{2+}$. Rovee and Miller [132] studied the tensile strength of healing isolated epidermis in guinea pig plantar wounds. The plantar skin was removed and placed in $2N$ sodium bromide at 37°C for 2 hr or in 0.1% trypsin solution at 14°C for 8–10 hr. The epidermis could then be easily split from the underlying dermis. The epidermal strength was measured after 3, 4, 5, 6, 7, 8, 10, 12, 14, and 20 days using 4-mm-wide strips and an Instron extensometer. The breaking strength of epidermal incisions rose rapidly from the third day on. At 8 days it was more than 50% of the control epidermal values and in 20 days it had reached the strength of control epidermis. This might well reflect the cohesive forces between epidermal cells. Desmosomes, intercellular "glue," plication of cell membranes with interdigitation, or any combination of these, might be factors responsible for producing epidermal tensile strength.

13.6 SUMMARY

To summarize present knowledge of factors responsible for tensile strength in wound healing it can be said that, during the first week of healing, neutral-salt soluble collagen and insoluble collagen together with mucopolysaccharides and noncollagenous proteins and some intercellular forces (not known in detail) are able to increase the tensile strength to such a level that the edges of most skin wounds remain in good apposition after removal of the stitches. Thereafter collagen alone is more and more responsible for tensile strength, and the effect of all other factors is restricted to stabilizing of collagen fibrils. Further work is necessary to help clarify, even from the mechanical point of view, the complicated interactions of various chemical components in wound healing.

ACKNOWLEDGMENTS

I wish to express my deep gratitude to my former Chief, Professor Eino Kulonen, M.D., Head of the Department of Medical Chemistry, University of Turku, for valuable guidance and laboratory facilities during the time I was working in his department.

I also wish to express my thanks to my teacher, Professor Sauli Vilkki, M.D., Head of the Department of Surgery, University of Turku, for untiring guidance in the problems of clinical surgery and for the active interest he showed in the field of experimental surgery.

My appreciative thanks are due to my present Chief, Docent Panu Vilkki, M.D., Head of the Department of Pediatric Surgery, for valuable help and instruction in clinical surgery throughout the past ten years and for useful criticism during preparation of this manuscript.

I am greatly indebted to my colleagues, Doctors J. Ahonen, K. Juva and J. Niinikoski, for kindly allowing me to present some of their results as original diagrams in this review.

Last but not least I owe my thanks to Miss Aino Wuolle, Mag. phil., for revising the language of the manuscript, and to Miss Tuula Rantanen for secretarial assistance.

REFERENCES

1. M. Allgöwer, *The Cellular Basis of Wound Repair*, Charles C. Thomas, Springfield, Ill., 1956.
2. F. R. Johnson and R. M. H. McMinn, *Physiol. Rev.*, **35**, 364 (1960).

3. J. Raekallio, *Ann. Med. Exptl. Biol. Fenniae* **39**, Suppl. 6 (1961).

4. J. Raekallio, *Die Altersbestimmung mechanisch bedingter Hautwunden mit enzymhistochemischen Methoden,* Schmidt-Römhild, Lübeck, 1965.

5. G. Asboe-Hansen, *Connective Tissue in Health and Disease,* Munksgaard, Copenhagen, 1954.

6. R. W. Chen and R. W. Postlethwait, *Monographs in Surg. Sci.,* **1**, 215 (1964).

7. L. C. Edwards and J. E. Dunphy, *New England J. Med.,* **259**, 224 (1958).

8. L. C. Edwards and J. E. Dunphy, *New England J. Med.,* **259**, 275 (1958).

9. W. Montagna and R. E. Billingham, *Advances in Biology of Skin,* Vol. 5, Pergamon Press, London, 1964.

10. P. S. Russell and R. E. Billingham, *Prog. Surg.,* **2**, 1 (1962).

11. J. A. Schilling, *Physiol. Rev.,* **48**, 374 (1968).

12. J. E. Dunphy and H. W. Van Winkle, Jr., *Repair and Regeneration. The Scientific Basis for Surgical Practice.* McGraw-Hill, New York, 1969.

13. J. Paget, *Lectures on Surgical Pathology,* Vol. 1, Longman, Brown, Green, and Longmans, London, 1853.

14. E. L. Howes, J. W. Sooy, and S. C. Harvey, *J. Amer. Med. Assoc.,* **92**, 42 (1929).

15. J. E. Dunphy and K. N. Udupa, *New England J. Med.,* **253**, 847 (1955).

16. J. E. Dunphy and D. S. Jackson, *Amer. J. Surg.,* **104**, 273 (1962).

17. J. C. Forrester, B. H. Zederfledt, T. H. Hayes, and T. K. Hunt, *Repair and Regeneration,* J. E. Dunphy and H. W. Van Winkle, Jr., Eds., McGraw-Hill, New York, 1969.

18. E. L. Howes, S. C. Harvey, and C. Hewitt, *Arch. Surg.,* **38**, 934 (1939).

19. S. M. Levenson, E. F. Geever, L. V. Crowley, J. F. Oates, C. W. Berard, and H. Rosen, *Ann. Surg.,* **161**, 293 (1965).

20. J. E. Dunphy, *Can. J. Surg.,* **10**, 281 (1967).

21. M. E. DeBakey, G. L. Jordan, A. C. Beall, Jr., R. M. O'Neal, J. P. Abbott, and B. Halpert, *Surg. Clin. North. Amer.,* **45**, 477 (1965).

22. D. W. James, *Advances in Biology of Skin,* Vol. 5, W. Montagna and R. Billingham, Eds., Pergamon Press, London, 1964.

23. M. Abercrombie, M. H. Flint, and D. W. James, *J. Embryol. Exp. Morphol.,* **2**, 264 (1954).

24. J. E. Dunphy, *Ann. Roy. Coll. Surg. England,* **26**, 69 (1960).

25. A. A. Glaser, R. D. Marangoni, J. S. Must, T. G. Beckwith, G. S. Brody, G. R. Walker, and W. L. White, *Med. Elect. Biol. Eng.,* **3**, 411 (1965).

26. R. A. Milch, *J. Surg. Res.,* **5**, 377 (1965).

27. S. C. Harvey, *AMA Arch. Surg.,* **18**, 1227 (1929).

28. N. Huu and H. M. Albert, *Amer. Surg.,* **32**, 421 (1966).

29. D. J. Preston, *Amer. J. Surg.,* **49**, 56 (1940).

30. D. M. Douglas, *Lancet,* **2**, 497 (1949).

31. B. Löfström and B. Zederfelt, *Acta Chir. Scand.,* **112**, 152 (1956).

32. R. J. Adamsons and I. F. Enquist, *Surg. Gynecol. Obstet.,* **117**, 396 (1963).

33. J. Viljanto, *Acta Chir. Scand. Suppl.,* **333**, (1964).

34. T. W. Botsford, *Surg. Gynecol. Obstet.*, **72**, 690 (1941).

35. S. A. Localio, W. Casale, and J. W. Hinton, *Surg. Gynecol. Obstet.*, **77**, 376 (1943).

36. Ph. Sandblom, *Acta Chir. Scand. Suppl.*, **89**, (1944).

37. J. Fast, C. Nelson, and C. Dennis, *Surg. Gynecol. Obstet.*, **84**, 685 (1947).

38. Ph. Sandblom, P. Petersen, and A. Muren, *Acta Chir. Scand.*, **105**, 252 (1953).

39. E. D. Savlov and J. E. Dunphy, *New England J. Med.*, **250**, 1062 (1954).

40. B. Zederfeldt, *Acta Chir. Scand., Suppl.*, **224**, (1957).

41. R. W. Postlethwait, J. F. Schauble, M. L. Dillon, and J. Morgan, *Surg. Gynecol. Obstet.*, **108**, 555 (1959).

42. J. F. Prudden, O. Gabriel, and B. Allen, *Arch. Surg.*, **86**, 157 (1963).

43. R. D. Harkness, *Biol. Rev.*, **36**, 399 (1961).

44. J. B. Herrmann, S. C. Woodward, and E. J. Pulaski, *Surg. Gynecol. Obstet.*, **119**, 269 (1964).

45. T. S. Nelson and C. J. Anders, *Arch. Surg.*, **93**, 309 (1966).

46. F. T. Caldwell, Jr., P. Donohue, and B. Rosenberg, *J. Amer. Med. Assoc.*, **179**, 773 (1962).

47. Y. Sako and O. H. Wangensteen, *Surg. Forum*, **2**, 117 (1951).

48. K. Cronin, D. S. Jackson, and J. E. Dunphy, *Surg. Gynecol. Obstet.*, **126**, 747 (1968).

49. N. N. Fellows, J. Burge, C. S. Halch, and P. B. Price, *Surg. Forum*, **2**, 111 (1951).

50. T. M. Scheinin and J. Viljanto, *Ann. Med. Exptl. Biol. Fenniae*, **44**, 49 (1966).

51. F. J. Gray and F. H. Caldwell, *Brit. J. Surg.*, **54**, 761 (1967).

52. P. Zink, *Deut. Z. Ges. Ger. Med.*, **56**, 349 (1965).

53. E. F. Geever, J. M. Stein, and S. M. Levenson, *J. Trauma*, **5**, 624 (1965).

54. R. H. Adler, M. Mendez, and C. Darby, *Surgery*, **52**, 898 (1962).

55. D. M. Douglas, *Wound Healing*, D. Slome, Ed., Pergamon Press, Oxford, 1961.

56. M. E. Nimni, E. deGuia, and L. A. Bavetta, *J. Invest. Dermatol.*, **47**, 156 (1966).

57. P. G. Nelson, D. J. Breen, and J. L. Bremner, *J. Surg.*, **37**, 75 (1967).

58. J. K. Narat, J. P. Cangelosi, and J. V. Belmonte, *Surg. Forum*, **7**, 176 (1956).

59. S. A. Mendoza and R. A. Milch, *Gerontologia*, **10**, 42 (1964/65).

60. W. M. Bryant and P. M. Weeks, *Plastic Reconstruc. Surg.*, **39**, 84 (1967).

61. J. Pikkarainen, *Acta Physiol. Scand., Suppl.*, **309**, (1968).

62. P. Bornstein and K. A. Piez, *J. Clin. Invest.*, **43**, 1813 (1964).

63. V. N. Orekhovitch and V. O. Shpikiter, *Recent Advances in Gelatin and Glue Research*, G. Stainsby, Ed., Pergamon Press, London, 1958.

64. D. A. Hall and R. Reed, *Nature*, **180**, 243 (1957).

65. B. J. Rigby, *Biochim. Biophys. Acta*, **62**, 183 (1962).

66. B. J. Rigby, *Biochim. Biophys. Acta*, **133**, 272 (1967).

67. K. H. Gustavson, *Svensk Kem. Tidskr.*, **65**, 70 (1953).

482   Tensile Strength of Healing Wounds

68. S. A. Mendoza and R. A Milch, *Surg. Forum.*, **15**, 433 (1964).
69. J. Viljanto and J. Ahonen, *Acta Chir. Scand.*, **134**, 183 (1968).
70. S. Kullander and A. Olsson, *Acta Endocrinol.*, **41**, 314 (1962).
71. M. D. Sussman, *Proc. Soc. Exptl. Biol. Med.*, **123**, 38 (1966).
72. J. E. Craik and I. R. R. McNeil, *Nature*, **209**, 931 (1966).
73. A. A. Ferris and F. E. Henry, Jr., *J. Amer. Osteopath. Assoc.*, **65**, 1082 (1966).
74. K. T. Wu, P S. Chopra, and P. N. Sawyer, *Invest. Surg.*, **64**, 605 (1968).
75. M. B. Williamson and H. J. Fromm, *J. Biol. Chem.*, **212**, 705 (1955).
76. H. C. Grillo and J. Gross, *Proc. Soc. Exptl. Biol. Med.*, **101**, 268 (1959).
77. A. Schmidt, *Acta Chir. Scand.*, **121**, 176 (1961).
78. A. Saxén and P. I. Tuovinen, *Acta Chir. Scand.*, **96**, 131 (1948).
79. R. C. Curran and J. S. Kennedy, *Nature*, **175**, 435 (1955).
80. M. Wolman and B. Wolman, *AMA Arch. Path.*, **62**, 74 (1956).
81. G. Hass, *Amer. J. Path.*, **16**, 549 (1940).
82. J. A. Schilling and L. E. Milch, *Proc. Soc. Exptl. Biol. Med.*, **89**, 189 (1955).
83. B. N. White, M. R. Shetlar, H. M. Shurley, and J. A. Schilling, *Proc. Soc. Exptl. Biol. Med.*, **101**, 353 (1959).
84. W. van B. Robertson and B. Schwartz, *J. Biol. Chem.*, **201**, 689 (1953).
85. D. S. Jackson and J. P. Bentley, *J. Biophys. Biochem. Cytol.*, **7**, 37 (1960).
86. L. A. Saikku, *Ann. Med. Exptl. Biol. Fenniae*, **34**, Suppl. 10 (1956).
87. I. E. Bush and R. W. Alexander, *Acta Endocrinol.*, **35**, 268 (1960).
88. J. H. Grindlay and J. M. Vaugh, *AMA Arch. Surg.*, **63**, 288 (1951).
89. R. J. Boucek and N. L. Noble, *AMA Arch. Path.*, **59**, 553 (1955).
90. J. F. Woessner Jr. and R. J. Boucek, *Arch. Biochem.*, **93**, 85 (1961).
91. R. W. Ehen and R. W. Postlethwait, *Surg. Gynecol. Obstet.*, **112**, 667 (1961).
92. J. E. Salvatore, W. S. Gilmer, M. Kashgaran, and W. Barbee, *Surg. Gynecol. Obstet.*, **112**, 463 (1961).
93. J. Viljanto and E. Kulonen, *Acta Pathol. Microbiol. Scand.*, **56**, 120 (1962).
94. J. Viljanto and A. Kivikoski, *Ann. Med. Exptl. Biol. Fenniae*, **40**, 118 (1962).
95. J. Viljanto, H. Isomäki, and E. Kulonen, *Acta Pharmacol. Toxicol.*, **19**, 191 (1962).
96. J. Viljanto, H. Isomäki, and E. Kulonen, *Acta Endocrinol.*, **41**, 395 (1962).
97. E. Vänttinen and J. Viljanto, *Ann. Med. Exptl. Biol. Fenniae*, **43**, 257 (1965).
98. J. Viljanto, *Scand. J. Clin. Lab. Invest.*, **19**, Suppl. 95, 88 (1967).
99. T. M. Scheinin and J. Viljanto, *Ann. Med. Exptl. Biol. Fenniae*, **45**, 373 (1967).
100. J. Viljanto, *Acta Chir. Scand.*, **135**, 297 (1969).
101. A. Lehtonen, *Acta Physiol. Scand. Suppl.*, **310**, (1968).
102. J. Ahonen, *Acta Physiol. Scand. Suppl.*, **315**, (1968).
103. E. Heikkinen and E. Kulonen, *Experientia*, **20**, 310 (1964).
104. E. Heikkinen, *Acta Physiol. Scand. Suppl.*, **317**, (1968).
105. J. Josse and W. F. Harrington, *J. Mol. Biol.*, **9**, 269 (1964).

106. N. V. Rao and W. F. Harrington, *J. Mol. Biol.,* **21,** 577 (1966).

107. H. B. Bensusan and S. O. Nielsen, *Biochemistry,* **3,** 1367 (1964).

108. W. Traub and A. Yonath, *J. Mol. Biol.,* **16,** 404 (1966).

109. K. Kühn, K. Bräumer, B. Zimmermann, and J. Pikkarainen, in press.

110. K. Juva and D. J. Prockop, *Biochim. Biophys. Acta,* **91,** 174 (1964).

111. K. I. Kivirikko and D. J. Prockop, *Biochem. J.,* **102,** 432 (1967).

112. K. Juva, *Acta Physiol. Scand. Suppl.,* **308** (1968).

113. J. J. Hutton, Jr., A. L. Tappel, and S. Udenfriend, *Arch. Biochem.,* **118,** 231 (1967).

114. T. K. Hunt, P. Twomey, B. Zederfeldt, and J. E. Dunphy, *Amer. J. Surg.,* **114,** 302 (1967).

115. K. Lampiaho and E. Kulonen, *Biochem. J.,* **105,** 333 (1967).

116. E. Kulonen, J. Niinikoski, and R. Penttinen, *Acta Physiol. Scand.,* **70,** 112 (1967).

117. J. Niinikoski, *Acta Physiol. Scand. Suppl.,* **334** (1969).

118. P. Fry, M. L. R. Harkness, and R. D. Harkness, *Amer. J. Physiol.,* **206,** 1425 (1964).

119. J. H. Fessler, *Biochem. J.,* **76,** 124 (1960).

120. H. R. Elden, *Biochem. Biophys. Acta,* **79,** 592 (1964).

121. J. Gross, J. H. Highberger, and F. O. Schmitt, *Proc. Soc. Exptl. Biol. Med.,* **80,** 462 (1952).

122. J. Gross, *J. Exptl. Med.,* **107,** 247 (1958).

123. D. S. Jackson, *Biochem. J.,* **54,** 638 (1953).

124. A. Clerici, A. Bairati, Jr., and P. Mocarelli, *Experientia,* **18,** 241 (1962).

125. M. K. Keech, *J. Biophys. Biochem. Cytol.,* **9,** 193 (1961).

126. E. Kodicek and G. Loewi, *Proc. Roy. Soc. London,* Ser. B, **144,** 100 (1955).

127. K. Kühn, *Leder,* **13,** 156 (1962).

128. G. Loewi and K. Meyer, *Biochim. Biophys. Acta,* **27,** 453 (1958).

129. M. Németh-Czóka, *Acta Histochem.,* **9,** 282 (1960).

130. S. M. Partridge, *Biochem. J.,* **43,** 387 (1948).

131. E. F. Geever, S. M. Levenson, and G. Manner, *Surgery,* **60,** 343 (1966).

132. D. T. Rovee and C. A. Miller, *Arch. Surg.,* **96,** 43 (1968).

14

Mechanism of Water Uptake by Skin

J. R. YATES

Division of Protein Chemistry, CSIRO, Parkville, Victoria 3052, Australia

Compared with other organs, the skin is not particularly rich in water under normal physiological conditions, and Lepore [1] found that of the soft tissues, the skin contains least water per unit weight. Skelton [2] also shows, for example, that skeletal muscles contain more water both relatively and absolutely than skin. In man, the skin constitutes 16–18% of the total body weight, and contains 18–20% of the total water of the body, whereas skeletal muscles constitute 41–42% of the body weight and contain about half the total body water.

485

There is considerable evidence that the skin acts as a reservoir both in receiving excess water and making water available according to the physiological needs of the organism. In spite of its lower water content compared to the other soft tissues of the body, a considerable mass of water is accumulated in the skin, a man of 65 kg having about 8.4 kg [2], and unlike most other organs this amount can change considerably without causing any functional disturbance [3, 4]. About 75% of the total available (i.e., extracellular) water of the body is contained in the muscles and the skin, and skin contains between four and five times as much available water per unit weight of tissue as the muscles [3]. On an absolute basis, however, because the total mass of muscle is about twice that of skin, the latter contains approximately twice as much available water as the muscle. In moderate dehydration all tissues lose water (per unit weight) in approximate proportion to their available water content [2, 4]. However in excessive hydration or severe dehydration, the role of skin is disproportionately high in changing its water content to offset both effects [2–9]. The ability of skin to act as a reservoir is seen most prominently in various pathological states, uptake being prominent in kidney insufficiency, obesity, acromegaly [10], and various intestinal deficiencies [11], and dehydration occurring in diabetes insipidus [12] and in parathyroid insufficiency [13].

Water contents of various animal skins have been determined by numerous workers, although a great amount of the work does not refer to fat-free skins, and consequently the figures display much greater variation than is actually the case. The problems of estimation of water content of skins have been discussed by Hermann [14], and by Wynn and Haldi [15]. The work of Eichelberger et al. [16, 17, 18] clearly shows that reproducible results can be obtained only if water contents are expressed relative to the weight of fat-free skin. Eichelberger et al [16, 18], under carefully controlled experimental conditions, found the water content of fat-free adult dog skins to be 71%, and surgical skin specimens from man give an average value of 72%. Values for other skins have been reported as 63.9% for dog [1], 61% for ox, 63% for calf [19], 60% for rat [20], and 67% for sheep [21], all calculated without prior fat extraction. These figures are only fairly typical because substantial variations in water content, over the surface area of a skin, and between different skins have been reported by a number of workers [1, 21, 22, 23]. Rothman [3] advances several reasons apart from differences in fat content to account for these variations. One reason is the heterogeneity of skin with different proportions of epidermis and corium, and also differences in arrangement of the fibers in skin over the various parts of the body. Differences in physical properties of skin depending on sampling position are well-known [24], as are variations in fiber weave with position [25]. Rothman [3], however, believes that the main reason for the variation in water content is the ease with which water is moved to and from the corium according to metabolic needs, and states that measured variations can be eliminated somewhat if the animal is kept under constant conditions for several days, followed by a definite period of fasting, before excision.

Variations in water content of skin with age are well-known, as is the decrease in water content from the embryo stage to adulthood, increasing again in senescence [26–30]. Meyer [31] shows that average values of the water content of skin are 80% in the foetus, 68.4% in the newborn, and 62.1% in adolescents and adults. Differences due to sex and diet have also been reported [32].

Small differences in water content between the various layers of the dermis have been reported [19, 22], but these are probably due to differences in fat content. An average value for epidermal water content has been given at 64.5% [33], but since the horny layer of the epidermis has a low water content, it becomes clear that the water content of the non-cornified layers of the epidermis alone is considerably higher. Eichelberger [in 3], on the basis of suggestions made by Manery and Haege [34] calculated that of the average 715 g of water in 1 kg of fat-free skin, 390 g are associated with fibrous and 325 g with nonfibrous proteins. Later work has indicated that the latter amount largely consists of water in the hyaluronic acid-protein complexes of the "ground substance" [4, 8, 35]. It is important to note that the maximum swelling capacity of the skin, (i.e., the maximum amount of water that the skin can hold), is not fully utilized under normal physiological conditions [8, 21].

14.1   STRUCTURE OF SKIN

Before considering the skin-water relationships in detail, it is desirable to look briefly at the structure of the material being dealt with. The structure of collagen at both molecular and electron microscope level is adequately reviewed by Ramachandran and Hodge, respectively [36]. The basic structural unit is the polypeptide chain in the poly-L-glycine II conformation, three of which are coiled together to constitute the tropocollagen macromolecule. Linear aggregates of tropocollagen macromolecules form the protofibrils, and fibrils consist of different numbers of these protofibrils aligned in parallel to give a fibrillar diameter of between 200–2000 Å. Great differences are found in the strength of the lateral bonding of protofibrils in different types of collagen. Fibrils from fish skins fray easily and dissolve in dilute acid solution, whereas bovine skin collagen does not fray and only swells in dilute acids. One reason for these differences may be the interweaving of the fibrils [37], combined with lateral cohesion due to covalent bonding between the tropocollagen macromolecules. The unit of connective tissue structure may be regarded as a fibril. Many fibrils associate laterally to form the fiber bundles, which may never branch, but may break up into smaller bundles. The fibers are interwoven into a pattern, the compactness of which varies according to both the type of animal, and the location on the animal [25]. Various levels of structure in the build up of connective tissue are represented diagrammatically by Gross [38]. It is apparent that differences in interweaving of fibers will impose varying restrictions on water uptake of the skin. In addition to the overall restrictions imposed by fiber weave, there is considerable evidence that individual fibers are enclosed in a reticulin sheath or by reticulin bands, the exact nature of which is unknown, and further that the intact sheaths or bands impose severe limitations on interfibrillar swelling [39–41]. Kwon et al. [42] have conclusively demonstrated the presence of a similar membrane in kangaroo-tail tendon, and have shown the restrictions that are imposed on swelling.

The spaces between the fibers are filled by "ground substance," a semigel continuum which may be regarded basically as a transudate of plasma containing metabolic-exchange products, and containing an important protein component, changes in which affect the permeability of the skin [43]. However one of the most important constituents of the "ground substance" is the mucopolysaccharide hyaluronic acid; the importance of this substance in the water relationships of skin will be dealt with later. Day [43] considers the "ground substance" of skin to have an organized structural network of protein macromolecules with the interstices of this network filled with aggregates of hyaluronic acid. Considered as a water-uptake system then, skin may be regarded as a heterogeneous system consisting of an irregular network of one phase in a continuum of another [44]. Due to the difficulty of defining the required parameters such as the geometry of the disperse phase, and the exact composition and properties of both phases, a rigorous mathematical treatment of water uptake by skin is virtually impossible.

14.2 HOW WATER IS HELD IN THE SKIN

A large proportion of the water in skin is found interstitially in the "ground substance," in dynamic equilibrium with the water in the rest of the organism [4, 8, 9, 35]. Both skin proteins and mucopolysaccharides, especially hyaluronic acid, play an important part in controlling the water content of skin. Skin connective tissue is able to take up large amounts of water which has often been referred to as belonging to one of two types, "free water" and "bound water." It is a matter of common observation that when fresh detached skin is cut, no water oozes from the skin substance, suggesting that the water is chemically bound. Only in certain pathological conditions, for example, visible oedema, may free water occur in connective tissue [8]. The actual definition of bound water is very vague, and the amount of "bound" water varies according to the particular definition adopted [45]. The most frequently used definition is that "bound water" is that part of the total which is not available to dissolve water soluble nonelectrolytes. Eilers and Labout [45] found that about 80% of the water in skin is "free" water (depending partly on the nonelectrolyte used), while the remaining 20% will not dissolve even the smallest molecule of nonelectrolyte. An indication of the difference of binding energies of various forms of water in skin is given by the data of Lloyd and Shore [46] who state that for water held by gelatin in the isoelectric state, a pressure of 8,000 lbs in.$^{-2}$ is required to remove loosely bound water, and 30,000 lbs in.$^{-2}$ to remove firmly bound water. Water taken up in the acid pH region, on the other hand, requires only 1500 lbs in.$^{-2}$ for its removal. Yates [47], working with fresh sheepskins, and fresh sheepskins that had been soaked in water, shows that only 35% in the former case and 55% in the latter case, of the water is removed by application of a centrifugal force equal to 10,000 G, and an increase in centrifugal force to more than ten times that value only results in the expression of a few more per cent of water. Yates suggests that this easily expressible water is simply held in spaces between the fiber bundles, and that water held in the interfibrillary spaces is not being removed by the application of a centrifugal force. Studies on the removal of water from sheepskins [48] have shown that the "apparent activation energy" of the drying process remains approximately constant over a range of skin-water content values from approximately 600% to 10% (both measured on a dry-weight basis) suggesting that a similar mechanism of water binding by skin may operate over the above range. Below 10% water content, stronger bonding is apparently involved since the "apparent activation energy" for removal of this water is increased markedly. Jahn and Witnauer [49] from differential thermal analysis studies of hides also show that at regains below about 15%, water is bound over a whole spectrum of binding energies. Similar results have been obtained by Watt et al. [50] for the desorption of water by wool keratin, and it is suggested that at low moisture levels, water is held to high-energy binding sites such as —OH, —COOH, or —NH$_3^+$ groups. The suggestions made from the kinetic data are confirmed by thermodynamic studies on the heats of sorption of collagen [51–53]. These show that the initial differential net heat of sorption is very high, indicating a high binding energy for the water at the low regain. The net heat of sorption rapidly drops as more water is absorbed, indicating weaker binding energies. Mellon et al. [54] have demonstrated that peptide groups are responsible for a considerable part of the water uptake from the vapor phase in proteins, and McLaren and Rowan [55] have reviewed the part played by various chemical groups in the adsorption of water vapor by polymers.

There have been many attempts to produce a theoretical isotherm for the uptake of water by swelling, polar systems, most of which give good agreement with experiment for a selected range of substrates (see Refs. [56, 57, 58] for example). White and Eyring [56] propose an isotherm derived by the method of statistical mechanics which gives excellent agreement with experiment for a range of substrates. In a detailed analysis of sorption isotherms of nonhomogeneous sorbents from the vapor phase, D'Arcy and Watt [58] suggest that the sorption isotherm is a composite curve comprised of component isotherms arising from three separate processes (a) monolayer adsorption by strongly bonding sites, (b) monolayer adsorption by weakly bonding sites, and (c) the formation of a multilayer, the extent of which is limited by the properties of the substrate. Kanagy [59] in this context states that adsorption of water vapor by collagen is entirely a function of available surface below 75% relative humidity, whereas above 75% relative humidity other factors exert an influence. It is largely the uptake of water from the liquid phase that is considered in this chapter. At this stage of water uptake most of the water molecules are associated only with other water molecules and not directly with the collagenous sorbent. This is a point of difference from (c) above, since water in the multilayer is not to be considered as liquid water [60], nor does the multilayer necessarily approach infinity at saturation vapor pressure. This is important from the point of view of liquid water uptake as it may dictate the mode of adsorption of the first few molecules from the liquid phase.

The large decrease in entropy on water uptake by a dry protein [52, 61–64] is indicative of an ordering of the water molecules taking place. As the water content of the substrate increases, the differential entropy change decreases. This together with the fact that the differential net heat of sorption is very low at high water contents, and that the free-energy change must become zero for the water content in equilibrium with liquid water, indicate that the final molecules of water taken up by the protein are thermodynamically almost identical with liquid water. However, there is considerable evidence for the existence of several phases of ordered water (as distinct from free water) in the water surrounding protein molecules [65–70], and Haly and Snaith have demonstrated that there are in tendon collagen four calorimetrically distinguishable types of water, but that at least a proportion of the water has the calorimetric properties of bulk water [71]. Ward [72] suggests that a layer of water three molecules thick is the maximum above which

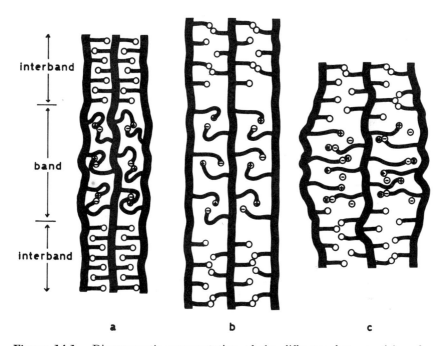

Figure 14.1. Diagrammatic representation of the difference between (a) a dry fibril; (b) a fibril swelling in water at neutrality; and (c) the result of acid swelling. Only polar side-chains are shown, with open-circled heads representing uncharged side chains, + and − signs designating correspondingly charged heads or ions, and H indicating hydrogen ions. The long charged side chains at bands normally distort the vertical main chain helices from a straight course. Neutral water (not shown) penetrates first bands and then interbands, separating main chains to an extent limited by hydrogen bonds between polar heads at interbands, and simultaneously more room becomes available for the charged side chains at bands, which now permit straightening of the main chains. Addition of acid discharges the negative side chains by means of hydrogen ions, and the equal number of free negative ions required to remain at the bands produce local osmotic swellings, which contract the structure axially. Reprinted with permission from R. S. Bear, *Advan. Protein Chem.*, **7**, 149 (1952).

the forces of adsorption are sufficient to cause any modification to the normal structure of water, but Ling [66] calculates that eight layers of water molecules sandwiched between two polar surfaces are in a polarized state. It is this polarized water which is not capable of dissolving small molecules or ions.

The actual location of water in skin, and the amounts associated with various levels of collagen organization (e.g., molecular, inter- and intrafibrillar), and with various components such as collagen and noncollagenous proteins are not known. It is known that water is an integral component of the collagen structure, and there is considerable evidence that the presence of some water is essential for maintaining the fibrillar structure of collagen [73, 74]. Removal of this water alters the intra- and intermolecular bond arrangement, an effect which is, however, reversible on rewetting the collagen [73, 75]. Rougvie and Bear [76] give a detailed account of the changes in the x-ray diffraction pattern of tendon collagen which occur when the dry tendons are wetted.

The swelling of a polymer network by water is dependent both on the polar groups it contains and on the number and situation of cross-links between the chains. The small number of covalent cross-links and the long polar side chains of collagen account for its much greater water uptake compared with the highly cross-linked wool keratin, for example, where chain separation and hence swelling is limited. Figure 14.1 shows a diagrammatic representation of swelling of fibrils under different conditions, and the reason for the increase in length of collagen fibers in neutral swelling is clearly seen.

14.3   STRATUM CORNEUM AND PERMEABILITY

It has long been known that diffusion of water through the skin is limited primarily by the stratum corneum, and the noncornified part of the epidermis offers little resistance to water transport. It has also been shown that the water present in the stratum corneum is essential for a normal functioning of this part of skin, and that the greater the water content of the outer layers the more permeable they become [77, 78]. Water in the stratum corneum is, of course, in dynamic equilibrium with that in the underlying epidermal layers and that in the atmosphere. It is of interest with regard to the uptake of water by skin in physiological conditions that Buettner [79] found a marked difference in permeability of skin between the liquid and vapor form of water. The resistance was about one-tenth as great for liquid contact as for vapor contact. Later workers [80, 81] postulate that because the chemical potential of water vapor is the same as that of liquid water with which it is in equilibrium, it is likely that the permeability of the skin is the same for both the liquid and the vapor form of water, and the discrepancies observed between the two for other polymer systems are probably due to the experimental difficulties of maintaining the saturation vapor pressure. The effectiveness of the stratum corneum as a water barrier, and its permeability after various treatments, will be dealt with elsewhere in this volume, as will the more general problem of the permeability of the skin as a whole. Within the context of the water-uptake mechanism it is sufficient to say that agents which influence the skin permeability will affect the rate of uptake but not the amount of water taken up at equilibrium. Astbury [82] working with hyaluronidase solution comments "diffusing solutions of (hyaluronidase) of bacterial or testicular origin, did not alter the type of swelling, but only the rate at which swelling took place. Maximum swelling is attained more quickly in the presence of diffusing solutions, but the amount and final equilibrium are unaltered."

14.4   QUANTITATIVE ASPECTS OF WATER UPTAKE

Although studies on water uptake of skin after removal from the animal are of no direct physiological importance, they can lead to a better understanding of the factors governing the water relationships of the skin. Because of the importance of water uptake by dried skins in the leather industry a number of workers have investigated the factors involved in uptake of water in the isoelectric pH range (i.e., pH 4.5–8.5). Stubbings and Theis [22], Cassell and McKenna [83], and Gustavson [84] have all drawn attention to the distinction between water uptake in this range and that at pH extremes. A large amount of work on this topic is empirical in nature but studies by Yates [21, 85] have elucidated certain quantitative aspects. Figure 14.2 shows water uptake curves for fresh skin (sheep) and skins that have been dried for varying lengths of time. After the drying process the capacity for taking up water decreases—a process very familiar in the leather industry [86–88]. It is also apparent from Fig. 14.2 that in the physiological state of skin, the full potential for water uptake is not utilized. These studies emphasized the tremendous variation in water uptake, both between and within skins. In a statistical analysis of the measurable skin parameters which may influence water uptake, Yates [21] finds that 90% of the variability between skin samples can be accounted for by variations in three parameters, density of skin sample, dry thickness of sample,

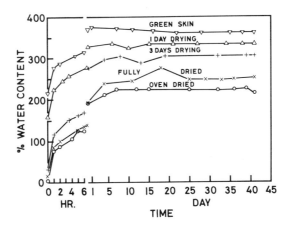

Figure 14.2. Water content against time of soaking for sheepskins dried to various levels. The water contents are measured on a dry weight basis. Approximate water contents at the commencement of soaking can be seen from the graph. Fully dried in this context means a commercially acceptable level (i.e., 15–25% water content). Soaking was carried out in a large excess of water in the presence of a bactericide [21]. (Reprinted from J. R. Yates, *J. Amer. Leather Chemists' Assoc.*, **60**, 712 (1965), by permission of the publishers.)

and amount of swelling of sample, (in this case swelling simply refers to the increase in thickness between wet and dry states). Of these three factors 55% of the total variation is accounted for by the latter factor, that is the capacity of skin to open up. In addition to variations in skin weave, a large part of this variation may be due to changes in interfibrillary proteins and mucopolysaccharides brought about in the drying process.

The quantity and nature of the proteins and mucopolysaccharides existing in the "ground substance" of skin very profoundly affect the extent of water uptake [87–90]. The physicochemical properties of these components change during drying and the skin no longer opens up to its full extent on soaking [87, 91, 92]. Cooper [88] found that even the least drastic of dehydration methods, freeze-drying, will cause some denaturation of interfibrillary proteins. For sheepskins dried in air, Yates [48] has shown that there is a highly significant linear relationship between the initial water content of the sample and the final water content after soaking in water for 72 hours. Extrapolation of this line to zero initial water content indicates that a completely dry skin on soaking should take up between 170–200% water (measured on a dry weight basis) at equilibrium [48].

The effect of various additives on the rate and extent of water uptake has been investigated [85] on the basis that agents which solubilize or disperse denatured "ground substance" components should restore the water-absorbing capacity of skin. It seems likely that changes in both proteins and mucopolysaccharides of the "ground substance," or possibly a complex of the two, are responsible for the reduction in water-uptake capacity on drying. Neither treatment with a protease (trypsin) [85], nor hyaluronidase separately [88] affect the extent of water uptake by dried skins, whereas a limited amount of free bacterial growth, where there is likely to be production of both protease and mucopolysaccharases, loosens the skin structure and largely restores the water-uptake capacity. It is apparent that the actual process of drying per se, causes changes in the "ground-substance" components because treatment of fresh skin with 10% sodium chloride solution [88] and hyaluronidase [93] prior to drying, produce a dry skin which has a similar uptake capacity to fresh skin, whereas treatment with the same reagents after drying has no effect. Yates [85] has shown that neither hydrogen bonding nor hydrophobic bonding is principally responsible for restricting the water uptake of dried skins. Mild techniques of dehydration (e.g., acetone dehydration at low temperature, freeze-drying, and vacuum dehydration at low temperature) cause less denaturation of the "ground-substance" components [47] and less compaction of the skin structure (as judged by thickness and density measurements). Consequently a much greater uptake of water compared to similar air-dried controls is observed. Acetone dehydration, in particular, produces an open-textured, sponge-like product, which absorbs water very rapidly and to a greater extent, especially in the presence of detergents, than skins dried by the other techniques.

14.5   MUCOPOLYSACCHARIDES AND WATER OF SKIN

Collagen fibers of skin are embedded in and surrounded by a continuous phase, and electron microscope studies show it to consist of a meshwork of extremely fine collagen fibers [37] associated with acid mucopolysaccharides and glycoproteins which can be demonstrated by histological techniques [94]. Diffusion studies have shown that the continuous matrix is a gel in which the hyaluronate molecule is an important component [95]. The nature of this "ground substance" has been the subject of a considerable amount of work, and Gersh and Catchpole [96] give an excellent account of its structure and function. These authors state that "basic to an understanding of the functional aspects of ground substance of connective tissue is its submicroscopic organization as a two-phase system. The water-rich (less dense) phase exists as submicroscopic vacuoles enclosed and separated from each other by the denser (colloid-rich) phase. The phases were assumed to be in thermodynamic equilibrium." Calculations indicate that about 45% of the water in skin is associated with the proteins and mucopolysaccharides of the "ground substance" [3].

There is a large volume of evidence that the hyaluronate molecule is involved in the water relationships of the skin [30, 97–100]. Hyaluronic acid consists of long chains of alternating units of D-glucuronic acid, and N-acetyl glucosamine, and its molecular weight has been variously estimated between 2×10^6 and 8×10^6 depending on its origin [101–104]. The polymeric chains consist of expanded, highly hydrated random coils in which all the carboxyl groups have a negative charge at physiological pH values. The precise distribution of hyaluronic acid in the skin is not clear. Toole and Lowther [105] have shown that only between 5–31% of the total hyaluronic acid is extractable from skin by homogenization in water, while 59–84% is extractable by homogenization in 1 M NaCl. They suggest that a considerable proportion of the hyaluronic acid is physically trapped in the gel structure, and Fessler [104] has shown that hyaluronic acid can be incorporated into the gel structure formed on warming solutions of tropocollagen and that this results in a gel which binds considerably more water than the collagen alone. Indeed it is highly probable that it is the hyaluronic acid-protein complex which is responsible for binding water in the ground substance and not hyaluronic acid alone, because hyaluronic acid forms only a viscous solution and not a gel [3, 43, 106–108]. The physical chemistry of hyaluronic acid has been summarized by Pigman et al. [109] and Balazs [103].

The actual amount of hyaluronic acid in skin is difficult to estimate due largely to the problems of separation from other skin components, especially the proteins which form part of the complex [110]. Rienits [99] gives values of from 20–40 mg/100 g dry weight of tissue, which because of the method of isolation may be low. Dorfman and Schiller [111] by an isotope-dilution method find a value of 215 mg/100 g of acetone-defatted, dry bovine skin, a figure which decreases with age [30]. There are several theories as to the nature of the complexing of the hyaluronate with the protein in the skin. Partridge [112] believes that the polyuronides have an orienting effect on proteins upon complexing, a view which presupposes certain stereospecific interactions beside electrostatic forces. Noguchi, however, believes that the interaction is purely electrostatic [113].

The most important feature of hyaluronic acid with respect to the water relationships of skin, is its large hydrodynamic specific volume, calculated to lie usually between 200–500 ml g^{-1} [100–104, 114, 115]. The actual value depends on the molecular weight [102], and in the case of low-molecular weight hyaluronic acid prepared from vitreous humor, can be as low as 6 ml g^{-1}, while values as high as 1000 and 1860 are quoted by Balazs [103] for hyaluronic acid prepared by electrodialysis from synovial fluid and umbilical cord. The dependence of the specific hydrodynamic volume on the molecular weight of hyaluronic acid is an important factor in the part played by hyaluronic acid in water-content regulation of connective tissue. The large volume of water associated with hyaluronic acid coils is not bound to the polysaccharides by long-range forces, and Laurent [116] showed that the x-ray diffractogram of water does not change in the presence of 2% hyaluronic acid as might be expected if water in the amount suggested by the hydrodynamic volume was bound to the polysaccharide chain. However Ogston and Phelps [117] state that much of the water surrounding the hyaluronic acid is not available as a solvent, and calculate that each gram of hyaluronic acid immobilizes about 300 ml of solvent, but also observe that this value varies with the concentration of the polymer.

From investigation of tissues in the physiological and pathological states, it is apparent that the hyaluronic acid of the "ground substance" plays an important part in binding extracellular—tissue water, and further that both its quantity and its degree of polymerization are important in determining the amount of water held (27, 43b, 97, 99, 108, 118–123]. Rienits [99] working on the sexual skin of baboons first demonstrated that a relationship exists between hyaluronic acid content and water content, but was not able to demonstrate any changes in degree of polymerization of hyaluronic acid with changing water content. Subcutaneous connective tissue plays a significant part in regulating the water balance of the organism, and in permitting water in the connective tissue to be in dynamic equilibrium with water in the rest of the organism [2, 4, 8, 9, 16, 108, 124, 125]. Hence the water-binding mechanism of the connective tissue must be an essential link in water mobilization of the total organism.

Hvidberg and Jensen [126] and Hvidberg [108] suggest that for long-term adaptation to prevailing water conditions, the amount of hyaluronic acid may vary, but this is necessarily a slow process and is limited by the "turn over" of hyaluronic acid which is estimated by Schiller et al. [127] to be of the order of 2 days. On the other hand, rapid adaptation to changing water requirements may possibly be brought about by alteration in the physicochemical condition, especially the de-

gree of polymerization of hyaluronic acid [108]. It is possible that alteration of a relatively few glycosidic bonds in the hyaluronic acid molecule
can occur rapidly and that this would be sufficient to cause substantial
changes in water binding. However it is of great significance in this
respect that Meyer [128] and Pigman et al. [109] indicate that some
linkages of a more labile character may be present in highly polymerized
hyaluronic acid. It is possible that these more labile linkages are broken
or reformed on rapid adaptation of "ground substance" to a new water
environment, a larger polymeric molecule being associated with increased
water content. The factors responsible for bringing about changes such
as those mentioned are not clear. Electrolyte conditions may be of importance, and at least in some cases the state of the "ground substance"
is under hormonal control [8, 97, 111, 121, 129–131]. That the situation
is not as straight-forward as that outlined above is indicated by the
work of Hvidberg and Jensen [126] and Cooper and Schmidt [7] who
were not able to demonstrate any decrease in water content of hyaluroni-
dase-treated areas in animals. In addition the changes in the state and
content of the hyaluronic acid in the skin brought about by dehydration
should theoretically alter the permeability, but experiments have failed
to demonstrate this [7, 8, 132].

Very little is known about the part played by the individual connective-tissue components in controlling hydration, but it is known that
in tissues which are highly hydrated the prominent mucopolysaccharide
is hyaluronic acid [123]. When sulphated mucopolysaccharides, for example, chondroitin sulphate, wholly or largely replace hyaluronic acid,
there is a lower degree of hydration. In the swelling of connective tissue
there is increased hydration both of "ground substance" and collagen
fibers, but it is suggested, however, by Slack [123] that an increase
of hydration of the mucopolysaccharide-protein complex occurs before
the swelling of the collagen fibers. Conversely under normal physiological
conditions it is most unlikely that dehydration affects the water content
of the collagen fibers, being largely confined to the ground substance.
Hvidberg [8] and Slack [123] both consider that the "ground substance"
probably constitutes by far the most important element in regulating
the water content of the skin in accord with the needs of the rest of
the body.

14.6 KINETICS OF WATER UPTAKE

There has been no published work on the kinetics of water uptake
by skin. However a series of unpublished experiments carried out in

the author's laboratories, in conjunction with Dr. I. C. Watt, has shown that the kinetics of water uptake by samples of air-dried sheepskin are dependent upon the concentration range of the sorption step, and on the initial water content of the material. Working with wool fibers, Watt [133] has shown that uptake of water to a regain level of 2.5% occurs entirely by a diffusion mechanism obeying Fick's laws. For regain levels between 2.5% and 19%, water uptake can only be partially described using Fick's laws [134], and at higher regain levels Fick's laws do not adequately describe any part of the water uptake by keratin. Above the 2.5% level of water content, water still enters by diffusion, but a second phenomenon begins to assume a more dominant role, and the overall mechanism is not diffusion-controlled. This phenomenon is one of stress-relaxation involving a rearrangement of the bonds holding together the particular molecular configuration. The initial inrush of water puts a strain on the weak interchain bonds, which therefore break and cause an expansion of the polymer network, permitting the entry of more water. As the water content increases, the molecular stress-relaxation mechanism assumes a greater importance. The kinetics of both the first and second stages of water absorption by keratin have been worked out in a series of papers by Watt [133–135]. The second stage of absorption has been shown to be temperature-dependent, and the proportion of uptake in this stage over various regain levels between 0% and 74% relative humidity has been determined. This coupled diffusion-relaxation mechanism was also demonstrated by Long and Watt [136] using a cellulose acetyl-bi-acetyl system.

It seems likely that a similar situation prevails in water uptake by collagen, but with a highly expanded water-content scale. The bulky side chains and the smaller number of covalent cross-links between chains in collagen compared to keratin, permit a much greater opening up of the structure (Fig. 14.1) and hence a greater water uptake than by keratin at the higher relative humidities [58]. These latter factors also suggest that a simple diffusion mechanism may be the controlling process in water uptake by collagen to a higher regain than in keratin. Elden and Feldman [137] studied the kinetics of liquid water uptake by rat-tail tendon and observed that diffusion is probably the main transport basis for swelling, although there exists an anomalous dependance of diffusion on time of swelling. Skin, of course, is a more complex system than tendon collagen, for example, and the actual sequence and precise nature of the events taking place during uptake of water by air-dried skins are not known. Slack [123] suggests that in the rehydration of dried tissue, the protein-mucopolysaccharide gel is hydrated before the collagen fibers, and whether or not a similar two-stage process to that outlined by Watt for keratin, occurs in this process can only be speculated. Until there has been a more detailed analysis of the kinetics of the water uptake by skin, the finer details of the process will not be elucidated.

Water uptake from the liquid phase by air-dried sheepskins has been investigated by Yates [21, 85], who showed that only for the first half-hour of uptake is the process temperature-dependent, higher temperatures giving a more rapid uptake. After this time temperature is without effect on either the rate, or the equilibrium uptake. As the uptake of water by both keratin and collagen is an exothermic process, it would be expected on thermodynamic grounds that at higher temperatures the final amount of water taken up would be less. This has been demonstrated for keratin by Watt [135]. The large sample variations with the sheepskin system may well prevent the detection of any temperature effect in the final stages of water uptake by this system, especially at the very high regain levels involved. It might be hypothesized by analogy with the keratin system, that in the first half-hour of uptake the simple diffusion process is the rate-controlling one, while after this time the stress-relaxation mechanism becomes predominant. The initial water contents of the skins used in this work were between 15–20% (dry-weight basis), and after half an hour are approximately double this. These figures give some idea of the difference in water-content scales between keratin and collagen. For obvious thermodynamic reasons the final level of water uptake is the same from both the liquid and the saturated vapor phase. It has been demonstrated by Watt [138] that the uptake of alcohols by keratin from the liquid and the saturation vapor phases give the same results as far as both rate and equilibrium uptake are concerned, and Watt states that it is justifiable to consider the liquid phase as the limiting case of vapor absorption, that is, saturation vapor pressure.

The relative complexities of skin and tendon systems are reflected in the times taken to reach equilibrium swelling in liquid water. Yates [21] has shown that approximately 48 hours is required to reach equilibrium swelling with air-dried sheepskins, whereas Elden and Feldman [137] demonstrated that rat-tail tendons (dried to equilibration with air at 25°C and 70% relative humidity), reach equilibrium water content in about ten minutes. Rat-tail tendons are a highly organized form of connective tissue, which furthermore contain minimum amounts of "ground substance" [139]. The organizational complexity of skin together with the large amounts of ground substance doubtless combine to make water uptake a relatively difficult and slow process.

14.7   ENERGETICS OF WATER UPTAKE

In the uptake of liquid water by a polymer system, dry polymer molecules absorb solvent and if there are no constraints the polymer swells without limit and finally passes into solution. In such a simple case swelling is merely a transient phenomenon. In skin where there are severe constraints imposed upon the system both at the fibrillar level, and the macroscopic level imposed by the interweaving of the fiber network, solvent absorption is not without limit and swelling is restricted.

McLaren and Rowen [55] discuss in general terms the thermodynamics of the sorption of water vapor by proteins. The driving force for uptake of water by skin is the tendency for the partial-molar free energy of the water in the polymer-water phase, to equal that in the liquid-water phase. At equilibrium swelling the solvent in both phases must have the same total partial-molar free energy [140].

In the polymer network $\Delta \bar{G}_1$ on swelling is composed of several contributions, mainly those due to the solvent-polymer mixing terms which include all the heat and entropy changes involved, $\bar{G}_{1,m}$ and those from the elastic-force contributions resisting swelling $\bar{G}_{el}$. At equilibrium

$$\Delta \bar{G}_1 = \Delta \bar{G}_{1,m} + \Delta \bar{G}_{el} \tag{1}$$
$$\Delta \bar{G}_1 = \Delta \bar{H}_1 - T\Delta \bar{S}_{1,m} - T\Delta \bar{S}_{el} \tag{2}$$

In Equation 2, $\Delta \bar{H}_1$ represents all the enthalpy changes and $\Delta \bar{S}_{el}$ represents the entropy change due to expansion of the polymer network at temperature T. For a given solvent-polymer system, which defines ΔH_1, the extent of equilibrium swelling is directly related to the number of cross-linkages or interchain constraints in the polymer network. Consideration of the heat and entropy changes involved in uptake of water by polymers gives valuable information concerning the precise nature of the process at a molecular level [55, 61, 141–145]. Measurements of the vapor pressures, and the heat involved when water vapor is added to and removed from natural fibrous protein polymers have made it possible to calculate in some detail the thermodynamic properties of such polymer-water systems [55, 61–64].

Kanagy [52] measured the differential heats of adsorption of water vapor by collagen and calculated the free energy and entropy changes involved in the process, but did not attempt any detailed interpretation of the results. Bull [51] published data on the water-vapor uptake curves for collagen, and calculated the free energy and heat changes from a dry to a saturated condition. From the data an attempt was made to explain the mechanism of adsorption. Dole and McLaren [53] refined some of Bull's data, and recalculated the differential net heat of sorption for collagen. The initial differential heat of sorption of water by collagen is of the order of -6000 cal mole^{-1}, a value much higher than that for other proteins studied and it is suggested that the stereochemistry of the proline and hydroxyproline rings facilitates chain separation, hence requiring less heat to separate the chains with consequent liberation of a larger quantity of heat. The net heat of sorption drops rapidly with increasing water content and this levels off at values of water content consistent with the formation of a monolayer according to the Brunauer, Emmett, and Teller theory [146]. There have been no detailed calculations of the entropy changes involved over the entire uptake range in the collagen-water system, but McLaren and Rowen [55] comment on the differences in the entropy changes during hydration between collagen and gelatin. At low vapor pressures, gelatin absorbs water with a positive net entropy, indicating that the process is not one of pure adsorption, but that a configurational change due to local solubilization is occurring. Collagen does not show this effect. There has been no work done on the thermodynamics of water uptake by skin, information which would be invaluable in determining the precise details of the uptake mechanism. Although the qualitative information obtained from Bull's data would doubtless still hold, it is highly likely that with the more refined calorimetric techniques available today for measuring heat changes, and with greater refinement in measuring small weight changes, the quantitative results may be slightly different.

14.8   NONPHYSIOLOGICAL UPTAKE OF WATER

There are two other circumstances under which uptake of water must be considered, neither of which are important physiologically, but both of which are interesting theoretically and are of practical consequence in the leather industry, for example. These are water uptake in pH regions outside the isoelectric region, and water uptake in the presence of neutral salts. The outward manifestations of these two types of water uptake are well-known in the leather industry. Soaking in acid or alkaline solutions in the absence of salts produces a turgid, translucent skin, and microscopic examination shows that the collagen fibers decrease in length but increase in diameter (Fig. 14.1). On the other hand, lyotropic swelling, that is, soaking in the isoelectric range in the presence of neutral salts produces a skin which remains flaccid and opaque. Examination of the fibers under the latter conditions shows them to be wider, and split into fibrils with the skin as a whole showing a much looser fiber weave. Unless, of course, treatment is so prolonged that chemical changes have occurred, acid-base swelling is completely reversible by application of a tensile load. Lyotropic swelling cannot be reversed by applying a tensile stress to the fibers, and normally is not completely reversible even after removing the lyotropic agent, a permanent swelling effect being produced. Both types of water uptake can of course occur simultaneously as in the case of acetic acid at pH values in the vicinity of 2 [147].

14.8.1   Uptake of Water Outside the Isoelectric pH Range

Figure 14.3 shows the variation in water uptake of skin as a function of the pH value of the solution with which it has become equilibrated. As Gustavson [147] correctly points out, the water associated with the skin proteins due to the acquisition of positive and negative charges in the acid and basic ranges respectively (i.e., due to osmotic effects), should be measured using the water-uptake curve in the isoelectric range as the base level, as this extra water is present in addition to both the structural water and the water held in the "ground substance" of

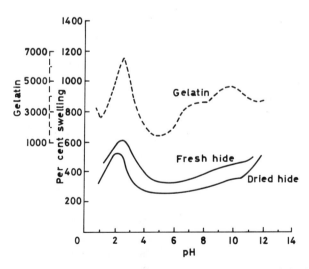

Figure 14.3. The water uptake of gelatin compared with that of fresh and dried hides at different pH values. (Reprinted with permission from K. H. Gustavson, *Chemistry and Reactivity of Collagen,* Chapter 7.)

the skin in the isoelectric range. The amount of water taken up by skin in the extreme regions of pH is controlled by two opposing factors, osmotic forces tending to cause water to pass into the skin, and cohesive forces of skin proteins together with the structural restraints tending to oppose uptake. The effect of fiber weave in opposing water uptake is clearly demonstrated at acid pH values in two ways. Isolated fiber bundles from oxhide have been shown to take up about twenty times their own weight of water at the pH of maximum swelling, while the intact hide takes up only three or four times its own weight [40, 148]. Moreover a gelatin gel takes up about ten times as much water as a piece of native hide of corresponding protein content ([147, 149] and Fig. 14.3). It is interesting to note that the water uptake by dried skins at pH values in the acid and isoelectric range is approximately one-fifth less than that of fresh skins, while the proportionate effect in the alkaline range is a great deal less [40, 147]. These acid-base effects on dried hides are accompanied by a smaller increase in width of the fiber and a smaller decrease in length than is the case with fresh hides. The lower uptake of dried skins is probably due, as in the isoelectric range, to physicochemical changes in the interfibrillary substances causing increased fiber cohesion. Alkalies have a greater solubilizing effect on this interfibrillary material, hence the less restricting effect on water uptake of dried skin in the alkaline range [40]. Measurements of water uptake by skin are normally made by observing changes in weight, but this does not distinguish between uptake caused by an increased osmotic pressure and that caused by reduction in cohesion. However it is possible to ascertain which type of swelling is dominant from direct visual and, if necessary, microscopic evidence.

When collagen reacts with acid or base the conditions exist for the establishment of a Donnan-membrane equilibrium between the collagen and the external solution, because there are nondiffusable ions in the collagen and diffusable ions in the liquid. The presence of the nondiffusable ions leads to an unequal distribution of the diffusable ions between the solid and the external solution, which in turn leads to an inflow of water for equalization of the ionic concentration inside the substrate and in the external solution. The application of the Donnan-equilibrium concept to the explanation of osmotic water uptake in extreme pH regions is dealt with in detail elsewhere [150, 151], but it should be pointed out that there are a number of very important effects concerned with the swelling of skin proteins that are not explained by this theory [147], and in particular the agreement between theory and experiment in the range of alkaline swelling is less satisfactory than in the acid range. This is perhaps not surprising since the Procter-

Wilson application of the Donnan equation was worked out for relatively simple systems, and as soon as structural factors come into play, the simple calculations based on the Donnan concept no longer apply. As Gustavson [147] points out, "the higher the restraints imposed on the structure of the solid phase, the less free water will be present, which accordingly implies introduction of new and unknown factors into the simple equation." The alternative theories of Gilbert and Rideal [152] and Steinhardt [153] which are able to account for uptake of acid by solid proteins, are no more able to completely explain the osmotic swelling of skin proteins than the Procter-Wilson theory. Gustavson [147] suggests that the electrostatic theory of Katchalsky et al. [154, 155] for swelling of polymethacrylates may be of greater value than the Donnan concept for explaining the swelling of collagen. In this theory the repulsive forces due to the high net positive or negative charges acquired by the proteins under acidic or basic conditions respectively cause some distortion in the molecules tending to form extended filaments. This tendency is opposed by structural limitations in the skin preventing complete extension, but possibly the separation of the adjacent collagen molecules permits the access of water to a much greater degree than in the system at the isoelectric point, that is, where there is no charge (see Fig. 14.1).

What is happening at a molecular level in osmotic swelling is not absolutely clear. However certain changes in the x-ray diffraction patterns have been observed in acid-swollen collagen from various sources. Nutting and Borasky [156] reported that acid-swollen fibrils exhibit an axial repeat distance shortened to 540 Å as compared to 650 Å in normal, dry collagen. Burge et al. [157] showed that the equatorial spot in the x-ray diffraction picture of rat-tail tendon collagen which is attributed to the intertropocollagen chain spacing perpendicular to the fiber axis increases from about 13.5 Å at minimum swelling in salt-free water to above 15 Å at pH 2 in the absence of neutral salts, indicating that some additional solvent was entering the fundamental fibrillar structure and the tropocollagen molecules. However, the sensitivity of this spacing to hydration is well-known [76], and from their work with lightly cross-linked rat-tail tendon collagen, Puett et al. [158] conclude that after the initial lattice adjustment brought about by water in crystalline tendon, no further alteration takes place either in the conformation of the individual chains in the crystalline region or in the lateral spacings of the tropocollagen units, on adjustment to the maximum osmotic swelling at pH 2. However there is considerable solvent absorption as shown in the weight uptake increase, the fiber volume and cross-sectional area increase, and the length decrease [159]. It is also of considerable importance that this solvent absorption reduces the structural stability of the fiber as indicated by changes in shrinkage temperature [159]. It is also interesting to note that the high-angle diffraction pattern is lost in collagen at the point of maximum swelling [147].

14.8.2 Uptake of Water in Lyotropic Swelling

Lyotropic swelling of collagen, and the lyotropic properties of various molecules, ions, and compounds are discussed in some detail by Gustavson [147] and von Hippel [160]. It is well-established that mammalian collagen is stabilized by cross-links of the hydrogen-bond type [160], mainly supplemented by salt links, and the evidence suggests that salt and acid solutions interact with collagen in such a way that various intermolecular forces are disturbed. This causes a decrease in stability of the collagen-type helix as manifested by a decrease in shrinkage temperature, often considerable solubilization of the collagen, and an increased amount of water uptake.

Although there is a great deal of phenomenological data on the effects of various chemical entities on the stability of the collagen helix in solution, there is considerable controversy about the mechanism of these effects. It is apparent that each type of reagent produces its own characteristic effects, and von Hippel [160] states "the generality of these (lyotropic) effects transcends any specific chemical or conformational aspect of macromolecular structure, and no explanation based on any special feature of a specific macromolecule is likely to be correct." Factors which may play a part in the mechanism of lyotropic swelling are discussed by a number of workers [160–166].

Within the context of the present considerations, however, it is sufficient to say that the disordering of the polypeptide chains by the lyotropic agents, results in a greater uptake of water than would otherwise be the case. This disordering of the chains with widening of the distance between interchain cross-linking groups, cannot be completely reversed by the application of a tensile load, unlike swelling due to osmotic effects.

As previously stated, lyotropic and osmotic swelling can occur simultaneously, and Gustavson [147] presents data showing the increased lyotropic effect of acetic acid compared to its purely osmotic effect when contrasted with hydrochloric acid both at pH 2. Acetic acid produces about 50% more water uptake, and about eight times the amount of collagen solubilization compared to hydrochloric acid. It produces a larger amount of permanent swelling in the skin, compared to hydrochloric acid which produces virtually none. The degree of disorganization of the molecular structure is shown by the respective reduction in shrinkage temperature, acetic acid causing a reduction of 12°C compared to 5°C for hydrochloric acid, and this data conclusively shows that the swelling produced by acetic acid is fundamentally different to that produced by hydrochloric acid. Ciferri et al. [158, 159, 167] have made detailed studies of the effects of salts on various physical properties of tendon collagen, including swelling, and conclude that their observations are not reconcilable with swelling taking place in interfibrillar spaces or structural voids. Following the work of Bear [168] and Schmitt [169] they postulate that at the ends of the tropocollagen units there are regions of reduced organization which are able to interact with the diluent in a manner characteristic of an amorphous region. Figure 14.1 shows diagrammatically how the changes in shape of the collagen fibril with lyotropic and osmotic changes can be accounted for. Since the collagen molecules are matched at band and interband levels of the fibril, this would seem to suggest that these regions are a gross reflection of the amino acid sequences in the molecules themselves. Bands probably represent levels rich in the larger acidic and basic side chains sticking out from the main coil, while interbands contain the average-sized hydroxyl containing side chains. Corresponding to the chemical contents, intrafibrillar stabilization at bands is accomplished largely by salt-type linkages and by hydrogen bonds at the interbands. As a consequence of this, osmotic swelling in acid or alkaline solution is largely at bands, causing a fibrillar shortening, while in neutral environments the protofibrillar separation is increased at all levels, removing the necessity for main-chain distortion at bands, and causing a slight lengthening of the fibril. It might be expected, from an inspection of Fig. 14.1 that when the fibrils have taken up water, they lose to a certain extent the differentiation between band and interband regions, and there is evidence for this from both x-ray diffraction and electron microscope studies [37, 170–172]. In addition, uptake of water by dry collagen produces an increase in the low-angle axial repeat spacing from 628 Å at 2% relative humidity to 672 Å at 100% relative humidity [172].

REFERENCES

1. M. J. Lepore, *Arch. Internat. Med.,* **50,** 488 (1932).
2. H. P. Skelton, *Arch. Internat. Med.,* **40,** 140 (1927).
3. S. Rothman, *Physiology and Biochemistry of the Skin,* University of Chicago Press, 1954, Chapter 21, p. 493.
4. L. J. Flemister, *Amer. J. Physiol.,* **135,** 430 (1942).
5. S. Sakata, *Arch. Exptl. Pathol. Pharmakol.,* **105,** 11 (1925).
6. H. P. Skelton, *Proc. Soc. Expt. Biol. Med.,* **23,** 499 (1926).

7. D. J. Cooper and A. Schmidt, *Acta Pharmacol. Toxicol.*, **13**, 169 (1957).
8. E. Hvidberg, *Acta Pharmacol. Toxicol.*, **16**, 28 (1959).
9. B. Hamilton and R. Schwartz, *J. Biol. Chem.*, **109**, 745 (1935).
10. E. Urbach, *Arch. Dermatol. Syphilis*, **156**, 73 (1928).
11. J. Haldi, G. Giddings, and W. Wynn, *Amer. J. Physiol.*, **141**, 83 (1944).
12. E. Urbach, *Arch. Dermatol. Syphilis*, **150**, 52 (1926).
13. H. Konigstein, *Arch. Dermatol. Syphilis*, **154**, 352 (1928).
14. F. Herrmann, *Ges. Expt. Med.*, **76**, 780 (1931).
15. W. Wynn and J. Haldi, *Amer. J. Physiol.*, **142**, 508 (1944).
16. L. Eichelberger, C. W. Eisele, and D. Wertzler, *J. Biol. Chem.*, **151**, 177 (1943).
17. L. Eichelberger and M. Roma, *J. Invest. Dermatol.*, **12**, 125 (1949).
18. C. W. Eisele and L. Eichelberger, *Proc. Soc. Expt. Biol. Med.*, **58**, 97 (1945).
19. G. D. McLaughlin and E. R. Theis, *J. Amer. Leather Chemists' Assoc.*, **19**, 428 (1924).
20. A. Bornstein and J. Kerb, *Biochem. Z.*, **126**, 120 (1921).
21. J. R. Yates, *J. Amer. Leather Chemists' Assoc.*, **60**, 712 (1965).
22. R. L. Stubbings and E. R. Theis, *J. Amer. Leather Chemists' Assoc.*, **45**, 138 (1950).
23. G. H. Green, *J. Soc. Leather Trades' Chemists*, **38**, 198 (1954).
24. C. L. Ornes and W. T. Roddy, *J. Amer. Leather Chemists' Assoc.*, **58**, 4 (1963).
25. G. O. Conabere, M. Dempsey, and B. W. Raymond, *Progress in Leather Science 1920–45*, British Leather Manufacturers' Research Association, 1948, Chapter 2, p. 28.
26. L. G. Lowrey, *Anat. Record*, **7**, 143 (1913).
27. N. F. Boas and J. B. Foley, *Proc. Soc. Expt. Biol. Med.*, **86**, 690 (1954).
28. E. Urbach, *Haut- Geschlechtskrankh.*, **26**, 217 (1928).
29. M. Ishizawa, H. Anabuki, and H. Ikawa, *Med. and Biol.* (*Japan*), **28**, 207 (1953).
30. E. Hvidberg, *Acta Pharmacol. Toxicol.*, **16**, 55 (1959).
31. A. Meyer, *Kinderheilk.*, **50**, 596 (1931).
32. J. Haldi, G. Giddings, and W. Wynn, *Amer. J. Physiol.*, **135**, 392 (1942).
33. H. E. C. Zheutlin and C. L. Fox, *Arch. Dermatol. Syphilis*, **61**, 397 (1950).
34. J. F. Manery and L. F. Haege, *Amer. J. Physiol.*, **134**, 83 (1941).
35. N. F. Boas, *Arch. Biochem. Biophys.*, **57**, 367 (1955).
36. G. N. Ramachandran, Ed., *Chemistry of Collagen*, Vol. I of *Treatise on Collagen*, Academic Press, 1967.
37. J. Gross and F. O. Schmitt, *J. Expt. Med.*, **88**, 555 (1948).
38. J. Gross, *Sci. Amer.*, **204**, 121 (1961).
39. M. Kaye, *J. Internat. Soc. Leather Trades' Chemists*, **13**, 73 (1929).
40. M. Kaye and D. Jordan Lloyd, *Proc. Roy. Soc. London*, Ser. B. **96**, 293 (1924).

41. D. Jordan Lloyd and R. H. Marriott, *Proc. Roy. Soc. London,* Ser. B. **118,** 439 (1935).

42. D. S. Kwon, P. Mason, and B. J. Rigby, *Nature,* **201,** 159 (1964).

43. T. D. Day, *J. Physiol. (London),* **109,** 380 (1949); **117,** 1 (1952).

44. R. M. Barrer, *Diffusion in Polymers,* J. Crank and G. S. Park, Eds., Academic Press 1968, Chap. 6, p. 165.

45. H. Eilers, and J. W. A. Labout, *Soc. Dyers Colourists, Symp. on Fibrous Proteins,* Leeds, 1946, p. 30.

46. D. Jordan Lloyd and A. Shore, *Chemistry of the Proteins.* J. & A. Churchill Ltd. 1938, Chap. 11, p. 370.

47. J. R. Yates, *J. Amer. Leather Chemists' Assoc.,* **61,** 235 (1966).

48. J. R. Yates, *J. Amer. Leather Chemists' Assoc.,* **61,** 171 (1966).

49. A. S. Jahn, and L. P. Witnauer, *J. Amer. Leather Chemists' Assoc.,* **62,** 334 (1967).

50. I. C. Watt, R. H. Kennett, and J. F. P. James, *Textile Res. J.,* **29,** 975 (1959).

51. H. B. Bull, *J. Amer. Chem. Soc.,* **66,** 1499 (1944).

52. J. R. Kanagy, *J. Res. Nat. Bur. Std.,* **44,** 31 (1950).

53. M. Dole and A. D. McLaren, *J. Amer. Chem. Soc.,* **69,** 651 (1947).

54. E. F. Mellon, A. H. Korn, and S. R. Hoover, *J. Amer. Chem. Soc.,* **70,** 3040 (1948).

55. A. D. McLaren and J. W. Rowen, *J. Polymer Sci.,* **7,** 289 (1951).

56. H. J. White and H. Eyring, *Textile Res. J.,* **17,** 523 (1947).

57. H. J. White and P. B. Stam, *Textile Res. J.,* **19,** 136 (1949).

58. R. L. D'Arcy and I. C. Watt, *Trans. Faraday Soc.* **66,** 1236 (1970).

59. J. R. Kanagy, *J. Res. Nat. Bur. Std.,* **38,** 119 (1947).

60. I. C. Watt and J. D. Leeder, *J. Textile Inst.,* **59,** 353 (1968).

61. S. Davis, and A. D. McLaren, *J. Polymer Sci.,* **3,** 16 (1948).

62. H. B. Dunford and J. L. Morrison, *Can. J. Chem.,* **33,** 904 (1955).

63. J. L. Morrison and J. F. Hanlan, *Nature,* **179,** 528 (1957).

64. J. L. Morrison and J. F. Hanlan, *Proc. 2nd Internat. Cong. Surface Activity,* London, 1957, Vol. 2, p. 322.

65. I. M. Klotz, *Science,* **128,** 815 (1958).

66. G. N. Ling, *Fed. Proc.,* **25,** 958 (1966).

67. F. W. Cope, *Biophys. J.,* **9,** 303 (1969).

68. C. F. Hazelwood, B. L. Nichols, and N. F. Chamberlain, *Nature,* **222,** 747 (1969).

69. A. R. Haly and J. W. Snaith, *Biopolymers,* **7,** 459 (1969).

70. P. L. Privalov and G. M. Mrevlishvili, *Biofizika,* **12,** 22 (1967).

71. A. R. Haly and J. W. Snaith, Unpublished data.

72. A. G. Ward, *Recent Advances in Food Science,* Vol. 3, *Biochemistry and Biophysics in Food Research,* J. M. Leitch and D. N. Rhodes, Eds., Butterworths, London, 1963, p. 207.

73. V. Mohanaradhakrishnan and N. Ramanathan, *Leather Sci.*, **14**, 220 (1967).

74. P. H. von Hippel and W. F. Harrington, *Protein Structure and Function*, Brookhaven Symposia on Biology, No. 13, 213 (1960).

75. H. J. C. Berendsen, *J. Chem. Phys.*, **36**, 3297 (1962).

76. M. A. Rougvie and R. S. Bear, *J. Amer. Leather Chemists' Assoc.*, **48**, 735 (1953).

77. O. Jacobi, *J. Appl. Physiol.*, **12**, 403 (1958).

78. F. A. J. Thiele and K. Schuetter, *Fette, Seifen, Anstrichmittel*, **64**, 625 (1962).

79. K. Buettner, *J. Appl. Physiol.*, **6**, 229 (1953).

80. J. Stannett and H. Yasuda, *J. Polymer Sci.*, B. **1**, 289 (1963).

81. J. Sivadjian and D. Ribeiro, *J. Appl. Polymer Sci.*, **8**, 1403 (1964).

82. D. McClean, *J. Pathol. Bacteriol.*, **42**, 477 (1936).

83. J. M. Cassel and E. McKenna, *J. Amer. Leather Chemists' Assoc.*, **49**, 553 (1954).

84. K. H. Gustavson, *Chemistry and Reactivity of Collagen*, Academic Press, New York, 1956, Chap. 3, p. 53.

85. J. R. Yates, *J. Amer. Leather Chemists' Assoc.*, **61**, 25 (1966).

86. G. D. McLaughlin and E. R. Theis, *J. Amer. Leather Chemists' Assoc.*, **18**, 324 (1923).

87. M. Kaye and D. Jordan Lloyd, *Biochem. J.*, **18**, 1043 (1924).

88. D. R. Cooper, *J. Soc. Leather Trades' Chemists*, **41**, 387 (1957).

89. C. C. Kritzinger, *J. Amer. Leather Chemists' Assoc.*, **43**, 243 (1948).

90. D. R. Cooper and R. L. Sykes, *J. Soc. Leather Trades' Chemists*, **40**, 401 (1956).

91. —— *Brit. Leath. Man. Res. Ass. Ann. Report*, **3**, 6 (1923).

92. A. Kuntzel, Collegium No. 650, p. 212 (1924).

93. J. H. Bowes, J. E. C. B. Cave, and R. G. Elliott, Quoted by D. R. Cooper, *J. Soc. Leather Trades' Chemists*, **41**, 387 (1957).

94. J. F. A. McManus, *Connective Tissue in Health and Disease*, G. Asboe-Hansen Ed., Munksgaard, Copenhagen, 1954, p. 31.

95. F. Duran-Reynals, *Connective Tissue in Health and Disease*, G. Asboe-Hansen, Ed., Munksgaard, Copenhagen, 1954, p. 103.

96. I. Gersh and H. R. Catchpole, *Perspec. Biol. Med.*, **3**, 282 (1960).

97. A. W. Ludwig, N. F. Boas, and L. J. Soffer, *Proc. Soc. Exptl. Biol. Med.*, **73**, 137 (1950).

98. A. W. Ludwig, *Proc. Soc. Exptl. Biol. Med.*, **85**, 424 (1954).

99. K. G. Rienits, *Biochem. J.*, **74**, 27 (1960).

100. H. J. Rogers, *Biochem. Soc. Symp.*, Cambridge, England, **20**, 51 (1961).

101. B. S. Blumberg and G. Oster, *Science*, **120**, 432 (1954).

102. J. H. Fessler, A. G. Ogston, and J. E. Stanier, *Biochem. J.*, **58**, 656 (1954).

103. E. A. Balazs, *Federation Proc.*, **17**, 1086 (1958).

104. J. H. Fessler, *Biochem. J.*, **76**, 124 (1960).

105. B. P. Toole and D. A. Lowther, *Biochim. Biophys. Acta*, **121**, 315 (1966).

106. S. H. Bensley, *Anat. Record*, **60**, 93 (1934).

107. W. A. Loeven, *Acta Physiol. Pharmacol. Neerl.*, **5,** 121 (1956).

108. E. Hvidberg, *Acta Pharmacol. Toxicol.*, **17,** 267 (1960).

109. W. Pigman, G. Matsumura, and A. Herp, *Proc. Fourth Intern. Cong. on Rheol.*, Providence, 1963; *Symp. on Biorheol.*, A. L. Copley, Ed., John Wiley and Sons, New York, 1965, pp. 505–519.

110. F. A. Bettelheim, *Nature*, **182,** 1301 (1958).

111. A. Dorfman and S. Schiller, *Recent Progr. Hormone Res.*, **14,** 427 (1958).

112. S. M. Partridge, *Biochem. J.*, **43,** 387 (1948).

113. H. Noguchi, *Biochim. Biophys. Acta*, **22,** 459 (1956).

114. A. G. Ogston and J. E. Stanier, *Biochem. J.*, **49,** 585 (1951).

115. B. S. Blumberg and A. G. Ogston, *Biochem. J.*, **66,** 342 (1957).

116. T. C. Laurent, *Arkiv. Kemi*, **11,** 513 (1957).

117. A. G. Ogston and C. F. Phelps, *Biochem. J.*, **78,** 827 (1961).

118. G. C. Heringa, *Proc. Sixth Intern. Congr. Exptl. Cytol.*, Stockholm, (1947), *Exptl. Cell Res. Suppl.*, **1,** 366 (1949).

119. R. H. Pearce and E. M. Watson, *Can. J. Res.*, E, **27,** 43 (1949).

120. C. Ragan and K. Meyer, *J. Clin. Invest.*, **28,** 56 (1949).

121. N. R. Joseph, M. B. Engel, and H. R. Catchpole, *Biochim. Biophys. Acta,* **8,** 575 (1952).

122. O. Wegelius and G. Asboe-Hansen, *Expt. Cell Res.*, **11,** 437 (1956).

123. H. G. B. Slack, *Amer. J. Med.*, **26,** 113 (1959).

124. J. R. Robinson and R. A. McCance, *Ann. Rev. Physiol.*, **14,** 115 (1952).

125. J. R. Elkinton and T. S. Danowski, *The Body Fluids*, Williams and Wilkins, Baltimore, 1955.

126. E. Hvidberg and C. E. Jensen, *Acta Chem. Scand.*, **13,** 2047 (1959).

127. S. Schiller, M. B. Mathews, L. Goldfaber, J. Ludowieg, and A. Dorfman, *J. Biol. Chem.*, **212,** 531 (1955).

128. K. Meyer, *Federation Proc.*, **17,** 1075 (1958).

129. E. Kulonen, *Acta Endocrinol.*, **12,** 147 (1953).

130. D. J. Cooper and A. Schmidt, *Acta Pharmacol. Toxicol.*, **13,** 155 (1957).

131. A. Schmidt, *Acta Pharmacol. Toxicol.*, **14,** 350 (1958).

132. D. H. Sprunt, *J. Expt. Med.*, **75,** 297 (1942).

133. I. C. Watt, *Textile Res. J.*, **30,** 443 (1960).

134. I. C. Watt and J. E. Algie, *Textile Res. J.*, **31,** 793 (1961).

135. I. C. Watt, *Textile Res. J.*, **30,** 644 (1960).

136. F. A. Long and I. C. Watt, *J. Polymer Sci.*, **21,** 554 (1956).

137. H. R. Elden and M. Feldman, *J. Polymer Sci.*, **A1,** 23 (1963).

138. I. C. Watt, *J. Appl. Polymer Sci.*, **8,** 1737 (1964).

139. K. Meyer, E. Davidson, A. Linker, and P. Hoffman, *Biochim. Biophys. Acta,* **21,** 506 (1956).

140. A. Veis, *Treatise on Collagen*, Vol. 1, "Chemistry of Collagen," G. N. Ramachandran, Ed., Academic Press, 1967, Chapter 8, p. 367.

141. A. B. D. Cassie, *Soc. Dyers Colourists, Symp. on Fibrous Proteins*, Leeds, 1946, p. 86.

142. F. A. Bettleheim and D. H. Volman, *J. Polymer Sci.*, **24**, 445 (1957).
143. J. L. Morrison and M. A. Dzieciuch, *Can. J. Chem.*, **37**, 1379 (1959).
144. F. A. Bettelheim and S. H. Ehrlich, *J. Phys. Chem.*, **67**, 1948 (1963).
145. R. Jeffries, *J. Textile Inst.*, Trans., **51**, 399 (1960).
146. S. Brunauer, P. H. Emmett, and E. Teller, *J. Amer. Chem. Soc.*, **60**, 309 (1938).
147. K. H. Gustavson, *Chemistry and Reactivity of Collagen*, Academic Press, New York, 1956, Chapters **7** and 8.
148. J. H. Bowes, *J. Soc. Leather Trades' Chemists*, **33**, 176 (1949).
149. D. Jordan Lloyd and H. Phillips, *Trans. Faraday Soc.*, **29**, 132 (1933).
150. H. R. Procter and J. A. Wilson, *J. Chem. Soc. (Trans.)*, **1**, 307 (1916).
151. J. A. Wilson, *Chemistry of Leather Manufacture*, 2nd Ed., Chemical Catalogue Co., New York, Vol. 1, 1928, Chapter 5, p. 129.
152. G. A. Gilbert and E. K. Rideal, *Proc. Roy. Soc. London*, A, **182**, 335 (1944).
153. J. Steinhardt, *Ann. N.Y. Acad. Sci.*, **41**, 287 (1941).
154. A. Katchalsky, O. Kunzle, and W. Kuhn, *J. Polymer Sci.*, **5**, 283 (1950).
155. A. Katchalsky, *J. Polymer Sci.*, **7**, 393 (1951).
156. G. C. Nutting and R. Borasky, *J. Amer. Leather Chemists' Assoc.*, **43**, 96 (1948).
157. R. E. Burge, P. M. Cowan, and S. McGavin, *Recent Advances in Gelatin and Glue Research*, G. Stainsby, Ed., Pergamon Press, 1958, p. 25.
158. D. Puett, A. Ciferri, and L. V. Rajagh, *Biopolymers*, **3**, 439 (1965).
159. A. Ciferri, L. V. Rajagh, and D. Puett, *Biopolymers*, **3**, 461 (1965).
160. P. H. von Hippel, *Treatise on Collagen*, Vol. 1, *Chemistry of Collagen*, G. N. Ramachandran, Ed., Academic Press, 1967, Chapter 6, p. 253.
161. J. Bello, H. C. A. Riese, and J. R. Vinograd, *J. Phys. Chem.*, **60**, 1299 (1956).
162. W. F. Harrington, and P. H. von Hippel, *Arch. Biochem. Biophys.*, **92**, 100 (1961).
163. L. Mandelkern, J. C. Halpin, A. F. Diorio, and A. S. Posner, *J. Amer. Chem. Soc.*, **84**, 1383 (1962).
164. D. R. Robinson and W. P. Jencks, *J. Amer. Chem. Soc.*, **87**, 2470 (1965).
165. P. H. von Hippel and K. Y. Wong, *J. Biol. Chem.*, **240**, 3909 (1965).
166. P. H. von Hippel and T. W. Schleich, *Biological Macromolecules*, Vol. II, S. N. Timasheff, and G. D. Fasman, Eds., Marcel Dekker Inc., New York, 1969.
167. L. V. Rajagh, D. Puett, and A. Ciferri, *Biopolymers*, **3**, 421 (1965).
168. R. S. Bear, *Advan. Protein Chem.*, **7**, 69 (1952).
169. F. O. Schmitt, *Rev. Mod. Phys.*, **31**, 5 (1959).
170. R. S. Bear, *J. Amer. Chem. Soc.*, **66**, 1297 (1944).
171. R. S. Bear, O. E. A. Bolduan, and T. P. Salo, *J. Amer. Leather Chemists' Assoc.*, **46**, 107 (1951).
172. B. A. Wright, *Nature*, **162**, 23 (1948).

15

Electrical Properties of Skin

ROBERT EDELBERG, Ph.D.

Rutgers Medical School

An adequate description of the electrical characteristics of skin must take into account both the spatial heterogeneity of this structure and

513

its temporal variability, two characteristics which permit it to serve in the preservation of internal homeostasis in the face of marked variations in ambient conditions. In addition to its role in thermoregulation and water-balance, the skin is also a tactile sensory organ, and its mechanical characteristics greatly influence the nature of the neural pattern which occurs where it makes contact with an object. They also modify the resistance of the skin to abrasion. These three roles are intimately associated with the activity of the sweat glands whose neurally controlled secretion influences both thermal balance through evaporative heat loss and mechanical characteristics by hydration of the corneum. An additional dynamic aspect of skin function is seen in the activity of the vasculature of the corium. Electrical measures taken from the skin may, as a consequence, reflect the level of sweat secretion, the state of the blood vessels of the corium, and the state of one or more living cell layers.

Since thermoregulatory and tactile requirements vary in different parts of the body, it is to be expected that the electrical characteristics of skin may show a topographical specificity. Moreover, in view of the changes in the integument of fur-bearing animals in response to seasonal variations, it is not surprising that electrical properties of human skin should also show an annual periodicity. In addition to short-term (phasic) variations and longer (periodic) variations in electrical properties, there are also changes as a function of age. The obvious change in the appearance of skin with development and aging suggests that the concomitant electrical changes may be related to structural rather than neural factors. Finally, because of the dependence of electrical properties on morphology and functional state, the electrical properties may change with cutaneous pathology.

In the light of the dynamically changing characteristics of skin, the treatment of its electrical properties should appropriately focus upon their relation to functional state as well as structure. Such a treatment is intimately related to the physiology of the skin, but detailed consideration of that subject is outside the focus of the present volume. In order to provide a basis for rational interpretation of electrical measures, however, certain aspects of functional relations in the skin will be briefly considered. For an earlier treatment of the electrical characteristics of the skin in relation to function as well as structure, the reader is referred to the excellent discussion by Rothman [1], and to subsequent discussions by Darrow [2], Martin and Venables [3], Wilcott [4], and Edelberg [5]. The methodology of electrodermal measurement has also been covered repeatedly in other sources, representative treatments being those of Barnett [6], Grings [7], Montagu [8], Montagu and Coles [9], Hume [10], Venables and Martin [11], and Edelberg [12].

15.1   MORPHOLOGICAL AND FUNCTIONAL DETERMINANTS OF ELECTRICAL PROPERTIES

15.1.1   Resistance or Conductance

Skin is a mosaic in which a relatively uniform laminated structure is perforated by structures having markedly different characteristics, namely the sweat ducts and hair follicles. The various layers of skin also differ among themselves in their electrical properties, some of which can only be surmised from indirect evidence. These various structures account for at least 90% of the resistance measured between two electrodes, approximately 1 to 2 cm² in area, placed at any two spots on the body surface. If the electrodes are considerably larger, the skin's resistance becomes a proportionately smaller fraction of the total, since the deep tissue resistance is essentially of constant magnitude, while the skin's resistance decreases with increasing area. Skin also accounts for essentially all of the potential difference measured between the two electrodes. Puncture of the skin at each electrode site reduces the resistance to a small fraction of its original value and essentially obliterates the potential difference between the two sites.

The electrical conductivity of any structure is directly related to its ionic permeability. The major thickness of the corneum has been considered by Rein [13] to be freely permeable to ions since he was able to demonstrate that large ionic dye radicals can diffuse as far as the compact layer of corneum near the germinating layer. Others such as Rushmer and his colleagues [14] regarded the corneum as an ion-impermeable layer. This author has shown by infiltration of skin with silver nitrate followed by chemical reduction [15] that the silver ion penetrates the corneum freely. Electron-micrographic examination showed that the silver is not uniformly distributed but concentrates in narrow channels (Fig. 15.1). Further evidence that the greater part of the corneum is freely permeable to ions is seen in the demonstration by Fleischmajer and Witten [16] that radioactive thorium (thorium-X) diffuses passively as far as the stratum conjunctum. Witten and his co-workers [17] demonstrated a similar result using phosphate ion containing radioactive phosphorus. There appears to be little doubt that ions readily penetrate most of the corneum. Whether the stratum conjunctum (and for the palmar and plantar surfaces the stratum lucidum) has appreciably ion-permeability is less clear. Much of the work on the "barrier" layer has concerned its impermeability to water [18, 19, 20] and one might expect, unless some form of active transport mecha-

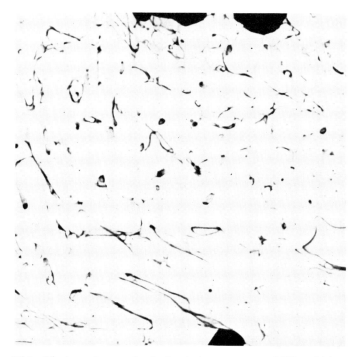

Figure 15.1 Electronmicrograph of pig stratum corneum, 0.250 μ thickness, showing areas infiltrated with silver nitrate. Micrograph by Dr. Benjamin Mosier.

nism exists in the corneum (an unlikely prospect), that these results hold for ions as well. Fleischmajer and Witten showed that although thorium-X does not diffuse passively through the stratum conjunctum, it does, if driven iontophoretically, invade the germinating layer to the dermoepidermal boundary and even penetrates the corium though to a lesser extent. The exosomatic current used in resistance measurements may, therefore, be effective in driving ions across the outer barrier, whence areas other than sweat glands and hair follicles would contribute to total skin conductance.

The preceding discussion refers to cases in which the corneum is at least moderately hydrated. Dry corneum is a poor conductor and the conductivity of the stratum disjunctum is markedly altered by the state of its hydration [21]. A dramatic demonstration of this may be observed if one touches a dry microelectrode (silver-silver chloride) tip to the skin surface. Resistance may be above 100 MΩ for a 10-μ tip. If one now places a microdroplet of saline beside the tip, resistance promptly falls (e.g., to 10 to 20 MΩ). These observations at first glance seem to imply that the corneum must contribute appreciably to total conductance, but conductance of current by the upper layers need not imply a path through the barrier layer. An obvious alternative is a lateral path from the stratum disjunctum to the spiral sweat duct and through the duct down to the dermis.

Observations by several investigators indicate the existence of a second barrier in the region of the dermoepidermal junction, possibly at the basement membrane of the germinating layer or the basal cell layer itself. Witten and his coworkers [22] had already shown that after longer exposures (48 hr) to thorium-X without iontophoresis, radiation tracks may be found in the germinating layer but *not* in the dermis. The dermoepidermal boundary thus appears to be an effective barrier against this ion as it is against some inorganic compounds [23]. These findings reinforce the conclusions reached by Pease [24] using electromicrographs that an intact membrane made up in part of basal cell membranes separates the dermis from the epidermis. The fact that iontophoretic driving did cause penetration of the stratum germinativum in the experiments of Fleischmajer and Witten would indicate that this is a route which may contribute to the conductance of the skin in conventional measurements.

Direct observation of an electrical-barrier layer in the deeper layers of the corneum or in the germinating layer may be also observed with microelectrode measurements. Suchi [25] and this author [26] have pushed pipette microelectrodes through the dry corneum while recording resistance. As the deeper layers of the stratum corneum are reached, resistance decreases appreciably, but not suddenly, probably as a consequence of increasing hydration. At a certain point the subject reports the first sensation of mild pain and as the pipette is pushed slightly further the resistance suddenly falls essentially to the magnitude of the electrode resistance alone. Suchi found this to occur at a depth of 50 μ on the forearm and 350 μ on the palm. The probe has apparently penetrated a discrete ionic barrier layer, possibly the same barrier layer demonstrated by Szakall [27, 28] and by Buettner [18] for water permeability. Whether the sudden fall in resistance occurs at the level of the stratum conjunctum or at the dermoepidermal boundary is not known. The experiments with radioactive thorium, cited earlier, would indicate that the stratum conjunctum is the predominant of the two possible barriers, but it should be stressed that experiments with a large ion such as thorium may not necessarily generalize to the Na^+, and Cl^- ions which probably account for most of the electrical transfer in the skin. Steric factors have been demonstrated to be of considerable importance in their effect on electrical measurements [28, 15, 29] and it is possible that the barrier for smaller ions is at a different locus than that for larger ones.

The germinating layer except perhaps for the more densely packed granular layer contains intercellular canaliculi through which ions move freely as evidenced by the demonstrated free diffusion of ferritin [30] and of the iontophoretic migration of ferrous ion through these passages [31]. The ferritin experiments showed that the dermoepidermal boundary at the basal layer of the germinating layer is permeable to ferritin since the ferritin had been injected intradermally. Pinocytosis had not been observed in the basement membrane. The experiments by Suchi [31] showed that iron is driven downward by iontophoresis as far as the dermoepidermal boundary and then appears to stop, although it may in fact enter the corium and disappear due to rapid diffusion. The canaliculi do not perforate the basal layer and if one is seeking the site of a contiguous living-cellular barrier layer, this is a likely choice, especially in view of the electronmicrographic observations by Pease [24]. The granular layer may also constitute such a site, but since these cells are in a transitional state their membranes may not be as impermeable to ions as are the living cells of the basal layer. There are then three candidates for the locus of a discrete barrier layer, the stratum conjunctum with the stratum lucidum, if present, and the granular and basal cell layers of the stratum germinativum. Actually, since a penetrating microelectrode passes through these areas rapidly, the discrete location of the electrical barrier may be apparent rather than real, and may in fact be comprised of a number of *relatively* impermeable layers which collectively in a series arrangement, constitute an effective electrical "barrier."

The innermost layer, the corium is relatively rich in intercellular spaces through which ions may pass freely. Its ready permeability to ions has been observed by Papa and Kligman [32] who found that the cationic dye, methylene blue, when driven into the sweat gland by strong electrical currents, migrates down the duct to the level of the corium whence it passes laterally. Its diffusion through the connective tissue is so rapid that its coloration can barely be seen in the neighborhood of the duct. Once the ionic current has reached the corium, one may regard it essentially as being inside the body. Free passage through this volume conductor means that most of the potential drop in the current path occurs in the layers above the corium. This is confirmed by microelectrode observations. Once the electrical barrier has been "punctured," further penetration of the corium has no effect on total R.

Other than hair follicles, the sweat glands constitute a major conductive path through the barrier layer. The lumen of the duct and secretory portion is a good conductor when filled with sweat, so that a secreting sweat gland affords a freely conducting current path from the surface to the secretory portion deep in the corium. This path is in series with the epithelial cells of the duct at the dermal level and of the gland proper. The cells of the duct wall where it spirals through the corneum are possibly permeable to ions since they are nonliving but this question is still unsettled. Contrary to earlier belief, the spiral duct does have a well-defined wall [33]. The portion of the duct passing through the germinating layer is permeable to ions, at least when a driving potential is applied as shown by Suchi's experiments with $FeSO_4$. The duct lining in the corium is also ion-permeable as demonstrated by the observation of movement of methylene blue from the duct into the connective tissue. Added evidence for the ion-permeability of the duct is to be found in the demonstration of reabsorption of salt by the duct lining [34]. Flesch and his co-workers [35] have apparently demonstrated that the sweat gland is not a ready route of access for solutes diffusing into the body even with the help of a strong potential gradient. This would at first glance seem to indicate that the lining of the glandular and ductal portions of the sweat gland are impermeable, but more likely indicates that the sweat ducts remain collapsed unless they are secreting; when they do secrete, any solutes tending to enter would be washed out by the emerging sweat. That this view is true is indicated by the observation that a microelectrode inserted into the pore of a filled sweat duct finds a low-resistance pathway to the interior. The high conductance of the sweat gland is consistent with the observation that electrical conductance is very high on those areas having highest concentration of sweat glands, namely the palmar and plantar surfaces, this despite the unusually thick corneum and the presence of a stratum lucidum in these areas. It is of interest that considerable penetration of the sweat duct was found for thorium-X [22] and for radioactive phosphate [17]. Thus the conclusions reached by Rothman [36] and by Flesch et al. [35] that solutes do not readily penetrate the sweat gland seems to be in doubt. The resolution of this paradox may be that penetration of the duct is accomplished only by very long exposures to strong electrical driving potentials. The possibility must also be considered that given enough time, these ions enter the sweat duct by lateral diffusion from the stratum disjunctum.

The hair follicle undoubtedly constitutes a low-resistance pathway through the skin. It is commonly recognized that this structure represents a preferred route for penetration of the skin by various solutes [37]. Moreover, the scalp was found to be the most conductive of a large number of tested areas on the body surface, its conductance being four times as high as palmar skin and more than ten times as high as the volar forearm [12]. Since the forehead also has a relatively high conductance, about four times the conductance of the forearm, there is some question as to whether one may attribute all of this high conductivity to hair follicles. Additional evidence for the preferential conductivity through the follicles is seen in microelectrode observations by this author. Skin on the dorsum of the skin close to a hair follicle had considerably lower resistance than skin some distance away from the hair.

The vascular plexuses of the corium may also contribute to the electrical properties of the skin. Since these are freely permeable to salts and are highly conductive, vasodilation causes a decrease in the resistance of tissue and conversely [38]. The maximum change, however, is usually less than 1 ohm [39]. Since internal-tissue resistance, including the corium, is less than 1 kΩ [6, 58] out of a total resistance which may be 20 kΩ cm^2, the maximum vascular contribution to variation in skin resistance is negligible as compared with the epidermal contribution. Evidence for this is seen in the independence of vasomotor activity in the skin and electrical conductance changes [41, 42]. When a fall in resistance occurs as a result of sudomotor reflex activity, the cutaneous vessels commonly constrict. Thus, any contribution from vasomotor activity would tend to reduce rather than increase the magnitude of the reflex change. Occasionally when an electrode is fastened tightly to the skin of the finger so that the subject senses a pulsation, a very small fluctuation may be observed superimposed on the normal conductance trace. This artifact may be induced by a local potential change of mechanical origin as will be discussed in Section 15.2.2, or by a pulsatile change in contact at the electrode-skin interface.

The above description in a general way pertains to skin as it is found over most of the body. The chief topological variants are the thickness of the corneum, the presence or absence of the stratum lucidum, the concentration and arrangement of sweat glands, and the presence or absence of hair, all of which influence the electrical properties. Not all differences in electrical properties are to be attributed to structural effects, however, since neural activity also influences the values of the various electrical measurements, and efferent neural activity varies considerably over various parts of the body. Thus the ratio of resistances from two different sites on the body may change considerably over the course of an hour, for example, from a ratio of 1.3 to 1 to a ratio of 0.8 to 1. Surface potential relations between loci may likewise vary over time.

The resistance of the skin up to this point has been treated as an ohmic resistance, that is, one in which the voltage generated by the current is a linear function of current strength and independent of frequency. In fact, neither of these two requirements hold for the skin. Gildemeister [46] held that the resistance of the skin is largely a reflection of a counter-EMF generated by the current as a result of membrane polarization (i.e., as a result of differential mobilities of oppositely charged ions). This view requires examination in more detail but will be more appropriately discussed in conjunction with impedance and capacitance.

15.1.2 Potential

Origins

Although a potential difference exists at the phase boundary between most biological structures and the surrounding fluid, this fixed charge (the eta potential) influences but does not constitute the potential difference measured between the surface of the skin and the inside of the body. The measureable potential differences across the skin are presumably membrane potentials and, although they could in special cases originate in an oriented-dipole layer, they typically arise from diffusion processes in which ionic components possess different mobilities [44]. They may develop at the interface between two layers of solution of different concentration or composition, but the interposition of a membrane usually enhances the differences in ionic mobilities either by virtue of the fixed charge on the membrane structure [45] or due to steric effects. Larger ions may be disproportionately retarded. Since diffusion potentials can develop even in the absence of a membrane, it becomes apparent that structures not ordinarily viewed as membranes, may by virtue of a selective action upon the ionic population, behave as "semipermeable" membranes. Thus the barrier layer of the corneum, although a mass of compacted cell carcasses, may exert a degree of selectivity if some of its channels are so narrow as to offer steric hindrance to ionic passage. If the channels are too wide to offer significant steric impedance they may still exert a selective action as a consequence of the fixed charge on the solid structure, whose electrostatic effects extend some distance out into the aqueous channels. Such a "membrane" would behave much like a collodion membrane in that potentials could develop across it, but these would depend passively on the concentration of the external and internal medium and not upon any dynamic processes which may modify the concentration gradient and which may transiently alter the characteristics of the membrane as occurs in the case of nerve, muscle, or epithelium. Other "passive" structures across which diffusion potentials could develop would be the spiral portion of the sweat duct, the stratum lucidum and perhaps the granular layer. Membrane potentials could develop across active living-cell layers in the secretory portion of the sweat gland, its duct up to the level of deeper regions of the corneum, and finally the basal layer of the germinating layer. All of these latter structures are innervated (although there is some doubt about the portion of the sweat duct which traverses the germinating layer) and the permeabilities of these sites may perhaps be altered by neurosecretory activity, thereby producing an alteration of the diffusion potential. Moreover, active ionic transport mechanisms in these membranes may generate electromotive driving forces which would contribute to the overall membrane potential. It is noteworthy that microelectrode measurements by Schulz and her co-workers [34] showed the lumen of the sweat duct to be about 40 mV negative with respect to the surrounding dermal tissue. The smooth muscle of the blood vessels, the myoepithelial cells and the piloerectile cells, when they contract, may set up dipoles in the volume conductor such that a contribution to surface potential may be made, but this effect, because of the multiplicity of shunt conduction paths in the corium compared with the high transepidermal resistance, can be expected to be low.

Since steric effects are not likely to account for an appreciable diffusion potential when the dominant ions are Na^+ and Cl^-, the possibility of electrostatic selectivity may be of importance, and it becomes of interest to know the polarity of the fixed charge of the various ionic screens. The specific location of structures having a fixed charge has been somewhat clarified by the use of staining reactions with electropositive or electronegative dye radicals. Thus Sulzberger and his co-workers [46] found the pore and spiral portion of the sweat duct to have a negative charge as indicated by its affinity for thioflavin-S and acriflavin. The basement membrane of the germinating layer is argyrophilic [47] and would, therefore, also be expected to have, at least in some portions, a net negative charge. The barrier layer of the corneum on the other hand has a strongly acidic reaction on its outer surface and a slightly alkaline reaction on its inner surface [1]. One could from these observations construct various models to explain skin potentials, but without additional experimental data, such attempts would be purely speculative.

Direct evidence for the difference in the polarization properties (and hence potential) of sweat gland and nonsweat gland areas is to be seen in microelectrode measurements which demonstrate differential effects of current upon the sweat gland as opposed to epidermal areas [48]. When constant currents of high density were passed through these respec-

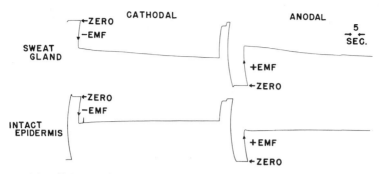

Figure 15.2. Polarization of sweat glands and areas between sweat glands with high current densities applied via pipette microelectrodes. Upper and lower strips are simultaneous recordings.

tive areas, the subsequent polarization curves were opposite in direction. At the sweat gland, cathodal currents (in which the cations were moving outward) caused a progressive increase in EMF, and an anodal current caused a progressive decrease, over a 1-min period (Fig. 15.2). In areas between sweat glands the opposite occurred. Suitable controls in these experiments demonstrated this to be cutaneous phenomena rather than evidence of electrode polarization. These results would be consistent with a model in which an electrical current may enter the body either via the sweat gland or through the epidermis according to the point on the surface at which the current enters. The epidermal structure producing differential polarization would in this instance be the corneum or some cell layer or layers in the germinating layer. Alternatively these findings could imply that the current entering at surface loci *be-tween* sweat pores, traverses the corneum but eventually enters the sweat duct when an ionic barrier is reached in the stratum corneum. Because of volume conductor effects such currents would likely be distributed over two or more sweat glands, and one might be primarily observing polarization effects in the upper corneum where current density is highest. The resolution of this question requires similar measurements made on sites from which the corneum has been largely removed by skin-stripping. Other experiments on gross sites have shown that there is essentially no rectification effect when currents of relatively low density (8 μA cm^{-2}) are used. This could reflect a cancelling effect of the two areas but more likely is evidence that such polarization is evidenced only at very high densities, since the discrete microelectrode placements did not show opposite effects when lower current densities were used.

Potential Measures

The skin surface is normally negative with respect to the inside of the body, the palmar and plantar surfaces being most negative. The mean transcutaneous potential at the palm was found to be −39.0 mV [12]. The mean value for forearm was −15.2 mV. The difference between these values, −23.8 mV, is typical of commonly reported measurements between the hand and arm. Surwillo [49] reports palm to arm potentials ranging from −12.3 to −56.8 mV (mean value −31.5 mV). This wide range in a population of subjects is typical and probably more representative of variation on the palm than on the arm, as suggested by the wide range of transcutaneous palmar potential, −10 to −60 mV reported by Davis and his co-workers [50]. It is noteworthy that the right hand has been found to be consistently more negative than the left, by approximately 5 to 7 mV in both right- and left-handed subjects [51], a finding probably related to the higher conductance found on the right hand [52].

Skin potential becomes more negative when the sweat glands are active, an observation consistent with the greater negativity and higher sweat gland concentration of the palmar as compared with nonpalmar surfaces. These observations together with microelectrode measurements of potential at the sweat pore and on the nearby corneum [53] lead to the view that the sweat gland is a source of negative potential. The nearby epidermal area is also negative with respect to the inside of the body, but less so than is the sweat gland. It is of interest that while areas rich in sweat glands (the palmar and plantar surfaces) become more negative with increasing activation, other areas of the body may become more positive (unpublished observations). This could mean either that the sweat glands in these areas are qualitatively different or that potentials originating in nonsweat gland areas of the skin become more positive with activation. A third explanation hinges upon an analysis of internal-circuit currents [53]. According to this model the deeper regions of the corneum are the site of a potential which is less negative than that of the interior of the sweat gland. A current therefore flows between the two; the potential measured at the surface is a function of the relative resistance of the sweat duct and the corneum (Fig. 15.3). Decreasing the resistance of the sweat duct (i.e., by filling) causes the surface to become more negative; decreasing the resistance of the corneum (i.e., by hydration) causes the surface to become more positive. Thus, depending upon the initial state of the tissue, increased sweating may cause either an increase or decrease in surface potential.

The microelectrode measurements of a difference of potential between sweat glands and epidermis and the evidence for an internal current flow between the two areas [53] may have special significance as an adaptive mechanism. Negatively charged bacteria accidently entering the sweat pore would be moved outward along the potential gradient between the duct and the surrounding tissue. Lykken [40] has suggested that such a mechanism could be effective at an injured area, but in that case the relative positivity of the damaged area would tend to attract rather than repel negatively charged bodies.

Solutions of certain electrolytes placed on the skin surface often, though not always, alter the potential. Increasing concentrations of either

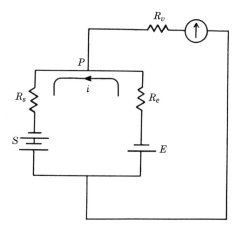

Figure 15.3. Circuit for internal currents in skin. Abbreviations: R_v, resistance of voltmeter; P, potential measured at surface; R_s, resistance of the sweat duct and internal resistance of the sweat-gland "battery;" S, potential of sweat-gland generator; R_e, resistance of epidermis other than sweat duct; E, potential of the epidermal generator. Value of P is determined by ratio of $R_s:R_e$. From Edelberg, *Ann. N.Y.A.S.*, 1968.

NaCl or KCl render the site more negative. Consistent with this is the observation that a potential develops between two similar sites each in contact with a solution of KCl of different concentration. The site in contact with the more concentrated solution is found to be negative with respect to the other [13]. Since the effective radii of K^+ and Cl^- in aqueous solution are the same, this effect is most likely a function of a fixed negative charge on the skin structure making it selectively cation-permeable. This selectivity is rather imperfect, however; a pair of sites in contact with 0.1 N and 0.01 N KCl shows a potential difference of the order of 10 to 25 mV [48] as compared with a theoretical value of 58 mV for a highly selective membrane. This potential develops very rapidly, and, in view of the compelling evidence that surface solutions do not enter the sweat duct unless driven in with high-potential gradients or allowed long periods for diffusion, the sites of these diffusion potentials likely resides in some portion of the corneum.

An important qualification of the above effect was the finding that in many cases, changing the surface concentration by a factor of 50 induced little or no change in the surface potential of the site. In such cases the surface potential in the very dilute solution was highly negative to begin with and it is supposed that the open sweat duct may account for the negative potential. In cases where the ducts are closed and the extraductal areas make a stronger contribution to the total surface potential (see Fig. 15.3) one may expect the diffusion potential through the epidermis to be well represented, resulting in a net change of surface potential as electrolyte concentration is varied.

15.2 PHASIC AND TONIC VARIATIONS IN RESISTANCE AND POTENTIAL

The previous discussion of the conducting pathways and sites of endogenous EMF in the skin sets the stage for interpretation of variation in these properties. A voluminous literature exists describing the variation in electrical properties of the skin when an individual is startled or frightened, or when he is engaged in various tasks, some involving motor behavior, others purely intellectual, such as problem solving. This literature has been reviewed repeatedly. In addition to references cited in the introduction, the reader is referred to meaningful discussions by Darrow [54], Richter [55], McCleary [56], Fujimori [57], Nakayama and Takagi [58], Wang [59, 60], Lader and Montagu [42], and Wilcott [61].

15.2.1 Responses of Central Origin

When central stimulation is adequate, and it should be appreciated that this system is exquisitely responsive, a discharge of sympathetic impulses to the skin causes a sudden change in skin resistance and surface potential known as the electrodermal response (EDR). The gross changes may be briefly described as follows. At a point about 1.5 to 2 sec after a brief stimulus, for example an 85 dB tone, a reduction in skin resistance starts, most easily measured on the palmar or plantar surfaces. This reaches a peak usually in less than 1 sec and may amount to as much as a 20% decrease, although it is more commonly of the order of 0.5 to 5%. Base levels range from 10 kΩ to 500 kΩ cm², even within the same individual. For discrete stimuli the response usually has a well-defined wave form as seen in Fig. 15.4a. Resistance is shown as decreasing upwards and after reaching peak (i.e., minimum) immediately starts to recover along an approximately exponential curve which has a time constant varying from 1 to 15 sec, most typically of the order of 4 to 6 sec [62]. In other cases the initial stimulus sets up a succession of neural bursts resulting in multiple responses as seen in Fig. 15.4b. In some instances, especially following a multiple response, the resistance level remains lower for an extended period, as, for example, when a subject is suddenly awakened. If one at the same time observes

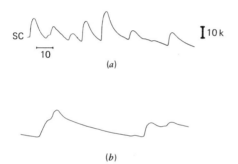

SC

10

(a)

10 k

(b)

Figure 15.4.   (a) Skin resistance responses from a palmar site. Time line represents 10 sec. Vertical calibration is 10 Ω. (b) Multiple skin resistance responses from same subject.

endogenous potentials at another site referred either to the dermis or to a relatively inactive area such as the inner aspect of the earlobe, there is a monophasic change of potential having a similar but not identical time course. The most common response is a negative shift of potential at the active site as shown in Fig. 15.5a. Somewhat less commonly seen is a biphasic response (Fig. 15.5b) in which an initial negative wave (the a-wave) is followed about one second after onset by a positive component (the b-wave). In some cases, the response is triphasic, the positive response being followed by a slow, high-amplitude negative component, the c-wave or γ-wave. Occasionally one observes monophasic positive waves, but in most instances if adequate amplification is used, a slight negative wave may be observed at the point of onset. The amplitudes of these various responses and component responses varies from minor perturbations of the baseline (e.g., 0.05 mV) to waves of 20 to 25 mV. Amplitude is commonly of the order of 0.5 to 5 mV.

15.2.2   Responses of Local Origin

In addition to responses of central origin one may elicit localized responses by mechanical stimulation in the immediate region of the electrode. Ebbecke [63] reported a reduction of resistance on nonpalmar surfaces in response to local stimulation with pressure, alternating current or heat. He interpreted these as due to direct stimulation of excitable cells, resulting in their depolarization. Several years later Rein [64]

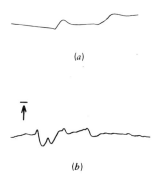

(a)

(b)

Figure 15.5.   (a) Negative skin potential responses from a palmar site referred to an inactive reference on the forearm. (b) Biphasic responses from the same site, some time later. Negative deflections are upwards.

demonstrated that these local responses were attended by positive potential waves. Although Richter [55] confirmed Ebbecke's report that such responses were not obtainable from the palmar surfaces, the present author has been able to obtain both resistance and potential local responses from the palmar as well as other surfaces using pressures of 120 to 180 mm Hg, or preferably stretch of the skin in the area of the electrode. The local decrease in resistance is of the order of 1 to 2%, while the positive potential shift is from 0.2 to 5 mV, depending upon the magnitude of the applied pressure or stretch (Fig. 15.6). The magnitude and polarity of these responses may be altered by varying the species of electrolyte solution on the surface. Local responses apparently originate in the epidermis, since they may be recorded from a

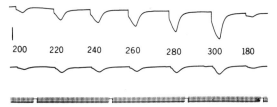

Figure 15.6. Simultaneous recordings of local positive potential responses to graded stretch stimulation. Numbers refer to pressure (mm Hg) in bladder used to exert stretch. Larger signals on time trace (bottom) are at 1-min intervals.

microelectrode on the surface, but not from one whose tip is situated in the dermis.

15.2.3   Determinants of Variation in Resistance and Potential

A wealth of experimental evidence leads to the conclusion that the EDR is related to an increase in sudomotor activity under the influence of cholinergic sympathetic fibers. It is not certain whether the attending evolution of sweat is caused by increased rate of secretion or by myoepithelial contraction superimposed on a tonic secretory rate. For the present purposes it need only be recognized that the sweat duct, if partially empty, tends to fill, that sweat may exit at the sweat pore and increase the hydration of the nearby epidermis or that it may perhaps diffuse laterally through the walls of the spiral portion into the corneum. In view of the fact that in miliaria a plugged orifice may cause considerable distension of the duct, one is tempted to regard the duct lining as impermeable to sweat. Sweat may, however, be produced at a much faster rate than that at which it diffuses into the surrounding tissue, especially if this is already wet to some extent, and during such conditions distention may persist. This suggests, in view of the tendency for sweating to be induced by emotional disturbances that miliaria may at times be exacerbated by emotional experiences.

The electrical concomitants of these movements of sweat seem apparent. As sweat rises up the ducts and reaches the surface, highly conductive pathways from the surface to the body of the sweat gland are opened. Thomas and Korr [65] have measured skin conductance and counted the total number of filled sweat ducts in an area and have shown an excellent linear relation between the two. It must be realized, however, that these measurements were made with dry electrodes held in place for only 1 to 4 sec per reading. Under such conditions the corneum probably remains dry and makes little or no contribution to total conductance. If the dry electrode is allowed to remain on the surface for an extended period, the corneum gradually becomes hydrated [21] and contributes to the total conductance. An estimate made by this author [26] based on a microelectrode survey of a circumscribed area of palmar skin, indicates that the entire population of sweat glands, when full, can account for less than 50% of the total conductance of a hydrated site. If the surface layer is permitted to dry, it becomes highly resistant (electrically) and even though deeper layers may be moistened by lateral diffusion from the duct, the dry surface layer in series acts as an effective electrical barrier.

Adams, in a series of elegant experiments on cats and humans, has accumulated evidence that the hydraulic capacitance of the corneum plays a major role in accounting not only for skin conductance but for the skin-conductance response as well [66, 67]. He holds that the assumption of a variable membrane is not necessary to explain either phenomenon and that apparent membrane characteristics of human skin may be possessed by the corneum. Most of his evidence is derived from cat and model experiments and it is possible that his conclusions are valid for the cat but hold only partially for the human.

An assortment of evidence suggests that the electrodermal response, although having a prominent ohmic component, is in large part of membrane origin. There is little doubt that the rise of sweat in the duct accounts for an ohmic change in skin conductance. The subsequent moistening of the corneum although slower also accounts for an ohmic effect. Its time course is such that its effects may not appear during the initial decrease in resistance, although they may alter the recovery limb by counteracting the rate of recovery of resistance. Adams [68] has shown that a secondary wave, which often appears as an inflection in the recovery limb after the initial peak of conductance has been reached, is probably due to this effect. These effects can also account for both negative and positive skin potential responses as has already been discussed, despite the absence of any change in diffusion potentials in the skin. Thus, phasic changes in conductance, potential, or impedance can all be produced by the effects of changes in duct-filling or by wetting of the corneum.

There are other properties of the skin, however, which are more difficult to explain without postulating the presence of an active membrane. One of these is seen in the specific effect of certain chemical agents upon the skin resistance response. If one uses a solution of 1 M $CaCl_2$ as an electrode medium for a finger site, the skin conductance response is found to be markedly potentiated as compared to the same site in tap water or dilute saline [29]. Moreover, the degree of potentiation is dependent upon the polarity of current at this site. If the direction of current (flow of positive ions) is inward, the potentiation is about 240%, but if current flow is reversed, the potentiation is only about 115%. Surprisingly, the recitification ratio for base resistance in this same solution is only 1.06. It appears that while the variable element responsible for phasic responses does have membrane characteristics, the base level itself depends mostly on ohmic elements. It is difficult to attribute the apparent membrane characteristics of the phasic change to the corneum, since any change in this dead structure would almost certainly be that due to hydration and this would be of an ohmic nature. Change in hydration does not, at any rate, seem to be involved since the electro-dermal response is obtained even more easily after the skin has soaked in $CaCl_2$ for 30 min, than when the site is dry. Moreover, the potentiating effect is seen in the rapidly ascending limb, which, if not of membrane origin, is almost certainly due to the rise of sweat in the ducts. The corneal hydration effect would come appreciably later.

Other chemical solutions effect the skin conductance response differently, 1 M KCl causing a reduction to about 45% of the magnitude in dilute saline, 1 M $AlCl_3$ potentiating it by about 600%. The cationic detergent, sodium benzalkonium chloride (Zephiran) in low concentration (0.005 M) depresses it to 45% of the magnitude in tap water [29]. This last is of special significance in view of the well recognized lytic effects of surface active agents upon membranes [69]. Again, while it is perhaps possible to explain these specific effects on a nonmembrane basis, it seems that the assumption of a selective membrane as the site of electrodermal responses would be a parsimonious explanation.

The effects of chemical agents upon the potential response also suggest the involvement of a membrane [5]. For example, 1 M $AlCl_3$ enhances the positive component of the skin potential response by 750% while having a negligible effect upon the negative wave. Solutions of 5 M NaCl essentially extinguish the positive wave and produce a dramatic potentiation of the slow negative or c-wave. Again one is reminded of the specific effects of various ions and of high concentrations upon cell-membrane potentials and action potentials.

As has been indicated earlier, there are two structures likely to serve as the locus of an active membrane, the ductal or secretory portions of the sweat gland and the germinating layer. The approximate locus of a sweat duct region which may be involved in the electrodermal response can be inferred from experiments by Shaver and his co-workers [70]. They inserted pipette microelectrodes into sweat ducts of the cat footpad and observed the potential change after stimulation of the plantar nerve. Potential responses were observed along the duct at the level of the germinating layer, but not below it. One would, therefore, tend to locate an active membrane in the duct wall at this level. It is possible that this participates in a salt- or water-reabsorption reflex which is part of the electrodermal response. Evidence for such a reflex was seen in continuous measurements of the hydration of the skin surface [71, 62]. These showed a sudden reduction in surface hydration in response to a variety of external stimuli. The response, when it occurred, was accompanied by a fast, positive-going potential change.

The alternative locus of an active membrane is in the stratum germinativum. If an active membrane exists here it may also function as part of a reflex mechanism controlling the reabsorption of water or salts. The route would presumably be from the sweat ducts through the canaliculi of this layer and through the dermoepidermal junction, that is, along the path observed by Suchi for the ferrous ion. The most likely place for a control over this process, if not at the duct, would be at the dermoepidermal boundary, possibly in the basal-cell layer.

An alternative suggested by studies on changes in tactile sensitivity attending the electrodermal response [26] is that part of the electrodermal reflex represents the byproduct of the arrival of neural impulses to tactile receptors in the germinating layers. Nerve endings found in this layer by Arthur and Shelley [72] were regarded by those authors as likely having a tactile function. Loewenstein [73] demonstrated the existence of an efferent system which served to sensitize peripheral receptors, and Wilcott [74] showed a relation between local skin-potential level and local sensitivity to pain. While a tactile mechanism might account for the occurrence of a potential response, its role in producing the conductance response commonly associated with the positive-potential response seems obscure and this appears to be a less likely explanation than that which takes the reabsorption processes into account.

In attempting to select which of the three, the upper sweat duct, the germinating layer, or the dermoepidermal boundary is the most likely site of the membrane effects, one may ask which of the three is readily accessible to the chemical agents affecting the electrodermal response. On the basis of the observations by Fleischmajer and Witten [16], one can almost discount the germinating layer because of the relatively high impermeability of the stratum conjunctum. Aluminum chloride has been shown to enhance the reabsorption of water, presumably by affecting part of the sweat duct [32]. Thus the sweat duct in the region of the germinating layer represents an excellent candidate for the site of an active membrane if it exists. In view of the demonstrated association of the reabsorption reflex with the positive skin-potential response [71] and of the dramatic potentiation of the positive response by $AlCl_3$ it is tempting to consider that these events are related and reflect a common effect upon sweat-duct function.

15.3   CAPACITANCE, TRANSIENTS, AND IMPEDANCE

15.3.1   Capacitance

In addition to the electrical characteristics already described, the skin has capacitance properties, indicated by the observation that its impedance decreases as the frequency of the measuring current is increased. The presence of a capacitance in the skin presents a great complication to the interpretation of ac measurements, since there are a number of electrical arrangements which may have a common equivalent resistance and capacitance in a parallel or series-parallel arrangement, and it is difficult to identify the actual circuit arrangement in the skin. Moreover, as Lykken has emphasized, the circuit model used to represent the skin in the bridge circuit used for measurement will, to a large extent, determine the apparent behavior of the skin as measuring frequency is varied.

Capacitance in tissue may arise when a thin structure in the current path interrupts the flow of ions, but, because of its dielectric property and thin dimension, allows interaction of the electrical potentials on either side of it. Frequently, in living tissue, sites of capacitance are in parallel with "ohmic" conductance pathways. Such a condition can exist at numerous loci, even in the corneum, where aqueous channel are distributed in a reticular arrangement within a nonconducting material. These nonconductive materials possess an appreciable dielectric constant, and can, therefore, constitute effective separators between the "plates" which are the aqueous areas. These miniature condensors are in parallel with other portions of these aqueous channels and are sometimes in parallel with each other, sometimes in series, as implied in Tregear's model [75]. Another likely locus of capacitance is the stratum conjunctum where the highly compact nature of this thin layer is probably associated with low leakage. The cells of the germinating layer constitute yet another locus of capacitance, as do the epithelial cells lining the secretory and ductal portions of the sweat gland.

One major source of capacitance in biological systems is polarization capacity which is not due to the static dielectric properties of structures in the current path, but is generated by the effect of current passage upon ionic distribution. This form of capacitance requires special treatment and will be discussed in Section 15.3.2.

15.3.2 Polarization and Polarization Capacitance

Gildemeister [76] measured the resistance of the skin with alternating currents and found that impedance at 5 to 6 kHz was only 2 to 3% of the dc value, and further that variations in response to stimulation of the subject could no longer be observed. In accordance with membrane theory of the time he regarded this as a demonstration that the electrical resistance of the skin was apparent rather than real, and that it was in fact a counter-EMF generated by the passage of current through an ion-selective membrane. In effect unequal mobilities of the ions gen-

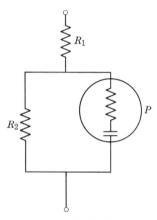

Figure 15.7. Representation of electrical circuit of the skin by a polarization model. R_1 is the ohmic resistance in series with the membrane. R_2 is the ohmic resistance in parallel with the polarization element, P. After Cole, *Cold Spring Harbor Symp.*, 1933.

erates an electrostatic drag, which is greater as current density increases. The increase in this counter-EMF is proportional to the increase in current, and, therefore, behaves much the same as the potential difference generated across an ohmic resistor, that is, as a capacitor in parallel with a resistor. Cole [77] expanded on this view and suggested an electrical model of the skin made up as shown in Fig. 15.7. The capacitor in this case is part of a polarization element, a capacitor in series with a resistor, as has been described by Fricke [78] for the case of polarization at the phase boundary of an electrode, but applicable to membranes as well. The capacitance and resistance of the polarization element vary with frequency such that the ratio of reactance to resistance, that is, the phase angle, remains constant. At higher frequencies, the phase angle is determined almost entirely by the polarization element, since its reactance becomes much lower than R_2. Cole calculated the phase angle of this polarization element from various data in the literature and obtained constant values in the neighborhood of either 55 or 90°. Barnett [6] recalculated these data in another way and found mean values from 65 to 82°. This is essentially an indictment of the unreliability of bridge measurement rather than an indication of skin variability. Barnett [6] argued that this was primarily due to the inclusion of the fixed-series resistance of the body in these measurements. Using a 3-electrode method for measuring the separate impedances of the "sheath" and of the deeper tissues, he found the phase angle of the skin to be constant over a frequency range from 2 kHz to 42 kHz and to vary from 64 to 78° across individuals.

Barnett and Cole regarded these results as evidence of a polarization element in a membrane. Lykken [40], however, argues that conclusions about the skin capacity are always inferential and depend upon an assumption about the nature of the equivalent circuit. He points out that the use of an impedance bridge having a parallel R-C pair to balance the skin will result in an apparent decrease in capacity with frequency even if the capacity of Fig. 15.7 is fixed. This is a viable criticism if the impedance measurement also includes the deep-tissue resistance, but in Barnett's experiments, that component was allegedly excluded. However, Lykken's findings imply that a second series ohmic resistor is present in the skin itself, probably in the corneum. If true his criticism of the prevalent methods of measurement are well-taken. Montagu [8] also argues for treating the skin as a *fixed* rather than a polarization capacitance in parallel with a resistor. This conclusion is based in good part upon the demonstration by Yokota and Fujimori [79] that the change in impedance during an electrodermal response is due solely to change in the parallel resistance, capacitance remaining constant. Whether the skin's capacitance is static or is a polarization phenomena is still uncertain. Various measurements of the magnitude of this capacitance, whatever its nature, have been made and seem in general agreement, ranging between 0.02 and 0.06 μF cm^{-2}, usually about 0.03.

If the capacitance of the skin is in fact a static one, there is reason to question Gildermeister's assumption that the dc skin resistance is actually a counter-EMF, since membrane polarization would by its very nature be associated with a polarization capacitance. Support for the view that the resistance element of the skin may be almost purely ohmic is seen in some recent experiments by the present author. Teorell [80], in a brilliant analysis of the origin of potentials in membranes during the passage of current, points out that a *selective* membrane behaves as a nonlinear system, since as current is increased a readjustment of concentrations occurs in the membrane and at its phase-boundary interfaces. When the current reaches an adequate value, the membrane channels become "saturated" with ions and from that point on measurements conform to the predictions of Teorell's equation. At very low currents, membrane polarization does not occur, and a measurement of membrane resistance in terms of the voltage generated by the current yields a true measure of ohmic resistance. As current increases polarization should become increasingly apparent and should show as an increase in apparent resistance of the membrane, that is, as an increase in the voltage generated by the passage of current. The relation of the total voltage developed across a membrane to the imposed current strength had been previously investigated by Fujimori [57] and by Edelberg and his co-workers [79], but neither observed effects at extremely low levels of current. The present author, in more recent experiments, examined the voltage-current curve at extremely low currents, that is, as low as 0.008 μA cm^{-2} and up to 2 μA cm^{-2}. The relation was linear over the entire range. These results conflict with those of Davis and Kennard [81] who found that the skin of the forearm behaved as an ohmic resistor only up to a current density of 0.1 μA cm^{-2}, but deviated from linear behavior above this value. The cause of the discrepancy between the measurement by Davis and Kennard and those by this author is not apparent. It is conceivable that the duration of the test exposure to each level of current may be different in the two studies. If the observations of this author are valid, they would indicate that the limiting membrane is nonselective.

At higher currents, the apparent resistance of the skin decreases [29, 82, 61]. This effect is opposite to that predicted by Teorell's formulation and may reflect an alteration in barrier-membrane structure, rendering it more permeable. It is time-dependent [12] and is observable in the curves of Davis and Kennard [81] and in Kryspin's phoreographic patterns [83].

15.3.3 Site of Capacitance

The localization of the site of the skin's capacitance is a matter of some importance since it has bearing not only on the nature of the circuitry to be used in the measurement of the phase angle, but also on whether it is a static or a polarization capacitance. Lawler and his associates [84] have adduced evidence which may indicate that it resides in the corneum. In their experiments, the impedance and capacitance of the skin was determined at each step in a stripping procedure, a process which removes layers of corneum by pressing a strip of pressure-sensitive tape to the surface and pulling it away. Both conductance and capacitance were found to increase progressively as successive strips were removed. As stated by Lawler, the increase in capacitance could have been caused either by decreasing the distance across the dielectric between the electrode and the underlying conducting zone or by removing successive capacitors originally in a series arrangement. In either case, the corneum would appear to be the dielectric material of a capacitance or series of capacitances. This would imply that at least some of the so-called "membrane" electrical properties of the skin may in fact be explained by the corneum.

In reality the likelihood that the capacitance of the skin as measured by Barnett [6] and by Lawler can be attributed to the corneum is remote. Consider, for example, the dry corneum which may have a thickness of as little as 0.1 mm. Even at this optimum thickness for capacitance and allowing a generous value of 10 as a dielectric constant, a value suggested by McClendon [85] for all membranes, the maximum capacitance per square centimeter of corneum would be far too low. It can be calculated from the expression

$$C = 0.089 \frac{KA}{t} \times 10^{-6} \; \mu\text{F}$$

where K is the dielectric constant, A the area in square centimeters and t the thickness in centimeters. This expression gives a maximum value of 0.00009 μF cm^{-2}, which is only a fraction of 1% of the capacitance value of 0.02 to 0.06 μF found for skin [6, 77]. If the corneum is considered to be broken into a series of much thinner capacitors whose total interplate distance is less than the total thickness of the corneum (due to aqueous channels) the capacitance may be higher but would still be unlikely to account for the observed value.

The approximate maximum thickness of the involved capacitor may be estimated if one assumes a high value for the dielectric constant, for example, 10, and a low value for capacitance, such as, 0.02 μF cm^{-2}. This gives a maximum thickness of 0.5 micron. For a dielectric constant of 5 and a capacitance of 0.05 μF cm^{-2}, the maximum thickness would be 0.1 micron. These thicknesses, while considerably greater than the estimated thickness of a cell membrane, imply that if the capacitance of the skin is of a static character, as opposed to a polarization capacity, it resides in a structure which is probably not greater than one or two cell layers in thickness.

In the light of this, one wonders why Lawler found the capacitance of the skin to increase from 0.02 to almost 0.04 μF as stripping of the corneum continued, since this would imply that the capacitance of the removed corneum in series with the final one was of the order of 0.04 μF. This possibility, as has been shown, is remote unless all of the capacitance of the corneum resides in a very thin layer or layers within it. It is not likely to be confined to a single layer, since in Lawler's experiment, capacitance increased regularly as each layer was removed. One likely explanation is that as the corneum is stripped away, more conductive channels to the underlying capacitor are opened, thus effectively increasing its area. The conclusion of the above reasoning is that the corneum as a hydration-dependent conductor does not contain appreciable shunt capacitance. The argument holds whether the resistance and capacitance of the corneum is treated as a whole or is broken into small serial R-C units as in Tragear's treatment. It would further follow that a change in corneal hydration could, in conjunction with a change in sweat-duct filling, account for reflex electrical impedance changes at high frequencies.

15.3.4   Transients

Although the most common method of investigating the skin's capacitance properties is by the use of ac measurements over a range of frequencies, another method was used very effectively by Hozawa [86] and more recently by Lykken [40, 59]. In this method a step voltage is applied to the skin and the current strength measured during the initial transient and in the subsequent steady-state region. Assuming the circuit to be represented by that in Fig. 15.8 [8], during the initial "infinite" rate of change of voltage the capacitor offers essentially no reactance and the current strength is determined purely by R_1. When after a few milliseconds the capacitor is fully charged, the current is determined by R_1 plus R_2. From calculations based on this approach, Hozawa determined the value of R_1, which he attributed to inner-tissue resistance, to be of the order of 380 ohms. This compares well with the value of 500 ohms found by Lykken, but is considerably higher than the 102 to 190 ohms found by Barnett [6] for deep tissue alone. The difference is of the order of the value of the series-ohmic resistance found by Barnett for the skin alone. Unfortunately, it is difficult to make precise comparisons of the various measures because different electrode areas were involved, and, as pointed out by Barnett, the ohmic resistance of the deep tissues is a constant, while that of the skin varies

reciprocally with area. Lykken has varied the electrode area to determine
the fixed portion of R (500 ohms) and has thereby calculated that the
portion of R_1 to be found in the skin was of the order of 8kΩ for 0.7
cm². Stripping of the corneum resulted in a reduction of only 3 kΩ,
and from this Lykken concluded that a sizeable series-ohmic resistance
lies in tissue beneath the stratum corneum but close enough to the surface
to show an area effect. It seems that this third component of R may
likely reside in the germinating layer.

The results with skin-stripping in Lykken's experiment led him to
modify Tregear's model [75] in which the corneum is represented as
a large number of parallel resistance-capacitance units in series. In order

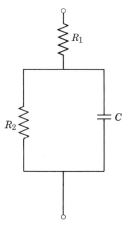

Figure 15.8.   Representation of the electrical circuit of the skin using a static
capacitance. R_1 represents the series ohmic resistance. R_2 is the ohmic resistance in
parallel with the fixed capacitance, C. After Montagu, *J. Psychosom. Res.,* **1964.**

to account for the change in R_1 with stripping, Lykken added a resistor
between each of the R-C units. In conventional dc measurements it
would be these interposed resistances which would be changed by hydration and which would, therefore, contribute to the ohmic component of
the EDR.

Values of R_2 can be obtained from comparison of the peak and
steady-state currents. Hozawa calculated values ranging from 57 to 440
kΩ cm². Montagu [8] reports values of the order of 32 to 710 kΩ
cm². Lykken found R_2 to be 78 kΩ cm² but this did not represent a
range of subjects. It should be appreciated that these values are close

to those measured by conventional dc techniques, the difference being in the small series-ohmic contribution of the skin.

The value of the capacitance in this model can be calculated by the transient method, if the time constant of the exponential decay is determined. Hozawa found a value of 0.02 μF cm^{-2} by this technique, a figure which compares favorably with estimates obtained from ac bridge measurements.

15.3.5   Impedance Measures

As a result of the skin's capacitance its impedance decreases with increasing frequency of the measuring current. The associated measures of resistive and capacitative components would depend upon the type of measuring system used and its relation to the actual arrangement of electrical elements in the skin. Thus, the impedance of the skin can be balanced out by a series resistance-capacitance circuit or by a parallel one. Each gives the equivalent adequate but not necessary circuit to represent its properties. However, at high frequencies (e.g., above 10 kHz) there is little doubt that the reactance of the shunt capacitance in the skin is very low and after subtracting deep-tissue resistance, the impedance should be essentially equal to the ohmic resistance of the skin. Impedance data have been reported by Gildemeister [88], Hozawa [89], Forbes [90], Barnett [6], Gerstner and Gerbstadt [91], Lawler et al. [84], Plutchik [92], and Montagu [8] among others. Their data cover a variety of frequency ranges and electrode size, the latter making it difficult to compare results, unlike the case for dc measurements. They are in rather good agreement, however, on the value for the skin's capacitance which has been placed for the most part between 0.02 and 0.04 μF cm^{-2}. If one uses as a representative value, 0.025 μF cm^{-2}, assuming it is a static capacitance, the reactance of a 1 cm^2 capacitative element may be calculated for various frequencies as follows:

1 Hz	6,300,000 ohms
10 Hz	630,000 ohms
100 Hz	63,000 ohms
1 kHz	6,300 ohms
10 kHz	630 ohms
100 kHz	63 ohms

The ohmic resistor in parallel has a value ranging from 20 to 500 kilohm cm^2. Thus, although the phase angle is less than 90°, it can be appreciated that at frequencies much above 1 kHz, the impedance will be determined almost entirely by the reactance of the capacitative element.

Lawler and his co-workers [84] obtained mean impedance values of 6,500 and 861 ohms at frequencies of 1 kHz and 10 kHz respectively, using 2 electrodes in series, each 2 cm in diameter. Subtracting the typical value of 500 for area independent deep-tissue resistance, gives values of 9,400 and 570 ohm cm^2 for the skin at these two frequencies. These are roughly of the same order as the values (6,300 and 630) estimated for the reactance element. Barnett [6] reported values of 2,400 ohm cm^2 and 720 ohm cm^2 at frequencies of 2 kHz and 10 kHz, respectively. These refer to the skin alone and do not include deep tissue. Again they are of the same order as the estimated values of 3,150 and 630 ohm cm^2 for the reactive element alone. At the upper frequency range, Gildemeister's [88] values were 500 to 1500 ohm cm^2 at 100 kHz in comparison with 63 ohms for the reactance element. This would indicate that an ohmic resistor sometimes as high as 1,000 ohms must be located in the skin, since the deep-tissue resistance would only account for about 500 ohms or less.

Impedance changes during an electrodermal response have been reported by Forbes and Landis [93], Forbes [90], Takagi and Nakayama [94], Yokota and Fujimori [79], Montagu [8], and Lykken et al. [87]. Gildemeister [76] had previously contended that at high frequencies, because polarization does not occur, the electrodermal response does not appear. His recordings at 5 to 6 kHz show only slight signs of a response. This was possibly a consequence of his use of liquid electrodes which kept the skin well hydrated. When pastes are used, hydration of the corneum may be changed by sweating, and any ohmic changes would be measurable as well with ac as with dc. Such changes would be independent of the frequency of measuring current unless the resistance of the corneum were shunted by appreciable capacitance. As has been indicated earlier, this is not likely.

It is therefore not surprising that the upper-frequency limit at which electrodermal responses may still be observed is consideraly higher than that indicated by Gildemeister. Forbes and Landis [93] reported EDRs as high as 10 kHz, and in one instance at 15 kHz. Their skin-electrode contact was made by means of blotters moistened with saturated ZnSO$_4$, a technique which would result in a relatively dry condition of the corneum and could account for their successful registration of EDRs. The present author using a paste contact has recorded EDRs at 20 kHz.

There is some question as to whether capacitance changes during an EDR. Forbes and Landis found changes in capacitance of the order of 0.5 to 1% in general agreement with earlier results by McClendon and Hemingway [95]. Yokota and Fujimori [79], however, found no evidence of a change in capacitance and concluded that the EDR depended entirely on a change in the parallel resistance. If valid, this result would imply that skin resistance is truly ohmic, since a polarization capacity would tend to change with change in membrane permeability. This conclusion would not preclude an active membrane as the site of the ohmic changes. An observation by Lykken et al. [96] is relevant to this issue. These authors found that the electrical behavior of the skin is well-represented by a model in which a variable voltage source is in series with a variable resistor. This might be interpreted as evidence that the two are in separate structures, but in fact the series resistor could be the internal resistance of the diffusion potential "battery." In the light of the findings by Yokota and Fujimori, the location of these elements in separate structures seems more plausible.

15.4   CHANGE IN ELECTRICAL PROPERTIES WITH AGING AND PATHOLOGY

15.4.1   Aging

If the sympathetic innervation of a cutaneous area is interrupted there may or may not be a change in skin resistance, depending upon the location. Richter [55] sectioned the nerves of the arm in the monkey and found that palmar resistance immediately rose to very high levels while that on the dorsum was essentially unaffected. This implies that tonic discharge to the palmar areas maintains an appreciable level of conductance. A similar conclusion may be inferred from the observation that a person at rest in the waking state has a considerably lower palmar resistance than when asleep.

Since the few reports to be found on the relation of aging to electrical characteristics deal with palmar sites, the above is pertinent. Any difference in resistance between young and old could as likely reflect differences in tonic neural activity as in morphology of the skin. Similarly, any differences in phasic electrical responses in the two age groups could as easily be of central neural as of cutaneous origin [97]. With this important source of ambiguity, any attempt to interpret changes in electrical properties with age is precarious. However, some scattered findings may be briefly summarized.

Van der Walk and Groen [98] reported that elderly persons had a significantly higher palmar-skin resistance than younger ones, the average at 60 to 69 years being 32.7 ±4.2 kΩ as compared with 18.9 ±0.8 kΩ at 20 to 29. Electrode areas were not reported. As previously discussed, there is a relation between skin resistance and the degree of filling of sweat ducts. When the sweat ducts are completely full a droplet of sweat may be seen emerging from the pore. A plastic impression of the skin will show a clear area wherever such a droplet has emerged [99]. Using this method, MacKinnon [100] demonstrated a regular decrease in the count of active (i.e., filled) sweat glands in the relaxed subject with increasing age and suggested that this was related to changing corticosteroid level. Her findings were confirmed by Ferreira and Winter [101] who used densitometer readings of the densest area of sweat prints as a measure of sweat production. They incidentally found that females have denser sweat prints than males at all ages. These findings are consistent with those of Burch, Cohn, and Neumann [102] who found the rate of water loss from the fingertips considerably reduced in old age. The observation by Van der Walk and Goren of an increase of resistance may be a consequence of these demonstrated structural alterations, such as those reported by Andrew [103].

The reduced sweat-gland count in the elderly would, on the basis of earlier discussion, lead to a prediction that their surface potential should be less negative. However, Surwillo [49, 104] in a careful study of skin potential levels from the palm referred to the forearm, found a progressive *increase* in surface negativity of the palm with age. The correlation between age and potential level was low (-0.23, $p < .02$) as was the regression coefficient -0.15), and it is therefore easily possible that another factor was masking the expected relationship. The increase in negativity with age is all the more difficult to explain in view of the increase in skin resistance and the finding by Venables and Martin [105] that as palmar-skin potential becomes more negative, resistance falls.

Investigations of phasic electrical changes in the elderly are even more difficult to interpret because of the likely difference in central processing of the stimuli used to elicit the reflex response. Thus Botwinick and Kornetsky [106] found that elderly subjects gave smaller resistance changes than the younger, but interpreted this as a central effect since the eye-blink reflex showed a similar age effect. In contrast to this, Surwillo [104] found that elderly subjects showed the same shift of skin-potential level during an extended-vigilance task as did younger subjects, but their cutaneous blood vessels did not show as much activity as in younger subjects.

The observable tissue changes of aged individuals do not seem consistent with the finding of higher skin resistance. Most of the pronounced changes are in the dermis [47] which contributes only slightly to skin resistance. The epidermis is essentially unchanged except on the dorsum of the hand, the face and sometimes the genitalia. The thickness of the epidermis if anything decreases with age [107, 108]. There is one observation which could account for an increased resistance. Andrew [103] reported that the lamellae of keratin in the aging rat become more eosinophilic and more adherent to each other. It is conceivable that this physicochemical change could have an effect on the ion impermeability of the stratum conjunctum. If the increasingly eosinophilic reaction reflects a tendency for fixed charge of the corneum to become more positive with age, one would expect the selective cation permeability to decrease. This could perhaps explain a change in surface negativity with age, although the polarity of such an effect cannot be predicted without a knowledge of the concentration gradients.

Clearly, available data on change in electrical properties during aging are at present uninterpretable. It is unfortunate that the few reported studies have used direct currents or have measured endogenous potentials. Impedance and microelectrode measures in conjunction with these would do much to clarify the likely structures responsible for the changing properties.

15.4.2   Injury and Pathology

Injury

In view of the evidence that the epidermis is the site of the skin's resistance, it is not surprising that puncturing it reduces the resistance to 10 to 20% of its original value. Recovery to 50% of the resistance of intact skin took 4 days on the average for the rat [15]. Skin-drilling, that is, abrading away the corneum to the level of the mucous layer with a dental burr [107], caused a similar fall and took 3 days for half recovery, 5 days for full recovery in these animals. Barnes [110] sanded the skin of humans to the point of bleeding and found surface negative potential to drop by 10 to 40 mV. This could signify that the site of the skin's potential is in the epidermis, but similar results would occur even if it resided solely in the sweat glands, since removal of the epidermis would effectively short circuit these potentials. These damaged areas took 43 hr (average) to recover their potential completely, a somewhat surprising finding since Lykken [40] using 30 skin strippings found that the potential showed no recovery up to 80 hours and took about 160 hr for complete recovery. According to Pinkus [109] who used 28 strippings, the granular layer is consolidated in 36 hr, and by 72 hr is double its normal thickness and is laying down the first layers of keratinized cells. Since Lykken and Pinkus used the same technique, this would imply that the potential does not recover until the corneal-barrier layer has formed. Such is not necessarily the case, however. Lykken found, using transient analysis, that the value of the parallel resistance fell to about 10% of the intact state and also failed to show signs of recovery for the first 80 hr. It then rose together with the negative potential but somewhat more slowly. The course of reduction and recovery of surface potential could therefore be explained by a model in which a negative potential source in the sweat gland is initially short-circuited by destruction of the corneal barrier and reappears when the latter is reestablished. Similar considerations may explain changes in the reflex skin-potential response after removal of the corneum by blistering [94]. In this case the negative skin-potential response is eradicated but a small positive component persists. The negative potential response reappears about two days later when partial regeneration has occurred.

Pathology

While it is clear that changes in electrical properties of the skin accompany various dermatoses, there is, as in the case of aging, a question of the extent to which they are caused by change in structure as opposed to change in nervous activity. Emotional factors are frequently accompanied by change in sympathetic discharge, as well as by dermatoses. Moreover, the emotional consequences of skin disfigurement may cause emotional reactions which change sympathetic (sudomotor) activity and hence skin resistance and potential. For this reason high-frequency measurements which are somewhat more indicative of structural changes than of tonic neural activity are preferred.

Measurements of potential or resistance of lesioned areas may be of use if compared with measurements on the healthy skin of the same individual, but even this cannot be accepted without question. As an example, Gougerot [112] found both the dry lesions and the "healthy" skin of psoriasis patients to be different from that of normals in terms of phase angle and impedance. Nevertheless, the magnitude of the difference between measurements in the lesioned area and on intact skin is often meaningful. Thus the finding by Barnes [110] that dermaphytotic lesions were 25 mV less negative than intact skin is evidence either that the site of the diffusion potential has been injured or that the sweat-gland potential has been short-circuited via the epidermis. Once again, interpretation is ambiguous until the site of origin of skin potentials is clearly defined.

Unfortunately, as in the case of aging, impedance studies of pathologic skin are considerably rarer than those using resistance or potential, probably because of the greater technical difficulty involved in impedance measurement. Gougerot [112] used an AC bridge in studies of eczema and psoriasis. In the course of this work he demonstrated that larger electrodes produce smaller phase angles, probably as a consequence of the constant resistance of the deep tissues. The impedance and phase angles of active eczematous lesions were both considerably lower than similar measures on healthy skin of the same individuals, a finding consistent with the common reduction of capacitance and parallel resistance in the face of a constant series resistance. This is equivalent to reduction in the "polarization" element. In cases of psoriasis, the phase angle and impedance of dry-lesioned areas were less than for healthy skin of normal subjects, but the healthy skin of psoriasis patients had higher impedances and larger phase angles than did the healthy controls. These findings were true for both small and large electrodes. At higher frequencies, however, such as, 7 kHz, the results varied considerably depending on whether large or small electrodes were used. This would again be explained by the fact that at higher frequencies, the fixed-series resistance of the deeper structures exerts a much greater effect on measurements than at lower frequencies, and that its effect is greater for larger electrode areas. These considerations argue for the use of a relatively small electrode in impedance measurement, or preferably the use of Barnett's 3-electrode technique [6] for separate measurement of the skin impedance. It is noteworthy that Gougerot has, since his earlier work, adopted the Barnett 3-electrode configuration [113].

Impedance measurements have been made by Gerstner and Gerbstadt [91] in various disease states, but their choice of 200 Hz as a bridge frequency implies that their measurements were reflecting essentially the same variables as DC measurements. Barnett used higher frequencies in studies on mental patients [114] and on cases of thyrotoxicosis [115]. He found impedance to be lower but the phase angle to be unchanged, and attributed this to a reduction in the thickness of the dielectric. It should be pointed out, however, that if impedance and capacitance of the skin are to a large part determined by the state of a polarization element as argued by Gildemeister [88] and by Cole [77], a change in permeability (perhaps as a result of change in neural activity) could also produce such a result.

REFERENCES

1. S. Rothman, *Physiology and Biochemistry of the Skin*, University of Chicago Press, Chicago, 1954. Chapter 2.

2. C. W. Darrow, *Psychophysiology*, **1**, 31 (1964).

3. I. Martin and P. H. Venables, *Psychol. Bull.*, **65**, 347 (1966).

4. R. C. Wilcott, *Psychol. Bull.*, **67**, 58 (1967).

5. R. Edelberg, "The Electrodermal System," In *Handbook of Psychophysiology,* N. Greenfield and R. Sternback, Eds., Holt, Rinehart and Winston, New York (in press) 1971.

6. A. Barnett, *J. Physiol.,* **93,** 349 (1938).

7. W. W. Grings, *J. Psychol.,* **35,** 271 (1953).

8. J. D. Montagu, *J. Psychosom. Res.,* **8,** 49 (1964).

9. J. D. Montagu and E. M. Coles, *Psychol. Bull.,* **65,** 261 (1966).

10. W. I. Hume, *J. Psychosom. Res.,* **9,** 383 (1966).

11. P. H. Venables and I. Martin, "Skin Resistance and Skin Potential," in *A Manual of Psychophysiological Methods,* P. H. Venables and I. Martin, Eds., John Wiley and Sons, New York, 1967.

12. R. Edelberg, "Electrical Properties of the Skin," in *Methods in Psychophysiology,* C. C. Brown Ed., Williams and Wilkins, Baltimore, 1967.

13. H. Rein, *Zeitschr. Biol.,* **85,** 195 (1926).

14. R. F. Rushmer, K. J. K. Buettner, J. M. Short, and G. F. Odland, *Science,* **154,** 343 (1966).

15. R. Edelberg, *NASA Manned Spacecraft Center Contract,* Report NAS 9-445, September 1963.

16. R. Fleischmajer and V. H. Witten, *J. Invest. Dermatol.,* **25,** 223 (1955).

17. V. H. Witten, E. W. Brauer, R. Loevinger, and V. Holmstrom, *J. Invest. Dermatol.,* **26,** 437 (1956).

18. K. J. K. Buettner and G. F. Odland, *Federation Proc.,* **16,** 18 (1957).

19. F. D. Malkinson and S. Rothman, "Percutaneous absorption," in J. Jadassohn, Ed., *Handbuch der Haut—und Geschlechtskrankheiten,* Suppl. Vol. 3, Springer, Berlin, 1963.

20. A. Szakall, *Berufsdermatosen,* **6,** 171 (1958).

21. I. H. Blank and J. E. Finesinger, *Arch. Neur. Psychiat.,* **56,** 544 (1946).

22. V. H. Witten, M. S. Ross, E. Oshry, and A. B. Hyman, *J. Invest. Dermatol.,* **17,** 311 (1951).

23. R. L. Ferguson and S. D. Silver, *Amer. J. Clin. Pathol.,* **17,** 35 (1947).

24. D. C. Pease, *Amer. J. Anat.,* **89,** 469 (1951).

25. T. Suchi, *Jap. J. Physiol.,* **5,** 75 (1955).

26. R. Edelberg, *J. Exp. Psychol.,* **62,** 187 (1961).

27. A. Szakall, *Arch. Dermatol. Syphil.,* **194,** 376 (1952).

28. A. Belouss, *Pfl. Arch. f. d. ges. Physiol.,* **162,** 507 (1915).

29. R. Edelberg, T. Greiner, and N. R. Burch, *J. Appl. Physiol.,* **15,** 691 (1960).

30. R. E. Nordquist, R. L. Olson, and M. A. Everett, *Arch. Dermatol.,* **94,** 482 (1966).

31. T. Suchi, in Y. Kuno, *Human Perspiration,* Charles C Thomas, Springfield, Ill. 1956, p. 311.

32. C. M. Papa and A. M. Kligman, *J. Invest. Dermatol.,* **49,** 139 (1967).

33. S. Takagi, *Jap. J. Physiol.,* **3,** 65 (1952).

34. I. Schulz, K. J. Ullrich, E. Fromter, H. Holzgreve, A. Frick, and U. Hegel, *Pfl. Arch. f. d. ges. Physiol.,* **284,** 360 (1965).

35. P. Fleisch, S. B. Goldstone, and F. Urbach, *Arch. Dermatol. Syphil.*, **63**, 228 (1951).

36. S. Rothman, *Physiology and Biochemistry of Skin,* University of Chicago Press, Chicago, 1954. Chapter 3.

37. G. M. MacKee, M. B. Sulzberger, F. Herrman, and R. I. Baer, *J. Invest. Dermatol.*, **6**, 43 (1945).

38. J. Nyboer, *Electrical Impedance Plethysmography,* Charles C Thomas, Springfield, Ill., 1959.

39. R. V. Hill, J. C. Jansen, and J. L. Fling, *J. Appl. Physiol.*, **22**, 161 (1967).

40. D. T. Lykken, *Psychophysiology,* **7**, 262 (1970).

41. C. W. Darrow, *Amer. J. Physiol.*, **88**, 219 (1929).

42. M. H. Lader and J. D. Montagu, *J. Neurol. Neurosurg. and Psychiat.*, **25**, 126 (1962).

43. M. Gildemeister, *Pfl. Arch. f. d. ges. Physiol.*, **200**, 278 (1923).

44. W. Nernst and E. H. Risenfeld, *Ann. phys.*, **8**, 600 (1902).

45. L. Michaelis, *J. Gen. Physiol.*, **8**, 33 (1925).

46. M. B. Sulzberger, F. Herrmann, R. Keller, and B. V. Pisha, *J. Invest. Dermatol.*, **14**, 91 (1950).

47. A. C. Allen, *The Skin, a Clinicopathological Treatise,* 2nd Ed., Grune and Stratton, New York, 1967.

48. R. Edelberg, *USAF School of Aerospace Med., Tech. Doc.,* Report 63-95, 1963.

49. W. W. Surwillo, *J. Gerontol.,* **20**, 519 (1965).

50. J. F. Davis, H. S. Morton, and B. Markland, *Proc. Nat. Biophysics Conf.,* **79**, Yale University Press, New Haven, Conn., 1957.

51. R. Wyatt and B. Tursky, *Psychophysiology,* **6**, 133 (1969).

52. P. A. Obrist, *Science,* **139**, 227 (1963).

53. R. Edelberg, *Ann. N.Y. Acad. Sci.,* **148**, 252 (1968).

54. C. W. Darrow, *J. Exp. Psychol.,* **10**, 197 (1927).

55. C. P. Richter, *Amer. J. Physiol.,* **88**, 596 (1929).

56. R. A. McCleary, *Psychol. Bull.,* **47**, 97 (1950).

57. B. Fujimori, *Jap. J. Physiol.,* **5**, 394 (1955).

58. T. Nakayama and K. Takagi, *Jap. J. Physiol.,* **8**, 21 (1958).

59. G. H. Wang, *Amer. J. Phys. Med.,* **36**, 295 (1957).

60. G. H. Wang, *Amer. J. Phys. Med.,* **37**, 35 (1958).

61. R. C. Wilcott and L. J. Hammond, *Psychophysiology,* **2**, 39 (1965).

62. R. Edelberg, *Psychophysiology,* **6**, 527, 1970.

63. U. Ebbecke, *Pfl. Arch. f. d. ges. Physiol.,* **190**, 230 (1921).

64. H. Rein, "Die Elektrophysiologie der Haut," in J. Jadassohn, Ed., *Handbuch der Haut—und Geschlechtskrankeiten,* Vol. **1**, Springer, Berlin, 1929.

65. P. E. Thomas and I. M. Korr, *J. Appl. Physiol.,* **10**, 505 (1957).

66. T. Adams, *J. Appl. Physiol.,* **21**, 1104 (1966).

67. T. Adams and J. A. Vaughan, *J. Appl. Physiol.,* **20**, 980 (1965).

68. T. Adams, *Federation Proc.,* **26**, 446 (1967).

69. R. Höber, *J. Gen. Physiol.*, **30**, 387 (1947).

70. B. A., Shaver Jr., S. W. Brusilow, and R. E. Cooke, *Bull. Johns Hopkins Hosp.*, **116**, 100 (1965).

71. R. Edelberg, *J. Comp. Physiol. Psychol.*, **61**, 28 (1966).

72. R. P. Arthur and W. B. Shelley, *J. Invest. Dermatol.*, **32**, 397 (1959).

73. W. R. Loewenstein, *J. Physiol.*, **132**, 40 (1956).

74. R. C. Wilcott, *Psychophysiology*, **2**, 249 (1966).

75. R. T. Tregear, *Physical Functions of the Skin*, Academic Press, London, 1966.

76. M. Gildemeister, *Pfl. Arch. f. d. ges. Physiol.*, **162**, 489 (1915).

77. K. S. Cole, *Cold Spring Harbor Symp. Quant. Biol.*, **1**, 107 (1933).

78. H. Fricke, *Philos. Mag. J. Sci.*, **14**, 310 (1932).

79. T. Yokota and B. Fujimori, *Jap. J. Physiol.*, **12**, 200 (1962).

80. T. Teorell, *Zeitschr. Electrochem.*, **55**, 460 (1951).

81. D. R. Davis and D. W. Kennard, *Nature*, **193**, 1186 (1962).

82. M. A. Wenger and L. A. Gustafson, "Some Problems in Psychophysiological Research, Part II, in *Physiological correlates of Psychological Disorder*, R. Roessler and N. S. Greenfield, Eds., University of Wisconsin Press, Milwaukee, 1962, p. 100.

83. J. Kryspin, *J. Invest. Dermatol.*, **44**, 227 (1965).

84. J. C. Lawler, M. J. Davis, and E. C. Griffith, *J. Invest. Dermatol.*, **4**,

85. J. F. McClendon, *Science*, **84**, 184 (1936).

86. S. Hozawa, *Pfl. Arch. f. d. ges. Physiol.*, **219**, 141 (1928).

87. D. T. Lykken, R. D. Miller, and R. F. Strahan, *Psychon. Sci.*, **4**, 355 (1966).

88. M. Gildemeister, *Pfl. Arch. f. d. ges. Physiol.*, **219**, 89 (1928).

89. S. Hozawa, *Zeitschr. Biol.*, **92**, 209 (1932).

90. T. W. Forbes, *Amer. J. Physiol.*, **117**, 189 (1936).

91. H. Gerstner and H. Gerbstadt, *Pfl. Arch. f. d. ges. Physiol.*, **252**, 111 (1949).

92. R. Plutchik and H. R. Hirsch, *Science*, **141**, 927 (1963).

93. T. W. Forbes and C. Landis, *J. Gen. Psychol.*, **13**, 188 (1935).

94. K. Takagi and T. Nakayama, *Jap. J. Physiol.*, **9**, 1 (1959).

95. J. F. McClendon and A. Hemingway, *Amer. J. Physiol.*, **94**, 77 (1930).

96. D. T. Lykken, R. D. Miller, and R. F. Strahan, *Psychophysiology*, **5**, 253 (1968).

97. B. M. Shmavonian, L. H. Miller, and S. I. Cohen, *Psychophysiology*, **5**, 119 (1968).

98. J. M. Van der Walk and J. Groen, *Psychosom. Med.*, **12**, 303 (1950).

99. M. L. Sutarman, *J. Physiol.*, **117**, 51 (1952).

100. P. C. B. MacKinnon, *J. Neurol., Neurosurg. and Psychiat.*, **17**, 124 (1954).

101. A. J. Ferreira and W. D. Winter, *Psychosom. Med.*, **27**, 207 (1965).

102. G. E. Burch, A. E. Cohn, and C. Neumann, *Amer. Heart J.*, **23**, 185 (1942).

103. W. Andrew, *Amer. J. Anat.*, **89**, 283 (1951).

104. W. W. Surwillo, *J. Gerontol.*, **21**, 257 (1966).

105. P. H. Venables and I. Martin, *Psychophysiology*, **3,** 302 (1967).

106. J. Botwinick and C. Kornetsky, *J. Gerontology*, **15,** 83 (1960).

107. R. Evans, E. V. Cowdry, and P. E. Neilson, *Anat. Record*, **86,** 545 (1943).

108. J. M. Thuringer and Z. K. Cooper, *Anat. Rec.*, **106,** 89 (1950).

109. B. Shackel, *Amer. J. Psychol.*, **72,** 114 (1959).

110. T. C. Barnes, *Amer. J. Surg.*, **69,** 82 (1945).

111. H. Pinkus, *J. Invest. Dermatol.*, **19,** 431 (1952).

112. L. Gougerot, *Ann. Dermatol. et de Syphilig.*, **7,** 101 (1947).

113. L. Gougerot and N. Marstal, *C. R. Soc. Biol. (Paris)*, **153,** 990 (1959).

114. A. Barnett, *Proc. Soc. Expt. Biol. Med.*, **40,** 697 (1939).

115. A. Barnett, *W. J. Surg.*, **45,** 540 (1937).

16

Dependence of Electrolyte Balance on Growth and Aging of Cells and Tissues

NORMAN R. JOSEPH

University of Illinois, Chicago, Illinois

The connective tissues of the body, including dermis, cartilage, and tendon, form a continuous structural matrix, which supports all the organs and most of the cells in their normal anatomical arrangements. The ensemble of cells, tissues, and fluids forms a physicochemical system that is heterogeneous at all levels—macroscopic, microscopic, and submicroscopic. It includes coexistent structures in many different states of aggregation, liquid, solid, and semisolid. Homogeneous liquids constitute a *milieu intérieur*, consisting of blood plasma, lymph, aqueous humor, synovial fluid, and peritoneal fluid. Other intercellular phases include submicroscopic water-rich phases of the ground substance of connective tissue [1–7]. All liquid and solid phases contain characteristic proteins and other macromolecular substances in soluble or insoluble forms, and as components of various complex physicochemical aggregates. Water and electrolytes are distributed throughout the cellular and extracellular structures, and may be treated as normal components of each kind of phase. Mineral and water balance is based on the laws of thermodynamics, and is governed by phase-rule principles of invariance and constraint [8, 9].

Physiological invariance in any organism requires a physicochemical steady state that implies almost perfect energy and electrolyte balance. The principles of animal ·calorimetry and basal metabolism show that the adult human organism, like all adult mammals, remains in such a state of day-to-day balance. The energy requirement of an adult man in a state of basal metabolism is of the order of 1,500 kcal per day. If this is met by an equal intake of nutrient calories, the body remains in a state of energy balance, and behaves as an almost perfect calorimeter. All the nutrient energy is converted to heat, and none remains to bring about internal changes in the body itself. This connotes that the principles of animal calorimetry and basal metabolism are governed by the First Law of Thermodynamics [10–12]. It signifies an invariant steady state in all cells and tissues; this implies constant chemical composition, constant physicochemical, thermal, and mechanical energy, and a state that approaches perfect electrolyte balance. Electrolyte and energy balance depends on steady states that are maintained by thermodynamic conditions of stability.

In periods of prenatal and postnatal growth and development, the chemical composition of many mammalian cells and tissues may be quite variable [13–16]. Before puberty, such cells may be considered to be univariant. The chemical composition and cellular states of aggregation vary in time, but the variations depend on only one independent variable—the formation and organization of the characteristic set of intracellular macromolecular substances, which determines chemical morphology and the state of intracellular water and electrolytes. In the period of development, the total energy content of the body depends on the growth curve for each individual; constant energy content and chemical composition are attained only with a state of maturity and constant weight. In that state, the organism may behave as a perfect calorimeter, which quantitatively converts nutrient energy to heat.

Physiological homeostasis, in the following treatment, is founded on the principles of thermodynamic stability and invariance, as applied to various kinds of open and closed systems. The state of aggregation of each kind of colloidal matrix is regarded as fundamental in determining physicochemical state. Under invariant physiological conditions, each kind of adult mammalian structure may be assigned a standard state, which is constant under specified conditions. Any state, however, may be physiologically adaptive, and may change under conditions of stress, muscular activity, and neural or hormonal stimulation. The fact that the adaptive responses are biological is not assumed to contradict physicochemical principles, as they are applied to the living organism.

16.1 ORGANISM AND ENVIRONMENT

16.1.1 Open, Closed, and Restricted Systems

All higher organisms inhabit environments that are characteristic for each species. The habitats of terrestrial mammals, for example, are confined to certain ranges of temperature, pressure, and chemical composition of the atmosphere. In both phylogenetic and ontogenetic development, strict limitations apply to the physicochemical states of internal and external environments [17]. Biological adaptations of organism to environment connote not only a fitness of the species for survival, but also a reciprocal "fitness of the environment" [18]. The edaphic and biotic requirements of any species determine the permissible variations of environmental conditions.

All species enter into physicochemical and biological relationships with the environment. Intracellular processes of combustion and respiration, in the case of mammals, require an external source of atmospheric oxygen within the range of pressures and temperatures to which the organism is adapted. Species that exchange heat energy, oxygen, carbon dioxide, nutrients, and waste products are classified as "biological open systems." But the openness of such systems is far from absolute. In all relationships with the environment, the animal organism retains its identity as a closed physicochemical system, with its characteristic anatomy and chemical morphology. Permanent structures and forms of internal energy are maintained. Enduring kinds of relationships with the environment are preserved. Human beings, for example, require air that is relatively free of toxic contaminants, such as carbon monoxide, chlorine, or radioactive gases. Each of us recognizes the importance of pure natural air. This is air of a limited number of degrees of freedom. A homeostatic organism in an environment with a restricted number of degrees of freedom is a physicochemical system with a large number of fixed conditions of state. In many ways it is equivalent to a closed system with fixed internal and external boundaries. In many cases, the surface of the skin or outer integument may be defined as the limiting boundary of the closed system. Energy requirements are met by environmental sources of oxygen and a relatively limited number of nutrient substances. Homeostasis requires simultaneous disposal of metabolic end products and in homoiotherms the control of body temperature.

In view of the specific conditions of constraint that control the interactions of organism and environment, it is necessary to qualify the definition of organisms as "open systems." In all cases, the organism is restricted with respect to the variability of essential internal and external conditions. The application of thermodynamics to biological variability involves the question of homeostasis or control of the *milieu intérieur* of the animal organism [17–19]. Certain distinctions must be made between purely physicochemical modes of control and physiological controls that depend on highly evolved neural and hormonal adaptations. Physicochemical interactions between organism and environment are common to all species. Highly developed physiological responses and adaptations always connote a complicated array of forces that may be integrated by the nervous and endocrine systems. These integrations are most highly developed in mammals and other higher vertebrates.

16.1.2   Application of the Phase Rule

The most general principles that govern the distribution of chemical substances and energy in heterogeneous systems were developed on the basis of thermodynamics by J. W. Gibbs [20]. These principles were applied by L. J. Henderson to mammalian blood [21]. Gibbs' method of reasoning was adapted to the complex equilibrium between blood plasma and the erythrocytes. Under physiological conditions, blood may be treated as a system that alternates cyclically between an arterial and a venous state. Its state is determined by the tensions of oxygen and carbon dioxide, each of which changes as blood travels from lung to the active cells and tissues. Blood samples *in vitro* may be kept in invariant states if they remain in equilibrium with a gas phase at constant tensions of O_2 and CO_2. In the living animal, blood is univariant when the oxygen and carbon dioxide tensions are coordinated both in lungs and in the tissues. Henderson applied the principles of heterogeneous equilibrium to blood that functions as a univariant system, as well as to the limiting state, where it behaves *in vitro* as an invariant closed system. In this methodology, he was influenced by Claude Bernard's ideas regarding the constancy of the *milieu intérieur* [17]. In particular, he was impressed by the respiratory function of blood in transporting maximal quantities of oxygen and carbon dioxide, with minimal fluctuations of the acid-base and electrolyte equilibrium.

Serum proteins, hemoglobin, and electrolytes are treated as constants for a given individual in a normal state. Blood is regarded as a closed system with respect to cells and proteins, and as an open system with respect to transport of oxygen and carbon dioxide. Transport of the gases between lung and active cells is irreversible. On the other hand, transport of inorganic electrolytes between blood plasma, erythrocytes, and other cells and tissues is reversible. The reason for this is that the inorganic ions do not enter into any irreversible reactions in cells or tissues [8, 9]. Unlike carbon dioxide and oxygen, they are neither produced nor consumed by living organisms; this signifies that under conditions of physiological invariance, they are not transported irreversibly. With respect to most inorganic electrolytes and proteins, the cardiovascular system behaves as if it were closed and invariant; with respect to oxygen and carbon dioxide, it behaves as an open system which remains in a steady state. The conditions for invariance of arterial and venous blood require that the rate of irreversible transport of CO_2 from active cells to lung must be the same as the rate of its formation in the cells. At the same time, oxygen must be taken up irreversibly in the lung at the same rate at which it is consumed in active cells. These conditions of irreversible transport of carbon dioxide and oxygen are required to maintain homeostasis. As Henderson demonstrated, an invariant open system may be treated by the same thermodynamic principles that apply to closed heterogeneous systems. Phase-rule principles of variability and invariance apply as well to open as to closed systems, and to systems in which both reversible and irreversible processes operate simultaneously to maintain a steady state.

Absorption of isotonic saline solutions from connective tissue spaces by the blood vessels was studied by Starling [22], who concluded that the process was determined by the osmotic pressure of the serum proteins (about 30 to 40 mm Hg). The direction of flow also depends on capillary pressure, and is therefore reversible. In a normal steady state, the distribution of the physiological ions between connective tissue and blood plasma has generally been regarded as a case of reversible osmotic equilibrium. Since the normal tissue fluid is approximately isotonic with blood, it functions as an extension of the circulating fluid in transporting, under invariant conditions, nutrients and oxygen to metabolizing cells. At the same time, carbon dioxide and other end products are irreversibly removed. The functions of the fluid are supplementary to those of the circulating blood in maintaining a steady state in cells and tissues [9].

Irreversible transport of carbon dioxide and oxygen is a necessary condition for invariant states of cells and connective tissues [8, 9]. Cellular respiration is accompanied by the irreversible formation of carbon dioxide and heat, and by the irreversible consumption of oxygen. Irreversible transport of water also occurs in the form of H_2CO_3. Connective tissue thus functions as a closed system with respect to inorganic electrolytes and its own characteristic fixed-colloidal components, and as an open system with respect to nutrients, oxygen, waste products, and heat. A normal resting state of respiration causes no change of chemical composition, energy, or physicochemical state. The invariant and restricted open system comprised by connective tissue and blood is therefore equivalent thermodynamically to a closed system in which chemical composition, state, and temperature are constant. Starling's concept of osmotic equilibrium between connective tissue and blood plasma, like Henderson's treatment of blood as a physicochemical system, is susceptible to theoretical generalizations that are based on the phase rule.

16.1.3   Definitions of Homeostasis

In the following statement, W. B. Cannon carefully distinguished his conception of physiological homeostasis from simple physicochemical equilibrium. "The constant conditions which are maintained in the body might be termed *equilibria*. That word, however, has come to have fairly exact meaning as applied to relatively simple physicochemical states, in closed systems, where known forces are balanced. The coordinated physiological processes which maintain most of the steady states in the organism are so complex and so peculiar to living beings—involving, as they may, the brain and nerves, the heart, lungs, kidneys, and spleen, all working cooperatively—that I have suggested a special designation for these states, *homeostasis*" [19]. This represents a definite contrast with Henderson's study of blood as a physicochemical system, in which water and electrolyte balance, acid-base equilibrium, and transport of the respiratory gases are treated as coordinated equilibria involving plasma and erythrocytes, as well as connective tissue and lung. The equilibria apply not only to blood treated as a closed system *in vitro*, but also to the varying physicochemical states represented by arterial, venous, and capillary blood.

In the general physiology of blood, neural and hormonal controls of homeostasis are evoked. These operate, as Cannon observed, on the heart, lungs, kidneys, and spleen. Cannon has also shown that the system of coordinated higher physiological controls is called into play in adaptations to situations involving "pain, hunger, fear, and rage" [23]. In mammals these are recognizable emotional states. In the normal resting organism, when it is possible to eliminate emotional stimuli, the neural and hormonal responses may approximate a neutral condition. This approaches what we have defined as the "physiological standard state," in which the *milieu intérieur* and the various aggregations of cells and connective tissues are as nearly as possible in states of constant chemical composition and temperature [8, 9, 24–29]. Although, in this state, heart, lungs, and kidneys cooperate to maintain homeostasis, they do so by the coordination of a steady play of *constant* neural and hormonal stimulation. The adaptive responses to extreme emotional stimuli such as fear and rage are not evoked.

In the physiological standard state, the prevailing states of body fluids, cells, and the colloidal *substratum* of extracellular aggregates remain constant. The states depend on the equilibrium that is maintained in a system of constant composition, temperature, and respiratory rates. The colloidal matrix behaves as an open system with respect to carbon dioxide, oxygen, nutrients, waste products, and heat. With respect to inorganic electrolytes and fixed macromolecular components, it behaves as a closed system. A constant interplay of neural and hormonal stimuli is imposed on coordinating organs and tissues, to maintain normal electrolyte balance. Nerves and endocrine glands, themselves, are cellular structures, for which standard states require definition. For a given kind of nerve or gland, the standard state could be defined as that which tends to maintain the physiological standard state in the cells and tissues that are under control. Thus in the final analysis, homeostasis depends on a coordinated system of stimuli and responses both physiological and physicochemical. Constant neural and hormonal stimuli result in constant physiological states. Changes of physiological stimuli would then produce specific responses in cells, tissues and the *milieu intérieur*.

In the standard state, carbon dioxide and heat are formed at constant rates from a steady input of nutrients and oxygen. The condition for invariance connotes quantitative conversion of heat energy, which is transported to the environment. No energy is available for internal changes that are not converted to heat. Homeostasis depends on a perfect balance between nutrient energy and metabolic heat. This implies the property of perfect calorimetry and constant internal energy of cells and tissues.

Homeostasis is here defined as a self-identity. It is a class of states that do not vary in time. This identifies it with the properties of the *milieu intérieur* which are invariant with respect to ontogenetic and phylogenetic development [8, 9, 29]. The most constant of these properties are the chemical potentials of water and electrolytes in mammalian blood at any period of life. Constant chemical potentials imply constant composition and freezing points of blood plasma.

16.2   THERMODYNAMICS OF CELLS AND TISSUES

16.2.1   The Chemical Potential

Among the most important thermodynamic functions introduced by Gibbs into the theory of heterogeneous equilibrium is the "potential" of a chemical substance [20]. Conforming to more recent usage, it is now called the "chemical potential." It is closely related to many other thermodynamic functions, and it plays an important role in all derivations related to the phase rule. In biological systems the distribution of electrolytes and water in cells, tissues, and blood depends on the chemical potentials of the ions in various phases. Since electrical potentials in cells and tissues are also correlated with the chemical potentials, they are directly related to the ion distributions [8, 9, 25–29].

Gibbs defined the potential in the following way [Ref. 20, p. 93]. "*Definition*—If to any homogeneous mass we suppose an infinitesimal quantity of any substance to be added, the mass remaining homogeneous and its entropy and volume remaining unchanged, the increase of the energy of the mass divided by the quantity of the substance added is the *potential* for that substance in the mass considered." In modern notation, energy is denoted as E and entropy as S. The chemical potential is denoted as μ, enthalpy as H, Helmholtz free energy as A, and Gibbs free energy as G. These are related by the following definitions:

$$H = E + PV \tag{1a}$$
$$A = E - TS \tag{1b}$$

and

$$G = H - TS \tag{1c}$$

where P, V, and T denote respectively pressure, volume, and absolute temperature.

Commenting on his definition of μ, Gibbs continued: ". . . we may evidently substitute for entropy, volume, and energy, respectively either temperature, volume, and the function A; or entropy, pressure, and the function H; or temperature, pressure, and the function G." Here I have substituted the modern symbols A, H, and G for the rather obsolete Greek symbols used by Gibbs.

In his equation, Gibbs stated the generalized formulation of μ_1 for the substance 1 in relation to E, A, H, and G.

$$\mu_1 = \left(\frac{dE}{dm_1}\right)_{S,V} = \left(\frac{dA}{dm_1}\right)_{T,V} = \left(\frac{dH}{dm_1}\right)_{S,P} = \left(\frac{dG}{dm_1}\right)_{T,P} \tag{2}$$

When μ_1 is expressed as a function of m_1, two other parameters are held constant; these pairs are represented by (S, V), (T, V), (S, P), and (T, P). A system in which entropy and volume are held constant is *closed*. The condition of constant entropy permits no heat energy to cross the boundary. The condition of constant volume signifies that no mechanical work of expansion or contraction is possible. Thus the conditions of constant entropy and volume forbid any exchange of heat or mechanical energy with the environment. There are similar conditions of constraint that apply to A and H. The condition of constant entropy closes a system with respect to heat exchanges, while constant volume closes it with respect to mechanical work. Only when μ is defined in relation to E are the conditions those of a completely closed or isolated system. The Gibbs free energy G is unique in that it applies to systems at constant temperature and pressure. Such systems are open both with respect to entropy changes, ΔS, and volume changes, ΔV. When water is converted to steam at 100°C and 1 atmosphere pressure, the free-energy change, ΔG, is zero. It is related to $P\Delta V$ and $T\Delta S$ by the equation,

$$\Delta G = \Delta E + P\Delta V - T\Delta S \tag{3}$$

This is a two-phase equilibrium between liquid and vapor. ΔH (or $\Delta E + P\,\Delta V$) represents the molal enthalpy of vaporization (about 9700 cal), and ΔS is the entropy of vaporization (26.0 cal mole^{-1} deg^{-1}).

In the open system, ΔE, ΔH, and ΔS are positive quantities because of increases of energy, volume, and entropy. However, ΔG is zero for a reversible two-phase equilibrium under conditions of constant temperature and pressure. The reversible equilibrium can also be expressed in relation to the chemical potential of water. Thus:

$$\mu'_{H_2O} = \mu''_{H_2O} \tag{4a}$$
$$\text{or} \qquad \Delta\mu_{H_2O} = 0 \tag{4b}$$

where μ' refers to the liquid, and μ'' refers to the vapor phase. Equation 4a was given general form as Gibbs' Equation 77 [20]. Although these equations hold for any of the kinds of systems referred to in Equations 2, the usual phase-rule conditions apply to systems at constant temperature and pressure. The general criteria of equilibrium are usually expressed in relation to G in open systems at constant temperature and pressure. Such systems are free to exchange heat and chemical substances with the surroundings, under certain fixed conditions of invariance or constraint. They are also free to undergo changes of volume, but these are usually small in "condensed systems," that is, liquids and solids.

Many biologists have hesitated to apply thermodynamics to living cells and tissues. This was not true in the period from Helmholtz to Rubner or Atwater, when the First Law was applied to animal calorimetry and basal metabolism [10–12]. These studies referred to the relationships between nutrient energy, metabolic heat, and external work. Second Law principles, relating to electrolyte distribution and phase equilibrium in the animal organism, seem not to have developed to a comparable extent. The prevailing explanations have tended to be mechanical, and cannot be related to the Second Law or to the phase rule. In fact, it has been shown that current explanations are incompatible with both the First and Second Laws, and with the principles of animal calorimetry [8, 9, 27].

The theory of active transport, for example, relies on various hypotheses of ion pumps, carriers, and other kinds of "transport mechanisms." It has been shown that such entities, even if existent, can do no irreversible work in an invariant system at constant temperature and composition. Performance of actual work, as postulated, would result in physicochemical changes that contradict the principles of homeostasis and invariant steady states. It is required by phase rule and by Carnot's principle that reversible processes in invariant systems involve no expenditure of energy or work. Electrolytic balance is independent of mechanisms [8, 9, 16, 27, 29].

Many authors have thought that the increase of entropy formulated by the Second Law applies only to the entire Universe, or to closed isolated systems. Biological "open systems" have been considered to present exceptions, not accessible to thermodynamic reasoning. It has often been overlooked that in physical chemistry, the phase rule is usually applied to open systems rather than to closed or isolated systems. The most familiar applications refer to descriptions of pressure-temperature curves of liquids and vapors, solubility or miscibility relationships between two liquids, solubilities of solids in liquids, or freezing-point diagrams of various systems. These relationships are generally studied under conditions of varying energy, entropy, and composition in open systems. To limit the phase rule to closed systems is to restrict the number of degrees of freedom to zero.

It is true that in the earlier pages of his treatise, Gibbs developed equations for closed systems at constant energy and entropy. However, in Equation 87, he introduced the function A, and defined H and G in Equations 89 and 91. In Equations 99 to 103, he showed the equivalence of five different kinds of fundamental equations, only one of which refers to a closed system (Equation 99). Equations 99 to 103 represent the fundamental equations in the general form; these impose no limitations on the phase rule. The chemical potential as defined for any system was expressed in Equation 104, and applies to all the possible kinds of closed and open systems (see Equation 2, above).

16.2.2   Phases and Degrees of Freedom*

In any phase of a physicochemical system, the Gibbs free energy G is related to T, P, and the composition in the following way (Gibbs' Equation 92):

$$dG = -S\,dT + V\,dP + \Sigma\mu_1\,dm_1 \qquad (5)$$

where the summation is made over n independently variable chemical substances. When T and P are constant:

$$dG = \Sigma\mu_1\,dm_1 \qquad (6)$$

The phase rule follows from these equations. The system exists in two or more phases if the chemical potentials μ_1, μ_2 . . . μ_n have constant values:

$$\mu_1' = \mu_1'' \cdots = \mu_1{}^p$$
$$\cdots\cdots\cdots\cdots$$
$$\mu_n' = \mu_n'' \cdots = \mu_n{}^p \qquad (7)$$

* A general treatment of the phase rule applicable to developing cells and tissues has been given in Chapter VI of *Physical Chemistry of Aging*, H. T. Blumenthal, Ed., Karger, Basel, New York (1971).

If p different phases are ordered in this way, there are $n(p-1)$ independent equations of this form. However, there are $(n-1)$ variable concentrations $(c_1 \ldots c_{n-1})$ of the n masses in each phase. Therefore, the total number of variable concentrations is $p(n-1)$. At constant temperature and pressure, the number of independent variables, or arbitrary parameters, is

$$p(n-1) - n(p-1) = n - p$$

If temperature and pressure are variable, there are 2 additional degrees of freedom. The total number of degrees of freedom f is given by:

$$f = n + 2 - p \qquad (8)$$

If f is zero, the system is invariant, and the composition of each phase is independent of time. If f is 1, the system has one degree of freedom, and the composition of one or more of the phases is then a function of one independently variable parameter. A biological system, for example, may have one degree of freedom if in the development of a certain kind of cell or tissue, the state of a phase is determined by the synthesis of its characteristic colloids. Physicochemical state can then be expressed by relating any one of the dependent variables (c_1, $c_2 \ldots$) to the formation of the independent variable, c_k. This would be of the nature of a growth curve, in which the state of the phase is a function of time. Such a system has one degree of freedom. This is characteristic of simple types of growth curves [8, 9].

16.2.3 Electrolyte Balance

Two main types of inorganic electrolytes are treated: those that are transported reversibly between two invariant phases, and those that are transported irreversibly. The first group includes NaCl, KCl, $CaCl_2$, and $MgCl_2$. These comprise four cations and one kind of anion, and are denoted as the inorganic physiological ions. They are of environmental origin, and are neither produced nor consumed in cells or tissues. They are of practically universal occurrence in mammalian structures. The second kind of electrolyte may be produced intracellularly in metabolic processes, and is of cellular origin. However, extracellular or environmental origins are not excluded. The example to be treated in the following is CO_2 (or H_2CO_3), which are produced in respiration. The conditions for reversible equilibrium of the physiological electrolytes between blood plasma (phase 1) and a cellular or tissue phase (phase

2) are as follows:

$$\mu'_{NaCl} = \mu''_{NaCl}; \quad \mu'_{KCl} = \mu''_{KCl}; \quad \mu'_{CaCl_2} = \mu''_{CaCl_2}; \quad \mu'_{MgCl_2} = \mu''_{MgCl_2} \quad (9)$$

These equations represent the phase-rule conditions for invariance (Equation 8). For a binary electrolyte such as NaCl, the value of μ_{NaCl} is equal to the sum of μ_{Na} and μ_{Cl}. It follows that:

$$\mu''_{Na} - \mu'_{Na} = \mu'_{Cl} - \mu''_{Cl}$$

and that:

$$\Delta\mu_{Na} = -\Delta\mu_{Cl} \quad (10)$$

where $\Delta\mu$ denotes the change of chemical potential between two phases. Similar conditions of stability apply to the other ions in states of reversible equilibrium:

$$\Delta\mu_{Na} = \Delta\mu_{K} = \frac{1}{2}\Delta\mu_{Ca} = \frac{1}{2}\Delta\mu_{Mg} = -\Delta\mu_{Cl} = \delta \quad (11)$$

where δ is defined as the equivalent change of chemical potential of each of the five ions. It depends on the standard physicochemical state of phase 2, and is a function of age, growth and development, when the state of phase 1 is constant. When the value of δ is fixed, the system is invariant. Otherwise, the number of degrees of freedom f is determined by the number of independent variables necessary to establish δ, when the state of phase 1 is fixed.

In respiratory metabolism, CO_2 is produced continuously and irreversibly. The condition for intracellular and extracellular invariance is that it must be transported at the same rate to blood, and expired from the lung [8, 9]. This distinguishes the bicarbonate ion from sodium, potassium, and chloride, which are not transported irreversibly when cells are in the invariant standard state. The condition for irreversible transport of H_2CO_3 in the standard state is

$$\mu'_{H_2CO_3} \leq \mu''_{H_2CO_3} \quad (12)$$

In the limit, for very low rates of respiration, the equality sign is applied. Then:

$$\Delta\mu_{H_2CO_3} = 0 \quad (13)$$

and

$$\Delta\mu_{HCO_3} = \Delta\mu_{Cl} = -\delta \quad (14)$$

In general Equations 9, 10 and 11 are the conditions of maximal stability of ion distributions in homeostasis. Equation 12 is the condition for a steady state of CO_2 distribution and transport in the normal invariant state. In a state of perfect invariance, the intracellular and extracellular concentrations of the metabolite would remain constant.

16:2.4   Water Balance

The condition for perfectly reversible water balance between blood plasma and an intracellular or extracellular phase is:

$$\mu'_{H_2O} = \mu''_{H_2O} \tag{15}$$

This is similar to Equation 4a, which was applied to the equilibrium between water and steam at constant temperature and pressure. It is thus a general condition for water balance in any heterogeneous system. The value of μ_{H_2O} is independent of the physicochemical state of water in either phase. Thus Equations 4 and 15 are applicable to phases in which water may coexist in any possible states; there are no restrictions constraining the equilibrium to any particular kinds of phases. The condition of phase-rule invariance is in its most general form. The classical Donnan equilibrium applies to water as a solvent in the liquid state [30]. In biological systems, however, water is not necessarily limited to that form of existence. When intracellular water is structured to form an integral part of the cell, its physicochemical behavior is different from that of pure liquid water [8, 9, 29, 31, 32]. It is in a different state of aggregation, and its functions as a solvent or dispersion medium are altered.

The chemical potential of water is related to the chemical potentials and concentrations of all chemical substances in a state of solution. The relationship is given by Gibbs' Equation 97:

$$-S\,dT + V\,dP = \Sigma m_1\,d\mu_1 \tag{16}$$

where the summation is taken over all substances. In an aqueous electrolyte solution at constant temperature and pressure:

$$-m_{H_2O}\,d\mu_{H_2O} = \Sigma m_i\,d\mu_i \tag{17}$$

where μ_i is the chemical potential of the ith species of ion, and m_i is the mass expressed as moles. The mass of water in moles is expressed as m_{H_2O}. Expressing the relationship with respect to ion concentrations in moles per kg water:

$$-d\mu_{H_2O} = 0.018\Sigma c_i\,d\mu_i \tag{18}$$

where c_i denotes the concentration of the ith kind of ion, and 0.018 is the molecular weight of water divided by 1000.

In any phase, the chemical potential of water is related to the concentrations and potentials of all the dissolved ions. For a two-phase invariant system that contains the five physiological ions and water, there are six independent conditions of stability. These include four equations among the five ions (Equations 11, which define δ). In addition, δ must satisfy Equations 15 and 17. The state of the system, if univariant, is then determined by δ. There is an additional condition (Equation 12) that refers to the state of H_2CO_3. In an invariant standard state of constant respiration, $\mu''_{H_2CO_3}$ would be a constant that depends on the state of each kind of cell or tissue. If that state depends on growth, aging, or development, the standard value of δ would depend on the composition and state of intracellular and extracellular colloids. The system would be univariant if the state at any time conforms to a univariant growth curve.

16.2.5   Reversible Electromotive Force

The equivalent change of chemical potential, δ, represents a force function that tends to drive inorganic cations from a cellular or tissue phase (phase 2) to blood plasma (phase 1). It connotes an "escaping tendency" for cations, and is measured in energy units (cal or joules per equiv). According to Equation 11, it also represents the escaping tendency of chloride ions from phase 1 to phase 2. The four equations among the five ions are conditions for a univariant system, when δ is a function of time, as in growth and aging. All processes of ion diffusion, exchange, or transport between two phases are restricted by these conditions of invariance or constraint, which are necessary to maintain an invariant steady state (homeostasis) at any point of the normal growth curve. At a boundary between two phases in the standard state, the electromotive force is denoted as E. Its value must satisfy the conditions for reversible transport of the two physiological ions in the standard state (Equation 11). Then the force function, or diffusion tendency, of the five ions is exactly balanced by E, which operates to prevent irreversible changes of concentration. These conditions are satisfied by Gibbs' Equations 687 and 688. In the present terminology:

$$FE + \delta = 0 \qquad (19)$$

where F is the Faraday constant (96,500 joules or 23,060 cal volt^{-1}). Here E and δ are constants that are characteristic of the standard state. The sum $(FE + \delta)$ represents the reversible work of transport for any ion or combination of ions; it is zero in homeostasis. This is in accordance with Carnot's principle, which requires the work yielded in an isothermal reversible process to be zero in an invariant system [27]. The stability and invariance of E and δ are predicated in Equation 11. At a phase boundary with unconstrained diffusion of the ions, Equations 7 and 11 would not hold; the system then acquires four degrees of freedom. It would then be impossible to maintain constant ion concentrations and potentials.

The conditions of homeostasis and invariance also require irreversible diffusion of CO_2 and H_2CO_3. According to Equations 12–14, this connotes that $\Delta\mu_H$ is positive with respect to $\Delta\mu_{Na}$, and that $\Delta\mu_{HCO_3}$ is positive with respect to $\Delta\mu_{Cl}$. Therefore:

$$FE + \Delta\mu_H \geq 0$$

and

$$FE - \Delta\mu_{HCO_3} \leq 0 \tag{20}$$

It follows that H_2CO_3 diffuses spontaneously and irreversibly from active cells under conditions that restrict the other ions to reversible diffusion [9].

The chemical potential of sodium ions is related to the concentration in any phase by the equation:

$$\mu_{Na} = \mu_{Na}{}^0 + RT \ln c_{Na} f_{Na} \tag{21}$$

where $\mu_{Na}{}^0$ is the standard chemical potential and f_{Na} is the activity coefficient. The value of $\mu_{Na}{}^0$ is related to the dielectric properties of the solvent or dispersion medium, while the value of f_{Na} is defined by means of a reference state. In ordinary salt solutions, this is always taken as infinite dilution, where f for any ion becomes 1.0. At any other concentration, the value depends on the ionic strength of the solution. In biological solutions, however, the reference state can only be the normal physiological standard state, where the ionic strength in any phase is a characteristic constant. In this state, f for all ions may be assigned the value of 1.0. All cells and tissues of the body are thus treated as restricted systems with a limited range of possible variations. They are not treated as true solutions or unrestricted systems, with a large number of possible degrees of freedom. All ion concentrations are confined within narrow limits. The value of μ^0 in any phase is thus a constant, which depends on the dielectric properties and interionic forces. In a change of standard chemical potential between any two phases, the predominant term is usually that produced by the change of dielectric constant; the effect due to a change of ionic strength is generally of a smaller order of magnitude [9].

When f is assigned the value of 1.0, the value of $\Delta\mu_{Na}$ becomes:

$$\Delta\mu_{Na} = \Delta\mu_{Na}{}^0 + RT \ln \frac{c''_{Na}}{c'_{Na}} \tag{22}$$

where c'_{Na} is the concentration in blood plasma, and where c''_{Na} refers to a cellular or tissue phase. These values refer to free or unbound ions. In the case of sodium, this is assumed to represent the total, implying complete ionization [8, 9, 16, 29]. According to Equation 19:

$$\Delta\mu_{Na} = -FE \tag{23}$$

When the values of c''_{Na} and c'_{Na} are known, the value of $\Delta\mu_{Na}^0$ can be calculated from an observed value of E. In connective tissue, calculated values of $\Delta\mu_{Na}^0$ have been found to be of the order of ± 0.2 kcal [9, 28, 29]. In adult cellular phases, values of the order of 2 to 3 kcal have been estimated.

The high intracellular values of $\Delta\mu_{Na}^0$ are mainly determined by low values of the intracellular dielectric constant. From the Born theory of ion-hydration energy, the following relationship has been derived:

$$\Delta\mu_i^0 = \frac{164z_i^2}{b_i}\left(\frac{1}{D''} - \frac{1}{80}\right) \tag{24}$$

where $\Delta\mu_i^0$ refers to an inorganic ion of radius b_i and charge z_i [34, 35]. The change of standard chemical potential is that between an intracellular or extracellular phase of dielectric constant D'' and an aqueous phase (blood plasma) of dielectric constant 80. This is the value for pure liquid water rather than that of the physiological fluid containing proteins and salts. It will be shown later that it also applies to various body fluids and to blood dialysates. The values of z_i^2/b_i for the various ions are as follows: Cl, 0.44; K, 0.6; Na, 0.8; Ca, 3.0; and Mg, 4.1 [16, 29]. These are expressed as reciprocal Angstrom units. The values of b_i were estimated by Laidler and Pegis [35] from the crystallographic results of Goldschmidt [36].

16.2.6   Standard Free Energies of Ion Distribution

The following relationship is applicable to any of the five ionic species:

$$\Delta\mu_i = \Delta\mu_i^0 + RT\ln\frac{c''_i}{c'_i} \tag{25}$$

where $\Delta\mu_i^0$ is determined by z_i, b_i, and D'', as shown in Equation 24. In general, the concentration of free ions, c''_i, is related to the total concentration, $(c_i)''$, by an ionization constant, α''_i, which measures the ratio of c''_i to $(c_i)''$. Hence:

$$\Delta\mu_i = \Delta\mu_i^0 + RT\ln\frac{\alpha''_i}{\alpha'_i} + RT\ln\frac{(c_i)''}{(c_i)'} \tag{26}$$

The quantity $(\Delta\mu_i^0)'$ is defined by the relationship:

$$(\Delta\mu_i^0)' = \Delta\mu_i^0 + RT \ln \frac{\alpha_i''}{\alpha_i'} \tag{27}$$

Then:

$$\Delta\mu_i = (\Delta\mu_i^0)' + RT \ln \frac{(c_i)''}{(c_i)'} \tag{28a}$$

or

$$\Delta\mu_i = (\Delta\mu_i^0)' + RT \ln (r_i) \tag{28b}$$

where $(\Delta\mu_i^0)'$ is the *apparent change of standard chemical potential*. The ion distribution ratio is denoted as (r_i). The values of $\Delta\mu_i$ for the five kinds of ions are related by Equation 11. When these *conditions of maximal stability* are applied:

$$(\Delta G_{K,Na}^0)' = -RT \ln \frac{(r_K)}{(r_{Na})}$$

$$(\Delta G_{\frac{1}{2}Ca,Na}^0)' = -RT \ln \frac{(r_{Ca})^{\frac{1}{2}}}{(r_{Na})}$$

$$(\Delta G_{\frac{1}{2}Mg,Na}^0)' = -RT \ln \frac{(r_{Mg})^{\frac{1}{2}}}{(r_{Na})}$$

and

$$(\Delta G_{Na,Cl}^0)' = -RT \ln (r_{Na})(r_{Cl}) \tag{29}$$

These represent the *apparent standard free energies* of ion distribution. The values may be determined from chemical analysis. The individual values of $(\Delta\mu_i^0)'$ require estimation of the dielectric constant and the ionization constants. Special assumptions regarding the relationships between ionization constants and the standard chemical potentials of the ions are necessary [8, 9].

16.2.7   Calculation of Standard Chemical Potentials from Electrolyte Composition

The total intracellular electrolyte concentration in moles per kg water is denoted as $\Sigma(c_i)''$, and the total in blood plasma is represented as $\Sigma c_i'$. The latter value may be estimated from the freezing point [8, 9]. The chemical potential of water in blood plasma can also be calculated from the freezing point. The relationship is:

$$\mu_{H_2O(s)} - \mu_{H_2O}^0 = 5.26\Delta_s \tag{30}$$

where the freezing point Δ_s is measured in centigrade degrees. The constant 5.26 denotes the entropy of fusion of ice; it is given as calories per mole per degree. The chemical potential of pure liquid water is denoted as $\mu_{H_2O}{}^0$.

If one imagines an aqueous electrolyte solution of the same total molal concentration $\Sigma(c_i)''$ as that of an intracellular phase, its freezing point depression, $\bar{\Delta}$, would differ from Δ_s, because of the difference between $\Sigma(c_i)''$ and $\Sigma c_i'$. There would also be a difference between $\mu_{H_2O(s)}$ and $\bar{\mu}_{H_2O(c)}$, the chemical potential of water in the aqueous solution of total concentration, $\Sigma(c_i)''$. From Equation 30, it is evident that:

$$\mu_{H_2O(s)} - \bar{\mu}_{H_2O(c)} = 5.26(\Delta_s - \bar{\Delta}) \tag{31}$$

By integration of Equation 18:

$$\mu_{H_2O(s)} - \bar{\mu}_{H_2O(c)} = 0.018RT[\Sigma(c_i)'' - \Sigma c_i'] \tag{32}$$

In general, $\Sigma(c_i)''$ for intracellular phases is less than $\Sigma c_i'$ in blood plasma. It follows that the chemical potential of water in blood is less than the value of $\bar{\mu}_{H_2O}$ in an aqueous solution of total concentration $\Sigma(c_i)''$. The condition for equilibrium between blood plasma and an intracellular phase is

$$\mu_{H_2O(s)} = \mu_{H_2O(c)} \tag{33}$$

Therefore,

$$\mu_{H_2O(c)} - \bar{\mu}_{H_2O(c)} = 0.018RT[\Sigma(c_i)'' - \Sigma c_i'] \tag{34}$$

Accordingly, the value of $\mu_{H_2O(c)}$ is generally lower than that of the chemical potential of water in an aqueous eletcrolyte solution of the same composition. The difference depends on the change of *standard* chemical potential of the ions. According to Equation 18, in a system at constant temperature and pressure:

$$-d\mu_{H_2O}'' = 0.018\Sigma c_i'' \, d\mu_i'' \tag{35}$$

For any ion in an intracellular phase, an ionization constant α_i'' is defined in relation to the total concentration, $(c_i)''$:

$$-d\mu_{H_2O}'' = 0.018\Sigma\alpha_i''(c_i)'' \, d\mu_i'' \tag{36}$$

Accordingly,

$$\bar{\mu}_{H_2O(c)} - \mu_{H_2O(c)} = 0.018\int\Sigma\alpha_i''(c_i)'' \, d\mu_i'' \tag{37}$$

Then, from Equation 34,

$$RT[\Sigma c_i' - \Sigma(c_i)''] = \int\Sigma\alpha_i''(c_i)'' \, d\mu_i'' \tag{38}$$

The change of state from the aqueous solution of total concentration $\Sigma(c_i)''$ to an intracellular system of the same total concentration involves changes of dielectric constant and standard chemical potentials. For any ion, the differential $d\mu_i$ depends on a change of $\bar{\mu}_i$ and on a change of standard chemical potential $\mu_i{}^0$. The part of μ_i that depends only on c_i is denoted as $\bar{\mu}_i$. Hehce, for any ion,

$$d\mu_i = d\bar{\mu}_i + d\mu_i{}^0$$

and

$$d\mu_i = RT d \ln \alpha_i'' + RT d \ln (c_i)'' + d\mu_i{}^0 \qquad (39)$$

In the integration of Equation 38, if $(c_i)''$ is treated as a constant for each kind of ion, with α_K'' and α_{Cl}'' depending only on $\mu_K{}^0$ and $\mu_{Cl}{}^0$, the following relationships are obtained:

$$\int \alpha_K''(c_K)'' \, d\mu_K'' + \int \alpha_{Cl}''(c_{Cl})'' \, d\mu_{Cl}'' = 0 \qquad (40)$$

The condition for the two integrals to vanish is that

$$\alpha_K'' = \exp\left(-\frac{\Delta\mu_K{}^0}{RT}\right) \quad \text{and that} \quad \alpha_{Cl}'' = \exp\left(-\frac{\Delta\mu_{Cl}{}^0}{RT}\right) \qquad (41a)*$$

Then:

$$\ln \alpha_K'' = -\frac{\Delta\mu_K{}^0}{RT} \quad \text{and} \quad \ln \alpha_{Cl}'' = -\frac{\Delta\mu_{Cl}{}^0}{RT} \qquad (41b)*$$

Analogous expressions for α_{Ca}'' and α_{Mg}'' are applicable [8, 9]. When the above formulations are applied to the integrals of Equations 38 and 40, it is found for cellular phases that:

$$\Delta\mu_{Na}{}^0 = \frac{RT[\Sigma c_i' - \Sigma(c_i)'']}{c_{Na}''} \qquad (42)$$

Therefore, the value of $\Delta\mu_{Na}{}^0$ can be estimated from the intracellular and extracellular electrolyte concentrations. By means of the Born equation, as modified by Laidler and Pegis [34, 35], it is also possible to estimate the intracellular or extracellular dielectric constant D'' when the value of $\Delta\mu_{Na}{}^0$ is known:

$$D'' = \frac{128}{1.6 + \Delta\mu_{Na}{}^0} \qquad (43)$$

---

* According to Equations 41a and 41b, α_K'' and α_{Cl}'' approach 1.0 as $\Delta\mu_K{}^0$ and $\Delta\mu_{Cl}{}^0$ approach zero. These are conditions for the integrals of Equation 40 to vanish. Actually, α_{Cl}'' approaches 1.0 in connective tissues, where D'' is 70 or higher. On the other hand, α_K'' approaches values of the order of 0.1 to 0.2, and $(\Delta\mu_K{}^0)'$ is about -1.0 to -1.4 kcal [9]. Equations 41a and 41b yield approximate values for α_K'' only when D'' is 50 or less. Under these conditions, the corresponding integral of Equation 40 is of a small order of magnitude.

where 1.6 Kcal is the value of μ_{Na}^0 in blood plasma [8, 9]. It also follows that the reversible electromotive force E may be estimated from the electrolyte composition. In general

$$-FE = \Delta\mu_{Na}^0 + RT \ln \frac{c_{Na}''}{c_{Na}'} \qquad (44)$$

When the intracellular electrolyte composition is known, $\Delta\mu_{Na}^0$ is evaluated by Equation 42. The value of E is calculated from known values of c_{Na}' and c_{Na}''. In connective tissue, both sodium and chloride may be completely ionized. In that case $\Delta\mu_{Na}^0$ is estimated from the formula:

$$\Delta\mu_{Na}^0 = \frac{RT[\Sigma c_i' - \Sigma(c_i)'']}{c_{Na}'' + 0.55c_{Cl}''} \qquad (45)$$

The constant 0.55 denotes the ratio of $\Delta\mu_{Cl}^0$ to $\Delta\mu_{Na}^0$. Hence $\Delta\mu_{Cl}^0$ is equal to $0.55\,\Delta\mu_{Na}^0$. It is also possible to estimate $(\Delta\mu_K^0)$, and $(\Delta\mu_{Cl}^0)$, from the electromotive force. Thus

$$-FE = (\Delta\mu_K^0)' + RT \ln \frac{(c_K)''}{(c_K)'} \qquad (46a)$$

and

$$FE = (\Delta\mu_{Cl}^0)' + RT \ln \frac{(c_{Cl})''}{(c_{Cl})'} \qquad (46b)$$

Similar formulations apply to calcium and magnesium.

16.2.8   Equivalent Weight and Colloidal Charge

Colloids of adult cells are characterized by a negative charge x that is expressed as equivalents per kg cell water [8, 9]. From known values of x, and the weight W of total colloid per kg water, the mean equivalent weight of the colloid may be calculated:

$$\text{Equiv wt} = \frac{W}{x} \qquad (47)$$

For many kinds of adult cellular structures, the mean equivalent wt is of the order of 1800 to 3000 g. This signifies the weight of colloid that is required to yield 1 equivalent of negative charge at physiological pH. For an intracellular phase, the value of x may be estimated from the known electrolyte composition. This is also true of connective tissue phases, for which electrometric methods are also available [3, 9, 37–39]. The negative colloidal charge x is equal to the excess of inorganic cations over anions in a cellular or tissue phase. Thus

$$x + \Sigma(c_i)''z_i = 0 \qquad (48)$$

where z_i, the charge of any inorganic ion, is taken as negative for chloride and other anions. The total ion concentration $(c_i)''$ is expressed as moles per kg water. Then x is estimated as equiv per kg water. The equivalent weight in grams is estimated by Equation 47.

The electrometric method has been applied to the study of the titration curves of a large number of colloidal surfaces, including connective tissue [37, 38, 39], epidermis [40, 41], skeletal muscle [42], and tissue cultures (myocardial and lung cells [43]. The titration curve requires the determination of x as a function of pH between the isoelectric point of the tissue and physiological pH. The electrochemical theory has been described in detail [37, 40, 41]. It involves the study at a given pH of an irreversible EMF at the tissue surface established by the application of a 0.015 M NaCl solution. This is referred to the value of E previously observed with a 0.15 M NaCl solution at the same pH. The following expression is applicable, in general, both to reversible and irreversible phase boundary potentials of this kind:

$$FE + \int \sum \frac{t_i}{z_i} d\mu_i = 0 \qquad (49)$$

where t_i is the transport number of the ith kind of ion, and z_i is the charge. The general formulation, as applied to boundary potentials [44], has been discussed in relation to both irreversible and reversible potentials in cells and tissues [16]. In the limit, for reversible transport of all ions:

$$FE + \frac{\Delta\mu_i}{z_i} = 0 \qquad (50)$$

Reversible transport requires constrained diffusion of all ions. This is fulfilled when the equivalent change of chemical potential, δ, is the same for all ions (Equation 11). Irreversible transport implies an increase in the number of degrees of freedom. In the measurement of the irreversible value of E between a tissue surface and a 0.015 M NaCl solution, the value depends on the fractions of current carried by sodium n_{Na} and chloride n_{Cl} [37–41]. Thus:

$$E_2 - E_1 = 61.7(n_{Na} - n_{Cl}) \qquad (51)$$

where 61.7 mV is the proportionality factor at 37°C, $(E_2 - E_1)$ is the observed displacement of E obtained when the buffered isotonic NaCl solution is replaced by the 0.015 M solution. The difference $(n_{Na} - n_{Cl})$

depends on the density of colloidal charge, x, at the given pH. At low values of x, and at pH levels higher than 3.7, an approximation formula is applicable at 37°C:

$$E_2 - E_1 = -12.3 + 206x \tag{52}$$

At pH levels below 3, the simple linear formulation is corrected [37, 40, 41]. Corrections are also required at high values of x. The determination of x as a function of pH is equivalent to a titration curve of a tissue. It yields information as to the relative numbers and strength of the various dissociable acidic groups in any region of the curve. The curve depends on the nature and numbers of all the groups and on the state of aggregation of the colloidal aggregates.

16.3 ELECTROLYTE BALANCE IN CELLS AND TISSUES

16.3.1 Body Fluids

Interstitial body fluids in equilibrium with blood plasma represent extensions of the *milieu intérieur*. They are of similar compositions with respect to the diffusible electrolyte components. These fluids contain liquid water in similar or identical states of aggregation. If it is assumed that the dielectric constants are also similar or identical, it would follow that the values of $\Delta\mu_i^0$ for the various ions would approach zero (Equation 24). It also follows that the values for the apparent standard free energies of ion distribution would also approach zero. Accordingly, the distribution of ions approaches that of the classical Donnan equilibrium for extracellular phases in liquid states [8, 9, 24–29].

Values of the distribution ratios (r_i) for sodium, potassium, and chloride are given in Table 16.1, with values of $(r_i)^{1/2}$ for calcium and magnesium. By means of the analytical data of Bauer, Ropes, and Waine [45, 46], values of the standard free energies of ion distribution in various fluids of the *milieu intérieur* are compared. Ion-distribution ratios in tissues such as synovial fluid and edema fluid are similar to those of *in vivo* blood dialysates, and yield similar values for the apparent standard free energies. In general, these values are less than 0.2 kcal per equivalent. Of 15 values given in Table 16.1, 5 are between 0.11 and 0.2 kcal; the remaining 10 values are less than 0.10 kcal. Accordingly, these results can be interpreted by the generalization that all values of $(\Delta G^0)'$ tend to approach zero when extracellular phases are in the liquid state of aggregation.

Table 16.1   Electrolyte Balance in Body Fluids[a]

Ion Distribution Ratios and Standard Free Energies	Synovial Fluid	Edema Fluid	In Vivo Dialysate	Ascitic Fluid
(r_{Cl})	1.01	1.03	1.02	1.02
(r_{Na})	0.93	0.97	0.91	0.94
(r_K)	0.75	0.73	0.78	0.94
$(r_{Ca})^{1/2}$	0.83	0.80	0.76	0.84
$(r_{Mg})^{1/2}$	0.88	—	0.66	0.86
$(\Delta G_{K,Na}^0)'$	0.13	0.17	0.09	0.00
$(\Delta G_{1/2Ca,Na}^0)'$	0.07	0.12	0.15	0.10
$(\Delta G_{1/2Mg,Na}^0)'$	0.03	—	0.20	0.05
$(\Delta G_{Na,Cl}^0)'$	0.03	0.00	0.04	0.03

[a] Data of Bauer, Ropes, and Waine and of Ropes and Bauer [45, 46]. Standard free energies in kcal per eq. Calculated by Equations 29.

Extracellular fluids such as the exudate from the hormonally stimulated sexual skin of the rhesus monkey also tend to approach the composition of fluids of the *milieu intérieur* [47]. The values of the chloride-distribution ratio, referred to blood plasma, are of the order of 1.05; these are quite similar to the values given in Table 16.1 for other fluids. Values of this order of magnitude are accounted for by colloidal charge rather than by changes of standard chemical potential and ion binding [8, 9, 16, 24–29].

16.3.2   Solid-phase Connective Tissues

Similar calculations for connective tissues in solid and semisolid states of aggregation are given in Table 16.2. When the values of the apparent standard free energies are compared, they are found to fall within the range of -0.7 to -1.4 kcal per equivalent for potassium-sodium distribution. These values are of a different order of magnitude from the values for body fluids, which are usually less than 0.1 kcal per equivalent. Deviations of the magnitude found in solid or semisolid connective tissues are explained by changes of dielectric properties, standard chemical potentials, and ion-binding [8, 9, 16, 24–29]. Similar deviations are found for $(\Delta G_{1/2Ca,Na}^0)'$ and $(\Delta G_{1/2Mg,Na}^0)'$. Whereas these values are generally of the order of 0.1 kcal or less for body fluids, they may be of the order of -0.5 kcal for tissues such as dermis or cartilage (Table 16.2). Accordingly, the chemical potentials of ions in connective tissue depend strongly on states of aggregation, dielectric constant and ion-binding.

Table 16.2 Apparent Standard Free Energies of Ion Distribution in Connective Tissue[a]

Tissue	K, Na	Na, Cl	$\frac{1}{2}$Ca, Na	$\frac{1}{2}$Mg, Na	Ref.
Dermis					
Dog	−1.3	−0.07	−0.17	−0.46	49
Man	−1.4	0.14	−0.43	−0.40	13
Pig	−1.4	0.03	−0.43	−0.46	13
Rabbit	−1.4	0.04	—	—	50
Cornea					
Ox	−1.0	0.03	0.00	−0.14	51
Tendon					
Rabbit	−1.2	0.00	—	—	52
Rat	−1.0	−0.24	—	—	53
Monkey	−0.9	−0.31	—	—	54
Cartilage					
Dog (art.)	−0.9	−0.35	−0.42	—	55
Dog (cost.)	−1.0	−0.14	−0.35	−0.35	56
Beef trachea	−0.7	0.42	−0.25	−0.28	57
Beef septum	−1.2	0.17	−0.35	−0.25	57

[a] Calculated by Equations 29. Values in kcal per eq.

These properties are reflected by the standard free energies of distribution, the colloidal charge, and the equivalent weight of the colloids. Characteristic values for the apparent standard free energies of electrolyte distribution are of the order of -0.7 to -1.4 kcal for $(\Delta G_{K,Na}^0)'$, 0.4 to -0.4 kcal for $(\Delta G_{Na,Cl}^0)'$, and 0.0 to -0.5 kcal for $(\Delta G_{\frac{1}{2}Ca,Na}^0)'$ and $(\Delta G_{\frac{1}{2}Mg,Na}^0)'$. As is shown in Tables 16.1 and 16.2, these values depend on whether the tissue is in the liquid or solid state. They approach zero for extracellular fluids, but may be of the order of -1.0 to -1.5 kcal in solid or semisolid phases.

16.3.3 Growth and Development of Dermis

A detailed study of the progressive changes of electrolyte, protein, and water composition of human and pig dermis from the fetal period until maturity was described by Widdowson and Dickerson [13]. This was the basis of theoretical calculations of the dielectric properties and equivalent weights of the tissue during growth and development of the pig [9]. Comparative calculations describing electrolyte balance in human skin are given in Table 16.3.

From the 22-week fetus to the adult state, the water content of human

Table 16.3   Development of Human Skin

Observations and Calculations	Fetus	Newborn	3–6 Months	Adult
Water[a]	901	828	675	694
Na	0.1332	0.1052	0.1028	0.1142
K	0.0400	0.0543	0.0648	0.0342
Cl	0.1065	0.0805	0.1071	0.1029
Ca	0.0068	0.0121	0.0168	0.0137
Mg	0.0042	0.0057	0.0110	0.0045
$\Sigma(c_i)''$ (moles)[b]	0.2852	0.2489	0.2886	0.2604
$\Sigma c_i'$	0.306	0.306	0.306	0.306
$\Sigma(c_i)'' z_i$ (equiv)	0.0777	0.0968	0.0883	0.0637
$\Delta\mu_{Na}^0$ (kcal)[c]	0.06	0.23	0.10	0.16
D''[c]	76	70	75	73
$\Delta\mu_{Na}$ (kcal)[c]	0.03	0.06	0.00	0.02
E (mV)[c]	−1.3	−2.6	0.0	−0.9
Equiv wt[c]	1400	2130	5500	7000
Collagen N[d]	2.8	18.6	47.3	65.8

[a] Water in g per kg tissue. Ion concentrations in equiv per kg water [13].
[b] $\Sigma(c_i)''$ and $\Sigma c_i'$ in moles per kg water.
[c] $\Delta\mu_{Na}^0$ calculated by Equation 45, D'' calculated by Equation 43. $\Delta\mu_{Na}$, and E calculated by Equations 22 and 44; equivalent weight calculated by Equation 47.
[d] Collagen nitrogen in g per kg water.

dermis decreases from 90.1 to 69.4% on a weight basis. Over the same period, collagen nitrogen increases from 2.8 to 65.8 g per kg tissue water. In these two correlated changes of the growth period, protein synthesis may be regarded as the independent variable. The mean equivalent weight of the tissue colloids increases from 1400 to 7000 g. Calculated values of $\Delta\mu_{Na}^0$ range from 0.06 to 0.23 kcal per equiv; there is no definite correlation with equivalent weight or with the colloidal charge, x, as estimated by Equation 48. Likewise, no definite trend is found in the calculated values of the dielectric constant, D''. These range from 70 to 76, the minimal value being found at the time of birth. The dielectric properties are found to be independent of age, growth, and development. The nature and quantity of the colloidal components, as estimated from collagen nitrogen and mean equivalent weight, show great changes. The increase in equivalent weight is correlated with an increase in the relative proportion of collagen in the tissue. This protein is characterized by its high equivalent weight and by its low colloidal charge at physiological pH [2, 9, 28, 37, 39, 48]. Tissues that are rich in collagen have relatively low capacities to bind sodium and other cations.

From the foregoing results, it is evident that electrolyte balance in dermis is determined by the colloidal charge and mean equivalent weight of the tissue polyelectrolytes rather than by any significant change of the dielectric properties of the tissue water. The system is univariant; the independent variable is the formation and organization of the solid colloidal components. This is a function of time. In the adult period, collagen nitrogen approaches an upper limit, and water content approaches a lower. The system then becomes invariant, with zero degrees of freedom; skin then attains a characteristic adult state of electrolyte and water balance. As for all other tissues or cells, the properties at any time depend on the nature of the growth curve of the entire organism. The value of any cellular or tissue parameter is thus a function of time in a system with one degree of freedom.

16.3.4   Comparison of Connective Tissues

Calculations of electrolyte balance in other connective tissues in the adult state are given in Table 16.4. These include comparative values

Table 16.4   Electrolyte Balance in Connective Tissue

Observations and Calculations	Dog Dermis [49]	Ox Cornea [51]	Dog Cartilage Articular [54]	Costal [55]
Water[a]	708	779	748	700
Na	0.1363	0.1887	0.2714	0.3586
K	0.0318	0.0279	0.0282	0.0493
Cl	0.1224	0.1208	0.0928	0.0556
Ca	0.0042	0.0082	0.1176	0.1166
Mg	0.0042	0.0040	—	0.0494
$\Sigma(c_i)''$ (moles)[b]	0.02989	0.3435	(0.3924)	0.5465
$\Sigma c_i'$	0.309	0.315	0.309	0.309
$\Sigma(c_i)''z_i$ (equiv)	0.0625	0.1080	(0.3244)	0.5183
$\Delta\mu_{Na}^0$ (kcal)[c]	0.03	−0.06	−0.19	−0.35
D''	78	—	—	—
$\Delta\mu_{Na}$ (kcal)[c]	0.01	0.11	0.21	0.21
E (mV)[c]	−0.4	−4.8	−9.2	−9.2
Equiv wt[c]	6,600	2,640	1,040	830

[a] Grams water per kg tissue. Ion concentrations in equiv per kg water.
[b] Total ions in moles per kg water. (Ca and Mg not included in Column 3.)
[c] $\Delta\mu_{Na}^0$ calculated by Equation 45. $\Delta\mu_{Na}$ and E calculated by Equations 22 and 44.

for the following: dog dermis, ox cornea, articular and costal cartilage of the dog. The most striking difference among the tissues is in the sodium content, in the total ion concentration, $\Sigma(c_i)''$, and in the colloidal charge, $\Sigma(c_i^*)''z_i$. Dermis is at the lower level for these parameters. Articular and costal cartilage stand at the upper limit. The sodium content of dog dermis is 136.3 mequiv per kg water; this is similar to the level in blood plasma. On the other hand, costal cartilage contains 358.6 mequiv sodium per kg water, and the value of the colloidal charge is extremely high (518.3 mequiv). The total molal concentration is 546.5 mM per kg water, the highest for any of the tissues. Since this total is much higher than the total in blood plasma, $\Sigma c_i'$, the calculated value of $\Delta\mu_{Na}^0$ is -0.35 kcal. Negative values of this parameter are also found in cornea and articular cartilage. All these tissues are characterized by highly negative colloidal charge, high total concentrations of ions, and low colloidal equivalent weights. In adult dog dermis, the equiv wt is 6,600 g. The values for the other tissues in Table 16.4 range from 830 to 2640 g, and correspond to higher values of the colloidal charge than those found in dermis.

According to Equation 24, negative values of $\Delta\mu_{Na}^0$ connote values of D'' that are higher than 80. However, this is not necessarily true for tissues in which the electrolyte concentrations and colloidal charge are very high. In articular and costal cartilage, the respective values of $\Sigma(c_i)''z_i$ are 324.4 and 518.3 mequiv per kg water. In these tissues, the ionic strength is much higher than in blood plasma, where it is of the order of 0.15 in ion-concentration units.* Accordingly, the interionic attractions is cartilage are of a high order of magnitude. These attractions tend to counteract the effect of a low dielectric constant, which produce positive values of $\Delta\mu_{Na}^0$. Negative deviations occurring in tissues such as cornea and cartilage, are sufficient to counterbalance the effects of a lowered dielectric constant in these tissues. Accordingly, negative values of $\Delta\mu_{Na}^0$ may be attributed to the highly negative colloidal charge, and to the concomitantly high ionic strength. In none of these tissues are

---

* The ionic strength I of an electrolyte solution is defined as one-half the sum of all the ion concentrations c_i (moles per kg water), multiplied by z_i^2:

$$I = \frac{1}{2}\sum c_i z_i^2$$

In ordinary salt solutions, the activity coefficients are lowered by an increase of the ionic strength. This causes negative deviations of the chemical potentials, μ_i. Negative deviations are also caused by ion-binding as measured by α_i'' (Equations 26–28). No attempt is made at present to distinguish the negative deviations at high ionic strength (electrostatic attractions) from the deviations due to ion-binding. Deviations produced by lowered dielectric constants are positive (Equation 24).

highly positive values of $\Delta\mu_{Na}^0$ found. Accordingly lower limits of D'' are estimated as about 70, as is found in mammalian dermis (Tables 16.3 and 16.4).

A general summary of the fundamental parameters is given in Table 16.5. This includes the dielectric properties such as D'' and $\Delta\mu_{Na}^0$. It also includes values of $(\Delta\mu_i^0)'$ for potassium, calcium, magnesium, and chloride, together with equivalent weights. Calculated values of the reversible electromotive force E are also included, as in Tables 16.3 and 16.4. These are estimated from the calculated values of $\Delta\mu_{Na}$ and δ.

Observed values of the reversible electromotive force are given in Table 16.6. These represent experimental results for rabbit dermis, tendon, cornea, and cartilage, and for rat dermis and tendon [9]. The values for the various tissues are small. They range from about 0 or -1 mV in dermis and tendon to about -10 mV for rabbit costal cartilage. The effect of age on these values is small; this is also true of the values calculated in Table 16.3 for human dermis. In general, the magnitudes of the observed values are in agreement with the calculated values for the various kinds of connective tissue that are described in Tables 16.3 to 16.6. The highest value calculated for any connective tissue is -15.0 mV for beef trachea. This is comparable to the lower limit of E calculated for intracellular phases [9].

Values of the negative colloidal charge x in equivalents per kg water, are also given in Table 16.6. These were estimated at pH 7.4 from measurements at the tissue surface when a 0.015 M NaCl solution is placed in contact with the tissue after equilibration with a buffered isotonic NaCl solution. The change of EMF $(E_2 - E_1)$ is a measure of the colloidal charge (Equation 52). Values of x estimated electrometrically are comparable to the values of $\Sigma(c_i)''z_i$ obtained by chemical analysis [9]. For rabbit dermis, the electrometric value is 0.050 equiv per kg water. A value of 0.055 equivalents is estimated from the analytical results of Table 16.4. Comparable values of 0.063 and 0.065 equiv are estimated for human and pig dermis, respectively (Table 16.3 and Ref. 9). A source of error results from the fact that bicarbonate ions are not included in the analytical figures. Their inclusion would lower the analytical figure for $\Sigma(c_i)''z_i$. Another source of error is the inclusion of cellular material in all samples taken for analysis [9, 13]. In costal cartilage, the electrometric value of x is much lower than the value of $\Sigma(c_i)''z_i$ estimated in Table 16.4. In this case, a large fraction of the total cation concentration is probably bound and immobile. Costal cartilage represents an upper limit of all connective tissues with respect to cation concentrations. At such high values of x, a large fraction of sodium, in addition to the other cations, may become bound and im-

Table 16.5 Thermodynamic Properties of Connective Tissues[a]

Tissue	E	D''	Na	K	$(\Delta\mu_i^0)'$ Cl (kcal per mole)	Ca	Mg	Equiv Wt	Ref.
Rabbit tendon	−0.9	76	0.09	−0.67	−0.10	—	—	18000	52
Ox cornea	−4.8	—	−0.06	−1.08	−0.18	0.12	−0.40	2640	51
Human dermis	−0.9	73	0.16	−1.17	−0.02	−0.54	−0.48	7100	13
Pig dermis	−2.2	72	0.17	−1.30	−0.06	−0.52	−0.58	7000	13
Rabbit dermis	−1.3	72	0.17	−1.14	−0.03	—	—	8300	50
Dog dermis	−0.4	78	0.03	−1.16	−0.06	−0.28	−0.86	6600	49
Articular cartilage									
Dog (6–12 weeks)	−8.8	—	−0.19	−0.99	−0.06	−0.70	−0.62	970	55
Dog (21–25 weeks)	−9.2	—	−0.19	−1.00	−0.07	−1.26	—	1040	55
Costal cartilage:									
Dog (3–7 weeks)	−7.9	—	−0.24	−1.44	0.13	−0.64	−1.29	780	56
Dog (22–30 weeks)	−9.2	—	−0.35	−1.19	0.20	−1.40	−1.40	830	56
Beef trachea	−15.0	79	0.01	−0.66	0.41	−0.48	−0.54	1200	57
Beef nasal septum	−9.2	—	−0.04	−1.19	0.19	−0.78	−0.59	1360	57

[a] Calculated as in Tables 16.3 and 16.4.

Table 16.6   Electrical Potentials and Colloidal Charge in
Connective Tissue (9).

Tissue	Resting Potential, E (mV)	Dilution Potential[a] $E_2 - E_1$ (mV)	Colloidal Charge[b] x (equiv per kg water)
Rabbit:			
Dermis			
6–12 months	−0.0	−2.2	0.050
30–32 months	−0.9	−2.0	0.051
Tendon			
6–12 months	−0.1	−6.1	0.032
30–32 months	0.4	−5.0	0.036
Cornea			
6–12 months	−2.2	1.1	0.067
30–32 months	−2.8	1.9	0.072
Costal cartilage			
6–12 months	−9.6	16.8	0.166
30–32 months	−8.3	15.5	0.151
Rat:			
Dermis			
8 days	−1.1	−0.7	0.058
21–24 days	−0.2	−1.0	0.056
6–12 months	−0.5	−2.0	0.051
18–24 months	−0.4	−1.5	0.054
Tendon			
21–24 days	0.0	−2.7	0.048
18–24 months	−0.7	−5.6	0.033

[a] Defined by Equation 51.
[b] Calculated by Equation 52 for dermis, tendon, and cornea. Values for
cartilage calculated by method given for high values of x [37, 38, 40, 41].

mobile. The effect would produce low values of x, as compared with
$\Sigma(c_i)''z_i$. No such limitations are found in applying the electrometric
method to the other connective tissues that are described in Table 16.6.

16.3.5   Comparative Dielectric Properties

The greatest deviations of electrolyte distributions and potentials are
found in cellular structures such as skeletal muscle [8, 9, 16, 24–29].
The magnitudes of the deviations may be measured as apparent standard
free energies of ion distribution (Table 16.7). Four mammalian species
are compared with respect to the values of $(\Delta G_{i,\mathrm{Na}}{}^0)'$ in skeletal muscle,

Table 16.7   Apparent Standard Free Energies of Ion Distribution in Skeletal Muscle[a]

Species	K, Na	½Ca, Na	½Mg, Na	Na, Cl
Man	−3.0	−0.6	−1.6	1.6
Pig	−3.0	−0.5	−1.7	1.8
Rabbit	−3.2	−0.9	−1.6	1.9
Rat	−3.1	−1.0	−1.7	2.0

[a] Calculated by Equations 29, as in Ref. 16 and 29. (Kcal per equiv).

as calculated by Equation 29. The results are representative of ion distributions as calculated for mammalian skeletal muscle, as well as for values found for amphibia and invertebrates. For potassium-sodium distribution, the values are approximately −3 kcal, as compared with values of the order of −0.5 to −1.0 kcal for calcium-sodium, and −1.6 or −1.7 kcal for magnesium-sodium. Values of $(\Delta G_{Na,Cl}{}^{0})'$ range from 1.5 to 2.0 kcal, signifying low values of (r_{Na}) and (r_{Cl}), as referred to blood plasma. The values of $(\Delta G_{i,Na}{}^{0})'$ calculated for skeletal muscle are, in all cases, of a higher order of magnitude than those found in body fluids or other extracellular phases (Tables 16.1 and 16.2). The deviations from the classical laws of "membrane equilibrium" progress in the following order: fluids, solid-phase connective tissue, skeletal muscle, and other cells. This implies a progressive series of deviations from the true liquid state of water.

Calculations of the changes of dielectric properties of skeletal muscle from fetal to adult states are given in Table 16.8. The values of $\Delta\mu_{Na}{}^{0}$ and D'' are calculated by Equations 42 and 43; $\Delta\mu_{Na}$ and E are calculated by Equations 22 and 44. The analytical values for the various ions at different stages of pre- and postnatal development differ markedly from the corresponding values in dermis (Table 16.3). In skeletal muscle, sodium decreases from 111.3 mequiv to 28.7 mequiv per kg water; potassium increases simultaneously from 62.1 mequiv to 134.6 mequiv per kg water. Chloride and calcium also show decreases, as magnesium increases from 12.9 to 25.8 mequiv. The total concentration, $\Sigma(c_i)''$, decreases from 267.1 to 199.8 mmole per kg water. All these values are correlated with the dielectric constant and the standard chemical potentials of the ions. Every parameter is a univariant function of time and of the growth curve of the entire muscle. The primary process is cellular growth, as measured by protein synthesis. Water content decreases from

90.7 to 76.5% over the growth period. As the ratio of protein to water increases, the dielectric constant decreases from about 70 to 30, and the mean colloidal equivalent weight increases from 950 to 1,800 g. All these properties are functions of growth, and the system has one degree of freedom. Growth is the one fundamental mode according to which young organisms are free to change. Other functions such as the chemical potentials of water and electrolytes are restricted by thermodynamic conditions of invariance or constraint [8, 9]. After maturity, muscle cells may be invariant.

A comparison of calculated values of the dielectric constant D'' for various cells and tissues is given in Table 16.9. Results are given for skeletal muscle, heart, liver, brain, kidney, and dermis for two species (man and pig). Values are compared as in Tables 16.3 and 16.8 for fetal, newborn, and adult states. Additional values are given for adult rats at 603 and 988 days of age. The values of D'' are calculated as in Table 16.3 for dermis, and as in Table 16.8 for cellular structures. As the results show, the dielectric properties tend to be specific for each

Table 16.8 Development of Human Skeletal Muscle

Observations and Calculations	Fetus 13–14 Weeks	20–22 Weeks	Newborn	4–7 Months	Adult
Water[a]	907	887	804	785	765
Na	0.1113	0.0677	0.0623	0.0638	0.0287
K	0.0621	0.0638	0.0717	0.1140	0.1346
Cl	0.0842	0.0739	0.0530	0.0452	0.0220
Ca	0.0062	0.0080	0.0053	0.0040	0.0033
Mg	0.0129	0.0118	0.0184	0.0255	0.0258
$\Sigma(c_i)''$ (moles)[b]	0.2671	0.2153	0.1988	0.2372	0.1998
$\Sigma c_i'$	0.306	0.306	0.306	0.306	0.306
$\Sigma(c_i)'' z_i$ (equiv)	0.1083	0.0774	0.1047	0.1621	0.1704
$\Delta\mu_{Na}^0$ (kcal)	0.22	0.8	1.0	0.7	2.4
D''^c	70	53	50	55	32
$\Delta\mu_{Na}$ (kcal)[c]	0.08	0.4	0.7	0.4	1.4
E (mV)[c]	−3.5	−17.6	−30.8	−17.6	−61.6
Equiv wt[c]	950	1550	2330	1700	1800

[a] Water in g per kg tissue; ion concentrations in equiv per kg water. Analytical results of Dickerson and Widdowson [14].

[b] $\Sigma(c_i)''$ and $\Sigma c_i'$ in moles per kg water.

[c] $\Delta\mu_{Na}^0$ calculated by Equation 42, D'' calculated by Equation 43, $\Delta\mu_{Na}$ and E calculated by Equations 22 and 44.

Table 16.9 Dielectric Constants of Cells and Tissues[a]

Species	Skeletal Muscle	Heart	Liver	Brain	Kidney	Dermis
Pig Fetus	64	41	51	55	61	70
Newborn	46	48	41	51	61	74
Adult	26	42	40	58	51	72
Man Fetus	69	45	47	58	56	76
Newborn	51	49	57	58	61	70
Adult	32	51	48	58	67	73
Rat 603 days	30	41	39	53	64	—
988 days	40	40	38	56	67	—

[a] Calculated as in Tables 16.3, 16.4, and 16.8, Refs. 8, 9. Values for rat tissues calculated from results of Lowry et al. [58, 59].

type of structure; they also show specific aging characteristics. In skeletal muscle, the fetal values are of the order of 60 or 70; the adult values decrease to a level of about 30. Levels of D'' in kidney are of the order of 60 at all stages of development. In dermis D'' is 70 or higher at all periods. Lower values of D'' are found in heart, liver and brain; D'' in these structures shows no marked tendency to change with growth, development, or age [8, 9].

The relationship between electrical potentials and ion distributions is shown in Fig. 16.1, in which the properties of adult human dermis are compared with human skeletal muscle at three stages of development: fetal (20–22 weeks), newborn, and adult (Table 16.8). In adult dermis, the calculated value of E is -0.9 mV (Table 16.3), and this is similar to the observed values for adult rats and rabbits (Table 16.6). It is also similar to the value of -1.3 mV calculated for human skin in the fetus. In skeletal muscle, however, the calculated value of E changes from -3.5 mV in the fetus to -61.6 mV in the adult. The respective values of D'' are 70 and 32 (Tables 16.8 and 16.9). In dermis the respective values of D'' are 76 and 73. In Fig. 16.1, the ion distribution ratios are plotted on a logarithmic scale (upper abscissa). This is expressed as $1/z_i$ $\log_{10}(r_i)$. The deviations from the classical Nernst equation are plotted as $(\Delta\mu_i^0)'/z_i$ on the right-hand ordinate. This method of plotting is based on Equations 23, 46a, and 46b, in which the deviations are proportional to $\Delta\mu_{Na}^0$, $(\Delta\mu_K^0)'$, and $(\Delta\mu_{Cl}^0)'$. The magnitudes thus depend on D'' (Equation 24). The values of E in skeletal muscle become very high in the adult state, and the magnitude is largely determined by the high value of $\Delta\mu_{Na}^0$. This depends on the intracellular state of water, as re-

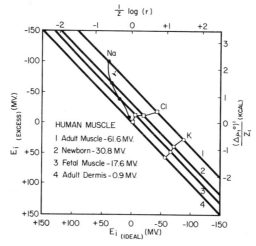

Figure 16.1. Distribution of ions in relation to reversible electromotive force in human skeletal muscle and dermis. Upper abscissa: ion ratios on logarithmic scale. Right hand ordinate: Values of $(\Delta\mu_i{}^{\circ}/z_i)'$ in kcal per equivalent. Left hand ordinate: deviation of EMF from classical Nernst equation (expressed as $E_{i'\text{excess}}$) in mV. Lower abscissa: EMF calculated from classical Nernst equation. Linear relationships are expressed by Equations 44 and 46. From top to bottom: human muscle (adult) -61.6 mV; human muscle (newborn), -30.8 mV; human muscle (fetal), -17.6 mV; human dermis (adult), -0.9 mV; calculated results from Tables 16.3 and 16.8.

flected by D''. In skeletal muscle D'' changes greatly with age (Table 16.9). No corresponding changes occur in dermis. Although the fetal values for dermis and muscle are similar (76 and 70), the adult values diverge widely (73 and 32).

Dielectric properties depend on intracellular or extracellular states of water, which in turn depend on the properties of the heterogeneous colloidal aggregates [8, 9]. Among biological phases, only the fluids of the *milieu intérieur* show dielectric constants of about 80 and standard free energies that approach zero (Table 16.1). The invariant colligative properties of blood plasma and other fluids show no tendency to change or develop with age. These fluids exist always in the same liquid states of aggregation, and are therefore invariant in time.

16.3.6 Acid-base Balance and Colloidal Charge

Acid-base balance in connective tissue, as well as in body fluids and intracellular phases, depends on the binding of hydrogen ions to the colloidal substances. At physiological pH, connective tissues are characterized by the colloidal charge x which can be measured electrometrically. According to the results of Table 16.6, the value for tendon is of the order of 0.03 equiv per kg water. In dermis it is 0.05 to 0.06 equiv, as compared to 0.07 equiv in cornea, and 0.16 equiv in cartilage. Recent measurements of x in the thoracic aorta of chickens range from 0.0617 equiv at two months to 0.0510 equiv at 24 months [60]. The comparable values in abdominal aorta are 0.0435 and 0.0412 equiv per kg water. In subcutaneous connective tissue, the ratio of charge to dry weight is 191 in immature, and 134 in adult chickens, where the ratio is expressed as mequiv per kg dry weight. As calculated from Equation 47, the equivalent weights are 5,200 for immature, and 7,500 for adult chickens. The adult value is similar to that found for various mammals (Table 16.5).

It has been shown that the value of x depends on pH. Exposure of tissue to solutions at pH 6.0 or lower results in a lowering of the negative colloidal charge [37–43]. Estimation of the value of x at a series of pH levels from 7.4 to 2.2 is equivalent to the measurement of a titration curve. The nature of the curve depends on the acid-base binding properties. At any level of pH in a buffered, isotonic saline solution, the hydrogen ions are in equilibrium with the dissociable acid groups of the tissue. As the pH is lowered and the hydrogen ion concentration is increased, the proton-binding groups become neutralized, and the immobile negative charge is decreased. As is shown in Table 16.10, the value of x for

Table 16.10 Titration Curves of Connective Tissue (Negative colloidal charge in equiv per kg water)[a]

pH	Rabbit[b] Tendon	Rabbit[b] Dermis	Guinea Pig[c] Dermis	Guinea Pig[c] Dermis (Scorbutic)	Rabbit[b] Cartilage
7.4	0.035	0.050	0.051	0.045	0.164
6.0	0.034	0.045	0.050	0.043	0.129
4.6	0.030	0.043	0.049	0.042	0.115
3.7	0.023	0.041	0.048	0.041	0.081
2.9	0.016	0.032	0.038	0.033	0.053
2.2	(0.008)	0.003	0.008	(0.005)	0.010

[a] Values in parentheses at pH 2.2 denote positive charge. The isoelectric points are higher than pH 2.2.
[b] Ref. 37.
[c] Ref. 39.

rabbit dermis at pH 7.4 is 0.050 equiv per kg tissue water. As the pH is progressively lowered from 6.0 to 2.2, the charge decreases from 0.045 to 0.003 equiv per kg water. At the isoelectric point of the tissue, the value of x becomes zero by definition. The isoelectric point of rabbit dermis is slightly lower than pH 2.2. A similar curve is found for rabbit tendon, which at every pH level shows a lower value of x than dermis. From pH 7.4 to 2.9, the value in tendon progressively decreases from 0.035 to 0.016 equiv per kg water. The sign of the charge changes in acid solutions. At pH 2.2 the positive charge is 0.008 equiv. The isoelectric point is in the neighborhood of pH 2.5.

Very high values of x are found in cartilage at pH 7.4. The value is of the order of 0.16 equiv, as compared with about 0.13 equiv at pH 6.0. Thus 0.03 equiv of hydrogen ions are bound between pH 7.4 and 6.0. Therefore cartilage is a more effective buffer than either dermis or tendon. This is due to its high content of chondroitin sulfate, which contains a dissociable carboxylic acid group in each disaccharide residue [61, 62]. About half of these groups are dissociable between pH 7.4 and 3.7. The other half occur between pH 3.7 and the isoelectric point, which is lower than pH 2.2.

In Table 16.10 results are also shown for dermis of the guinea pig. At pH 7.4 the value of x is 0.051 equiv per kg water. Between pH 7.4 and 2.2, the value decreases to 0.008 equiv. As in the rat, most of the titrable groups occur between pH 2.9 and 2.2. Normal guinea pigs, as compared with scorbutic animals (deprived of ascorbic acid), show higher values of x. In the scorbutic animals at pH 7.4, x decreases from 0.051 to 0.045 equiv per kg water. All points on the titration curve show changes of similar magnitudes. At pH 2.2 the colloidal charge is positive, and approximately 0.005 equiv per kg water. Acid-base balance as well as water and electrolyte equilibrium change in pathological states of connective tissue. The changes depend on the net colloidal charge and on the nature of the titrable groups. Pathological disorders such as scurvy and pellagra are caused by a lack of one specific dietary factor. Such a deficiency is due to one independent variable. In a state of this kind, there is an increase of one degree of freedom in the state of the tissue.

Changes of acid-base binding are also produced by the addition of many kinds of anions, cations, or uncharged molecules to connective tissue [37, 38, 63, 64, 65]. These include the normal physiological cations (potassium, calcium, and magnesium), as well as anions such as succinate, citrate, and lactate. When these combine with connective tissue or other biological phases, there are marked changes in proton binding. Combination of metabolic acids with ground substance of connective tissue or other biological phases would be an important factor in homeostasis; in active states, a fraction would be retained by connective tissue and withheld from blood.

Analogous binding of hydrogen ions to insoluble proteins such as collagen or keratin has been studied by pH titration curves [48, 66]. The binding of various kinds of anions strongly increases the binding of hydrogen ions to insoluble proteins. Acid-base equilibrium and electrolyte balance are reciprocally related.

16.4   CHEMICAL MORPHOLOGY AND PHYSICOCHEMICAL STATE

16.4.1   Phase-Rule Conditions of Invariance and Constraint

Under conditions of maximal stability in a heterogeneous biological system, the distribution of electrolytes is described by the equivalent change of chemical potential of the ions. When two phases are in the liquid state, electrolyte balance is described by the classical Donnan equilibrium [30, 45, 46]. This is true of the body fluids that are described in Table 16.1. In the classical theory, the dielectric constant of two liquid phases is the same on both sides of a semipermeable membrane. In that case $\Delta\mu_i^0$ is zero for each of the ions, and the standard free energies of ion distribution approach zero [24–27]. The distribution of all ions is then determined by one independent variable, the colloidal charge x which depends on acid-base equilibrium in the system. It is dependent on pH and the titration curve of the soluble protein [21, 66, 67, 68]. In a system that contains five kinds of diffusible ions, there are four thermodynamic conditions of constraint (Equations 11). A fifth equation is given by the condition of electrical neutrality (Equation 48), which establishes the relationship between x and $\Sigma(c_i)''z_i$. There are then five independent equations among six parameters, and the system has one degree of freedom.

When the state of aggregation and dielectric constant of a solid or semisolid phase differ from those of blood plasma, the values of $\Delta\mu^0$ of all the ions deviate from zero, as is shown by Equation 24. In that case, the system acquires an additional degree of freedom. When the electrolyte composition of blood plasma is constant, as in homeostasis, the composition of the second phase depends on two parameters, D'' and x. The dielectric constant describes the properties of water in a solid or semisolid state of aggregation. The colloidal charge depends on the net number of fixed negative charges of the immobile intracellular or extracellular aggregates. If D'' and x could vary independently, the system would be bivariant. However, if there is a fixed relationship between the two parameters, the system would be univariant.

In prenatal and postnatal periods of development, both the dielectric constant and the colloidal charge may vary to different degrees, depending on the nature of the cell or tissue. The mean equivalent weight of the colloid tends to increase with age and growth. It is inversely proportional to the negative colloidal charge and directly proportional to the weight of colloid, when both charge and weight are expressed in relation to the water content of the tissue. In human skeletal muscle, the mean equivalent weight increases from 950 to 1,800 g during the period of growth and development (Table 16.8). Simultaneously, the dielectric constant changes from about 70 in the fetus to 32 in the adult. Since there is no evidence that the two parameters can vary independently, skeletal muscle should be considered to be univariant. In human dermis, the changes during growth are quite different; the fetal dielectric constant is 76; the adult value is 73. In the same period, the colloidal equivalent weight increases from 1,400 to 7,000 g per equiv of negative charge (Table 16.3). This is caused by a large increase of collagen, a protein with a relatively low capacity to bind cations [48]. In general, connective tissues are characterized by high values of the dielectric constant (70 to 80), as is shown in Table 16.5. It should not be assumed, however, that the values of D'' are uniform throughout the tissue. In regions of great heterogeneity, the dielectric constant in certain tissues may be low. When the tissue water is homogeneous and unstructured, the dielectric constant would approach the normal value of water. In regions where water is structured and immiscible, considerable deviations may be possible, especially at heterogeneous phase boundaries [70].

Connective tissues differ greatly with respect to colloidal charge and equivalent weight. In Table 16.5, the values of equivalent weight range from about 800 in cartilage to 18,000 in tendon. Similarly, values of colloidal charge or $\Sigma(c_i)''z_i$ range from about 0.03 to 0.52 equiv per kg water (Tables 16.4 and 16.6). When the value depends on growth and aging, the system is univariant, whether or not the dielectric properties change. Human dermis, for example, is univariant (Table 16.3). The equivalent weight increases from 1,400 to 7,000 g from the fetal to the adult state, as D'' and its correlated properties remain nearly constant. These properties depend on the state of aggregation of tissue water.

16.4.2   Conditions for Intracellular and Extracellular Invariance

With respect to the tendency of muscle to concentrate potassium ions at the expense of sodium, Jacques Loeb [71] gave the following explanation: " . . . the potassium is used for the building up of more complex compounds in which the K cannot be dissociated as a free ion. If a tissue utilizes one kind of metal in this way, for example, K, while another metal, for example, Na, is chiefly used for the formation of dissociable compounds with Na as a free ion, the consequence will be that the ashes of a tissue contain K and Na in altogether different proportions from what they are contained in the surrounding solution. I think we may take it for granted that, at least, K forms a nondissociable constituent of the protoplasm of a number of tissues of animals and plants . . . ."*

Recent estimations of the ionization constants of potassium and sodium in the muscle of a number of mammals, amphibia and invertebrates have yielded values of the order of 0.02 for α_K'' and 1.0 for α_{Na}'', where α'' denotes the ratio of free to total ions [8, 16, 29]. In connective tissue, the value of $(\Delta\mu_K^0)'$ is usually of the order of -1.0 to -1.4 kcal (Table 16.5). Since the dielectric constant is of the order of 70 to 80, the value of α_K'' would vary from about 0.1 to 0.2. This value depends on the dielectric constant (Equations 41, 42, and 43), according to a statistical distribution of energy [8]. The apparent standard free energy of potassium-sodium distribution, $(\Delta G_{K,Na}^0)'$ yields the ratio of (r_K) to (r_{Na}). It depends on the dielectric constant, D'' of the dispersion medium and on the ionization constants. Since α_K'' is also a function of D'', there is only one degree of freedom. Similar considerations apply to the apparent standard free energies of calcium, magnesium, and chloride distribution, as referred to sodium [8, 16, 29].

For a given cell or tissue, D'' is a function of time in the growth period, or a constant in the adult period (Tables 16.3 and 16.8). Loeb's explanation of intracellular potassium accumulation is the "building up of more complex compounds" in which the ion is largely undissociated. This connotes that synthesis of intracellular colloidal substances is the independent variable. Over the period of a century or more, many kinds of intracellular and extracellular colloids have been described. These

---

* The fact that potassium is used in the building up of complex aggregates in plant cells while sodium is excluded to a large extent indicates that macromolecular synthesis (or growth) is the common factor in all electrolyte metabolism. This is emphasized by the fact that plants synthesize cellular and extracellular substances by absorption of photochemical energy, while animals obtain energy only from proteins, carbohydrates, and fats in the diet.

include proteins, nucleic acids, lipids of various kinds, polysaccharides, and complex aggregates that consist of two or more of these. If in any kind of tissue, the complex mixture of macromolecules is of constant composition at any given period, the system would be a univariant function of age or growth. It would depend on a growth curve that is characteristic of the whole organism.

If an intracellular phase is characterized by its composition with respect to a set of n different macromolecular substances, $S_1, S_2 \ldots S_n$, the mixture is univariant when each of the concentrations $C_1, C_2, \ldots C_n$ is a function of time. The system is then characterized by a set of n constant values of the concentrations at any point on the growth curve. In a system of this kind, the values of D'' and x are also univariant functions of state or of time. There is some kind of relationship, however complex, between D'' and x. The coordination of all electrolytes with cellular morphology and state depends on the relationship between dielectric properties and colloidal charge. The electrolyte distribution is invariant when the set of n macromolecules is fixed. In a univariant growth curve, the growth rate at any time depends on the existing morphological state; it is a function of age or weight. Energy balance also depends on the growth rate [72]. A state of perfectly quantitative conversion of nutrient energy to heat occurs only in adult organisms after the end of the growth period. The energy content of the body increases during the growth period, and the distribution of electrolytes changes with the synthesis of the characteristic sets of colloids in cells and tissues.

Univariance signifies that the colloidal composition is determined by a synchronized kind of synthesis, which determines the state as a whole, with reference to both cellular and extracellular morphology. Protoplasm behaves as a unit; this is also true of connective tissue ground substance. Anything that interferes with the synthesis of any of the intracellular or extracellular substances would cause an increase of the number of degrees of freedom f which measures the variability. Such changes may be pathological. In connective tissue, they could be produced by specific nutritional deficiencies, as in scurvy or pellagra. On the other hand, an increase of the degrees of freedom may result from physiological adaptations or from normal responses to hormonal stimulation [3, 63–65, 73]. Normal or adaptive homeostasis depends on the maintenance of a minimal number of degrees of freedom in the physicochemical system.

In addition to the characteristic set of macromolecular substances, any intracellular or extracellular phase is characterized by concentrations of the physiological ions: $(c_{Na})''$, $(c_K)''$, $(c_{Ca})''$, $(c_{Mg})''$, and $(c_{Cl})''$. The invariant set in the *milieu intérieur* establishes constant chemical potentials of the binary and ternary electrolytes (NaCl, KCl, CaCl$_2$, and

$MgCl_2$) throughout a system of p phases. The chemical potentials and standard chemical potentials of each kind of ion are coordinated by the dielectric properties of the dispersion medium, or the structuring of cellular and tissue water. If the macromolecular set $(S_1, S_2, \ldots S_n)$ is invariant in time, then the intracellular and connective tissue composition is invariant with respect to electrolytes and water. The state of a heterogeneous system with 1 or 2 degrees of freedom may be represented by either Cartesian or d'Ocagne nomograms. These have been described for blood [21] and for connective tissue [63–65].

16.4.3   The *milieu intérieur*

While cells and connective tissues may be mainly univariant or invariant with respect to normal growth and aging, blood plasma and body fluids tend to be invariant. The reason is that water in these tissues undergoes no change of state, and the dielectric properties remain constant. Changes of protein content are insufficient to cause measurable changes of colloidal charge or electrolyte balance. The freezing point and the chemical potential of water tend to remain constant. The standard value of μ_{H_2O} in the *milieu intérieur* of mammals is of the order of -3.2 cal per mole. In fresh water or marine invertebrates, however, the values of Δ range from about $-0.1°C$ to $-2.0°C$, depending on the nature of the species [29]. According to Equation 30, the corresponding values of μ_{H_2O} would be -0.526 to -10.52 cal per mole. Lower organisms in aqueous habitats are poikilotherms and are unable to control body temperature. In many species the control of electrolytes in the *milieu intérieur* is also limited; such organisms are poorly adapted to changes in temperature or salinity of the external environment. Higher organisms, which to a great extent, have become independent of the external environment are classed by Claude Bernard as *vie constante;* the lower forms of life are classed as *vie oscillante.* "In the variable state (*vie oscillante*) the living organism is not entirely subordinate to external conditions, yet it is so bound up in them that it is subject to all their variations. In the constant state of existence (*vie constante*) the living organism appears to be free and its manifestations of life seem to be produced by an internal vital principle, free from the restraint of external physicochemical conditions; this appearance is an illusion. On the contrary, it is in the mechanism of an existence characterized by freedom and independence that the close relationship between the organism and external conditions is particularly evident."

"We cannot therefore admit in living organisms a free vital principle which fights against physical conditions. The opposite has been proved

and thus it overthrows all the contrary conceptions of the vitalists"*
[17].

It seems evident that in the case of *vie oscillante,* the number of
degrees of freedom *f* is determined by temperature, pressure, and the
number of variable components in the environment. The internal composition and state of lower forms are not controlled by a "free vital
principle." In Henderson's theory the organism survives because of the
fitness of the environment [18]. Environmental changes of temperature
are known to change growth rates, metabolic rates, and longevity in
poikilotherms. Changes of external salinity also affect growth and metabolism [71]. These facts indicate that in *vie oscillante,* the organism
is affected by many kinds of external variations. No intracellular mechanisms exist which enable it to control its own internal state in the face
of external changes.

In highly evolved forms, the control of the *milieu intérieur* is the
function of lung and kidney, as influenced by neural and hormonal stimuli [19, 21, 73, 75]. Individual cells degenerate to a state of *vie oscillante*
when these functions fail. This corresponds to the fact that pathological
states connote an increase in the number of degrees of freedom [8, 9].
Under these circumstances, the cells of the body possess no internal
mechanisms to resist fluctuations in the internal environment.

Biological solutions must be assumed to have existed on Earth ante-
cedently to the existence of the first living forms [18]. This is implicit
in the idea of environmental fitness. Body fluids in mammals and many
forms of invertebrates and vertebrates are heirlooms from remote
paleozoic waters [75–77]. In most of these species, the characteristic
ratios of ion concentrations tend to remain constant. On a molal basis,
the ratios are roughly: Na/K, 35; Na/Ca, 60; Na/Mg, 100. Thus the
internal saline concentrations of mammalian body fluids, as a first approximation, correspond to dilutions of sea water of the present era.
Most body cells of mammals, amphibians, and marine organisms are
adapted to these ratios [71, 76, 77]. They are also adapted to the chemical potentials of water and electrolytes of the body fluids. In mammals
these properties are phylogenetic and ontogenetic invariants [8, 9, 16,
29]. They undergo only small changes during the life span; the differences among the species are also small. The fluids are invariant in time
because they undergo no changes of state which alter the dielectric
properties.

In cells, tissues, and body fluids, the chemical potentials and standard

---

* Translation in Ref 74. Claude Bernard's principle should be compared with
Carnot's principle that an invariant system can do no work [27].

chemical potentials of the various ions are correlated by thermodynamic conditions of stability and constraint. Chemical morphology and physico-chemical state of each kind of cell or tissue develop in time with the variable sets of macromolecular components. When the *milieu intérieur* is constant, the number of degrees of freedom is determined by the variability of these sets. When, however, the macromolecular sets are fixed, as in the normal adult state, variability is determined by the number of degrees of freedom of the *milieu intérieur*. In perfect homeo-stasis, this number is zero.

REFERENCES

1. I. Gersh and H. R. Catchpole, *Amer. J. Anat.*, **85**, 457 (1949).
2. I. Gersh and H. R. Catchpole, *Persp. Biol. Med.*, **3**, 282 (1960).
3. N. R. Joseph, M. B. Engel, and H. R. Catchpole, *Biochem. Biophys. Acta,* **8**, 575 (1952).
4. W. H. Chase, *AMA Arch. Pathol.*, **67**, 525 (1959).
5. J. B. Dennis, *AMA Arch. Pathol.*, **67**, 533 (1959).
6. W. Bondareff, *Gerontologia*, **1**, 222 (1957).
7. M. B. Engel, N. R. Joseph, D. M. Laskin, and H. R. Catchpole, *Ann. N.Y. Acad. Sci.*, **85**, 309 (1960).
8. N. R. Joseph, *Gerontologia*, **14**, 142 (1968).
9. N. R. Joseph, H. R. Catchpole, and M. B. Engel, *Gerontologia*, **15**, 31 (1969).
10. M. Rubner, *Z. Biol.*, **21**, 250 (1885).
11. W. O. Atwater and F. G. Benedict, *U.S. Dept. Agr. Bull.*, 136 (1903).
12. W. Dampier, *A History of Science*, 4th ed. Cambridge University Press, 1966.
13. E. M. Widdowson and J. W. T. Dickerson, *Biochem. Jr.*, **77**, 30 (1960).
14. J. W. T. Dickerson and E. M. Widdowson, *Biochem. J.*, **74**, 247 (1960).
15. E. M. Widdowson and J. W. T. Dickerson, *Mineral Metabolism*, C. L. Comar and F. Bronner, Eds., Chemical Composition of the Body, Vol. 2A, Academic Press, New York, 1964.
16. N. R. Joseph, *Gerontologia, Basel*, **12**, 155 (1966).
17. C. Bernard, *Leçons sur les Phénomènes de la Vie Communs aux Animaux et aux Vegetaux*, Ballière, Paris, 1878.
18. L. J. Henderson, *The Fitness of the Environment*, Macmillan, New York, 1913.
19. W. B. Cannon, *The Wisdom of the Body*, W. W. Norton Co., New York, 1932.
20. J. W. Gibbs, "On the Equilibrium of Heterogeneous Substances," In *Collected Works*, Vol. 1, Longmans Green, New York, 1928.
21. L. J. Henderson, *Blood. A Study in General Physiology*, Yale University Press, New Haven, 1928.

22. E. H. Starling, *J. Physiol.*, **19**, 312 (1896).

23. W. B. Cannon, *Bodily Changes in Pain, Hunger, Fear and Rage*, D. Appleton Co., New York, 1929.

24. N. R. Joseph, M. B. Engel, and H. R. Catchpole, *Nature*, **191**, 1175 (1961).

25. N. R. Joseph, M. B. Engel, and H. R. Catchpole, *Nature*, **203**, 931 (1964).

26. N. R. Joseph, M. B. Engel, and H. R. Catchpole, *Nature*, **206**, 6 (1965).

27. N. R. Joseph, *Nature*, **209**, 398 (1966).

28. H. R. Catchpole, N. R. Joseph, and M. B. Engel, *Federation Proc.*, **25**, 1124 (1966).

29. N. R. Joseph, *AAAS Symp. on Biology of the Mouth*, P. Person, Ed., Washington, D.C., 1968.

30. F. G. Donnan, *Z. Elektrochem.*, **17**, 572 (1911).

31. J. D. Bernal, *Soc. Expt. Biol. Symp.*, **19**, 17 (1965).

32. I. Klotz, Federation Proc. Suppl., **15**, S24 (1965).

33. G. N. Lewis and M. Randall, *Thermodynamics* K. S. Pitzer and L. Brewer, Eds. McGraw-Hill, New York, 1961.

34. M. Born, *Physik. Z.*, **1**, 45 (1920).

35. K. J. Laidler and C. Pegis, *Proc. Roy. Soc. London*, **A241**, 80 (1957).

36. V. M. Goldschmidt, *Skriften Norske Videnskaps Akad. (Oslo) I. Mat. Natur. Kl.*, **8** (1926).

37. N. R. Joseph, H. R. Catchpole, D. M. Laskin, and M. B. Engel, *Arch. Biochem. Biophys.*, **84**, 224 (1959).

38. M. B. Engel, N. R. Joseph, D. M. Laskin, and H. R. Catchpole, *Amer. J. Physiol.*, **201**, 621 (1961).

39. E. G. Goldin and N. R. Joseph, *AMA Arch. Surg.*, **97**, 753 (1968).

40. N. R. Joseph, R. Molimard, and F. Bourliere, *Gerontologia*, **1**, 18 (1957).

41. N. R. Joseph and M. B. Engel. *Arch. Biochem. Biophys.*, **85**, 209 (1959).

42. M. B. Engel, H. R. Catchpole, and N. R. Joseph, *Science*, **132**, 669 (1960).

43. M. B. Engel, R. W. Pumper, and N. R. Joseph, *Proc. Soc. Expt. Biol. Med.*, **128**, 990 (1968).

44. S. Glasstone, *Introduction to Electrochemistry*, Van Nostrand, New York, 1960.

45. W. Bauer, M. W. Ropes, and H. Waine, *Physiol. Rev.*, **20**, 272 (1940).

46. M. W. Ropes and W. Bauer, *Synovial Fluid Changes in Joint Disease*, Harvard University Press, Cambridge, 1953.

47. A. G. Ogston, J. St. L. Philpot, and S. Zuckerman, *J. Endocrin*, **1**, 231 (1939).

48. K. H. Gustavson, *The Chemistry and Reactivity of Collagen*, Academic Press, New York, 1956.

49. L. Eichelberger, C. W. Eisele, and D. Wertzler, *J. Biol. Chem.*, **151**, 177 (1943).

50. J. F. Manery and A. B. Hastings, *J. Biol. Chem.*, **127**, 657 (1939).

51. F. P. Fischer, *The Cornea*, C. I. Thomas, Ed., C. C. Thomas, Springfield, Ill., 1955.

52. J. R. Manery, I. S. Danielson, and A. B. Hastings, *J. Biol. Chem.*, **124**, 359 (1938).

53. M. R. Levitt, L. B. Turner, A. Y. Sweet, and D. Pandiri, *J. Clin. Invest.*, **35**, 98 (1956).

54. A. Y. Sweet, M. F. Levitt, H. L. Hodes, H. Haber, and B. Kurzman, *J. Clin. Invest.*, **37**, 65 (1958).

55. L. Eichelberger, W. H. Akeson, and M. Roma, *J. Bone and Joint Surg.*, **40A**, 142 (1958).

56. L. Eichelberger and M. Roma, *Amer. J. Physiol.*, **178**, 296 (1954).

57. L. Eichelberger, T. D. Brewer, and M. Roma, *Amer. J. Physiol.*, **166**, 328 (1951).

58. O. H. Lowry, A. B. Hastings, T. Z. Hull, and A. N. Brown, *J. Biol. Chem.*, **143**, 271 (1942).

59. O. H. Lowry, A. B. Hastings, C. M. McCay, and A. N. Brown, *J. Gerontol.*, **1**, 345 (1946).

60. S. P. Porterfield, T. B. Calhoon, and H. S. Weiss, *Amer. J. Physiol.*, **215**, 324 (1968).

61. K. Meyer, "Chondroitin Sulfates," In *Polysaccharides in Biology*, G. F. Springer, Ed., Josiah Macy Jr. Foundation, New York, 1958.

62. M. B. Mathews, *Biology of the Mouth*, AAAS Symp. P. Person, Ed., Washington, D.C., 1968.

63. M. B. Engel, N. R. Joseph, and H. R. Catchpole, *AMA Arch. Pathol.*, **58**, 26 (1954).

64. N. R. Joseph, M. B. Engel, and H. R. Catchpole, *AMA Arch. Pathol.*, **58**, 40 (1954).

65. H. R. Catchpole, N. R. Joseph, and M. B. Engel, *AMA Arch. Pathol.*, **61**, 503 (1956).

66. J. Steinhardt, *Ann. N.Y. Acad. Sci.*, **41**, 287 (1941).

67. J. Loeb, *Proteins and the Theory of Colloidal Behavior*, McGraw-Hill, New York, 1924.

68. E. J. Cohn, *Physiol. Rev.*, **5**, 349 (1925).

69. E. J. Cohn and J. T. Edsall, *Proteins, Amino Acids and Peptides*, Reinhold Publishing Corp., New York, 1943.

70. M. B. Engel and E. Zerlotti, *Amer. J. Anat.*, **120**, 489 (1967).

71. J. Loeb, *The Dynamics of Living Matter*, Columbia University Press, New York, 1906.

72. d'A. W. Thompson, *On Growth and Form*, Macmillan, New York, 1945.

73. H. R. Catchpole, *Federation Proc.* **25**, 1144 (1966).

74. J. F. Fulton, Ed., *Selected Readings in the History of Physiology*, Charles C Thomas, Springfield, Ill., 1930.

75. H. W. Smith, *From Fish to Philosopher*, Little, Brown Co., Boston, 1953.

76. A. B. Macallum, *Proc. Roy. Soc. London*, **B82**, 602 (1910).

77. A. B. Macallum, *Physiol. Rev.*, **6**, 316 (1926).

3. The molecule is not stabilized by intrapolypeptide-chain hydrogen bonds, which are common in protein molecules consisting of a single polypeptide chain, but is stabilized by interpolypeptide-chain (i.e, intrapolypeptide chain, but is stabilized by interpolypeptide-chain (i.e, intramolecular) hydrogen bonds and by the presence of proline and hydroxyproline, which have a limiting ring structure as part of the peptide bond, and lock the chain into a helical structure.

4. The molecular weight of soluble collagen is about 300,000, and its dimensions approximately $2{,}800 \times 15$ Å.

5. The three polypeptide chains of the molecule may all be different in amino acid content (α_1, α_2, and α_3 subunits) or two of the chains may be the same (i.e., two α_1 subunits and one α_2 subunit per molecule).

6. As the collagen molecule matures in the tissue, but still remains soluble, intramolecular (i.e., interchain) and intermolecular (i.e., interchain between chains of different molecules) covalent bonds are formed. These result in β-components (i.e., two covalently bonded α-subunits or chains) and γ-components (i.e., three covalently bonded α-subunits) being formed which can be detected by chromatography, electrophoresis, and ultracentrifugation in the thermally denatured collagen.

7. There is some evidence that the three polypeptide chains of the molecule contain nonhelical appendages of a limited number of amino acid residues (telopeptides), which differ in content and sequence from the typical part of the collagen molecule, and may be involved in stabilizing the molecular and fibril structures of collagen.

17.1.3 Preparation of Neutral-salt soluble and Acid-soluble Collagen

Soluble collagens are normally divided into two classes, namely, those extracted from the collagenous tissue with solutions of sodium chloride (neutral-salt soluble collagen, NSC) and those extracted with acidic solutions of organic acids after prior removal of the NSC (acid-soluble collagen, ASC). Most soluble collagens reported in the literature have been extracted by this basic method, with modifications in the strength of the salt solution, strength and type of organic acid, and repurification procedure, which may produce differences in the properties of the soluble collagen. The age, species, and organ site of the collagenous tissue used for the extraction may also alter the properties of the soluble collagen. In most of the work reported here the results are based on the soluble collagen from calf skin, which is a convenient source for bulk preparation.

A typical extraction procedure would be as follows: The skin of a 2-month-old Jersey bull calf was taken off immediately after slaughter.

17

Irradiation of Soluble Collagen

D. R. COOPER

Leather Industries Research Institute, Rhodes University, Grahamstown, Republic of South Africa

17.1 INTRODUCTION

The action of ultraviolet and γ-irradiation on structural tissue proteins such as collagen, keratin, and myosin is of wide theoretical and practical interest in biophysics, medicine, pathology, and in food, leather, and wool technology. Both forms of irradiation are used for sterilization in such fields as virology and bacteriology, and in the preservation of food for storage. While the prime function of this irradiation is to destroy bacteria, it may also irreversibly alter the properties of the proteins and other constituents of the material being sterilized. Natural ultraviolet light from the sun causes sunburn and irreversible changes in agricultural products such as wool and skin, while artificially-produced ultraviolet light from such industrial sources as welding plants causes skin burn. Further, γ-irradiation is used medically for the treatment of tumors and therefore the effect of this on body proteins in the path of these penetrating rays must be considered. Finally, ionizing radiation is a valuable research tool to facilitate the understanding of the structure of complex proteins and polymers. Radiation caused by charged and uncharged particles and electromagnetic waves has been widely used to determine structural vulnerability to high-energy impingement through bond rupture, free radical formation, cross-linking, decarboxylation, and deamination.

In many of the examples quoted above the material being irradiated by intent, or unintentionally, contains the structural tissue protein collagen. In order to accomplish its structural functions collagen exists mainly as an insoluble, relatively inert matrix of fibrils, for example, in tendon, cartilage, bone, skin, and teeth [1, 2, 3, 4], but is nevertheless in association with soluble forms of collagen [5, 6, 7], the metabolic intermediates produced by the collagen-forming fibroblasts [2]. Being in a soluble, less cross-linked form, this collagen is more susceptible to the action of chemicals, enzymes, and radiation. Therefore a study of the effects of irradiation *in vivo* or *in vitro* must account for both the soluble and insoluble forms of collagen. This chapter is therefore the natural sequel to the previous chapters on the irradiation of intact skin and insoluble collagen fibers.

17.1.1 Modes of Action of Radiation on Soluble Proteins

The action of irradiation on soluble proteins may take one or more of the following forms, depending upon the source and intensity of the radiation and the amino acid content and sequence in the three-dimensional arrangement of the polypeptide chain or chains of the protein molecule.

1. Scission of peptide bonds of the polypeptide chain without destroying the two adjacent amino acid residues forming the bond.

2. Scission of covalent intramolecular bonds (e.g., γ-glutamyl, β-aspartyl, and ϵ-amino peptide links, ester links, and carbohydrate links), with concomitant loss in stability of the specific three-dimensional native structure.

3. Scission of covalent intermolecular bonds in soluble, simple polymeric forms of the protein.

4. Scission of peptide bonds of the nonhelical telopeptides, which are peculiar to the collagen molecule.

5. Photolysis of the disulfide bonds of cystine, which is not of importance in the case of collagen since this does not generally contain the sulfur-amino acids [8, 9].

6. Destruction of individual amino acids, with consequent disruption of the polypeptide chain of the molecule.

7. Introduction of intermolecular cross-links.

It is evident from the above that the main consequence of irradiation is irreversible disruption of the native structure of protein molecules, with some reported instances of irradiation induced cross-linking (see for example, Refs. 10, 11, 12, 13, and 14). The irradiation of soluble proteins may be done in aqueous solution or using the dry protein. In the former case complications arise from the "indirect effect" involving attenuation of the available radiation intensity by the solvent with the accompanying production of free radicals from the solvent during exposure, although it has been reported that free radicals can also be formed during the irradiation of dry proteins [15].

17.1.2 Structure of the Collagen Macromolecule

In order to understand the action of ultraviolet and γ-irradiation on soluble collagen it is necessary to know the detailed structure of the collagen macromolecule. The current status of knowledge of this structure has been the subject of several excellent reviews [6, 7, 16, 17, 18, 19], and will not therefore be repeated in detail, but it is pertinent to record the highlights of this information. The main features of the molecular structure of soluble collagen relevant to the present discussion may be summarized as follows:

1. The collagen molecule (tropocollagen) consists of three polypeptide chains each of which occurs as a left-handed helix with 3.3 residues per turn. These three helical chains are in turn wound around each other in a right-handed triple helix.

2. Each polypeptide chain contains about 1000 amino acid residues, with every third residue being glycine and the sequence gly-prox-X (where X can be hydroxyproline) occurring regularly in the chain.

This was cooled in ice, cleaned free of blood, flesh and fat, and minced to a fine pulp in the presence of ice to keep the mincer and the skin cold.

Neutral-salt soluble collagen was prepared as follows. The skin pulp was extracted three times with five times its weight of 10% (wt/v) NaCl solution, each successive extraction being done at 0–4° for 96 hr. The extracts were clarified by centrifuging at 14000 g and —2° through the continuous-action rotor of a MSE model 18 centrifuge. The clear extracts were saturated with solid $(NH_4)_2SO_4$, and the precipitated proteins collected by centrifugation. The precipitate was dissolved in 1 M NaCl and dialyzed against a large volume of this solvent to remove excess salts. The protein solution was then filtered through paper pulp and brought to pH 3–4 with acetic acid. After standing overnight the precipitated protein was collected and redissolved in 0.5 N acetic acid. This solution was centrifuged at 32,000 g at —2° for 1 hr to remove insoluble material. The neutral-salt soluble collagen was precipitated by the addition of solid NaCl to give a final concentration of 5% (wt/v). The collagen was dissolved in 0.5 N acetic acid and the solution clarified by centrifugation at 32,000 g at —2° for 1 hr and dialyzed against three lots of 0.2 M Na_2HPO_4 until precipitation was complete. The precipitated collagen was redissolved in 0.15 N acetic acid, dialyzed against several changes of this solvent and then freeze-dried. The dry salt-free neutral-salt soluble collagen was stored over silica gel at 4°.

The acid-soluble collagen was prepared from the residual skin by adjusting the pH of this to 4.0, and extracting with three lots of 0.01 N acetic acid. The acid-soluble collagen was then purified as above. Except where stated all operations were carried out in a coldroom at 0–4°.

17.2   THE EFFECT OF ULTRAVIOLET IRRADIATION ON SOLUBLE COLLAGEN

Ultraviolet irradiation has been shown to cause peptide-bond fission and cross-linking in proteins in general (see for example, Refs. 13, 14, and 20) and collagen in particular [21, 22, 23, 11, 12, 24].

17.2.1   Ultraviolet Irradiation Method

In the work of the author reported here, the ultraviolet irradiation was done by preparing solutions of the soluble collagen in 0.15 M potassium acetate buffer, pH 4.8, and irradiating in a coldroom with a Hanovia UVS 220A lamp operated by a regulated power supply, the solution temperatures being 0–4°. The solutions were placed in fused-quartz tubes at a distance of 46 cm from the lamp, which is rated to give an ultraviolet intensity at 92 cm of 420–540 W cm^{-2} of radiation below 4000 Å.

Irradiations were either in the presence of air or oxygen-free nitrogen, the latter containing not more than 10 vpm of oxygen and no oxides of nitrogen or carbon. In the latter case the nitrogen, after passing through a solution of alkaline pyrogallol and a spray trap, was then bubbled through the protein solution for 30 min before irradiation was commenced, and during the whole period of irradiation. The bubbling rate was 100 ml min^{-1} and was kept low to avoid excessive frothing of the solution.

17.2.2   Viscosity of Ultraviolet-irradiated Collagen

The change in reduced viscosity for acid-soluble collagen as a function of time of irradiation for different collagen concentrations is shown in Fig. 17.1. Similar results were obtained for neutral-salt soluble collagen. The reaction-rate plots for the effect of ultraviolet irradiation on the

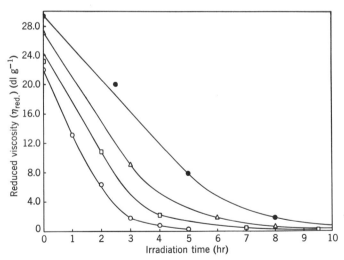

Figure 17.1. Effect of ultraviolet irradiation on the reduced viscosity of acid-soluble calf-skin collagen in 0.15 M HAc. ●, 0.041% (W/V); △, 0.033% (W/V); □, 0.017% (W/V); ○, 0.010% (W/V) [59].

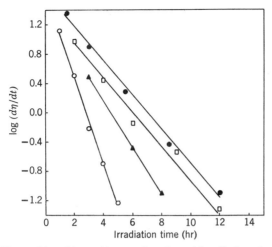

Figure 17.2.   Plots of log ($d\eta_{red}/dt$) as a function of irradiation time at a distance of 46 cm at 0–4°. ●, 0.080% (W/V) acid-soluble calf-skin collagen; □, 0.042% (W/V) neutral-salt soluble calf-skin collagen; ▲, 0.033% (W/V) acid-soluble calf-skin collagen; ○, 0.010% (W/V) acid-soluble calf-skin collagen [26].

reduced viscosity of collagen with time are obtained from the relationship between log ($d\eta/dt$) and t, as derived from Equation 1 [25]:

$$\ln \left(\frac{d\eta}{dt}\right) = \ln \left(-k\eta_0\right) - kt \cdot \cdot \cdot \tag{1}$$

where η is the reduced viscosity at time t, η_0 is the total change in reduced viscosity during the reaction, and k is the apparent first-order rate constant. The results (Fig. 17.2) show that the change in viscosity induced by irradiation is a first-order reaction, with a much greater rate constant k than that for optical rotation (see below). Rate constants of 8.5×10^{-3} and 10.5×10^{-3} min^{-1} were obtained for neutral-salt soluble and acid-soluble collagen respectively at concentrations of 0.042 g of protein 100 ml^{-1}. The fractional change in reduced viscosity for acid-soluble collagen as a function of time of irradiation is shown in Fig. 17.3.

17.2.3   Optical Rotation of Ultraviolet-irradiated Collagen

The change in the specific optical rotation for acid-soluble collagen as a function of time of irradiation is shown in Fig. 17.4 for different concentrations of collagen. Similar results were obtained for neutral-

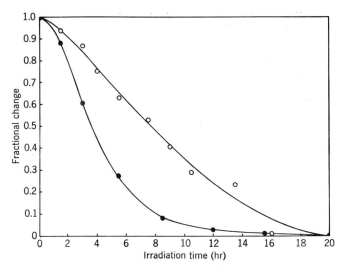

Figure 17.3.   Fractional change in specific rotation and reduced viscosity as a function of irradiation time at a distance of 46 cm and 0–4° for acid-soluble calf-skin collagen. ●, $(\eta_t - \eta_{20})/(\eta_0 - \eta_{20})$, where η_t is the reduced viscosity at time t, and η_0 and η_{20} are reduced viscosities at zero time and after irradiation for 20 hr respectively. ○, $([\alpha]_t - [\alpha]_{20})/([\alpha]_0 - [\alpha]_{20})$, where $[\alpha]_t$ is the specific rotation at time t, $[\alpha]_0$ is the specific rotation of the zero-time control, and is equal to −415°, and $[\alpha]_{20}$ is the specific rotation after irradiation for 20 hr, and is equal to −114° (0.08%, W/V) [26].

salt soluble collagen. The reaction-rate plots for optical rotation are obtained from the relationship between log $(d[\alpha]/dt)$ and t, as derived from Equation 2 that is similar to Equation 1:

$$\ln \left(\frac{d[\alpha]}{dt}\right) = \ln (-k[\alpha_0]) - kt \cdots \tag{2}$$

where $[\alpha]$ is the specific optical rotation. The results [26] show that the change in optical rotation induced by irradiation also follows a first-order reaction ($k = 2.6 \times 10^{-4}$ and 3.7×10^{-4} min⁻¹ for neutral-salt soluble and acid-soluble collagen respectively, at concentrations of 0.075 g of protein 100 ml⁻¹). The fractional change in specific rotation for acid-soluble collagen as a function of time of irradiation is shown in Fig. 17.3.

It has been reported [27, 28]; that when collagenase reacts with ichthyocol the viscosity changes faster with time of reaction than the optical rotation, as was found in the present case for irradiation (Fig.

17.3). Since viscosity is a function of the axial ratio of a molecule, whereas optical rotation is related more to spatial configuration, due either to the helical natures of the individual chains or interchain alignments [29, 30] this is interpreted as an initial scission of the collagen molecule into polypeptides with a relatively low axial ratio, having a helical configuration, followed by randomization of the polypeptide chains. The latter is probably due to thermal denaturation. Nishihara and Doty [31, 32] found similar changes in these physical properties on ultrasonic degradation of calfskin collagen, where viscosity and sedimentation indicated that the molecule was progressively fragmented into shorter segments.

17.2.4   Collagen-Fold Reformation of Ultraviolet-irradiated Collagen

In order to study the effect of ultraviolet irradiation on collagen-fold reformation, solutions of acid-soluble collagen (1.36 mg ml⁻¹) in 0.15 M potassium acetate buffer, pH 4.8, which is known to have the minimum effect on mutarotation [33], were irradiated in the presence of

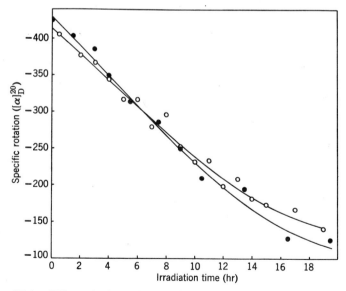

Figure 17.4.   Effect of ultraviolet irradiation on the specific rotation of soluble calf-skin collagen. ●, 0.080% (W/V) acid-soluble collagen; ○, 0.07% (W/V) neutral-salt soluble collagen. Collagen was irradiated at 46 cm at 0–4° [59].

air for periods of up to 19 hr and denatured at 45° for 15 min, and the helix formation followed by optical rotation while the solution was kept at 15° (Fig. 17.5). The results for a nonirradiated solution are included, showing a recovery of 80% of the helical content of the native collagen. This recovery for native acid-soluble collagen is considerably higher than the 59% recovery reported for neutral-salt soluble collagen [34], but is in agreement with other reported values (50–85%; [35]).

It is evident from the irradiation data (Fig. 17.5 and Table 17.1) that ultraviolet irradiation decreases the initial rate of mutarotation, that is, $(d[\alpha]/dt)_0$, and considerably decreases the amount of helix formation in the partial reformation on cooling of the collagen-fold or some modification of this structure [17, 36]. Further, with irradiation periods of about 19 hr, both the recovery of helical nature and the association of subunit chains virtually cease to take place. The specific rotation after 19 hr of irradiation followed by storage at 15° for 48 hr ($[\alpha]_D^{15} = -154°$; $[\alpha]_{365}^{15} = -550°$) was considerably lower than for the nonirradiated material, and approaches the mean-residue rotation of collagen in the denatured form ($[\alpha]_D^{15} = -90°$ to $-120°$; $[\alpha]_{365}^{15} = -450°$), indicating almost complete loss of the poly-L-proline II-type helix.

A parallel study was also made of the change in reduced viscosity

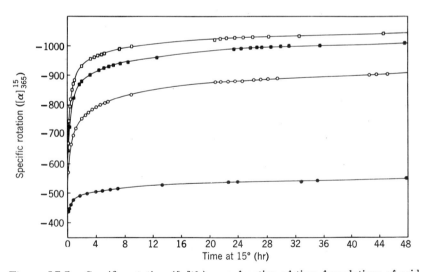

Figure 17.5. Specific rotation ($[\alpha]_{365}^{15}$) as a function of time for solutions of acid-soluble collagen (1.36 mg ml—l) irradiated with ultaviolet light at 0–4°, thermally denatured at 45° and then kept at 15°: □, Not irradiated; ■, irradiated for ½ hr; ○, irradiated for 3 hr; ●, irradiated for 19 hr [60].

Table 17.1   Rate of Collagen-fold Formation of Acid-soluble Collagen After Ultraviolet Irradiation, Thermal Denaturation, and Cooling to 15°[a]

Irradiation Time (hr)	Initial Rate of Mutarotation at 15° $(d[\alpha]/dt)_0$ (deg min^{-1}) 589 mμ	365 mμ	$10^{-2} \times$ Initial Rate of Reduced-viscosity Recovery at 15° $(d\eta_{red}/dt)_0$ (dl g^{-1}/min)
Not irradiated	0.80	7.0	2.0
½	0.59	4.3	1.2
1	—	—	0.7
3	0.45	3.3	0.4
19	0.02	1.5	0.0

[a] Solutions were irradiated at 0–4° for the specified times, and then thermally denatured at 45° for 15 min, before being cooled to 15°.

at 15° (Fig. 17.6 and Table 17.1). Ultraviolet irradiation caused a decrease in the initial rate of viscosity recovery, $(d\eta_{red}/dt)_0$, and the amount of chain association occurring parallels the regain in helical content. Fig. 17.7 illustrates the relationship between the reduced vis-

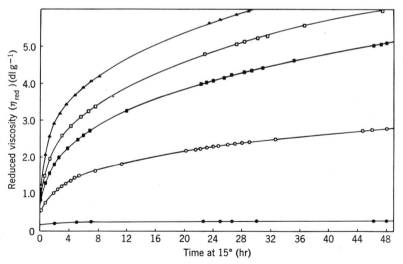

Figure 17.6.   Reduced viscosity (η_{red}) as a function of time for solutions of acid-soluble collagen (1.36 mg ml−1) irradiated with ultraviolet light at 0–4°, thermally denatured at 45° and then kept at 15°: ▲, Not irradiated; □, irradiated for ½ hr; ■, irradiated for 1 hr; ○, irradiated for 3 hr; ●, irradiated for 19 hr [60].

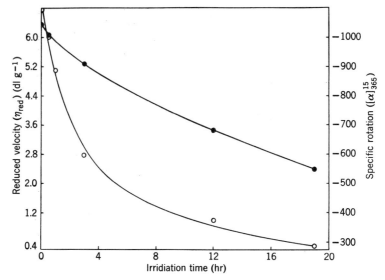

Figure 17.7. Specific-rotation (●) and reduced-viscosity (○) recoveries as functions of irradiation time at 0–4°, for solutions of acid-soluble collagen (1.36 mg ml—l) irradiated with ultraviolet light, heat denatured and then kept at 15° for 48 hr [60].

cosity attained on cooling heat-denatured solutions for 48 hr at 15° and the irradiation time. This relationship is thus a measure of aggregation or interchain association [17], which is directly related to irradiation damage. The main effect of irradiation would appear to be almost complete in the first 5 hr under the prescribed conditions, which indicates that the first breaks in the polypeptide chain are clearly more effective than subsequent breaks in reducing subunit chain association. The relationship between specific-rotation recovery and irradiation time is also illustrated in Fig. 17.7, representing the effect of irradiation damage on the helical content or interchain reaction [37, 38].

A similar relationship [34] was found for the irradiation of neutral-salt soluble collagen with ultraviolet light, indicating that the first breaks in the chain are more effective than later ones in decreasing the initial rate of mutarotation, and that the initial rate of mutarotation decreases as the chain length is diminished [38]. It is a reasonable assumption that the irradiation time is proportional to the number of breaks in the chain.

The order of reaction for the recovery of optical rotation and reduced viscosity at 15°, with and without irradiation, can be obtained by plotting log $(d[\alpha]/dt)$ and log $(d\eta_{red}/dt)$ against recovery time at 15°. A nonlinear relationship was obtained; as illustrated in Fig. 17.8 for reduced-viscosity recovery; showing that the random coil-to-helix transformation is not a first-order reaction [33, 17, 35]. Similar findings were noted with neutral-salt soluble collagen.

The accumulative effect of the irradiation, which also shows that the irradiation damage is not reversible, was illustrated as follows [34]. A solution of neutral-salt soluble collagen (1.36 mg ml⁻¹ of 0.15 M potassium acetate buffer, pH 4.8) was irradiated for 30 min, heat-denatured at 40° for 10 min and kept at 15° for 48 hr while the viscosity was measured at regular intervals. After this the solution was immediately irradiated again for a further 30 min, heat-denatured at 40° for 10 min and kept at 15° for 32 hr, while the viscosity was again recorded. After the first irradiation and 32 hr reformation time at 15° the reduced viscosity was 2.88 dl g⁻¹, whereas the reduced viscosity after the second irradiation and the same time for reformation was 1.64 dl g⁻¹. For a continuous irradiation interval of 60 min with 32 hr reformation time the reduced viscosity was 2.25 dl g⁻¹. The latter is not a strict comparison since the reduced viscosity had not reached equilibrium even after 48

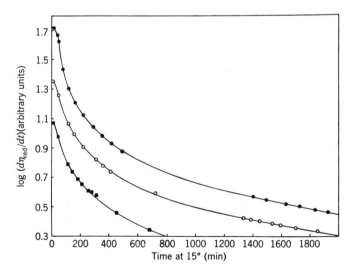

Figure 17.8. Plots of log (d_{red}/dt) as a function of time at 15°, for solutions of acid-soluble collagen (1.36 mg ml—1) irradiated with ultraviolet light at 0–4° and thermally denatured at 45°: ●, Not irradiated; ○, irradiated for 1 hr; ■, irradiated for 3 hr [60].

Table 17.2   Summary of Reduced-viscosity and Specific-rotation Recovery Values for Neutral-salt Soluble Collagen Subjected to Ultraviolet Irradiation[a]

Treatment	Reduced Viscosity (dl g^{-1})	Specific Rotation ($[\alpha]_D$)
Control: no irradiation and no heat-denaturation	15.94	−339°
Heat-denaturation but no irradiation	4.10	−235
Irradiated for ½ hr in air with heat-denaturation	3.16	−230
Irradiated for 1 hr in air with heat-denaturation	2.47	—
Irradiated for 3 hr in air with heat-denaturation	1.30	−204
Irradiated for 10 hr in air with heat-denaturation	0.55	−159
Irradiated for 19 hr in air with heat-denaturation	0.28	−89
Irradiated for ½ hr in N₂ with heat-denaturation	2.20	−202
Irradiated for 1 hr in N₂ with heat-denaturation	1.02	—

[a] Values were obtained after heat-denaturation and keeping solutions at 15° for 48 hr.

hr. It has been reported [33, 25] that viscosity can increase over a period of many days.

Experiments also showed the differences in helix formation and aggregation brought about by ultraviolet irradiation in air and nitrogen. Samples of the same collagen solution in 0.15 M potassium acetate buffer, pH 4.8, were irradiated for ½ hr and 1 hr in air and with pure oxygen-free nitrogen bubbling through the solution. The collagen, when irradiated in the presence of nitrogen, gave less recovery of optical rotation and viscosity at 15° than when the irradiation was done in the presence of air. It is apparent from the data in Table 17.2 that irradiation for 1 hr in air actually gives a greater recovery of reduced viscosity than ½-hr irradiation in the presence of nitrogen.

A summary is given in Table 17.2 of the reduced viscosity and specific rotation obtained for solutions of neutral-salt soluble collagen kept at 15° for 48 hr, after various irradiation treatments.

17.2.5   Amino Acid Analysis of Ultraviolet-irradiated Collagen

The amino acid compositions of neutral-salt soluble and acid-soluble collagen before and after irradiation for 19 hr at 4° are given in Table 17.3. The irradiated collagens were dialyzed against several changes of distilled water to remove any degraded protein before being freeze-dried for amino acid analysis. These analyses show that, though the α- and β-components are degraded into low-molecular-weight fragments by the irradiation, as shown by chromatography and ultracentrifugation (see below), only limited changes occur in the amino acid composition. Thus

Table 17.3   Amino Acid Composition of Native- and Ultraviolet-irradiated Neutral-salt Soluble and Acid-soluble Collagen[a]

| Amino Acid | Amino Acid Composition (g 100 g^{-1} of protein) | | | |
| | Nonirradiated | | Irradiated with Ultraviolet Light for 19 hr | |
	Neutral-Salt Soluble Collagen	Acid-Soluble Collagen	Neutral-Salt-Soluble Collagen	Acid-Soluble Collagen
Ala	8.32	9.13	8.95	8.33
Arg	8.20	7.35	8.54	7.66
Asp	5.06	5.61	4.37	5.70
Cys	Trace	None	Trace	None
Glu	10.88	10.06	11.50	9.85
Gly	19.46	21.22	21.08	21.48
His	0.71	0.48	0.51	0.44
Hyl	1.17	1.15	1.27	1.19
Hyp	9.60	11.15	10.00	12.75
Ile	1.70	1.33	1.70	1.05
Leu	3.38	2.87	3.43	2.05
Lys	3.89	3.40	3.99	3.74
Met	0.96	0.59	0.67	0.35
Phe	1.93	1.87	1.22	0.75
Pro	11.47	12.80	12.17	14.00
Ser	3.44	3.27	3.39	3.41
Thr	2.04	1.73	1.86	1.77
Tyr	0.65	0.51	0.34	0.14
Val	2.46	2.05	2.44	1.58
Amide N	(0.88)	(0.77)	(0.98)	(0.94)
Total	95.32	96.57	97.43	96.24
Total N	18.2	18.3	18.9	18.6

[a] The results for neutral-salt soluble collagen are based on a single analysis, and those for acid-soluble collagen are the averages of duplicate analyses.

the amounts of tyrosine and phenylalanine are decreased. Both collagen preparations, before and after irradiation, contained a small amount of 3-hydroxyproline [39], which appeared just before the methionine sulfoxide peak in the amino acid elution. After irradiation both preparations gave a ninhydrin-positive component appearing after leucine in very small amounts (about 0.1%).

17.2.6   Chromatography of Ultraviolet-irradiated Collagen

Chromatography was carried out to study the effect of ultraviolet irradiation on the subunit composition of acid-soluble collagen [39, 40]. The chromatography of unirradiated, thermally denatured acid-soluble collagen (Fig. 17.9) resulted in the recovery of approximately 21% α_1, 5% β_{11}, 13% β_{12}, and 61% α_2. Davidson and Cooper [40] have shown that the large amount of the α_2-subunit obtained by this chromatography method may be attributed to the presence of four additional components having similar elution characteristics to the α_2-subunit. These four additional components designated A, B, C, and D have been correlated with the dimeric subunits α_2-α_2, α_1-α_1, β_{11}-β_{11}, and β_{12}-β_{12} respectively.

The chromatography of acid-soluble collagen irradiated for 2, 6, and 17 hr. (Fig 17.10 and Table 17.4) indicates that the β_{12}- and α_2-fractions

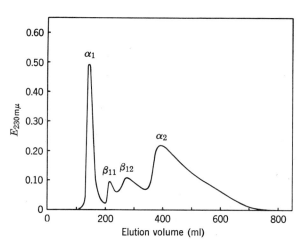

Figure 17.9.   Elution pattern of approximately 50 mg of acid-soluble calf-skin collagen on CM-cellulose at 40° after denaturation at 45° for 30 min. The column was eluted witha linear salt gradient using 500 ml, 1 = 0.06 acetate buffer and 500 ml, 1 = 0.16 acetate buffer [60].

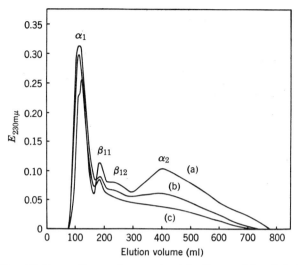

Figure 17.10. Elution patterns of approximately 50 mg of irradiated acid-soluble calf-skin collagen on CM-cellulose at 40° after denaturation at 45° for 30 min. The column was eluted with a linear salt gradient using 500 ml, l = 0.06 acetate buffer and 500 ml, l = 0.16 acetate buffer. (a) 2 hr irradiation; (b) 6 hr irradiation; (c) 17 hr irradiation [60].

together with components A, B, C, and D are most labile towards ultraviolet irradiation, resulting in the elution of degraded material close to the α_1-position.

Table 17.4 Effect of Ultraviolet Irradiation on the Subunit Composition of Acid-soluble Collagen

Irradiation Dose (hr at 0–4°)	Recovery of Soluble Protein After Irradiation (%)	Composition (%)		
		α_1	$\beta_{11} + \beta_{12}{}^a$	$\alpha_2{}^b$
0	100	21	18	61
2	96	23	20	57
6	80	37	20	43
17	70	49	20	31

[a] Poor resolution of the β_{11}- and β_{12}-subunits after irradiation made an individual assessment impossible.
[b] The α_2-fraction was found to be a composite of the α_2-subunit and components A, B, C, and D [40].

17.2.7 Ultracentrifugation of Ultraviolet-irradiated Collagen

The ultracentrifugation of thermally denatured acid-soluble collagen resulted in the separation of the α- and β-subunits with sedimentation coefficients $S_{20,w}$, 2.6s, and 3.4s, respectively [39]. The ultracentrifugation of thermally denatured acid-soluble collagen that had been irradiated for 2 hr resulted in a similar sedimentation pattern except for a considerable decrease in the β-peak (Fig. 17.11). The chromatographic analyses above show, however, a marked decrease in the composite α_2-fraction. Davidson & Cooper [40] have shown that their major components A and B are eluted with α_2-fraction by the method of Piez,

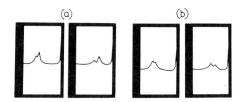

Figure 17.11. Sedimentation patterns of (a) thermally denatured acid-soluble calf-skin collagen; (b) thermally denatured acid-soluble calf-skin collagen irradiated for 2 hr. The photographs were taken after 80 and 120 min at 56, 100 rpm and 35°. The solutions contained 0.4% (W/V) of protein in sodium formate buffer (pH 3.75 and 1 = 0.15). Sedimentation is from left to right [60].

Eigner, and Lewis [39], but sediment with the β-subunits. The labile nature of these components A and B would explain the large decrease in the β-peak obtained after ultraviolet irradiation.

7.3 DISCUSSION

The effect of ultraviolet irradiation on the subunit composition of acid-soluble collagen has indicated the labile nature of the β_{12}- and α_2-subunits, as well as the components A, B, C, and D [40]. The labile nature of the β_{12}- and α_2-subunits may be expected, as the α_2-chain has been shown to be rich in both tyrosine and phenylalanine residues [39]. Although it has been suggested that components A, B, C, and D are terminally linked dimeric subunits their labile nature may also be expected, as tyrosine is thought to play a significant role in the intermolecular linkage of such subunits [41]. Cooper and Davidson [26] have shown that both tyrosine and phenylalanine residues in soluble collagens are labile under the prescribed conditions. The relative decrease in the subunit content, indicated by ultracentrifugation, would also suggest that depolymerization of the major components A (α_2-α_2) and B (α_1-α_1) takes place at an early stage in the ultraviolet-irradiation reaction.

Piez and Carrillo [33] regard the pyrrolidine ring content, the subunit content, and the solvent employed as being the prime factors that control the rate and extent of mutarotation in cooled solutions of soluble collagen after thermal denaturation. According to Harrington and von Hippel [17], and reformation of the collagen-type structure occurs in a three-stage mechanism. The primary step is considered to be a local intrachain configurational change involving the locking of proline residues into the poly-L-proline II-configuration which then leads to the development of a loose, poly-L-proline II-type helix along the polypeptide chain of the molecules, allowing specific interhelical association (i.e., lateral chain association through interchain hydrogen bonding) to form triple helical structures of the collagen-type. There is some doubt, however, as to the validity of this theory since it hinges on the formation of a stable single-chain intermediate in the form of a poly-L-proline II-type helix [42, 9]. Flory and Weaver [43] have proposed that the single-chain helix can only have transitory existence, therefore the formation of the triple helical-type structure stabilized by interhelical hydrogen bonding is necessary in the reformation of the collagen-type structure. Alternatively, the formation of a hydrogen-bonded, triple-helical collagen-type structure may occur by the reverse folding of a single polypeptide chain, or of a double polypeptide chain [30, 9]. This chain folding would allow intrachain hydrogen bonding, not possible in a single chain without folding, and equivalent in its stabilizing action to interchain hydrogen bonding in native tropocollagen. Another factor in this recovery mechanism is the role of interchain, random hydrogen bonding to yield a range of structures of varying stability, in addition to more specifically ordered collagen-type structures involving cooperative hydrogen bonding [44, 42, 45, 46].

Since ultraviolet irradiation affects both the rate and the extent of helix formation in acid-soluble collagen, it is necessary to consider which of the above factors are affected by the irradiation. The amino acid analyses show that no significant decrease in the hydroxyproline and proline content occurs after irradiation, and therefore the initial nucleation step involving the pyrrolidine ring cannot be affected by irradiation. The amino acid analyses also show that, apart from phenylalanine and tyrosine, which are present in small amounts, no great loss of amino acids occurs on irradiation. Although tyrosine and phenylalanine are thought to play a critical role in the intermolecular interaction resulting in fibril formation [47], the role played by these residues in controlling the rate and extent of mutarotation in solutions of cooled gelatins does not appear to have been considered [33, 34]. Although the main effect of irradiation has been shown to be the conversion of the α- and β-subunits into smaller peptide chains, destruction of tyrosine and penylalanine residues resulting in considerable depolymerization may well be a contributory factor.

Therefore the effect of ultraviolet irradiation on the collagen-fold formation would appear to be the formation of shorter peptide chains, in the random-coil form, which hinder the propagation of the helical structure starting at the pyrrolidine rings and proceeding along the single-chain random coils [38]. This would presumably also decrease the amount of lateral chain association between single helical chains, and any single-chain folding giving helices stabilized by intramolecular association [36]. Since the mutarotation studies of irradiated acid-soluble collagen and of neutral-salt soluble collagen [34] give very similar results, similar intramolecular structures for both acid-soluble and neutral-salt soluble collagens are suggested.

In conclusion, all these results indicate that the main effect of ultraviolet irradiation under the experimental conditions specified is to decompose the collagen molecule by peptide bond fission, with the minimum of amino acid destruction. No evidence was found for the formation of intermolecular cross-links.

17.4   THE EFFECT OF γ-IRRADIATION ON SOLUBLE COLLAGEN

Some physicochemical effects of γ-irradiation on collagen have been reported. Bowes and Moss [48] found a decrease in the tensile strength and shrinkage temperature of irradiated oxhide at 5 and 50 Mrad doses. They also reported a limited destruction of acidic and basic amino acids, as well as those having a ring structure. Relatively little hydrolytic scission of peptide bonds was indicated from terminal-group analysis. Ramanathan, Mohanaradhakrishnan, and Nayudamma [49] reported similar decreases in tensile strength and shrinkage temperatures for irradiated tail-tendon collagens at 10 and 30 Mrad doses, as well as modified electron micrographs, x-ray diffraction patterns, and optical birefringence. Cassel [50] irradiated tail-tendon collagen (5–220 Mrad doses) and found little damage to amino acid residues at doses less than 20

Mrads. Methionine, phenylalanine, and threonine were shown to be most labile at higher irradiation doses, and alanine, glycine, hydroxyproline, proline, and arginine were least affected. Strakhov and Shifrin [51] reported that at 10^4–10^5 rads of γ-irradiation cross-linking of collagen molecules occurs, whereas at irradiation doses above 10^7 rads the destructive effect predominates.

The exposure of collagen fibers to ionizing radiation has been shown to result in a progressive decrease in their shrinkage temperature [50, 52, 53] and in the formation of intermolecular cross-links [10]. The decrease in shrinkage temperature induced by irradiation is probably due to disorganisation of the secondary structure of the collagen triple helix. Similar effects have been noted for soluble collagen [54, 55].

When a solution is irradiated, the principal effect is to dissociate the solvent into free radicals, which may then attack the solute (the "indirect effect"). Most studies have been concerned with the irradiation of proteins in aqueous solution, when the "indirect effects" of irradiation are important. The present work concerns two fractions of collagen prepared from the skin of a newborn calf. Both fractions were freeze-dried and exposed to γ-irradiation in the absence of oxygen.

17.4.1   γ-Irradiation Method

Freeze-dried samples of the soluble collagen were dried under vacuum over P_2O_5 for 24 hr, sealed under vacuum into glass tubes and irradiated at 22° from a 300–400 c ^{60}Co source. The rate of irradiation was 1.2 krads min^{-1}.

17.4.2   Collagen-Fold Reformation of γ-Irradiated
Collagen: Mutarotation

To study the effect of γ-irradiation in the dose range 1 krad-10 Mrads, solutions of irradiated and nonirradiated acid-soluble collagen (1.2 — 1.4 mg ml^{-1} of 0.15 M potassium acetate, pH 4.8) were denatured at 45° for 15 min and helix reformation monitored by optical-rotation measurements at 15° [56, 57]. Typical optical-rotation recovery curves are shown in Fig. 17.12. This information is summarized in Tables 17.5 and 17.6, which show that both the initial rates of mutarotation and the actual recoveries after 48 hr decrease as the irradiation dose increases; a similar progressive decrease with irradiation dose was also observed in the specific rotation of the collagen solutions containing irradiated collagen before thermal denaturation (Table 17.6). Thus the mutarotation recovery, being the specific-rotation value attained after 48

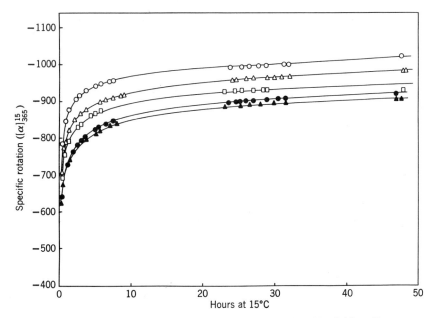

Figure 17.12. Specific rotation ($[\alpha]_{365}^{15}$) of γ-irradiated acid-soluble collagen as a function of time. Solutions (1.2–1.4 mg ml—1) were thermally denatured at 45° for 15 min and then kept at 15°: $\bigcirc$, Not irradiated; $\triangle$, 1 krad; $\square$, 10 krads; $\bullet$, 100 krads; $\blacktriangle$, 500 krads [56].

hr at 15° expressed as a percentage of the specific rotation of the corresponding original solution containing irradiated material with no history of heating, is remarkably constant at about 80% for all the doses of γ-irradiation (Table 17.6), whereas the mutarotation recovery expressed as a percentage of the specific rotation of the unirradiated native acid-soluble collagen decreased from 81 to 62% (Table 17.6).

The relationships between the amount of irradiation and the specific rotation at 15° of the solutions with no thermal history above this temperature, and the mutarotation values for heated solutions after 48 hr at 15°, are shown in Fig. 17.13. These results show a rapid decrease in the specific-rotation and mutarotation values with the initial relatively small doses of γ-irradiation, up to about 100 krads. As the dose is increased a steady decrease in these values occurs at a lower rate.

17.4.3 Viscosity Recovery

A parallel study was made of the regain in reduced viscosity at 15° after thermal denaturation. Increased doses of γ-irradiation caused a

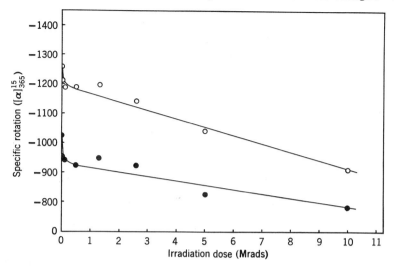

Figure 17.13. Specific rotation ($[\alpha]_{365}^{15}$) of γ-irradiated acid-soluble collagen as a function of irradiation dose. Solutions (1.2–1.4 mg ml—1) were measured before heating (○), and after heating at 45° for 15 min and keeping at 15° for 48 hr (●) [56].

decrease in the initial rate of viscosity recovery [56, 57] and in the reduced viscosity after 48 hr at 15° (Tables 17.5 and 17.7, and Fig. 17.14).

The recovery in reduced viscosity expressed as a percentage of the reduced viscosity of the corresponding collagen sample with no thermal history (Table 17.7) is not as constant as a similar relationship measured by specific rotation (Table 17.6), and has a much lower value of about 16%. The same recovery values expressed as a percentage of the reduced viscosity of the original unirradiated collagen ($[\eta]_{red}^{15} = 41.2$) decrease markedly from 16 to 2.5% (Table 17.7). Therefore the recovery in reduced viscosity on cooling thermally denatured solutions is very much lower than the recovery in specific rotation. Further, the irradiation has a bigger effect on viscosity than on the optical rotation of unheated solutions. Thus after 10 Mrads the specific rotation falls to 73% of the specific rotation of unirradiated collagen (Table 17.6), whereas the reduced viscosity falls to 12% of the reduced viscosity of unirradiated collagen (Table 17.7).

The relationships between the irradiation dose and the reduced viscosity ($[\eta]_{red}^{15}$ corrected to 1.2 mg mg⁻¹; see Fig. 17.16) for unheated solutions, and the viscosity recovery after 48 hr at 15° following thermal

Table 17.5 Rate of Collagen-fold Formation of Acid-soluble Collagen After γ-Irradiation, Thermal Denaturation, and Cooling to 15°[a]

Irradiation Dose (Mrads)	Initial Rate of Mutarotation $(d[\alpha]/dt)_0$ at 365 mμ and 15° (deg. min⁻¹)		Specific Rotation $[\alpha]_{365}^{15}$ After 48 hr at 15°		$10^{-2} \times$ Initial Rate of Recovery of Reduced Viscosity $(d\eta_{red}/dt)_0$ (dl g⁻¹ min⁻¹)		Reduced Viscosity After 48 hr at 15° (dl g⁻¹)	
	Neutral-Salt Soluble Collagen	Acid-Soluble Collagen	Neutral-Salt Soluble Collagen	Acid-Soluble Collagen	Neutral-Salt Soluble Collagen	Acid-Soluble Collagen	Neutral-Salt Soluble Collagen	Acid-Soluble Collagen
0	6.5	7.0	−974°	−1045°	2.5	2.0	5.68	6.76
1.3	2.8	5.4	−944	−950	1.0	0.9	3.98	4.08
2.6	2.1	4.9	−905	−927	0.9	0.8	3.27	3.59
5.0	1.2	3.1	−832	−827	0.3	0.3	1.49	1.65
10.0	0.9	1.4	−745	−783	0.2	0.2	0.86	1.04

[a] Solutions of irradiated collagen were thermally denatured at 45° for 15 min before being cooled to 15°.

Table 17.6 Optical-rotation Data for Collagen After γ-irradiation

	Specific Rotation at 15° of Collagen After Irradiation ($[\alpha]_{365}^{15}$)	Specific Rotation of Irradiated Collagen (% of That for Native Collagen)	Specific Rotation After Thermal Denaturation and Cooling to 15° for 48 hr ($[\alpha]_{365}^{15}$) (Mutarotation Recovery)	Mutarotation Recovery (% of Specific Rotation of Native Collagen)	Mutarotation Recovery (% of Specific Rotation of Corresponding Unheated Collagen)
ASC[a]	−1261°	100	−1025°	81	81
ASC + 1 krad	−1228	98	−991	79	81
ASC + 10 krads	−1215	96	−956	76	79
ASC + 100 krads	−1191	95	−944	75	79
ASC + 500 krads	−1192	96	−926	73	78
ASC + 1.3 Mrads	−1199	95	−950	75	79
ASC + 2.6 Mrads	−1145	91	−927	73	81
ASC + 5 Mrads	−1046	83	−827	66	79
ASC + 10 Mrads	−914	73	−783	62	86

[a] ASC, acid-soluble collagen.

621

Table 17.7 Viscosity Data for Collagen After γ-Irradiation

	Reduced Viscosity at 15° of Collagen After Irradiation ($[\eta]_{red}$[15] at 0.12 g 100 ml^{-1}) (dl g^{-1})	Reduced Viscosity of Irradiated Collagen (% of That for Native Collagen)	Viscosity Recovery After Thermal Denaturation and Cooling to 15° for 48 hr ($[\eta]_{red}$[16]) dl g^{-1}	Viscosity Recovery (% of Reduced Viscosity of Native Collagen)	Viscosity Recovery (% of Reduced Viscosity of Corresponding Unheated Collagen)	Limited Viscosity Number $\lim_{c \to 0} [\eta]_{red}$[15] (dl g^{-1})
ASC[a]	41.2	100	6.68	16.0	16	16.3
ASC + 1 krad	28.0	68	5.72	14.0	20	13.5
ASC + 10 krads	28.2	69	4.92	12.0	17	13.1
ASC + 100 krads	27.3	66	4.00	9.7	15	12.1
ASC + 500 krads	24.2	59	3.61	8.8	15	11.4
ASC + 1.3 Mrads	32.2	78	4.08	9.9	13	12.7
ASC + 2.6 Mrads	22.3	54	3.59	8.7	16	11.0
ASC + 5 Mrads	12.0	29	1.65	4.0	14	6.6
ASC + 10 Mrads	4.8	12	1.04	2.5	22	2.9

[a] ASC, acid-soluble collagen.

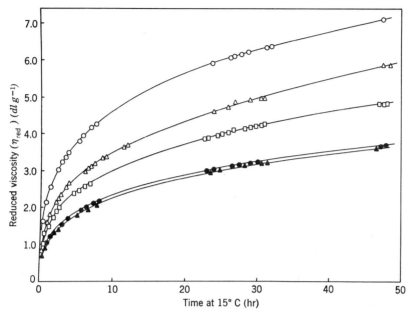

Figure 17.14. Reduced viscosity ($[\eta]_{red}^{15}$) of γ-irradiated acid-soluble collagen as a function of time. Solutions (1.2–1.4 mg ml—l) were thermally denatured at 45° for 15 min and then kept at 15°: ○, Not irradiated △, 1 krad; □, 10 krads; ●, 100 krads; ▲, 500 krads [56].

denaturation, respectively, are shown in Fig. 17.15. These relationships are comparable with similar studies carried out by specific-rotation measurements (Fig. 17.13), except that the reduced viscosity of the un-heated samples falls very rapidly with initial low doses.

The dependence of reduced viscosity on concentration at each irradiation dose is shown in Fig. 17.16. It is evident that, as the amount of irradiation is increased, the concentration-dependence of the reduced viscosity decreases very significantly. Since it is difficult to determine the reduced viscosity at zero concentration (i.e., the intrinsic viscosity or limiting viscosity number, $[\eta]$) from extrapolation of these curves, the inherent viscosity ($[\ln(\eta/\eta_0)]/c$) was plotted against concentration [58]. This gave a linear relationship and accurate extrapolation to zero concentration (Table 17.7). The relationship between limiting viscosity number and irradiation dose is recorded in Fig. 17.17. Once again these data show an initial rapid decomposition at doses below 100 krads.

The fractional changes in specific rotation and reduced viscosity for unheated solutions of acid-soluble collagen as a function of irradiation

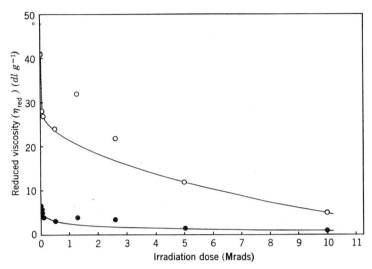

Figure 17.15.   Reduced viscosity ($[\eta]_{red}^{15}$) of γ-irradiated acid-soluble collagen as a function of irradiation dose. Solutions (1.2–1.4 mg ml−1) were measured before heating (○), and after heating at 45° for 15 min and keeping at 15° for 48 hr (●) [56].

time or dose [59] have the same form as those for ultraviolet irradiation (Fig. 17.3), with reduced viscosity decreasing at a greater rate than specific rotation. Similar results are reported for acid-soluble collagen from shark skin [55].

17.4.4   Melting Curves

The melting curves for unirradiated and irradiated acid-soluble collagen are given in Fig. 17.18, from which values can be obtained for T_m, the temperature at the midpoint of the transition (melting point) $\Delta[\alpha]_T$, the difference between the specific rotation at the high and low temperature ends of the transition, and ΔT, the difference in temperature between the points at which the helix-coil transition is one-quarter and three-quarters complete [38]. It is apparent that at the lower doses of irradiation the curves are biphasic, the lower melting point being attributable to the helix-to-coil transition of those molecules rendered thermally more labile by the irradiation, and the higher melting point to undamaged collagen molecules or molecules insufficiently damaged to show significant change [54].

The melting points are given in Table 17.8, together with the values for $\Delta[\alpha]_T$ and ΔT, the latter being uncorrected for the biphasic nature of the curves. The melting points of the more labile material as a function of irradiation dose are shown in Fig. 17.19. Comparable changes in the melting curves for acid-soluble collagen from rat-tail tendon irradiated in solution have been reported by Bailey [54], with the melting temperature decreasing with increasing irradiation dose.

17.4.5   Amino Acid Analysis of γ-Irradiated Collagen

In Table 17.9 the amino acid analyses of irradiated neutral-salt soluble and acid-soluble collagen are given. Comparison of these values with

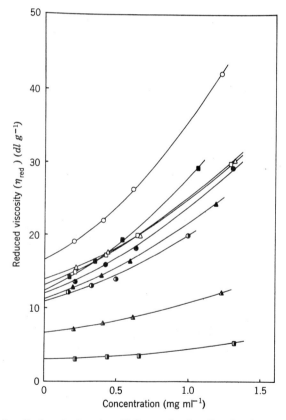

Figure 17.16.   Reduced viscosity ($[\eta]_{red}^{15}$) of γ-irradiated acid-soluble collagen as a function of concentration (mg ml—1): ○, Not irradiated; △, 1 krad; □, 10 krads; ●, 100 krads; ▲, 500 krads; ■, 1.3 Mrads; ◑, 2.6 Mrads; ▲, 5 Mrads; ◨, 10 Mrads [56].

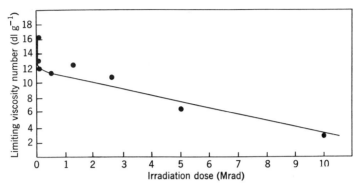

Figure 17.17. Limiting viscosity number $(\lim_{C \to 0} [\eta]_{red}^{15})$ of γ-irradiated acid-soluble collagen as a function of irradiation dose [56].

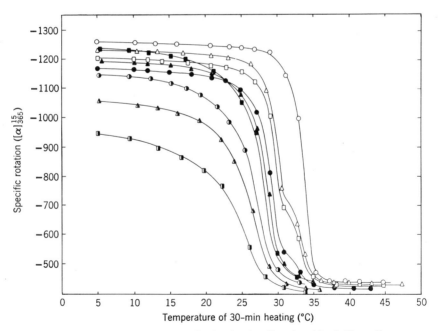

Figure 17.18. Specific rotation $([\alpha]_{red}^{15})$ of γ-irradiated acid-soluble collagen as a function of temperature: $\bigcirc$, Not irradiated; $\triangle$, 1 krad; $\square$, 10 krads; $\bullet$, 100 krads; $\blacktriangle$, 500 krads; $\blacksquare$, 1.3 Mrads; $\circleddash$, 2.6 Mrads; $\blacktriangle$, 5 Mrads; $\blacksquare$, 10 Mrads [56].

Table 17.8   Melting-Point Data for Collagen After γ-Irradiation

| | Melting Point, T_m | | | |
	Low	High	$(\Delta\alpha_{365})_T$	ΔT
ASC[a]	—	38.6°	−828°	1.2°
ASC + 1 krad	34.4°	38.6	−804	1.6
ASC + 10 krads	34.6	38.8	−786	2.0
ASC + 100 krads	33.8	—	−770	2.7
ASC + 500 krads	33.4	—	−765	2.9
ASC + 1.3 Mrads	32.8	—	−790	3.8
ASC + 2.6 Mrads	31.0	—	−736	3.2
ASC + 5 Mrads	30.6	—	−662	4.6
ASC + 10 Mrads	29.2	—	−563	7.0

[a] ASC, acid-soluble collagen.

those reported for nonirradiated neutral-salt soluble and acid-soluble collagen [26] shows that little if any destruction of amino acids occurs at the prescribed irradiation doses.

The published data on the amino acid analysis of various collagen preparations from skin (see, for example, Tristram and Smith, [8]) show quite wide variations in the content of hydroxyproline and tyrosine, due probably to variable contamination with noncollagenous proteins.

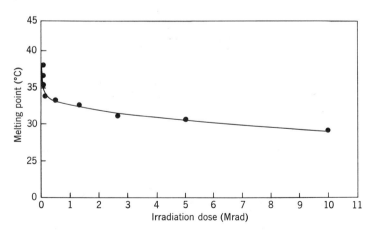

Figure 17.19.   Melting temperature (°C) of γ-irradiated acid-soluble collagen as a function of irradiation dose [56].

Table 17.9   Amino Acid Composition of γ-Irradiated
Soluble Collagen

| Amino Acid | Neutral-Salt Soluble Collagen | | Acid-Soluble Collagen | |
| | Irradiation Dose | | | |
	5 Mrads	10 Mrads	5 Mrads	10 Mrads
Ala	8.15	7.86	8.42	8.62
Arg	7.38	7.26	7.58	7.70
Asp	6.41	6.95	6.50	6.33
Glu	9.64	10.39	9.64	9.69
Gly	18.89	18.02	19.76	20.29
His	0.59	0.75	0.57	0.56
Hyl	0.84	0.78	0.89	0.58
Hyp	11.59	10.52	11.61	11.80
Ile	1.59	1.89	1.57	1.62
Leu	2.73	3.21	2.72	2.82
Lys	3.26	3.71	3.23	3.21
Met	0.54	0.71	0.42	0.78
Phe	1.76	1.95	1.78	1.81
Pro	11.21	10.52	11.57	11.89
Ser	3.37	3.52	3.39	3.48
Thr	1.86	2.04	1.77	1.81
Tyr	0.49	0.72	0.47	0.48
Val	2.08	2.34	2.09	2.13
Total	93.16	94.05	94.82	96.44

The neutral-salt soluble collagen used in the present study did have a relatively low hydroxyproline and high tyrosine content, which indicates the possible presence of noncollagenous impurities.

17.4.6   Chromatography of γ-irradiated Collagen

The chromatography of nonirradiated thermally denatured acid-soluble collagen (Fig. 17.20) may be compared with similar findings where different methods were used [60, 40]. The use of the Spectrochrom Analyzer gave improved resolution over that obtained by the method of Piez, Eigner, and Lewis [39]. The reasons for this are that a more exhaustive gradient involving the use of a buffer change to a higher ionic strength ($I = 0.26$) was used, and that the microcurvette of the Spectrochrom Analyzer has a much smaller volume (0.05 ml) compared with about 1 ml for most flow cells with a path length of 10 mm. Component

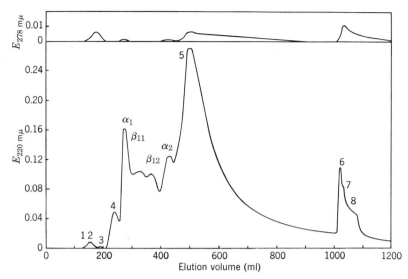

Figure 17.20. Elution pattern of approximately 50 mg of acid-soluble calf-skin collagen on CM-cellulose at 40° after denaturation at 45° for 30 min. The column was eluted with a linear salt gradient using 500 ml 1 = 0.06 acetate buffer and 500 ml, 1 = 0.16 acetate buffer followed by a change to 1 = 0.26 acetate buffer [57].

4 probably corresponds to the α_3-subunit reported by several authors (see, for example, Piez, [61]). The large component 5 was in some cases resolved into several peaks and it is concluded that this component consists of the dimeric subunits α_1-α_1, α_2-α_2, β_{11}-β_{11} and β_{12}-β_{12} described previously [40]. The resolution of the minor components 1,2,3,6,7, and 8 has not been reported in earlier findings, although components 1,2, and 3 may be the same as the E, F, and G components separated by a different chromatography procedure [40]. Since CM-cellulose is a weak cation-exchanger, the acidic nature of components 1,2, and 3 and the basic nature of components 6,7, and 8, together with their relatively high extinction at 278 mμ (Fig. 17.20), due to the presence of aromatic constituents, suggest that these components are telopeptide residues. Further evidence on the nature of these components has been reported elsewhere [62]. The chromatography of nonirradiated thermally de-natured neutral-salt soluble collagen gave a similar elution pattern to that of acid-soluble collagen, except for a slightly smaller peak contain-ing the α_1-α_1, α_2-α_2, β_{11}-β_{11} and β_{12}-β_{12} dimers.

The chromatography of γ-irradiated neutral-salt soluble and acid-soluble collagen at 1.3, 2.6, 5, and 10 Mrads showed the early breakdown

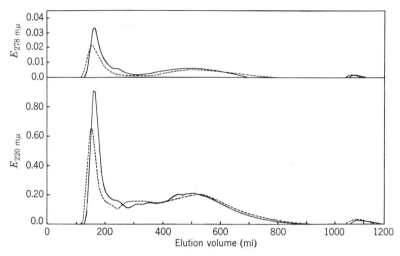

Figure 17.21. Elution patterns of approximately 50 mg of calf-skin collagen irradiated with 1.3 Mrad γ-irradiation: full-line-acid-soluble collagen; dotted-line-neutral-salt soluble collagen. The column was eluted with a linear salt gradient using 500 ml l = 0.06 acetate buffer and 500 ml l = 0.16 acetate buffer followed by a change to l = 0.26 acetate buffer [57].

at low doses of irradiation of the chromatographic component containing the dimeric subunits, resulting in the elution of degraded material just in front of the α_1-position. A typical chromatographic separation of acid-soluble collagen after 1.3 Mrads of irradiation is shown in Fig. 17.21. The relatively high extinction of this degraded material at 278 mμ was noted in all cases.

17.4.7 Ultracentrifugation of γ-Irradiated Collagen

The ultracentrifugation of thermally denatured neutral-salt soluble and acid-soluble collagen both resulted in the separation of the α- and the β-subunits with $S_{20,w}$ 2.6 and 3.4s, respectively [39]. The ultracentrifugation of thermally denatured neutral-salt soluble collagen that had initially been irradiated at 5 and 10 Mrads in an anhydrous condition resulted in single heterodisperse peaks with $S_{20,w}$ 1.86 and 1.71s, respectively. Thermally denatured acid-soluble collagen irradiated at 5 and 10 Mrads resulted in similar peaks with $S_{20,w}$ 1.95 and 1.81s, respectively (Fig. 17.22).

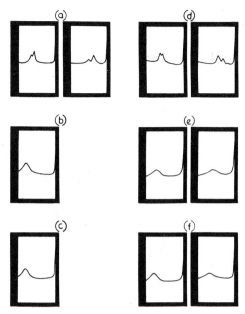

Figure 17.22. Sedimentation patterns of (a) thermally denatured acid-soluble collagen, (b) thermally denatured acid-soluble collagen + 5 Mrads, (c) thermally denatured acid-soluble collagen + 10 Mrads, (d) thermally denatured neutral-salt soluble collagen, (e) thermally denatured neutral-salt soluble collagen + 5 Mrads, (f) thermally denatured neutral-salt soluble collagen + 10 Mrads. The photographs were taken after 80 and 120 min at 56, 100 rev min—1 and 35°. Sedimentation is from left to right [57].

17.5   DISCUSSION

To discuss the optical rotation and viscometric data for γ-irradiated collagen, it is necessary to consider the contribution to these physical properties from the various structural elements of the collagen molecule. With optical rotation the primary structure contributes a value equivalent to the residue rotation of collagen in the fully denatured form ($[\alpha]_{365}{}^{43}$ —460°, [63]) which is the sum of the individual rotations of the amino acids in the molecule plus the structural contribution of the chain. The latter has a value of $[\alpha]_D{}^{40}$ —27° in the total rotation for calfskin collagen gelatin of $[\alpha]_D{}^{40}$ —140° [64] and represents a contribution of approximately 8% in the total rotation for calfskin of $[\alpha]_D{}^{15}$ —340°. The remaining rotation for collagen representing some 64% of the total (i.e., from $[\alpha]_{365}{}^{15}$ —450° to —1261°) is mainly due to the three helical chains which constitute the molecule, with some contribution from the conformation of these into the triple helix [37]. The primary structure being a random chain will contribute little to the overall viscosity. Thus Veis and Anesey [65] give a value of 0.57 dl g⁻¹ for the intrinsic viscosity at 40° of bovine γ-gelatin. The secondary structure of collagen will make some contribution to the viscosity, with the tertiary structure making the most contribution due to the rigidity of the triple helix.

The effect of relatively low doses of γ-irradiation is clearly evident in the reduction of specific rotation, and even greater decrease in reduced viscosity of the irradiated collagen with doses up to about 100 krads, as well as in the relationship between reduced viscosity and collagen concentration (Tables 17.5 and 17.6 and Fig. 17.16). This can be accounted for by a significant decrease in the rigidity of the collagen molecule, which must arise from breaks in one or more of the three individual polypeptide chains of the molecule, without necessarily destroying the amino acid residues involved in the peptide bonds [50, 48, 57]. This will also decrease the helical stability of these chains and the specific rotation of the molecule, but to a smaller extent (Fig. 17.13). The extent of the specific rotation recovery (Fig. 17.12 and Table 17.5) and viscosity recovery (Fig. 17.14 and Table 17.6) of thermally denatured solutions of the irradiated collagen support these conclusions. The second phase of the irradiation damage occurred above about 100 krads, where a steady decrease in the original and recovered values for specific rotation and reduced viscosity for the unheated and thermally denatured solutions, respectively, occurred at a lower rate than was the case below this dose range (Tables 17.5 and 17.6 and Figs. 17.13 and 17.15). The decrease in the rate may be due to the fact that the initial breaks in the polypeptide chains are more effective in decreasing these physical properties than later breaks, a finding that has been reported for other methods of chain scission [38].

These results are different from those of Welling and Bakerman [66], who concluded from their γ-irradiation of soluble collagen in solution that no change in the optical rotation or viscosity occurred below 90 krads, that above this the viscosity decreased rapidly and that above 130 krads the optical rotation began to fall slightly. The present results (Tables 17.5 and 17.6) show that changes in both optical rotation and viscosity were measurable at 1 krad after irradiation of the dry protein, suggesting that the screening effect of the solvent media in protein solutions considerably decreases the effective irradiation dose impinging on the protein. On this basis increased degradation by the "indirect" effect due to the production of free radicals would appear to be insufficient to offset the protective role of the solvent in decreasing the irradiation intensity. Yates [53] found that irradiation of intact skin in the dry state (13–17% water content) caused appreciably more damage than irradiation in the wet state (60–67% water content).

The γ-irradiation also appears to destroy the ordered polymeric forms of tropocollagen [57], which may account partially for the change in relationship between reduced viscosity and concentration [67]. Extracts of tropocollagen contain covalently linked polymeric molecules, which are reduced initially to monomeric molecules by such agents as sonic irradiation, and chemical and enzyme treatment [68, 67, 69]. These linear polymers may be formed through covalent telopeptide links [63], and depolymerization could occur through scission of these peptide links.

One of the features of these results is the degree of optical-rotation recovery during mutarotation. Thus the specific-rotation recovery expressed as a percentage of the specific rotation of native collagen ($[\alpha]_{365}^{15}$ 1261°) decreases from 81 to 62% with increased irradiation (Table 17.5). But the specific-rotation recovery, expressed as a percentage of the specific rotation of the corresponding sample with no thermal history, remains remarkably constant at about 80% for all irradiation doses (Table 17.5). On the assumption that the sites of irradiation damage can be expected to occur at random in individual molecules, the most general conclusion to be drawn from these observations appears to be that the nucleation sites important in renaturation are comparatively uniformly distributed along the polypeptide chains. Hence fragmentation of each molecule into lengths of damaged and intact structure does not prevent the subsequent nucleation and propagation of the collagen-type structure from occurring independently in all the undamaged portions simultaneously, provided that these segments contain the minimum number of residues required to stabilize a length of helical structure [38]. A comparatively uniform distribution of nucleating centers would be consistent with the observations of previous workers [35, 70].

Further, the recovery of a constant fraction of the optical rotation of the original exposed collagen even at high doses suggests that damage is restricted to scission of bonds between α-amino acid residues comprising the "band" regions of the molecule rather than the "interband" pyrollidine-rich regions normally responsible for nucleating the collagen-type structure. The "interband" regions, which consist largely of the sequence gly-pro-X (where X is often hyp), appear to remain largely intact. It has been estimated that the interband regions represent 60–70% of the collagen molecule and are 20–30 residues long, whereas the "band" regions are about 15 residues long [38]. The stability of these interband regions would explain the relatively high recovery of specific rotation in the gelatin-to-collagen transition, since these regions probably initiate collagen-fold reformation [25, 17, 38].

With regard to the data on reduced viscosities (Table 17.6), it is evident that the γ-irradiation has a greater effect on these than on specific rotation. Thus the reduced viscosity of the irradiated collagen, expressed as a percentage of the reduced viscosity of native collagen, showed decreases ranging from 68 to 12%. The reduced-viscosity recovery expressed as a percentage of the reduced-viscosity of the corresponding unheated sample is fairly constant at about 16%, whereas the reduced-viscosity recovery decreased from 16 to 2.5% with increasing irradiation. Breaks in the polypeptide chains in these band regions would significantly decrease the rigidity of the molecule without affecting the helical content to the same extent.

In the reversion of thermally denatured solutions of the irradiated collagens, it is evident that the relative rates and final-recovery values are greater for optical rotation than for viscosity (Tables 17.5 and 17.6). In these recovery experiments, the collagen solutions were heated at 45° to convert the tropocollagen, or irradiation-damaged tropocollagen, into individual α- and β-subunits, or fragments of these with the irradiated collagen. Therefore, where fragments of these chains occur in the cooled solutions of sufficient length to reform individual segments only of the collagen-fold type, optical-rotatory power remains high owing to additivity, specific rotation being practically independent of particle size. With reduced viscosity, however, values observed depend closely on hydrodynamic shape and size factors; reduced viscosity will thus be an average value for the various fragments present.

An important feature of the melting curves is their biphasic nature at the lower doses of irradiation, thus giving two denaturation temperatures. Similar results were found by Bailey [54] from the irradiation of solutions of acid-soluble rat-tail collagen between 3 and 30 krads, the lower melting point being due to the thermal disruption of a range of irradiation-damaged triple helices, and the higher melting point to the thermal denaturation of undamaged or marginally damaged triple helices. On this basis, it can be concluded from Fig. 17.18 that under the experimental conditions employed no intact collagen-type structure remains at doses above 100 krads, corresponding to the disappearance of the high-temperature "shoulder" region on the melting curve. For solutions of acid-soluble collagen Bailey [54] found that at 30 krads all the molecules were sufficiently damaged to be thermally labile below the melting point of the native collagen. Bearing in mind the different sources of collagen, quantitative differences in the amounts of irradiation required to produce comparable effects in the present study and previous studies by other workers would appear to be due to the protective screening of the solvent environment in the latter cases.

The melting curves (Fig. 17.18) give melting points for the damaged collagen that decrease rapidly with the initial low doses of irradiation, and then decrease at a much less rapid rate as the irradiation is increased (Fig. 17.19), which is consistent with a progressive loss in helical structure. The quantity $\Delta[\alpha]_T$ is proportional to the number of residues that pass from a helical to a random-coil conformation, and, as this value decreases as the irradiation dose is increased (Table 17.7), this would indicate a decrease in the helical content. Similarly the temperature difference (ΔT) which is directly related to the phase transition and serves as a convenient measure of the "degree of cooperativeness" of the helical structure [38] increases in proportion to the irradiation (Table 17.7).

Bailey, Rhodes and Cater [10], Bailey [54], and Tomoda and Tsuda [71] have shown that γ-rays can introduce intermolecular cross-links into collagen fibrils, soluble collagen, and gelatin in the presence of water, but this tendency is decreased in the presence of oxygen and radical scavengers [66], suggesting that these cross-links arise from the action of free radicals. It is evident that some of the experimental results for the dose range 5 krads–2.6 Mrads do not always fall into line with the rest of the results (see Figs. 17.15 and 17.16). It is possible therefore that in this range some cross-links are formed on irradiating dry collagen by a mechanism other than that involving the action of free radicals derived from the solvent.

The irradiation damage is not reversible, unlike the heat denaturation of collagen, which is at least partially reversible [42, 30], since the optical rotation and viscosity of solutions of irradiated collagen kept at 15° without any heating step remained constant over periods up to 30 hr and showed no tendency to recover the values of the native soluble collagen. This is further shown by the decrease in mutarotation and viscosity recovery at 15° for thermally denatured solutions of collagen of increasing irradiation dose.

The action of γ-irradiation on both neutral-salt soluble and acid-soluble collagen in the dry state causes significant changes in their subunit composition, even at relatively low doses. The resultant elution of these degraded components near the void volume of the chromatography column indicates either that low-molecular-weight components have been liberated by the irradiation, or that changes in the cationic character of particular components have taken place. The sedimentation studies show that degradation of the original collagen occurred on irradiation, resulting in material with a range of molecular weights generally lower than that of the α-subunits. The absence of the β-peak indicated by ultracentrifugation of irradiated collagen suggests that depolymerization of the major α_1-α_1 and α_2-α_2 dimers (component 5) takes place. As the collagen was irradiated in the dry state, the indirect action of free-radical formation from any solvent cannot be implicated in the degradation observed.

It is possible that the telopeptides, which are considered to be involved in both inter- and intramolecular bonding [63], and are susceptible to proteolytic enzymes, are likewise susceptible to γ-irradiation. This could account for the ready decomposition of the polymeric forms of collagen, shown by chromatography and ultracentrifugation, even at relatively low doses of irradiation.

In conclusion, ultraviolet irradiation acts on proteins by being absorbed by those amino acids containing a chromophoric group, namely, tyrosine, tryptophan, phenylalanine, and, to some extent cystine residues. This energy is transferred to the peptide bonds where it causes fission and decomposition of the molecule. Thus the primary chemical reaction of ultraviolet irradiation is photolysis of aromatic and disulfide residues [20, 14]. Since collagen does not contain disulfide bonds and tryptophan, but only phenylalanine and small amounts of tryosine, the primary chemical reaction must take place at the site of these two amino acids.

Since γ-rays are high-energy electromagnetic radiations they are extremely penetrative and interact with atoms or molecules by the ejection of electrons from these, causing ionization. The ejected high-speed electrons cause further ionizations which result in chemical changes. When the energy of the ejected electron is insufficient to cause ionization, excited molecules are produced. Free-radical formation is an important factor in the action of γ-irradiation. The net result of these reactions is of three general types, namely, scission of peptide bonds, disruption of hydrogen bonding, and the formation of cross-links.

Nevertheless, it is apparent from the results reported that ultraviolet and γ-irradiation appear to produce very similar effects on soluble collagen, although the two forms of irradiation are different and act via different mechanisms.

ACKNOWLEDGEMENTS

The author wishes to acknowledge discussions with, and the work done by, R. J. Davidson and A. E. Russell. This work was financed by the annual grants of the Livestock and Meat Industries Control Board and the Council for Scientific and Industrial Research.

REFERENCES

1. D. R. Cooper and A. E. Russell, *Clinical Orthopaedics and Related Research,* (1969a), No. 67, 188.
2. S. Fitton Jackson, *Treatise on Collagen,* G. N. Ramachandran, Ed., Vol. 2B, Chap. 1, Academic Press, London, 1968, p. 1.
3. M. J. Glimcher and S. M. Krane, *Treatise on Collagen,* G. N. Ramachandran, Ed., Vol. 2B, Chap. 2, Academic Press, London, 1968, p. 68.
4. A. Veis, *Treatise on Collagen,* G. N. Ramachandran, Ed., Vol. 1, Chap. 8, Academic Press, London, 1968, p. 367.
5. P. M. Gallop, O. O. Blumenfeld, and S. Seifter, *Treatise on Collagen,* G. N. Ramachandran, Ed., Vol. 1, Chap. 7, Academic Press, London, 1968, p. 339.
6. K. A. Piez, *Treatise on Collagen,* G. N. Ramachandran, Ed., Vol. 1, Chap. 5, Academic Press, London, 1968, p. 207.
7. P. H. von Hippel, *Treatise on Collagen,* G. N. Ramachandran, Ed., Vol. 1, Chap. 6, Academic Press, London, 1968, p. 253.
8. G. R. Tristram and R. H. Smith, *Advan. Protein Chem.,* **18,** 227 (1963).
9. O. W. Mc Bride and W. F. Harrington, *Biochemistry,* **6,** 1484 (1967).
10. A. J. Bailey, D. N. Rhodes, and C. W. Cater, *Radiation Res.,* **22,** 606 (1964).
11. E. Fujimori, *Biopolymers,* **3,** 115 (1965).
12. E. Fujimori, *Biochemistry,* **5,** 1034 (1966).
13. A. D. Mc Laren, *Advan. Enzymol.,* **9,** 75 (1949).
14. A. D. Mc Laren and D. Shugar, *Photochemistry of Proteins and Nucleic Acids,* Pergamon Press, London, 1964, p. 110.
15. E. S. Copeland, T. Sanner, and A. Pihl, *Radiation Res.,* **35,** 437 (1968).
16. G. N. Ramachandran, *Treatise on Collagen,* G. N. Ramachandran, Ed., Vol. 1, Chap. 3, Academic Press, London, 1968, p. 103.
17. W. F. Harrington and P. H. von Hippel, *Advan. Potein Chem.,* **16,** 1 (1961).
18. A. J. Hodge, *Treatise on Collagen,* G. N. Ramachandran, Ed., Vol. 1, Chap. 4, Academic Press, London, 1968, p. 185.
19. J. E. Eastoe, in G. N. Ramachandran, Ed., *Treatise on Collagen,* Vol. 1, Chap. 1, Academic Press, London, 1968, p. 1.
20. E. K. Rideal and R. Roberts, *Proc. Roy. Soc.* A, **205,** 391 (1951).
21. N. Ramanathan, *Bull. Cent. Leath. Res. Inst., Madras,* **8,** 511 (1962).
22. E. Bottoms and S. Shuster, *Nature,* **199,** 192 (1963).
23. F. S. LaBella and D. P. Thornhill, *Studies of Rheumatoid Disease,* Proc. of the Third Canadian Conf. on Res. in the Rheumatic Diseases, Toronto, 246 (1965).
24. M. Nishigai, (1964). *Proc. 12th Symp. Collagen Res. Soc. Japan, Odawara; Collagen Curr.,* **5,** 352 (1965).
25. P. H. von Hippel and W. F. Harrington, *Biochim. Biophys. Acta,* **36,** 427 (1959).
26. D. R. Cooper and R. J. Davidson, *Biochem. J.,* **97,** 139 (1965).

27. S. Seifter, P. M. Gallop, and E. Meilman, *Recent Advances in Gelatin and Glue Research*, G. Stainsby, Ed., Pergamon Press, London, 1958, p. 164.

28. P. H. von Hippel and W. F. Harrington, *Brookhaven Symp. Biol.*, **13**, 213 (1960).

29. A. Veis and J. Anesey, *Recent Advances in Gelatin and Glue Research*, G. Stainsby, Ed., Pergamon Press, London, 1958, p. 269.

30. M. P. Drake and A. Veis, *Biochemistry*, **3**, 135 (1964).

31. T. Nishihara and P. Doty, *Recent Advances in Gelatin and Glue Research*, G. Stainsby, Ed., Pergamon Press, London, 1958, p. 262.

32. T. Nishihara and P. Doty, *Proc. Nat. Acad. Sci., Wash.*, **44**, 411 (1958).

33. K. A. Piez and A. L. Carrillo, *Biochemistry*, **3**, 908 (1964).

34. D. R. Cooper and R. J. Davidson, *Biochem. J.*, **98**, 655 (1966).

35. W. F. Harrington and P. H. von Hippel, *Arch. Biochem. Biophys.*, **92**, 100 (1961).

36. A. Veis, *The Macromolecular Chemistry of Gelatin*, Academic Press, New York, 1964, p. 267.

37. P. H. von Hippel and K. Y. Wong, *Biochemistry*, **2**, 1387 (1963).

38. P. H. von Hippel and K. Y. Wong, *Biochemistry*, **2**, 1399 (1963).

39. K. A. Piez, E. A. Eigner, and M. S. Lewis, *Biochemistry*, **2**, 58 (1963).

40. R. J. Davidson and D. R. Cooper, *J. S. Afr. Chem. Inst.*, **20**, 69 (1967b).

41. A. L. Rubin, D. Pfahl, P. T. Speakman, P. F. Davison, and F. O. Schmitt, *Science* **139**, 37 (1963).

42. G. Beier and J. Engel, *Biochemistry*, **5**, 2744 (1966).

43. P. J. Flory and E. S. Weaver, *J. Amer. Chem. Soc.*, **82**, 4518 (1960).

44. K. Kuhn, J. Engel, B. Zimmermann, and W. Grassmann, *Arch. Biochem. Biophys.*, **105**, 387 (1964).

45. A. E. Russell and D. R. Cooper, *Biochem. J.*, **113**, 221 (1969).

46. A. E. Russell and D. R. Cooper, *Biochemistry*, (1969).

47. F. O. Schmitt, L. Levine, M. P. Drake, A. L. Rubin, D. Pfahl, and P. F. Davison, *Proc. Nat. Acad. Sci., Wash.*, **51**, 493 (1964).

48. J. H. Bowes and J. A. Moss, *Radiation Res.*, **16**, 211 (1962).

49. N. Ramanathan, V. Mohanaradhakrishnan, and Y. Nayudamma, *Biochim. Biophys. Acta*, **102**, 533 (1965).

50. J. Cassel, *J. Amer. Leather Chemists, Assoc.*, **54**, 8 (1959).

51. I. P. Strakhov and I. G. Shifrin, *Radiats. Khim. Polim., Mater Simp., Moscow*, 333 (1964).

52. A. J. Bailey, J. R. Bendall, and D. N. Rhodes, *Internat. J. Appl. Radiation Isotopes*, **13**, 131 (1962).

53. J. R. Yates, *Radiation Res.*, **34**, 648 (1968).

54. A. J. Bailey, *Radiation Res.*, **31**, 206, (1967).

55. M. Kubota, S. Kimura, and T. Ohashi, *Hikaku Kagaku*, **14**, 105 (1968).

56. D. R. Cooper and A. E. Russell, *Biochem. J.*, **113**, 263 (1969b).

57. R. J. Davidson and D. R. Cooper, *Biochem. J.*, **107**, 29 (1968).

58. J. T. Yang, *Advan. Protein Chem.*, **16**, 323 (1961).

59. R. J. Davidson, Rhodes University, Ph.D. Thesis, (1968).

60. R. J. Davidson and D. R. Cooper, *Biochem. J.,* **105,** 965 (1967a).

61. K. A. Piez, *J. Biol. Chem.,* **239,** 4315 (1964).

62. D. R. Cooper and R. J. Davidson, *J. Chromatog.* **34,** 332 (1968).

63. M. P. Drake, P. F. Davison, S. Bump, and F. O. Schmitt, *Biochemistry,* **5,** 301 (1966).

64. K. A. Piez and J. Gross, *J. Biol. Chem.,* **235,** 995 (1960).

65. A. Veis and J. Anesey, *Arch. Biochem. Biophys.,* **98,** 104 (1962).

66. L. Welling and S. Bakerman, *Nature,* **201,** 495 (1964).

67. P. Bornstein, A. H. Kang, and K. A. Piez, *Biochemistry,* **5,** 3803 (1966).

68. P. F. Davison and M. P. Drake, *Biochemistry,* **5,** 313 (1966).

69. O. O. Blumenfeld, M. Rojkind, and P. M. Gallop, *Biochemistry,* **4,** 1708 (1965).

70. W. Grassmann, K. Hannig, H. Endres, and A. Riedel, *Hoppe-Seyl. Z.,* **306,** 123 (1956).

71. Y. Tomoda and M. Tsuda, *Nature,* **190,** 905 (1961).

Index

Notes